Male Infertility

Diagnosis and Treatment

DEDICATION

This book is dedicated to our wives, Sanderina Kruger and Laura Oehninger, who were always there over the last decades, inspiring us to achieve and to contribute.

Male Infertility
Diagnosis and Treatment

Editors

Sergio C Oehninger MD PhD
Professor, Departments of Obstetrics and Gynecology, and Urology
  and
Division Director, The Jones Institute for Reproductive Medicine
Eastern Virginia Medical School, Norfolk, Virginia
USA

Thinus F Kruger MD FRCOG
Professor and Chairperson
Department of Obstetrics & Gynaecology, and Reproductive Biology Unit
Tygerberg Academic Hospital and Stellenbosch University,
Tygerberg
South Africa

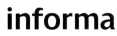

© 2007 Informa UK Ltd

First published in the United Kingdom in 2007 by Informa UK Ltd, 4 Park Square, Milton Park, Abingdon, Oxon OX14 4RN. Informa Healthcare is a trading division of Informa UK Ltd. Registered Office: 37/41 Mortimer Street, London, W1T 3JH. Registered in England and Wales Number 1072954.

Tel.: +44 (0)20 7017 6000
Fax: +44 (0)20 7017 6699
E-mail: info.medicine@tandf.co.uk
Website: www.informahealthcare.com

Although every effort has been made to ensure that all owners of copyright material have been acknowledged in this publication, we would be glad to acknowledge in subsequent reprints or editions any omissions brought to our attention.

A CIP record for this book is available from the British Library.

Library of Congress Cataloging-in-Publication Data

Data available on application

ISBN10: 0-415-39742-1
ISBN13: 978-0-415-39742-1

Distributed in North and South America by

Taylor & Francis
6000 Broken Sound Parkway, NW, (Suite 300)
Boca Raton, FL 33487, USA

Within Continental USA
Tel.: 1(800)272 7737; Fax: 1(800)374 3401
Outside Continental USA
Tel.: (561)994 0555; Fax: (561)361 6018
E-mail: orders@crcpress.com

Distributed in the rest of the world by
Thomson Publishing Services
Cheriton House
North Way
Andover, Hampshire SP10 5BE, UK
Tel.: +44 (0)1264 332424
E-mail: tps.tandfsalesorder@thomson.com

Composition by Parthenon Publishing

Printed and bound in India by Replika Press Pvt. Ltd.

Contents

Section 2 – Diagnosis of male infertility

Section 3 – Therapeutic alternatives for male infertility

Acknowledgments

We have been able to complete this work thanks to the devoted efforts of a few assistants. We wish to acknowledge the editorial assistance of Helena Krüger (from Tygerberg), who made a significant contribution to the textbook, but died sadly on 14 October 2005. We sincerely appreciate the excellent help of Madaleine du Toit, who took over the responsibilities for Helena. Irene Foy (from the Jones Institute) is thanked for her secretarial contributions.

We also wish to acknowledge clinicians, scientists and laboratory personnel of the Reproductive Biology Research Laboratory at the Department of Obstetrics and Gynaecology, Tygerberg Hospital, Stellenbosch University; the Vincent Palotti Hospital, Cape Town, Republic of South Africa; and the Jones Institute for Reproductive Medicine, Department of Obstetrics & Gynecology, Eastern Virginia Medical School, Norfolk, VA, USA.

We are truly indebted to all contributors for their enthusiasm in making this project a success.

Foreword

In about one-half of all couples who are plagued by infertility, the male partner has a deficiency in his sperm.

Infertility in the male has two very peculiar characteristics. First, even though details of the pathology of the sperm deficiency are not at all understood in most cases, there is a very good therapeutic modality which overcomes these problems and is still able to transmit the male partner's genetic message to the next generation. This therapeutic modality is, of course, intracytoplasmic sperm injection (ICSI). This successful therapy has made it seem less urgent to investigate the pathophysiology of male infertility. This is unfortunate, as there is an inner concern and some evidence that ICSI may transmit to succeeding generations the seeds of an increased incidence of sperm defects.

Section 1 and several chapters of Sections 2 and 3 of this book tell us what is known about this area and thus serve as a launching pad for the further necessary investigation of the pathophysiology of sperm deficiencies. These chapters also alert the clinician to our ignorance of the molecular details of at least some sperm problems, which may lead to the passing of these defects to the next generation by ICSI. There is no doubt, however, that ICSI is one of the major breakthrough 'blockbuster' treatments resulting in the enjoyment of children for couples who otherwise would not be able to.

The second peculiar characteristic of male infertility is that it is often diagnosed by a most unlikely specialist – the gynecologist – simply because it is this specialist who is most likely to be consulted first by those who are infertile. Thus, it is not surprising that the editors of this book are gynecologists who have specialized in problems of reproduction and superspecialized in problems of male infertility. Hence has come into existence the subspecialty of andrology, which has found a home most often within the broad field of obstetrics and gynecology. Special problems of infertility in the male are treated by the urologist, and in some countries by dermatologists, but the therapy of last resort, i.e. ICSI, is in the hands of reproductive endocrinologists who have at their fingertips the technology of *in vitro* fertilization (IVF).

It is noteworthy that *Male Infertility: Diagnosis and Treatment* is a synthesis of current knowledge about human andrology, and comes from two departments of obstetrics and gynecology where it was realized, even before the era of IVF, that a new perspective was required if true progress was to be made in solving the problems of male infertility.

Notwithstanding these considerations, the editors have assembled an outstanding list of contributors who thoroughly overview the approach to male infertility not only from the perspective of the reproductive endocrinologist but also from the urologist, dermatologist and medical scientist points of view.

Andrology is by no means a matured discipline, as indicated above. However, this book is a superb summary of our current understanding of the art and science of this dynamic approach to the solution of a major portion of infertility.

Howard W Jones Jr MD
Professor Emeritus, The Jones Institute for
Reproductive Medicine
Department of Obstetrics & Gynecology
Eastern Virginia Medical School
Norfolk, VA
USA

Preface

Physicians dealing with childless couples are well aware of the high incidence of male infertility. Recent estimates indicate that a male factor is present in up to 40–50% of cases consulting for infertility. While the causes of male infertility are multiple, the therapeutic options have traditionally been more limited. Urological and medical interventions have been, and continue to be, successfully implemented in defined clinical scenarios. But, undisputedly, the explosive growth and efficiency of assisted reproductive technologies (ART) has changed the direction of the field of andrology.

Without any doubt, the development of intracytoplasmic sperm injection (ICSI) constituted a significant advancement not only in the treatment of infertility but also in nurturing further development of the discipline of clinical andrology. As a microtechnique to assist fertilization, ICSI has allowed men with severely compromised semen parameters (patients with oligo-astheno-teratozoospermia, alone or in combination, presenting with antisperm antibodies and even with obstructive or non-obstructive azoospermia) to achieve their desire to establish a family.

Spermatozoa are highly differentiated cells that have an essential function to fertilize the oocyte, leading to embryo development. Functionally competent sperm cells are the result of the complex processes of spermatogenesis that involve cell differentiation, multiplication (mitosis), acquisition of the haploid stage (meiosis) and a dramatic metamorphosis (spermiogenesis). Spermatozoa are released into the epididymis (spermiation), where further maturational, structural, biochemical and functional changes (capacitation) take place. Gametogenesis and seminiferous tubule functions occur under strict endocrine and paracrine control. To fertilize the oocyte successfully, the spermatozoon must be able to perform the critical functions of migration, recognition and binding to the zona pellucida, penetration of the zona pellucida, binding to the oolemma, activation of the oocyte, nuclear decondensation and participation in pronuclear formation leading to syngamy. This complex sequence of events leads to multiple potential opportunities for errors and interference by a multitude of pathogenic mechanisms.

Current treatment options for male infertility include a large number of urological procedures (reconstructive surgery in cases of ductal obstruction, correction of varicocele and others), medical–pharmacological interventions (use of hormones, antibiotics), low-complexity assisted reproductive procedures (such as intrauterine insemination therapy) and the more advanced and complex ART. However, despite that contemporary therapies have enhanced the opportunities for conception in couples suffering from male infertility, often these solutions are raised in the absence of a defined etiological or pathophysiological diagnosis. Male infertility is unfortunately still considered 'idiopathic' in a large proportion of cases.

The first *in vitro* fertilization (IVF) child in the world, Louise Brown, was born in Bourn Hall, UK in 1978. She was followed by the first IVF birth in

Australia in 1980; in Norfolk, USA in 1981 (Elizabeth Carr); in continental Europe in 1982; and in 1984 in Tygerberg, South Africa (reviewed in Fauser and Edwards 2005)[1]. Since the early 1980s, the efficiency of IVF has improved dramatically, with clinical pregnancy rates per transfer cycle increasing from the mid-teens to 30–50%, according to the individual prognosis group. This accomplishment has been achieved by continuing efforts resulting in improved ovarian stimulation protocols, optimized gametes and embryo *in vitro* culture conditions, superior techniques of oocyte retrieval and embryo transfer, and development of more efficient embryo cryopreservation programs.

The field of andrology has grown exponentially in parallel to the developments in ART. A few of the most significant milestones and some relevant clinical papers are worth highlighting:

- Manual for the examination of semen (WHO 1980, fourth revised edition 1999)[2];
- First paper on IVF and male infertility (Wood 1984)[3];
- Aneuploidy in human sperm using fluorescence *in situ* hybridization (FISH) (Joseph *et al.* 1984)[4];
- Chromosomal abnormalities in human sperm (Martin 1985)[5];
- Male factor and IVF: first years of Norfolk experience (Van Uem *et al.* 1985)[6];
- First human pregnancy by IVF with epididymal sperm in obstructive azoospermia (Temple–Smith *et al.* 1985)[7];
- Sperm morphology as a prognostic factor for IVF (Kruger *et al.* 1986)[9];
- IVF and epididymal aspiration in congenital absence of the vas deferens (Silber *et al.* 1987)[8];
- Description and definition of the Tygerberg Strict Criteria (R Menkveld 1987 – PD thesis);
- Births after microsurgical sperm aspiration/ IVF in men with congenital absence of the vas deferens (Patrizio *et al.* 1988)[10];
- Definition of male factor in ART (Acosta *et al.* 1989)[11];

- First pregnancies following preimplantation genetic diagnosis (PGD) from biopsied embryos sexed by Y-specific DNA amplification (Handyside *et al.* 1990)[12];
- ICSI: first pregnancies (Palermo *et al.* 1992)[13];
- Place of ICSI in the management of male infertility (Oehninger 2001)[14];
- Pregnancy after testicular sperm aspiration/ ICSI (Schoysman *et al.* 1993)[15];
- Microsurgical epididymal sperm aspiration/ ICSI and congenital absence of the vas deferens (Tournaye *et al.* 1994)[16];
- The essential partnership between diagnostic andrology and ART (Mortimer 1994)[17];
- Intrauterine insemination for male subfertility (Ombelet *et al.* 1995)[18];
- Pregnancies after ICSI with testicular sperm (Silber *et al.* 1995)[19];
- Pregnancies after ICSI with testicular sperm in non-obstructive azoospermia (Devroey *et al.* 1995)[20];
- Deletions of the Y chromosome and severe oligospermia (Reijo *et al.* 1996)[21];
- Infertility in ICSI-derived sons (Kent-First *et al.* 1996)[22];
- Prospective follow-up study of ICSI children (Bonduelle *et al.* 1996)[23];
- Thresholds for semen parameters in fertile versus subfertile populations (Ombelet *et al.* 1997)[24];
- Approaching the next millennium: management of andrology diagnosis in the ICSI era (Oehninger *et al.* 1997)[25];
- Consensus workshop on diagnostic andrology (European Society of Human Reproduction and Embryology, ESHRE) (Fraser *et al.* 1997)[26];
- Detection of aneuploidy in human sperm using FISH (14 chromosomes) (Pang *et al.* 1999)[27];
- Forging a partnership between total quality management and the andrology laboratory (De Jonge 2000)[28];
- A meta-analysis of sperm function tests (Oehninger *et al.* 2000)[29];

- Testicular dysgenesis syndrome (Skakkebaek *et al.* 2001)[30];
- ICSI should not be the treatment of choice for all cases of *in vitro* conception (Oehninger and Gosden 2002)[31];
- Multiple gestations in ART: an ongoing epidemic (Adashi *et al.* 2003)[32];
- Identification of the subfertile male in the general population: suggested new thresholds (van der Merwe *et al.* 2005)[33].

The overall objective of this book is to deliver information in an approachable fashion about the most common pathogenic mechanisms involved in male infertility and the state-of-the-art diagnostic tools, and a detailed description of the current therapeutic options available for the infertile man. The organization of the book follows these goals. Objective evidence, supported by a thorough and updated list of references, is presented in each individual chapter. The contributing authors have presented easy-to-read chapters and the outlined information should be readily understood by a variety of readers, including medical and postgraduate students, physicians and scientists interested in reproduction.

Indeed, the main expectation is that a wide range of generalists and specialists (andrologists, reproductive endocrinologists, urologists, obstetricians and gynecologists, primary-care practitioners) will benefit from the information presented herein. It was not our aim to present a manual with recipes of screening tests or techniques, but rather to examine the rationale behind clinical management, always supported by evidence-based medicine. Notwithstanding these considerations, methods have been succinctly mentioned and the interested reader can access more technical details through the extensive cited bibliography.

We were fortunate to assemble an outstanding and international group of contributors: six of the seven continents are represented (Europe, North and South America, Africa, Australia and Asia). This multidisciplinary group of authors includes clinicians and scientists who have had a significant impact as pioneers and/or have made distinguished contributions to the field of male infertility.

Section 1 critically discusses 'Basic concepts: sperm physiology and pathology'.

In Chapter 1, CF Hoogendijk, TF Kruger and R Menkveld (from South Africa) provide a synopsis of the 'Functional anatomy and molecular morphology of the spermatozoon'. The authors outline the basic anatomy of the human spermatozoon through a light- and electron-microscopic approach. In addition, they introduce the concepts of chromosomal arrangement and the high degree of organization of the sperm nuclear chromatin.

In Chapter 2, M Luconi and E Baldi (from Italy) and GF Doncel (from the USA) present 'The physiology and pathophysiology of sperm motility'. The authors describe with accuracy the mechanochemical basis of sperm movement, placing special emphasis on the regulatory factors involved in the acquisition and maintenance of sperm motility, hyperactivation and chemotaxis. The authors also discuss the molecular defects associated with asthenozoospermia, a sperm pathology that represents one of the main causes of male infertility, as well as systemic and *in vitro* therapeutic approaches for this condition.

In Chapter 3, CF Hoogendijk and R Henkel (from Germany, now South Africa) delineate 'The pathophysiology and genetics of human male reproduction'. This chapter reviews in detail the genetic controls that are operative at different steps of spermatogenesis, the nuclear chromatin organization levels and the role of spermatozoa in early embryogenesis.

In Chapter 4, G Barroso (from Mexico) and S Oehninger (from the USA) describe the 'Contribution of the male gamete to fertilization and embryogenesis'. A large body of evidence demonstrates that: (1) the fertilizing spermatozoon plays a significant part in bringing about the development of the zygote, with its contributions being well beyond the delivery of the paternal DNA; and (2) infertile men with or without altered 'classic' semen parameters may have associated sperm dysfunctions that can result in aberrant embryogenesis. This review focuses on examination of the paternal effects that become manifest before and after the major activation of embryonic gene expression.

In Chapter 5, O Mudrak and A Zalensky (from the USA) present innovative work on 'Genome architecture in human sperm cells: possible implications for male infertility and prediction of pregnancy outcome'. The concepts of chromosome territories, architecture, compactness and position, telomeres localization and the dynamic modifications during fertilization in the normal and abnormal situations are elegantly set forth.

In Chapter 6, HE Chemes and VY Rawe (from Argentina) describe 'Sperm pathology: pathogenic mechanisms and fertility potential in assisted reproduction'. The authors define sperm pathology as the discipline that characterizes structural and functional deficiencies in abnormal spermatozoa. They accurately detail phenotypes associated with sperm motility and morphology disturbances and the impact of non-specific anomalies and systematic defects of genetic origin.

In Chapter 7, N Jørgensen, C Asklund, K Bay and NE Skakkebæk (from Denmark) present 'Testicular dysgenesis syndrome: biological and clinical significance'. It is proposed that testicular cancer, hypospadias, cryptorchidism and low sperm counts are symptoms of a disease complex, the testicular dysgenesis syndrome (TDS), with a common origin in fetal life. The knowledge of the etiology of TDS is still rather limited, but environmental and life-style factors are suggested as contributing factors. The authors present a sophisticated description of how genetic polymorphisms or aberrations may render some individuals particularly susceptible to these exogenous factors.

Section 2 discusses the 'Diagnosis of male infertility'. Notwithstanding the major impact of IVF and ICSI, the approach to the assessment and treatment of male infertility is much more than simply ART. An exhaustive anamnesis and a thorough physical examination of the male partner are of paramount importance in the initial screening of the infertile couple. The cornerstone of the andrological evaluation in all cases is repeated semen analysis. A urological, endocrine, genetic and/or imaging work-up should be implemented as appropriate.

In Chapter 8, AP Cedenho (from Brazil) describes the 'Evaluation of the subfertile male'. This chapter thoroughly delineates the clinical assessment of the male partner consulting for infertility, and how the work-up should be further individualized according to the findings of the anamnesis and physical examination.

In Chapter 9, R Menkveld provides an excellent state-of-the-art contribution on the 'The basic semen analysis', including laboratory performance, interpretation of results and quality-control guidelines.

In Chapter 10, K Coetzee (from New Zealand) and TF Kruger present their extensive experience in 'Advances in automated sperm morphology evaluation'. Automated systems have the power to increase the objectivity, precision and reproducibility of sperm morphology evaluations. As attractive as this option may seem, not many automated systems have been introduced into routine andrology laboratories. The majority of systems currently in operation are used in more experimental situations, because of the objective biological resolution of the systems.

In Chapter 11, DR Franken (from South Africa) and TF Kruger give a powerful insight into why 'Sperm morphology training and quality-control programs are essential for clinically relevant results'. The authors present prospective studies that clearly illustrate that an external quality-control program can be successfully implemented on condition that continuous monitoring is part of the program.

In Chapter 12, R Menkveld updates 'The role of the acrosome index in prediction of fertilization outcome'. Evidence is presented supporting the view that careful assessment of acrosome morphology provides extended information on the sperm fertilizing capacity.

In Chapter 13, DR Franken, HS Bastiaan (from South Africa) and S Oehninger give a thorough presentation of the 'Acrosome reaction: physiology and its value in clinical practice'. A simple and novel microassay using minimal volumes of solubilized zona pellucida is highlighted. The authors demonstrate that the use of a calcium ionophore or the natural solubilized zona pellucida in combination with fluorescent lectins constitute validated assays for assessment of the induced acrosome reaction in live sperm. The authors conclude that such tests should therefore be implemented in the functional evaluation of sperm from subfertile men, in order to guide clinical management properly.

In Chapter 14, S Oehninger, M Arslan (from Turkey) and DR Franken provide a detailed overview of 'Sperm–zona pellucida binding assays'. Clinical data have demonstrated that successful sperm–zona pellucida binding is essential for the achievement of *in vitro* fertilization, and that abnormalities of this binding step are frequently present in subfertile men. Human sperm–zona pellucida interaction under *in vitro* conditions reflects multiple sperm functions, including the acquisition and completion of capacitation, recognition and binding to specific zona pellucida receptors and induction of the physiological acrosome reaction. The authors provide unequivocal evidence supportive of the use of sperm–zona pellucida binding assays in the clinical setting.

In Chapter 15, R Henkel (from Germany, now South Africa) outlines 'Detection of DNA damage in sperm'. The author describes a variety of techniques developed to examine sperm DNA, and presents a compelling view that testing for DNA integrity and damage should be introduced into the routine andrological laboratory work-up.

In Chapter 16, P Patrizio, J Sepúlveda and S Mehri (from the USA) accurately review the 'Chromosomal and genetic abnormalities in male infertility'. The authors outline a multitude of genetic and chromosomal aberrations diagnosed in infertile men, as well as detection methods and clinical significance. Based on the evaluated data, the authors outline a defined algorithm for genetic evaluation of the infertile male/infertile couple prior to and after ICSI.

In Chapter 17, RJ Aitken and LE Bennetts (from Australia) elegantly describe 'Reactive oxygen species and their impact on fertility'. The authors unequivocally demonstrate that excessive production or exposure to reactive oxygen species is both statistically and causally associated with defective sperm function and DNA damage.

In Chapter 18, TI Siebert (from South Africa), FH van der Merwe (from South Africa), TF Kruger (from South Africa) and W Ombelet (from Belgium) outline 'How do we define male subfertility and what is the prevalence in the general population?'. The authors critically discuss present standards for the definition of male subfertility/infertility and their drawbacks, and introduce new thresholds based upon worldwide-derived experience.

In Chapter 19, R Henkel (from Germany, now South Africa) presents detailed information on 'DNA fragmentation and its influence on fertilization and pregnancy outcome'. Over the past few years, the interest of scientists and clinicians has focused on the influence and involvement of sperm DNA fragmentation on and in fertility, as this parameter may have a serious impact on fertilization and pregnancy. The author thoroughly describes the potential mechanisms that may lead to DNA damage during spermatogenesis and sperm maturation.

In Chapter 20, M-L Windt (from South Africa) extends these concepts with a detailed analysis of 'The impact of the paternal factor on embryo quality and development: the embryologist's point of view'. The author delineates the limitations of current methodologies used in the IVF laboratory to assess the impact of the male factor and to select embryos for transfer. Many studies have focused on embryo selection, and, especially since single-embryo transfer has become a goal in many countries, methods for selection of the genetically normal spermatozoon with the potential to contribute to normal embryo development are under current and active investigation.

Section 3 delineates the 'Therapeutic alternatives for male infertility'.

In Chapter 21, M Arslan, S Oehninger and TF Kruger carry out a thorough description of the 'Clinical management of male infertility'. The authors examine the causes and diagnostic and therapeutic management of the most common clinical scenarios, with emphasis on isolated and combined oligo-astheno-teratozoospermia. The chapter provides defined avenues to be pursued following a state-of-the-art diagnostic screening.

In Chapter 22, VM Brugh and DF Lynch (from the USA) present an update on 'Urological interventions for the treatment of male infertility'. This team of urologists elegantly describes varicocele repair, cryptorchidism and orchiopexy, disorders of ejaculation, ductal obstruction, vasovasostomy versus ICSI, congenital bilateral absence of the vas deferens and testis biopsy techniques.

In Chapter 23, G Haidl (from Germany) outlines 'Medical treatment of male infertility'. The author carefully presents medical options based on objective evidence as related to: (1) specific treatment (cases where hormonal supplementation is indicated in the form of gonadotropins, gonadotropin releasing hormone (GnRH), androgens, treatment of emission and ejaculatory disturbances and anti-infectious agents); and (2) empirical treatment (use of antiestrogens, aromatase inhibitors, purified/recombinant follicle stimulating hormone (FSH), antioxidants, carnitines, mast-cell blockers, phosphodiesterase inhibitors, zinc salts, kallidinogenase, adrenoceptor antagonists and antiphlogistic treatment).

In Chapter 24, FH Comhaire and AMA Mahmoud (from Belgium) share their extensive experience on 'Male tract infections: diagnosis and treatment'. The understanding of the link between infection of the accessory sex glands and reduced male fertility is scientifically acquired and diagnostic tools are available, but results of antibiotic treatment in terms of fertility remain disappointing. The latter is probably due to the irreversibility of functional damage caused by chronic infection/inflammation. The authors stress that prevention, early diagnosis and adequate treatment of infections of the male tract, both trivial and sexually transmitted, are of pivotal importance.

In Chapter 25, GS Nakhuda and MV Sauer (from the USA) describe 'Sperm-washing techniques for the HIV-infected male: rationale and experience'. The authors review the clinical aspects of providing fertility care for HIV-positive men and their uninfected female partners, focusing on the technical facets of sperm processing and options available for treatment.

In Chapter 26, AE Semprini and L Hollander present their extensive observations on 'Treatment of HIV-discordant couples – the Italian experience', and discuss the evidence regarding human immunodeficiency virus (HIV) transmission and safe parenthood in men infected with HIV. Reproductive counseling and semen washing with ART are the milestones in offering reproductive assistance to these individuals.

In Chapter 27, W Ombelet and M Nijs (from Belgium) outline the current status of 'Artificial insemination using homologous and donor semen'. The authors argue that there is clear evidence in the literature that this low-complexity therapy can be offered as a first-line treatment in most cases of mild and moderate male-factor infertility, resulting in acceptable pregnancy rates, before starting more invasive and more expensive techniques of assisted reproduction such as IVF and ICSI. A detailed description of indications, techniques, results and cost-efficiency is presented.

In Chapter 28, A van Steirteghem (from Belgium) reviews 'Intracytoplasmic sperm injection: current status of the technique and outcome'. Based on the pioneer work performed at his center, the author discusses the indications for and technique of ICSI, the outcome and children's health (including pregnancy complications, major malformations, possible causes of adverse outcome and multiple pregnancies).

In Chapter 29, V Vernaeve (from Spain) and H Tournaye (from Belgium) examine the techniques and indications of 'Sperm retrieval for intracytoplasmic sperm injection'. The authors present a sophisticated description of surgical sperm retrieval in patients with obstructive and non-obstructive azoospermia, and predictive factors for success and outcome. They present an in-depth discussion of clinical questions, including testicular sperm extraction (TESE) by open biopsy or by percutaneous fine needle aspiration, multiple testicular biopsies or a single testicular biopsy, microsurgical or conventional testicular sperm extraction, how many TESE procedures and adverse effects of testicular sperm extractions.

In Chapter 30, G Huszar, A Jakab, C Celik-Ozenci and GL Sati (from the USA) elegantly describe 'Hyaluronic acid binding by human sperm: andrology evaluation of male fertility and sperm selection for intracytoplasmic sperm injection'. This group of authors introduces the novel concept of an association between a testis-expressed chaperone protein, sperm cellular maturity and function, including fertilizing potential, and frequencies of aneuploidy in human spermatozoa.

In Chapter 31, R Sa, M Sousa, N Cremades, C Alves, J Silva and A Barros (from Portugal) outline '*In vitro* maturation of spermatozoa'. At present, the major goal of somatic cell–germ cell coculture systems is to establish a minimum of conditions that can artificially keep alive a more or less functional epithelium for a reasonable period of time. This group of investigators share their extensive experience with experimental studies of animal and human spermiogenesis *in vitro*. The objectives are directed not only to produce gametes *in vitro* for those cases where no spermatids are found, but also to enable a more controlled study of the mechanism of action of toxins, hormones and signal molecules on the seminiferous epithelium.

As a corollary, Chapter 32 by DA Paduch, M Goldstein and Z Rosenwaks (from the USA) presents a view to the future, with 'New developments in the evaluation and management of the infertile male'. The authors highlight the significance of the following topics: (1) advances of genetics in male infertility; (2) the reproductive health of survivors of childhood and adult malignancies; (3) hormonal manipulation in the treatment of idiopathic infertility; (4) the use of alternative and integrative medicine in male infertility; and (5) surgical treatment of male infertility. The authors conclude that, 'Over the next decade further developments in our understanding of the genetics and physiology of male reproduction, advances in stem cell research and better ways of measuring outcomes of surgical techniques, combined with novel therapeutic options, will allow us to offer treatment to patients who are considered sterile by today's standards.'

We are enthusiastic about the book in its content and presentation of the state-of-the-art of the discipline of andrology. We also remain hopeful that extended cellular–molecular–genetic investigations of the processes of human spermatogenesis and sperm capacitation and interaction with the female gamete, as well as the paternal contributions to embryogenesis, will lead to improved therapies to alleviate human infertility further. As the human genome project and the area of proteomics/metabonomics and translational research advance, their results and those of studies performed in combination with more classic reproductive biology–endocrinology techniques will bring us near to the achievement of these goals.

Sergio C Oehninger MD PhD
Thinus F Kruger MD FRCOG

REFERENCES

1. Fauser BC, Edwards RG. The early days of IVF. Hum Reprod Update 2005; 11: 437
2. World Health Organization. WHO Laboratory Manual for the Examination of Human Semen and Sperm–Cervical Mucus Interaction, 4th edn. Cambridge: Cambridge University Press, 1999
3. Wood C. Selection of patients. In Wood C, Trounson A, eds. Clinical In Vitro Fertilization. Philadelphia: Springer-Verlag, 1984: 31
4. Joseph AM, Gosden JR, Chandley AC. Estimation of aneuploidy levels in human spermatozoa using chromosome specific probes and in situ hybridization. Hum Genet 1984; 66: 234
5. Martin RH. Chromosomal abnormalities in human sperm. Basic Life Sci 1985; 36: 91
6. Van Uem JF, et al. Male factor evaluation in in vitro fertilization: Norfolk experience. Fertil Steril 1985; 44: 375
7. Temple-Smith PD, et al. Human pregnancy by in vitro fertilization (IVF) using sperm aspirated from the epididymis. J In Vitro Fert Embryo Transf 1985; 2: 119
8. Silber S, et al. New treatment for infertility due to congenital absence of vas deferens. Lancet 1987; 2: 850
9. Kruger TF, et al. Sperm morphologic features as a prognostic factor in in vitro fertilization. Fertil Steril 1986; 46: 1118
10. Patrizio P, et al. Two births after microsurgical sperm aspiration in congenital absence of vas deferens. Lancet 1988; 2: 1364
11. Acosta A, Oehninger S, et al. Assisted reproduction and treatment of the male factor. Obstet Gynecol Surv 1989; 44: 1
12. Handyside A, et al. Pregnancies from biopsied preimplantation embryos sexed by Y-specific DNA amplification. Nature 1990; 334: 768
13. Palermo A, et al. Pregnancies after intracytoplasmic injection of single spermatozoon into an oocyte. Lancet 1992; 34: 17
14. Oehninger S. Place of intracytoplasmic sperm injection in management of male infertility. Lancet 2001; 357: 2068
15. Schoysman R, et al. Pregnancy after fertilisation with human testicular spermatozoa. Lancet 1993; 342: 1237
16. Tournaye H, et al. Microsurgical epididymal sperm aspiration and intracytoplasmic sperm injection: a new effective approach to infertility as a result of congenital

bilateral absence of the vas deferens. Fertil Steril 1994; 61: 1445

17. Mortimer D. The essential partnership between diagnostic andrology and modern assisted reproductive technologies. Hum Reprod 1994; 9: 1209

18. Ombelet W, Puttemans P, Bosmans E. Intrauterine insemination: a first-step procedure in the algorithm of male subfertility treatment. Hum Reprod 1995; 10 (Suppl 1): 90

19. Silber SJ, et al. High fertilization and pregnancy rate after intracytoplasmic sperm injection with spermatozoa obtained from testicle biopsy. Hum Reprod 1995; 10: 148

20. Devroey P, et al. Pregnancies after testicular sperm extraction and intracytoplasmic sperm injection in non-obstructive azoospermia. Hum Reprod 1995; 10: 1457

21. Reijo R, et al. Severe oligozoospermia resulting from deletions of azoospermia factor gene on Y chromosome. Lancet 1996; 347: 1290

22. Kent-First MG, et al. Infertility in intracytoplasmic-sperm-injection-derived sons. Lancet 1996; 348: 332

23. Bonduelle M, et al. Prospective follow-up study of 877 children born after intracytoplasmic sperm injection (ICSI), with ejaculated epididymal and testicular spermatozoa and after replacement of cryopreserved embryos obtained after ICSI. Hum Reprod 1996; 11 (Suppl 4): 131

24. Ombelet W, et al. Semen parameters in a fertile versus subfertile population: a need for change in the interpretation of semen testing. Hum Reprod 1997; 12: 987

25. Oehninger S, Franken D, Kruger T. Approaching the next millennium: how should we manage andrology diagnosis in the intracytoplasmic sperm injection era? Fertil Steril 1997; 67: 434

26. Fraser L, et al. Consensus workshop on advanced diagnostic andrology techniques. ESHRE Andrology Special Interest Group. Hum Reprod 1997; 12: 873

27. Pang MG, et al. Detection of aneuploidy for chromosomes 4, 6, 7, 8, 9, 10, 11, 12, 13, 17, 18, 21, X and Y by fluorescence in-situ hybridization in spermatozoa from nine patients with oligoasthenoteratozoospermia undergoing intracytoplasmic sperm injection. Hum Reprod 1999; 14: 1266

28. De Jonge C. Commentary: forging a partnership between total quality management and the andrology laboratory. J Androl 2000; 21: 203

29. Oehninger S, et al. Sperm function assays and their predictive value for fertilization outcome in IVF therapy: a meta-analysis. Hum Reprod Update 2000; 6: 160

30. Skakkebaek NE, Rajpert-De Meyts E, Main KM. Testicular dysgenesis syndrome: an increasingly common developmental disorder with environmental aspects. Hum Reprod 2001; 16: 972

31. Oehninger S, Gosden RG. Should ICSI be the treatment of choice for all cases of in-vitro conception? No, not in light of the scientific data. Hum Reprod 2002; 17: 2237

32. Adashi EY, et al. Infertility therapy-associated multiple pregnancies (births): an ongoing epidemic. Reprod Biomed Online 2003; 7: 515

33. van der Merwe FH, et al. The use of semen parameters to identify the subfertile male in the general population. Gynecol Obstet Invest 2005; 59: 86

Contributors

R. John Aitken PhD ScD FRSE
ARC Centre of Excellence in Biotechnology and
  Development and Discipline of Biological
  Sciences
University of Newcastle
Callaghan, NSW
Australia

Cláudia Alves BSc
Department of Genetics
Faculty of Medicine
University of Porto
Portugal

Murat Arslan MD
Assistant Professor, Department of Obstetrics
  and Gynecology
Mersin University, Mersin, Turkey
  and
The Jones Institute for Reproductive Medicine,
Department of Obstetrics & Gynecology
Eastern Virginia Medical School
Norfolk, VA
USA

Camilla Asklund MD
University Department of Growth and
  Reproduction
Rigshospitalet
Copenhagen
Denmark

Elisabetta Baldi PhD
Associate Professor in Clinical Pathology
'DENOthe' Andrology Unit
Department of Clinical Physiopathology
University of Florence
Florence
Italy

Alberto Barros MD PhD
Cathedratic Professor and Director, Department
  of Genetics
Faculty of Medicine
University of Porto
Centre for Reproductive Genetics A Barros
Porto
Portugal

Gerardo Barroso MD
Professor, Departamento de Obstetricia y
  Ginecologia, and Director de la División de
  Reproducción Asistida
Instituto Nacional de Perinatologia
México DF
México

Hadley S Bastiaan PhD
Reproductive Biology Unit
Obstetrics and Gynaecology Department
Tygerberg Hospital and Stellenbosch University
Tygerberg
South Africa

Katrine Bay MSc
University Department of Growth and
  Reproduction
Rigshospitalet
Copenhagen
Denmark

Liga E. Bennetts
Discipline of Biological Sciences
University of Newcastle
Callaghan, NSW
Australia

Victor M Brugh III MD
Assistant Professor, Department of Urology
Eastern Virginia School of Medicine
and
Consultant Urologist
The Jones Institute for Reproductive Medicine
Norfolk, VA
USA

Agnaldo P Cedenho MD
Professor, Laboratory of Human Reproduction
Division of Urology
Paulista School of Medicine
Federal University of São Paulo
UNIFESP
São Paulo
Brazil

Ciler Celik-Ozenci PhD
The Sperm Physiology Laboratory
Department of Obstetrics and Gynecology
Yale University School of Medicine
New Haven, CT
USA

Hector E Chemes MD PhD
Laboratory of Testicular Physiology and
  Pathology
Center for Research in Endocrinology
National Research Council (CONICET)
Buenos Aires Children's Hospital, Buenos Aires
Argentina

Kevin Coetzee PhD
Fertility Associates Ltd
Newtown, Wellington
New Zealand

Frank H Comhaire MD
Professor, Center for Medical and Urological
  Andrology and Reproductive Endocrinology
University Hospital Ghent
Ghent
Belgium

Nieves Cremades BSc
Chief Embryologist, IVF Unit
Department of Gynecology
General University Hospital of Alicante
Spain

Gustavo F Doncel MD PhD
Professor of Obstetrics and Gynecology and
  Director, CONRAD Preclinical Research
Department of Obstetrics and Gynecology
Eastern Virginia Medical School
Norfolk, VA
USA

Daniel R Franken PhD
Professor, Department of Obstetrics and
  Gynaecology
Tygerberg Hospital
Tygerberg
South Africa

Marc Goldstein MD
Professor of Urology and Professor of
  Reproductive Medicine
Department of Urology
Weill Medical College of Cornell University
New York, NY;
The Population Council Center for Biomedical
  Research
New York, NY
  and
Center for Reproductive Medicine and Infertility
Weill Medical College of Cornell University
New York, NY
USA

Gerhard Haidl MD PhD
Department of Dermatology/Andrology Unit
University of Bonn
Bonn
Germany

Ralf Henkel PhD
Department of Urology
Friedrich Schiller University
Jena
Germany

Lital Hollander BSc
Clinica Ostetrica e Ginecologica
Università di Milano
Milan
Italy

Christiaan F Hoogendijk MSc
Reproductive Biology Unit
Department of Obstetrics and Gynaecology
Tygerberg Hospital
University of Stellenbosch
Tygerberg
South Africa

Gabor Huszar MD
Professor, The Sperm Physiology Laboratory
Department of Obstetrics and Gynecology
Yale University School of Medicine
New Haven, CT
USA

Attila Jakab MD
The Sperm Physiology Laboratory
Department of Obstetrics and Gynecology
Yale University School of Medicine
New Haven, CT
USA

Niels Jørgensen MD PhD
Certified Clinical Andrologist
Specialist in Medical Endocrinology and
  Consultant
University Department of Growth and
  Reproduction
Rigshospitalet
Copenhagen
Denmark

Michaela Luconi PhD
Associate Professor, 'DENOthe' Andrology Unit
Department of Clinical Physiopathology
University of Florence
Florence
Italy

Donald F Lynch Jr MD
Professor and Chairman, Department of Urology
  and Professor of Obstetrics and Gynecology
Eastern Virginia Medical School
Norfolk, VA
USA

Ahmed MA Mahmoud MD PhD
Center for Medical and Urological Andrology
  and Reproductive Endocrinology
University Hospital Ghent
Ghent
Belgium

Sepideh Mehri MD
Research Fellow
Yale Fertility Center
Yale University
New Haven, CT
USA

Roelof Menkveld PhD
Andrology Laboratory
Reproductive Biology Unit
Department of Obstetrics and Gynaecology
Tygerberg Hospital and Stellenbosch University
Tygerberg
South Africa

Olga Mudrak
The Jones Institute for Reproductive Medicine
Norfolk, VA
USA
and
Institute of Cytology
Russian Academy of Sciences
St Petersburg
Russia

Gary S Nakhuda MD
Assistant Professor, Division of Reproductive
  Endocrinology
Department of Obstetrics and Gynecology
College of Physicians and Surgeons
Columbia University
New York, NY
USA

Martine Nijs Mas Sc
Department of Obstetrics and Gynecology
Genk Institute of Fertility
St Jans Hospital
Genk
Belgium

Willem Ombelet MD PhD
Professor, Department of Obstetrics and
  Gynecology
Genk Institute of Fertility Technology
ZOL Campus St Jan
Genk
Belgium

Darius A Paduch MD PhD
Assistant Professor of Urology and Assistant
  Professor of Reproductive Medicine
Department of Urology
Weill Medical College of Cornell University
New York, NY;
The Population Council
Center for Biomedical Research
New York, NY
and
Center for Reproductive Medicine and Infertility
Weill Medical College of Cornell University
New York, NY
USA

Pasquale Patrizio MD
Professor of Obstetrics and Gynecology
  and Director
Yale Fertility Center
Yale University
New Haven, CT
USA

Vanesa Y Rawe
Laboratory of Biology, Research and Special
  Studies
Center of Studies in Gynecology and
  Reproduction
CEGyR
Buenos Aires
Argentina

Zev Rosenwaks MD
Professor of Obstetrics and Gynecology
and
Revlon Distinguished Professor of Reproductive
  Medicine
Center for Reproductive Medicine and Infertility
Weill Medical College of Cornell University
New York, NY
USA

Rosália Sá BSc
Lab Cell Biology
Institute of Biomedical Sciences Abel Salazar
and
Department of Genetics
Faculty of Medicine
University of Porto
Porto
Portugal

G Leyla Sati MS
The Sperm Physiology Laboratory
Department of Obstetrics and Gynecology
Yale University School of Medicine
New Haven, CT
USA

Mark V Sauer MD
Professor and Vice Chairman, Department of
  Obstetrics and Gynecology
Columbia University and Chief, Division of
  Reproductive Endocrinology
College of Physicians and Surgeons
Columbia University
New York, NY
USA

Augusto E Semprini MD
Clinica Ostetrica e Ginecologica
Università di Milano
Milan
Italy

Jose Sepúlveda MD
Clinical Assistant Professor, Instituto Estudio
  Concepcion Humana
Monterrey, México
and
Yale Fertility Center
Yale University
New Haven, CT
USA

T Igno Siebert MD
Department of Obstetrics and Gynaecology
Stellenbosch University
Tygerberg
South Africa

Joaquina Silva MD
Chief Embryologist, Centre for Reproductive
  Genetics A Barros
Porto
Portugal

Niels E Skakkebaek MD PhD
Professor, University Department of Growth and
  Reproduction
Rigshospitalet
Copenhagen
Denmark

Mário Sousa MD PhD
Professor, Director Lab Cell Biology
Institute of Biomedical Sciences
Department of Genetics
Faculty of Medicine
University of Porto
and
Scientific Director
Centre for Reproductive Genetics A. Barros
Porto
Portugal

Herman Tournaye MD PhD
Professor, Centre for Reproductive Medicine
Brussels Free University
Brussels
Belgium

F Haynes van der Merwe MD
Department of Obstetrics and Gynaecology
Stellenbosch University
Tygerberg
South Africa

André Van Steirteghem PhD
Professor and Director, Centre for Reproductive
  Medicine and Research
Centre for Reproduction and Genetics
Vrije Universiteit
Brussels
Belgium

Valérie Vernaeve MD PhD
Instituto Valenciano de Infertilidad (IVI)
IVI – Barcelona
Barcelona
Spain

Marie-Lena Windt PhD
Reproductive Biology Unit
Department of Obstetrics and Gynaecology
Tygerberg Hospital and Stellenbosch University
Tygerberg
South Africa

Andrei Zalensky PhD
Associate Professor, The Jones Institute for
  Reproductive Medicine
Norfolk, VA
USA
and
Institute of Cytology
Russian Academy of Sciences
St Petersburg
Russia

Color section

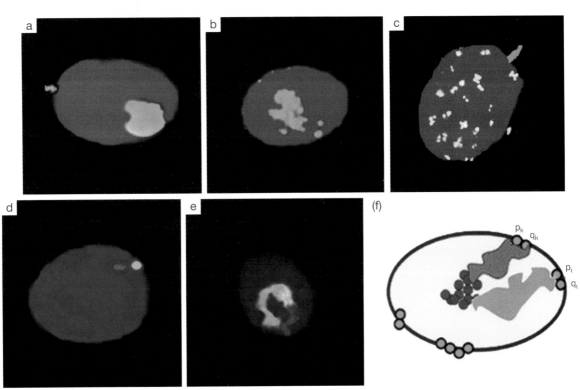

Color plate 1 (Figure 5.1) Chromosome organization in human sperm. (a) Chromosome territory: chromosome 6 (CHR6) (green) was localized using a painting probe. Total DNA counterstained with propidium iodide (PI) (red). (b) Centromeres (green) were visualized using immunofluorescence with antibodies against CENP-A (centromere protein A). Total DNA counterstained with PI (red). (c) Fluorescence *in situ* hybridization (FISH) using TTAGGG probe (yellow/green) shows that the majority of telomeres are joined as dimers and tetramers. Subtelomeric sequences located at the p and q arms of one chromosome are spatially close. Total DNA counterstained with PI (red). (d) Subtelomeric sequences located at the p and q arms of chromosome 3 (subTEL3q, pink; subTEL3p, emerald) are spatially close. Total DNA counterstained with diamidino-2-phenylindole (DAPI) (blue). (e) FISH using arm-specific probes microdissected from CHR1 (1q, green; 1p, red) indicates looping of this chromosome. Total DNA counterstained with DAPI (blue). (f) Schematic model of sperm nuclear architecture. Selected chromosome territories (pink and ocher), telomeres (TEL) (green circles) and centromeres (CEN) (red circles) are shown within a section through the nucleus. Non-homologous CEN are clustered into a chromocenter, while TEL interact at the nuclear periphery. Modified from Ward and Zalensky 1996 (reference 38)

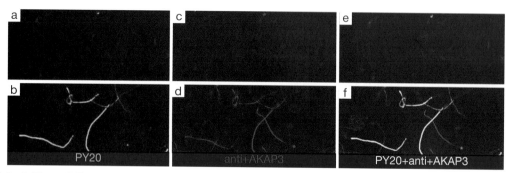

Color plate 2 (Figure 2.3)   Immunofluorescence analysis of fixed and permeabilized human spermatozoa. Confocal microscopy of double immunolabeling for tyrosine phosphorylated proteins ((b), PY20 antibody, green) and Akinase anchoring protein 3 (AKAP3) ((d), anti-AKAP3 antibody, red) reveals positivity for both antibodies in sperm tails. Simultaneous analysis of dual fluorescence confirms that tyrosine phosphorylation corresponds to AKAP3 in the tail ((f), double fluorescence, yellow). (a), (c), (e), negative controls without primary antibody. From reference 9, with permission

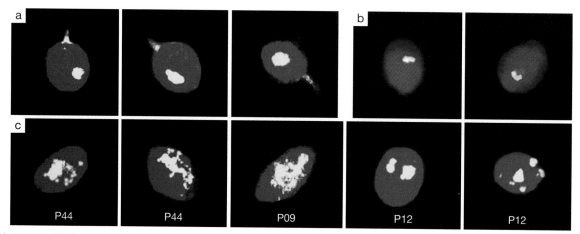

Color plate 3 (Figure 5.2)   Determination of chromosome intranuclear localization using fluorescence *in situ* hybridization (FISH) with painting probes. (a) Typical patterns of chromosome 1 (CHR1) painting probe hybridization (yellow) in normal sperm. (b) Typical patterns of CHR1 arm-specific probe hybridization (1p, green; 1q, red) in normal sperm. (c) Patterns of CHR1 hybridization in three samples of abnormal sperm.

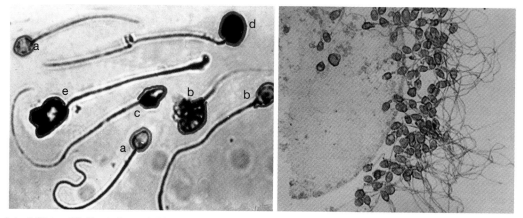

Color plate 4 (Figure 30.1)   Left panel: Mature (a) and diminished-maturity sperm with cytoplasmic retention (b–e) after creatine kinase (CK) immunostaining. Right panel: CK-immunostained sperm–hemizona complex. Observe that only the clear-headed mature spermatozoa without cytoplasmic retention are able to bind

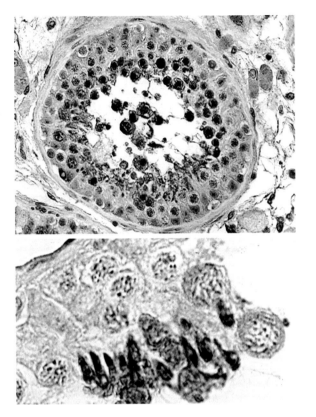

Color plate 5 (Figure 30.2)   Human testicular biopsy tissues immunostained with HspA2 antiserum. Sections represent lower (upper panel) and high (lower panel) magnifications to illustrate the tubular structure, and staining pattern of the adluminal area. HspA2 expression begins in meiotic spermatocytes, but is predominant during terminal spermiogenesis in elongated spermatids and spermatozoa

Color plate 6 (Figure 30.3)   A model of normal and diminished maturation of human sperm. In *normal* sperm, maturation HspA2 is expressed in the synaptonemal complex of spermatocytes, supporting meiosis. HspA2 is likely also involved in the processes of late spermiogenesis, such as cytoplasmic extrusion (represented by loss of the residual body, RB), plasma membrane remodeling and formation of the zona pellucida- and hyaluronic acid-binding sites (change from blue to red membrane and stubs). *Diminished-maturity* sperm lack HspA2 expression, which causes meiotic defects and a higher rate of retention of creatine kinase (CK) and other cytoplasmic enzymes, increased levels of lipid peroxidation (LP) and consequent DNA fragmentation, abnormal sperm morphology and deficiency in zona and hyaluronic acid binding

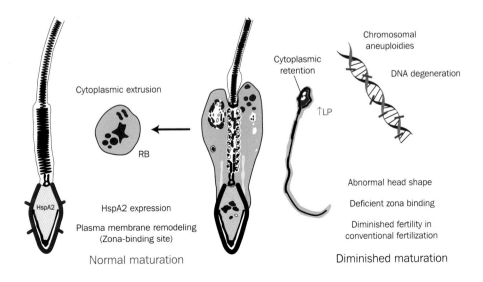

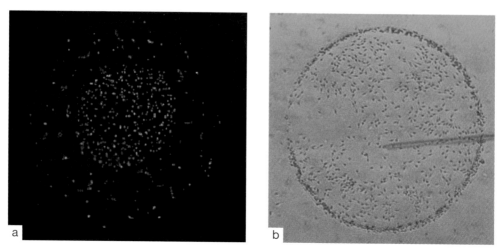

Color plate 7 (Figure 30.4)   Sperm movement patterns on the hyaluronic acid-coated spots used for sperm selection. Mature sperm are bound, and diminished-maturity sperm remain motile. Sperm are stained with cyber green DNA stain (Molecular Probes, Eugene, OR) that permeates viable sperm

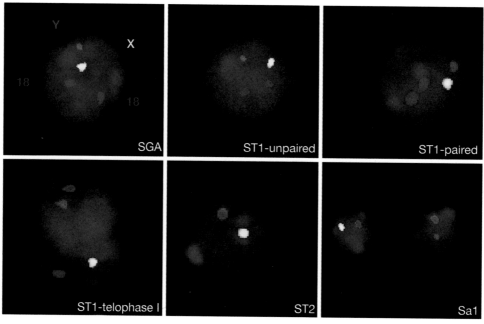

Color plate 8 (Figure 31.4)   Cocultures. Fluorescence *in situ* hybridization (FISH) analysis of spermatogonia A (SGA), primary spermatocytes (ST1), secondary spermatocytes (ST2) and early round spermatids (Sa1). 18 = violet, X = yellow, Y = red

Section 1

Basic concepts: sperm physiology and pathology

1

Anatomy and molecular morphology of the spermatozoon

Christiaan F Hoogendijk, Thinus F Kruger, Roelof Menkveld

INTRODUCTION

This chapter summarizes light and electronmicroscopic features that outline the basic characteristics of the anatomy of the human spermatozoon. Furthermore, sperm chromosomes are discussed in terms of the highly ordered and specific structure and packaging of the chromatin, together with the potential relationship between the increased incidence of numerical chromosomal aberrations and abnormal sperm morphology observed in infertile men.

LIGHT AND ELECTRON MICROSCOPIC MORPHOLOGICAL CHARACTERISTICS OF SPERMATOZOA

Spermatozoa are highly specialized and condensed cells that do not grow or divide. A spermatozoon consists of a head, containing the paternal heredity material (DNA), and a tail, which provides motility (Figures 1.1 and 1.2). The spermatozoon is endowed with a large nucleus, but lacks the large cytoplasm that is characteristic of most somatic cells. Men are unique among mammals in the degree of morphological heterogeneity of spermatozoa found in the ejaculate[1–3].

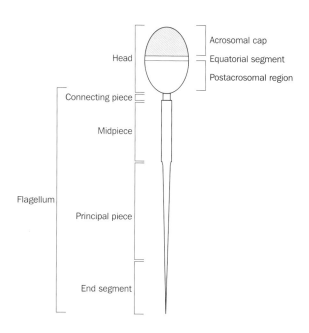

Figure 1.1   Schematic drawing of light microscopic human spermatozoon

Sperm head

Light microscopy

Human spermatozoa are classified using brightfield microscope optics on fixed, stained specimens[2,3]. The heads of stained human spermatozoa are slightly smaller than the heads of living

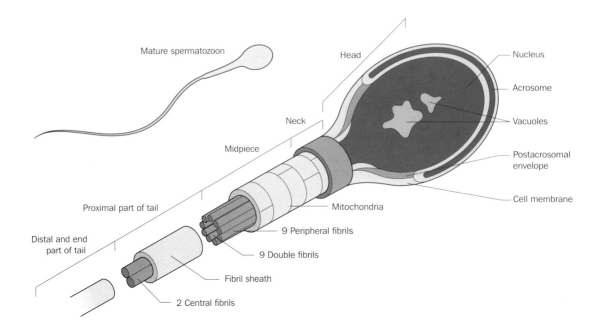

Figure 1.2   Light and electron microscopic diagrams of human spermatozoon

spermatozoa in the original semen, although the shapes are not appreciably different[4]. The normal head should be oval in shape. Allowing for the slight shrinkage that fixation and staining induce, the length of the head is about 3–5 µm, and the width 2–3 µm. These values span the 95% confidence limits of comparative data for both Papanicolaou-stained and living sperm heads[4]. Two slightly different types of normal spermatozoa head forms have been described, based on spermatozoa found in endocervical canal mucus after coitus[3]. The first and most common form, as identified under the microscope with bright-field illumination, is the perfectly smooth oval head; the second form is oval, still having a smooth or regular contour, but being slightly tapered at the postacrosomal end[3]. Since diversity is a fact of all biological systems, trivial variations must be regarded as normal[3].

The following head aberrations can be observed: head shape/size defects, including large, small, tapering, pyriform, amorphous, vacuolated (> 20% of the head surface occupied by unstained vacuolar areas), and double heads, or any combination of these[5]. Human spermatozoa have a well-defined acrosomal region constituting about two-thirds of the anterior head area[2,3,5]. They do not exhibit an apical thickening like many other species, but show a uniform thickness/thinning towards the end, forming the equatorial segment. Because of this thinning, the area is visualized as more intensely stained when examined with the light microscope. Depending on this staining intensity, the acrosome will appear to cover 40–70% of the sperm head.

Scanning electron microscopy

Scanning electron microscopy (SEM) is useful for demonstration of the surface structures of spermatozoa in great detail. Owing to its three-dimensional image, furthermore, it is possible to observe and interpret the complex structure of a human spermatozoon more easily and completely than with either light or transmission electron microscopy. The sperm head is divided into two unequal parts by a furrow that completely encircles the head, i.e. the acrosomal and postacrosomal regions. The acrosomal region can represent up to two-thirds of the head length and, in some cases, a depression is noted in this area, which is regarded as morphologically normal. The equatorial segment is not always clearly visible with SEM. Just after the equatorial segment is the beginning of the postacrosomal region, which is marked by maximal thickness and width of the spermatozoon. The postacrosomal region is divided into two parts by the posterior ring, forming two equal bands. The band closest to the acrosome stands out[1]. The surface of the human spermatozoon, washed free of seminal plasma, appears smooth, without coarse particles. The only exception is the acrosome, especially the anterior part, that may frequently appear rough[1].

Light and electron microscopic and molecular morphological characteristics of spermatozoa

The electron microscopic morphological characteristics of human spermatozoa are presented in Figures 1.2–1.6. The sperm head is a flattened ovoid structure consisting primarily of the nucleus. The acrosome is a cap-like structure covering the anterior two-thirds of the sperm head (Figures 1.2 and 1.3), which arises from the Golgi apparatus of the spermatid as it differentiates into a spermatozoon. Unlike in other mammalian species, the acrosome of the human spermatozoon does not exhibit apical thickening, but has an anterior segment of uniform thickness. The acrosome contains several hydrolytic enzymes, including hyaluronidase and proacrosin, which are necessary for fertilization[1].

During fertilization of the egg, the enzyme-rich contents of the acrosome are released at the time of acrosome reaction. During fusion of the outer acrosomal membrane with the plasma membrane at multiple sites, the acrosomal enzymes are released. The anterior half of the head is then devoid of plasma and outer acrosomal membrane and is covered only by the inner acrosomal membrane[6]. The equatorial segment of the acrosome persists more or less intact, since it does not participate in the acrosome reaction (Figure 1.3).

The posterior portion of the sperm head is covered by the postnuclear cap, which is a single membrane. The equatorial segment consists of an overlap of the acrosome and the postnuclear cap (Figure 1.3). The nucleus (Figure 1.3), constituting 65% of the head, is composed of DNA conjugated with protein. The chromatin within the nucleus is very compact, and no distinct chromosomes are visible. Sperm nuclei can have incomplete condensation with apparent vacuoles. The genetic information carried by the spermatozoon is 'encoded' and stored in the DNA molecule, which is made up of many nucleotides. The hereditary characteristics transmitted by the sperm nucleus include sex determination[1].

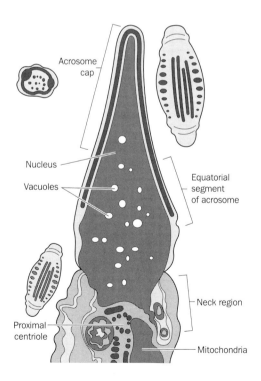

Figure 1.3 Schematic drawing of longitudinal section of sperm head

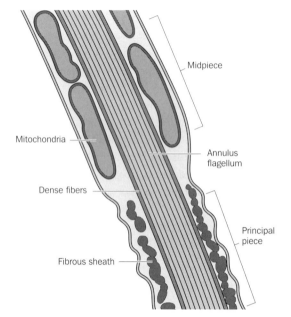

Figure 1.4 Longitudinal section of region between the midpiece and principal piece of human spermatozoon

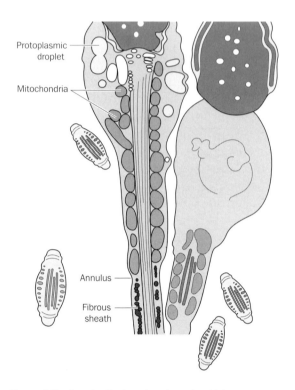

Figure 1.5   Longitudinal section through midpiece

Molecular morphology

The sperm chromosome structure is very complex. Some of the attributes are similar to somatic cell DNA organization and others are unique to spermatogenic cells. Sperm DNA packaging can be subdivided into four levels.

Level I: chromosomal anchoring by the nuclear annulus   The two strands of naked DNA which make up each chromosome are attached to a sperm-specific structure, the nuclear annulus. This represents a novel type of DNA organization, termed chromosomal anchoring, that is found only in spermatogenic cells. The nuclear annulus is shaped like a bent ring, and is about 2 μm in length. It is found only in sperm nuclei, although it is currently unknown at what stage of spermiogenesis it is first formed. So far there is no evidence for a nuclear annulus-like structure in any somatic cell type. In contrast, there is evidence of its existence in hamster[7], human[8], mouse and *Xenopus* sperm nuclei. Its existence in a wide variety of species suggests a fundamental role in sperm function.

Unique DNA sequences were found to be associated with the nuclear annulus. Ward[9] termed these sequences NA-DNA. The existence of these unique sequences suggests that the nuclear annulus anchors chromosomes according to particular sequences and not by random DNA binding. By organizing the chromosomes so that the NA-DNA sites of each chromosome are aggregated onto one structure, the nuclear annulus may also affect the determination of sperm nuclear shape. For example, in the hamster spermatozoon, the longer chromosomes may extend into the thinner hook of the nucleus, while a portion of every chromosome is located at the nuclear annulus. This is supported by image analysis of the distribution of DNA throughout the hamster sperm nucleus, which demonstrates that the highest concentration of DNA in the packaged sperm nucleus is at the base, where the nuclear annulus is located; in contrast, the lowest concentration of DNA is in the hooked portion[10].

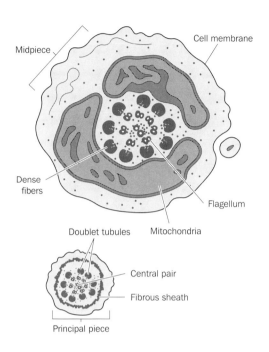

Figure 1.6 Cross-section of human sperm tail

This hypothesis is further supported by electron microscopic evidence that the chromatin near the implantation fossa is one of the first areas to condense during spermiogenesis[11]. Thus, the nuclear annulus may represent the only known aspect of sperm chromatin condensation that is specific for individual chromosome sites.

Level II: sperm DNA loop domain organization Anchored chromosomes are organized into DNA loop domains. Parts of the nuclear matrix, protein structural fibers, attach to the DNA every 30–50 kb by specific sequences termed matrix attachment regions (MARs). This arranges the chromosome strands into a series of loops. This type of organization can be visualized experimentally in preparations known as nuclear halos. Halos consist of loops of naked DNA, 25–100 kb in length, attached at their bases to the matrix. Each loop domain visible in the nuclear halo consists of a structural unit of chromatin that exists *in vivo* in a condensed form.

The organization of DNA into loop domains is the only type of structural organization resolved thus far that is present in both somatic and sperm cells. In somatic cells, DNA is coiled into nucleosomes, then further coiled into a 30-nm solenoid-like fiber and then organized into DNA loop domains. The corresponding structures in sperm chromatin have a very different appearance. Protamine binding causes a different type of coiling, and DNA is folded into densely packed toroids, but still organized into loop domains. Mammalian sperm nuclei contain a small amount of histones that are presumably organized into nucleosomes[12,13], but most of the DNA is reorganized by protamines. This means that with the evolutionary pressure to condense sperm DNA, all aspects of chromatin structure are sacrificed other than organization of the DNA into loop domains. This suggests that DNA loop domains play a crucial role in sperm DNA function.

Level III: protamine decondensation The binding of protamines condenses the DNA loops into tightly packaged chromatin. DNA protamine binding forms toroidal or doughnut-shaped structures in which the DNA is very concentrated[14]. During spermiogenesis, histones, the DNA-binding proteins of somatic spermatogenic precursor cells, are replaced by protamines. Since histone-bound DNA requires much more volume than the same amount of DNA bound to protamines[15], this change in chromatin structure probably accounts for some of the nuclear condensation that occurs during spermiogenesis. Protamines bind DNA along the major groove; this completely neutralizes DNA so that neighboring DNA strands bind to each other by van der Waals forces. Protamine binding leads to condensation and preservation of the DNA loop domain organization present in the round spermatid[9].

Level IV: chromosome organization The results of several studies[10,16,17] have led to the proposal of a model[18] in which there are limited constraints on the actual position of the chromosomes in the sperm nucleus. The NA-DNA sequences are located at the base of the nucleus, centromeres are located centrally and telomeres are located peripherally. Outside these three constraints, the folding of the chromosomal p and q arms is flexible.

Sperm tail

Light microscopy

Sperm tail formation arises at the spermatid stage. During spermatogenesis the centriole is differentiated into three parts: midpiece, main or principal piece and endpiece (Figures 1.1 and 1.2). The midpiece is of similar length to the head, and is separated from the tailpiece by a ring, the annulus (Figure 1.5). The following tail aberrations can be observed:

- Neck and midpiece aberrations include their absence (seen as 'free' or 'loose' heads), non-inserted or 'bent' tail (the tail forms an angle of about 90° with the long axis of the head), distended/irregular/bent midpiece, abnormally thin midpiece (i.e. no mitochondrial sheath) or any combination of these[5];

- Tail aberrations include short, multiple, hairpin, broken (angulation > 90°) tails, irregular width, coiling tails with terminal droplets or any combination of these[5];

- Cytoplasmic droplets greater than one-third of the area of a normal sperm head are considered abnormal. They are usually located in the neck/midpiece region of the tail, although some immature spermatozoa may have a cytoplasmic droplet at other locations along the tail[3,5]. The endpiece is not distinctly visualized by light microscopy.

Scanning electron microscopy

With SEM the tail can be subdivided into three distinct parts, i.e. midpiece, principal piece and endpiece. In the midpiece the mitochondrial spirals can be clearly visualized. This ends abruptly at the beginning of the midpiece. The midpiece narrows towards the posterior end. A longitudinal column and transverse ribs are visible. The short endpiece has a small diameter due to the absence of outer fibers[1].

Transmission electron microscopy

The midpiece possesses a cytoplasmic portion and a lipid-rich mitochondrial sheath that consists of several spiral mitochondria, surrounding the axial filament in a helical fashion (Figures 1.2, 1.5 and 1.6). The midpiece provides the sperm with the energy necessary for motility. The central axial core of eleven fibrils is surrounded by an additional outer ring of nine coarser fibrils (Figures 1.2 and 1.6). Individual mitochondria are wrapped around these outer fibrils in a spiral manner to form the mitochondrial sheath, which contains the enzymes involved in the oxidative metabolism of the sperm (Figures 1.2 and 1.4–1.6). The mitochondrial sheath of the midpiece is relatively short, being slightly longer than the combined length of the head and neck[1].

The principal piece (main piece), the longest part of the tail, provides most of the propellant machinery. The coarse nine fibrils of the outer ring diminish in thickness and finally disappear, leaving only the inner fibrils in the axial core for much of the length of the principal piece (Figure 1.2)[19]. The fibrils of the principal piece are surrounded by a fibrous tail sheath, which consists of branching and anastomosing semicircular strands or 'ribs' held together by their attachment to two bands that run lengthwise along opposite sides of the tail[1]. The tail terminates in the endpiece with a length of 4–10 μm and a diameter of < 1 μm. The small diameter is due to the absence of the outer fibers and sheath and distal fading of microtubules.

SPERM MORPHOLOGY AND CHROMOSOMAL ANEUPLOIDIES

Many authors have studied the association between abnormal sperm shape and increased frequency of aneuploidies. The conclusions of these studies are inconsistent; this is most probably because the sperm attributes were evaluated in the same semen sample, but not in the same sperm. As early as 1991, Martin studied sperm karyotypes[20]. She demonstrated that all chromosomes undergo nondisjunction during spermiogenesis, but that the G-group chromosomes (21 and 22) and the sex chromosomes have a significantly increased frequency of aneuploidy. Using fluorescence *in situ* hybridization (FISH), Spriggs and co-workers[21] determined that most chromosomes have a disomy frequency of approximately 0.1% (1/1000); in contrast, the sex chromosomes and chromosomes 21 and 22 have a significantly increased frequency of aneuploidy. Thus, the sex chromosome bivalent and the G-group chromosomes are more susceptible to nondisjunction during spermatogenesis.

Bernardini *et al.*[22] suggested a relationship between increased frequencies of aneuploidy and diploidy in semen samples containing spermatozoa with enlarged heads. Several other studies have concluded that morphologically abnormal sperm may also have a significantly increased risk for being aneuploid[23–27]. An interesting report, based on the examination of sperm injected into mouse oocytes, suggested that in semen samples with high incidences of amorphous, round and elongated sperm heads, there was an increased proportion of structural chromosome abnormalities, such as chromosome and chromatid fragments and dicentric and ring chromosomes, but no increase in numerical chromosomal aberrations[28]. Further, Ryu *et al.*[29] studied 120 normal and abnormal sperm (according to Tygerberg strict criteria) each in eight men, and concluded that normal morphology is not a valid indicator for the selection of sperm with haploid nuclei. Rives *et al.*[30] showed that although the disomy frequencies of infertile males were directly related to the severity of oligozoospermia, there was no relationship between aneuploidy frequency and abnormal

morphology. In men with increased levels of globozoospermia, shortened flagella syndrome or sperm with acrosomal abnormalities, no association was found between sperm shape and numerical chromosomal aberrations[31].

In another study, De Vos and co-workers[32] determined the influence of individual sperm morphology on fertilization, embryo morphology and pregnancy outcome after intracytoplasmic sperm injection (ICSI). With regard to the different morphological defects observed, they found the following fertilization rates: 63.4% (52 of 82) for spermatozoa with elongated heads; 63.3% (124 of 196) for spermatozoa with cytoplasmic droplets; 59.6% (223 of 374) for spermatozoa with amorphous heads; and 34.1% (15 of 44) for spermatozoa with broken necks. One hundred and one injected spermatozoa showed a combination of two morphological defects (overall fertilization rate, 57.4%). No fertilization ensued from six round-headed spermatozoa lacking acrosomes, and 12 spermatozoa showing vacuoles in their acrosomes provided a fertilization rate of 66.6%. These authors concluded that sperm morphology assessed at the moment of ICSI correlated well with fertilization outcome but did not affect embryo development. Furthermore, the implantation rate was lower when only embryos resulting from injection of abnormal spermatozoa were available.

Recently, Celik-Ozenci and co-workers[33] studied the relationship between sperm shape and numerical chromosomal aberrations in individual spermatozoa, using FISH, objective morphometry and sperm dimension and shape assessment, along with Tygerberg strict criteria. The results indicate that numerical chromosomal aberrations can be present in sperm heads of any size or shape, but the risk is greater with amorphous sperm. Even the most normal-appearing sperm with normal head and tail size could be disomic or diploid, although diploidy is less prevalent with normal sperm dimensions and shape.

CONCLUSIONS

Although many of the structures described here, especially the ultrastructural characteristics based on electron microscopy studies, are not visible by standard light microscopic examination, a basic knowledge of these structures is very important for the correct evaluation and interpretation of sperm morphology. In turn, this information will assist the clinician in the estimation of male fertility potential.

From the molecular structure of the sperm, it is evident that the sperm DNA is packaged within the nucleus in an extremely complex and ordered fashion; there is, however, some degree of flexibility to this organization. A detailed model of how chromosomes are packaged in the sperm nucleus is gradually emerging; implications of this knowledge are already having an impact upon the study of fertility, particularly in preparations of nuclei for ICSI, diagnosis of semen samples and understanding the fate of sperm DNA after fertilization. As our knowledge of sperm chromatin increases, it is becoming more evident that visual assessment is an unreliable method for selection of sperm for ICSI. More specific methods for sperm selection, such as hyaluronic acid binding[34], may alleviate the problem of fertilization with sperm of diminished maturity and genetic integrity during ICSI.

REFERENCES

1. Hafez ESE. Human Semen and Fertility Regulation in Men. St Louis: CV Mosby, 1976
2. Kruger TF, et al. Sperm morphological features as a prognostic factor in in vitro fertilization. Fertil Steril 1986; 46: 1118
3. Menkveld R, et al. The evaluation of morphological characteristics of human spermatozoa according to stricter criteria. Hum Reprod 1990; 4: 586
4. Katz DF, et al. Morphometric analysis of spermatozoa in the assessment of human male fertility. J Androl 1986; 7: 203
5. World Health Organization. WHO Manual for the Examination of Human Semen and Sperm–Cervical Mucus Interaction, 2nd edn. London: Cambridge University Press, 1992
6. Barros C, Franklin LE. Behavior of the gamete membranes during sperm entry into the mammalian egg. J Cell Biol 1986; 37: 13
7. Ward WS, Coffey DS. Identification of a sperm nuclear annulus: a sperm DNA anchor. Biol Reprod 1989; 41: 361
8. Barone JG, et al. DNA organization in human spermatozoa. J Androl 1994; 15: 139
9. Ward WS. DNA loop domain tertiary structure in mammalian spermatozoa. Biol Reprod 1993; 48: 1193
10. Ward WS, et al. Localization of the three genes in the assymetric hamster sperm nucleus by fluorescent in situ hybridization. Biol Reprod 1996; 54: 1271
11. Loir M, Courtens JL. Nuclear reorganization in ram spermatids. J Ultrastruct Res 1979; 67: 309
12. Tanphaichitr N, et al. Basic nuclear proteins in testicular cells and ejaculated spermatozoa in man. Exp Cell Res 1978; 117: 347
13. Choudhary SK, et al. A haploid expressed gene cluster exists as a single chromatin domain in human sperm. J Biol Chem 1995; 270: 8755
14. Hud NV, Downing KH, Balhorn R. A constant radius of curvature model for the organization of DNA in toroidal condensates. Proc Natl Acad Sci USA 1995; 92: 3581
15. Ward WS, Coffey DS. DNA packaging and organization in mammalian spermatozoa: comparison with somatic cells [Review]. Biol Reprod 1991; 44: 569
16. Zalensky AO, et al. Well-defined genome architecture in the human sperm nucleus. Chromosoma 1995; 103: 577
17. Haaf T, Ward WS. Higher order nuclear structure in mammalian sperm revealed by in situ hybridization and extended chromatin fibers. Exp Cell Res 1995; 219: 604
18. Ward WS, Zalensky A. The unique, complex organization of the transcriptionally silent sperm chromatin. Crit Rev Eukaryot Gene Expr 1996; 6: 139
19. White IG. Mammalian sperm. In Hafez ESE, ed. Reproduction of Farm Animals, 3rd edn. Philidelphia: Lea & Febiger, 1974
20. Martin RH. Cytogenetic analysis of sperm from a man heterozygous for a pericentric inversion, inv(3)(p25q21). Am J Hum Genet 1991; 48: 856
21. Spriggs EL, Rademaker AW, Martin RH. Aneuploidy in human sperm: the use of mulicolor FISH to test various theories of nondisjunction. Am J Hum Genet 1996; 58: 356

22. Bernardini L, et al. Study of aneuploidy in normal and abnormal germ cells from semen of fertile and infertile men. Hum Reprod 1998; 13: 3406

23. Colombero LT, et al. Incidence of sperm aneuploidy in relation to semen characteristics and assisted reproductive outcome. Fertil Steril 1999; 72: 90

24. Calogero AE, et al. Aneuploidy rate in spermatozoa of selected men with abnormal semen parameters. Hum Reprod 2001; 16: 1172

25. Rubio C, et al. Incidence of sperm chromosomal abnormalities in a risk population: relationship with sperm quality and ICSI outcome. Hum Reprod 2001; 16: 2084

26. Yakin K, Kahraman S. Certain forms of morphological anomalies of spermatozoa may reflect chromosomal aneuploidies. Hum Reprod 2001; 16: 1779

27. Templado C, et al. Aneuploid spermatozoa in infertile men: teratozoospermia. Mol Reprod Dev 2002; 61: 200

28. Lee JD, Kamiguchi Y, Yanagimachi R. Analysis of chromosome constitution of human spermatozoa with normal and aberrant head morphologies after injection into mouse oocytes. Hum Reprod 1996; 11: 1942

29. Ryu HM, et al. Increased chromosome X, Y, and 18 nondisjunction in sperm from infertile patients that were identified as normal by strict morphology: implication for intracytoplasmic sperm injection. Fertil Steril 2001; 76: 879

30. Rives N, et al. Relationship between clinical phenotype, semen parameters and aneuploidy frequency in sperm nuclei of 50 infertile males. Hum Genet 1999; 105: 266

31. Viville S, et al. Do morphological anomalies reflect chromosomal aneuploidies? Case report. Hum Reprod 2000; 15: 2563

32. De Vos A, et al. Influence of individual sperm morphology on fertilization, embryo morphology, and pregnancy outcome of intracytoplasmic sperm injection. Fertil Steril 2003; 79: 42

33. Celik-Ozenci C, et al. Sperm selection for ICSI: shape properties do not predict the absence or presence of numerical chromosomal aberrations. Hum Reprod 2004; 19: 2052

34. Huszar G, et al. Hyaluronic acid binding by human sperm indicates cellular maturity, viability, and unreacted acrosomal status. Fertil Steril 2003; 79: 1616

2

Physiology and pathophysiology of sperm motility

Michaela Luconi, Elisabetta Baldi, Gustavo F Doncel

INTRODUCTION

Mammalian spermatozoa become motile and acquire the ability to swim during their transit from the testis to the oviduct. These changes are initiated and controlled by several extra- and intracellular factors, which also play a pivotal role in regulating the acquisition of hyperactivated motility and chemotaxis.

This chapter summarizes the mechanochemical basis of sperm movement, placing special emphasis on the regulatory factors involved in acquisition and maintenance of sperm motility, hyperactivation and chemotaxis. It also covers the molecular basis of asthenozoospermia, a sperm pathology characterized by reduced sperm motility, which represents one of the main causes of male infertility. Finally, it presents systemic and *in vitro* therapeutic approaches for asthenozoospermia, along with the most recent findings on pharmacological and physiological molecules capable of stimulating sperm motility.

MECHANOCHEMICAL BASIS OF SPERM MOTILITY

Sperm swimming is characterized by a rhythmic, three-dimensional, asymmetric movement of the flagellum. This unique movement is assured by

the complex organization of the flagellum (Figure 2.1). With the exception of the distal part (endpiece) containing only the central couple of microtubules, the entire flagellum is organized in a cylindrical structure called the axoneme, consisting of nine pairs of tubulin A and B microtubules (doublets) connected to each other by nexin arms and to the central doublet by radial spokes. Each microtubule doublet is externally anchored to nine asymmetric outer dense fibers (ODFs), which are surrounded by the fibrous sheath in the principal piece and packed by mitochondria in the middle piece of the sperm tail (Figure 2.1). The base of the flagellum is thickened by a connecting piece consisting of nine segmented columns which distally fuse with the corresponding ODFs[2], and is responsible for the transmission of tail movement to the head. The reciprocal sliding of each pair of microtubules originates from the sequential anchoring of the dynein arms to the neighboring doublet and adenosine triphosphate (ATP)-dependent generation of sliding force. This sliding results in bends of alternating direction, which propagate the oscillation along the tail. The asymmetry of the axonemal structure as well as the outer microtubule connections to the central doublet and the ODF–fibrous sheath complexes confer a helical shape to the propagating flagellar beat. ODFs are essential for the development of forward motility in the mature sperm, and their

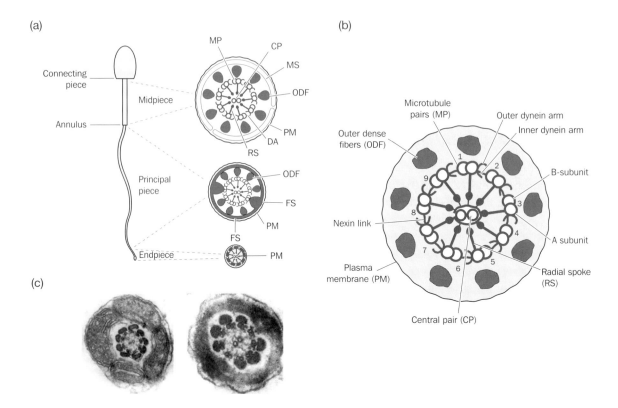

Figure 2.1 Schematic representation of a human spermatozoon. (a) Longitudinal section showing head, middle piece, principal piece and endpiece. The insets on the right show the cytoskeletal organization of the sperm tail in transverse sections at different levels: middle (top), principal (center) and endpiece (bottom). Electron microscopy of transverse sections of the sperm tail at the levels of the middle (left) and the principal piece (right) are presented in (c). (b) Drawing showing organization of the axoneme. CP, central pair; MS, mitochondria; ODF, outer dense fibers; PM, plasma membrane; DA, dynein arms; RS, radial spoke; MP, microtubule pairs; FS, fibrous sheath. Modified from reference 1, with permission

structure and number are highly conserved throughout evolution. In particular, their cross-sectional area correlates positively with the length of the flagellum[3].

Oscillations can originate in different regions of the flagellum; however, the beat frequency seems to be controlled by the basal region, which acts as a sort of pacemaker. Although different models have been proposed, the mechanism underlying the initiation of a new bend at the flagellar base is still unknown[4]. A recent paper on a knock-out mouse model for the functional dynein heavy chain has demonstrated the importance of these arms on the development of sperm motility[5]. In fact, mice in which the dynein inner-arm heavy

chain gene has been deleted show asthenozoospermic characteristics, with the majority of spermatozoa unable to achieve forward progressive motility. In such spermatozoa, the outer dense fibers retain their attachments to the inner surface of the mitochondria. These links are essential in normal spermatozoa for midpiece development, but disappear when spermatozoa acquire the ability to swim upon release from the epididymis. Conversely, disruption of dynein inner-arm heavy chains in knock-out mice results in insufficient force to overcome these bridges, and spermatozoa are unable to undergo normal tail bending.

Energy to support the sliding force of the microtubules is provided by ATP, which is hydrolyzed by the dynein ATPase arms associated with the outer doublets of the microtubules. Although oxidative phosphorylation in midpiece mitochondria has long been considered a major source of ATP, local production of energy in the sperm principal piece through an alternative glycolytic enzyme pathway has recently been proposed as the main source of energy for flagellar movement. In fact, albeit reduced, motility is still present when mitochondrial oxidative phosphorylation is uncoupled in sperm[6]. Moreover, these two metabolic processes are strictly compartmentalized to the middle and principal pieces of the sperm flagellum, and although oxidative phosphorylation is more efficient than glycolysis in producing ATP, it is unlikely that ATP diffusion from the former to the latter compartment could supply enough energy to support flagellar movement in the distal region of the flagellum. Miki *et al.*[7] elegantly demonstrated that the sperm-specific glycolytic enzyme glyceraldehyde-3-phosphate dehydrogenase-S (GAPDS, and its human ortholog GAPD2) is necessary for sperm motility and fertility, since sperm from Gapds(–/–) knock-out mice, in which oxidative phosphorylation is unaffected, generate only 10.4% of the ATP produced in wild-type controls. Moreover, sperm motility was impaired, with virtual absence of forward movement, and the mice were infertile[7]. Therefore, glycolysis seems to be the pivotal metabolism producing ATP for sperm motility. This concept is reinforced by the presence of sperm-specific isoforms of other glycolytic enzymes such as hexokinase and lactate dehydrogenase, which are selectively expressed in the sperm principal piece[8].

REGULATION OF SPERM MOTILITY

Upon release from the testis, human and all mammalian spermatozoa are immotile. In order to reach and fertilize the oocyte, they acquire the ability to swim during their transit through the epididymis and the female genital tract. Several extra- and intracellular factors are important for the development and maintenance of sperm motility (Figure 2.2). These two processes appear to be regulated in a similar way. However, the majority of *in vitro* studies have been focused on the maintenance of sperm motility, using ejaculated or caudal epididymal spermatozoa. The following are some of the main factors regulating sperm movement.

Calcium

Under physiological conditions, calcium is one of the most important ions regulating human sperm motility[10]. However, the role of calcium in activating spermatozoa has always been regarded as controversial. Indeed, voltage-gated, cyclic nucleotide-gated and transient receptor potential calcium channels have been described along the plasma membrane of the entire flagellum (for reviews see references 11 and 12), thus suggesting the importance of calcium entry for motility. Transient receptor potential calcium channels have recently been demonstrated in the sperm tail and are involved in stimulation of sperm motility by capacitation-dependent calcium entry[13]. Knock-out mice for the newly discovered CatSper calcium channel specifically expressed in the tail are infertile due to loss of progressive motility[14]. An increase in intracellular calcium levels is also indirectly implicated in the activation of intracellular calcium stores via inositol 1,4,5-triphosphate (IP3) signaling[15,16]. Upon entry, calcium activates phospholipases and modulates several enzyme activities. In particular, the activated calcium/calmodulin (CaM) complex has been shown to stimulate sperm motility through direct interaction with soluble adenylate cyclase (sAC)[17,18], protein kinases[19,20], phosphatases[21] and phosphodiesterases[22], finally leading to an increase in cyclic adenosine monophosphate (cAMP) and phosphorylation of sperm proteins. CaM has been characterized in sperm axonema and proposed as the intracellular calcium sensor regulating motility[23]. CaM levels are reduced in sperm from

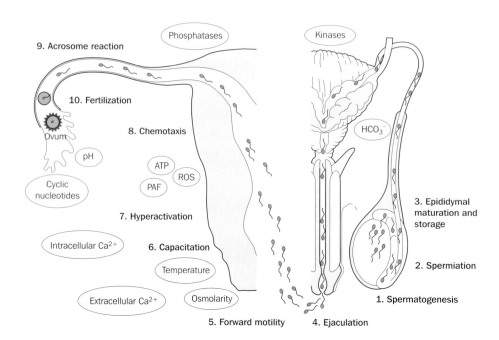

Figure 2.2   Factors regulating sperm motility during the 'sperm journey' from the testis (right) to the ovary (left). External and intracellular factors controlling sperm motility are indicated (oval labels) together with the activation processes (numbered) that spermatozoa undergo during their transit through the male and female reproductive tracts. ATP, adenosine triphosphate; PAF, platelet-activating factors; ROS, reactive oxygen species. Modified from reference 9, with permission

asthenozoospermic patients[24], and inhibitors of this enzyme negatively affect sperm motility[25]. Among CaM target enzymes, Marin-Briggiler *et al.*[19] characterized a CaM-dependent protein kinase. Inhibition of the isoform IV of this kinase results in a specific decrease in motion parameters and ATP levels without affecting sperm viability, protein tyrosine phosphorylation or acrosome reaction[19]. Incubation of motile sperm in the absence of calcium dramatically reduces motion parameters[19], suggesting the importance of calcium in the maintenance of human sperm motility.

Extracellular calcium has been demonstrated to be essential for sperm motility. Evidence also suggests that its intracellular concentrations must be strictly regulated to allow for precise timing of sperm activation[26,27]. Decreasing levels of external calcium between the caput and cauda of the epididymis are associated with progressive development of sperm motility and an increase in protein

tyrosine phosphorylation[28,29]. Calcium addition to demembranated human sperm suppresses motility[30], and increased intracellular calcium levels following cryopreservation negatively correlate with sperm motility and fertilizing ability[31].

Although many papers have focused on the role of calcium entry channels, very little is known about calcium extrusion from the cell. Recently, plasma membrane Ca^{2+}/calmodulin-dependent Ca^{2+} ATPases (PMCA) have been demonstrated to be essential for maintaining intracellular calcium homeostasis[32]. Indeed, homozygous male mice with a targeted gene deletion of PMCA isoform 4, which is highly enriched in the sperm tail, are infertile due to severely impaired sperm motility. Furthermore, this detrimental effect can be mimicked by inhibition of the enzyme in wild-type animals, thus supporting the hypothesis of a pivotal role of PMCA4 in the regulation of sperm function and intracellular Ca^{2+} levels[32].

The molecular mechanisms underlying such striking stimulatory and detrimental effects of calcium on sperm motility are still unclear; however, they seem to be linked to the activation of concurrent signaling pathways such as those involving protein kinases and phosphatases. Indeed, calcium levels must be kept low in order to prevent activation of phosphatases such as calcineurin[27], which dephosphorylates and inactivates tail proteins involved in sperm motility[27,33]. An alternative hypothesis developed by Aitken's group suggests that keeping internal calcium homeostasis in the presence of high extracellular calcium decreases ATP availability for tyrosine phosphorylation and sperm movement[34].

Bicarbonate and adenylate cyclases

Bicarbonate has long been demonstrated to enhance sperm motility in different species both *in vitro* and *in vivo*[35–38]. The importance of this molecule in regulating sperm activation *in vivo* is further suggested by the increasing millimolar gradient of HCO_3^- that spermatozoa encounter during their journey from the testis to the site of fertilization. The increased level of HCO_3^- in seminal plasma compared with the epididymal fluid may allow motility to develop in the ejaculate. Okamura *et al.*[39] showed a positive correlation between lower levels of HCO3- in the semen of infertile men with poor sperm motility. However, in male reproductive fluids, HCO3- levels must be kept low to prevent spermatozoa from undergoing premature activation and hyperactivated motility, processes that are stimulated by the 3–4-fold higher HCO_3^- concentrations present in the female reproductive tract[40].

The molecular mechanism by which HCO_3^- stimulates sperm motility involves a direct activation of sperm sAC, independent of intracellular pH[41]. sAC, which is insensitive to forskolin and G-protein regulation, and is selectively activated[42–44] by HCO_3^-, appears to be the main adenylate cyclase present in mature spermatozoa, although different isoforms of the membrane adenylate cyclase (mAC) have also been described[45–47]. In somatic cells, the precise compartmentalization of sAC in distinct subcellular microdomains provides the mechanism for localized cAMP rise specifically to activate protein kinase A (PKA) in different cellular compartments[48,49]. In fact, unlike mAC, sAC could diffuse and generate cAMP at the site where its target enzyme, PKA, is localized[50]. Sperm sAC activity, however, seems to be predominantly associated with the sperm particulate fraction[51].

Mice defective for sAC are infertile, apparently due to impairment of sperm motility[52]. Interestingly, motility can be restored in sAC knock-out mice by cAMP administration[52]. However, such treatment does not reverse hyperactivation and tyrosine phosphorylation defects or the sperm inability to fertilize, suggesting that sAC is also necessary for appropriate spermatogenesis and/or epididymal maturation[53]. Treating sperm with an inhibitor of sAC, KH7, the same authors were able to distinguish between sAC-dependent and independent processes during mouse sperm capacitation, showing that tyrosine phosphorylation of protein as well as sperm motility and hyperactivation are regulated by sAC, while the acrosome reaction is not[53]. A role played by mAC in controlling sperm motility, however, cannot be ruled out. In fact, selective knock-out of membrane olfactory adenylate cyclase 3 is associated with male infertility due to the sperm's inability to penetrate the zona pellucida. These spermatozoa show a significant reduction in both motility and acrosome reaction[54].

Kinases and phosphatases

Although abundant evidence indicates the importance of protein phosphorylation as one of the key processes in transducing the stimulatory signals governing motility, little is known about the specific kinases and phosphatases involved. Generally, sperm motility has been demonstrated to be associated with increased tyrosine phosphorylation of specific sperm-tail proteins following tyrosine and serine–threonine kinase activation. Furthermore, sperm motility is negatively associated with phosphatase activation[26,29,33,55]. Tyrosine phosphorylated proteins in response to sperm capacitation are mainly localized in sperm tails[56–58]. A defect in the tyrosine phosphorylation of specific sperm proteins in response to capacitation has been described in asthenozoospermic patients, associated with reduced motility and hyperactivation capacity[59,60]. This defect in protein tyrosine phosphorylation seems to be linked to membrane fluidity in spermatozoa from asthenozoospermic patients[60] and infertile men with varicocele[61]. Interestingly, even semen from normozoospermic men present distinct sperm subpopulations that show different plasma membrane fluidity and ability to undergo protein tyrosine phosphorylation and hyperactivation in response to capacitation[62].

Sperm protein phosphorylation is regulated by a finely tuned balance between kinase and phosphatase activities[33,63]. In particular, the adenylate cyclase/cAMP/PKA system has been demonstrated to be involved in tyrosine phosphorylation of different sperm proteins associated with motility[27,56,63–66]. cAMP produced by the activation of adenylate cyclase binds to PKA holoenzyme, inducing the release and activation of the catalytic subunit. Sperm treatments enhancing intracellular cAMP and PKA activity stimulate motility[64,67]. Since protein kinase A is a serine–threonine kinase, it is assumed that in order to stimulate tyrosine phosphorylation it activates some intermediate tyrosine kinases. An alternative pathway involving tyrosine kinase activation upstream to PKA has recently been reported by our groups[55,68,69]. In fact, both inhibition of phosphatidylinositol 3-kinase (PI3K) by LY294002 and physiological activation of sAC by bicarbonate stimulate an increase in intracellular cAMP levels in concurrence with enhanced tyrosine phosphorylation of the tail scaffolding protein, A kinase anchoring protein 3 (AKAP3). Confocal microscopy of fixed and permeabilized spermatozoa confirms that capacitation-induced tyrosine phosphorylation of sperm proteins occurs mainly at the tail and, in particular, on AKAP3 (Figure 2.3). The stimulated phosphorylation of AKAP3 results in an increased binding of PKA regulatory subunit RIIβ, which is thus selectively recruited and activated in the sperm tail, where it interacts with its targets, finally resulting in an increase in sperm motility. Disruption of PKA–AKAP3 interaction results in the inhibition of sperm motility[68]. Sperm treatment with the PKA inhibitor H89 results in the inhibition of sperm motility, but not of AKAP3 tyrosine phosphorylation[55,68], thus suggesting that PKA is involved in the regulation of sperm motility downstream to tyrosine kinases. Inhibition of motility and tyrosine phosphorylation following sperm treatment with H89 has been reported by other authors, conversely suggesting an upstream effect of PKA[70–72]. Such discrepancy could be explained either by differences in H89 concentrations and timing of H89 addition or by hypothesizing that tyrosine phosphorylation affects different targets upstream and downstream of PKA activation.

The importance of AKAP scaffolding proteins in regulating sperm motility has recently been highlighted by targeted disruption of the Akap4 gene, whose product, AKAP4, is closely related to AKAP3. These mutant mice show defects in sperm flagella and motility resulting in infertility[73]. Contradictory reports exist regarding the alteration of AKAP genes in men affected by dysplasia of the fibrous sheath[74,75]. However, defects in the ability of such scaffolding proteins to undergo tyrosine phosphorylation, thus affecting PKA recruitment, have not been excluded.

Cell volume and osmolarity

During their transit and maturation through the epididymis, spermatozoa acquire the ability to regulate cell volume, a very important process for the adequate development of motility. In fact, the osmolarity of the luminal fluid increases from the testis to the epididymis, and normal spermatozoa counteract shrinkage by increasing the uptake of organic osmolytes such as L-carnitine and amino

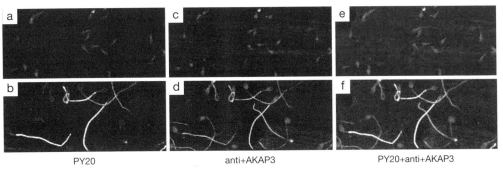

PY20   anti+AKAP3   PY20+anti+AKAP3

Figure 2.3   Immunofluorescence analysis of fixed and permeabilized human spermatozoa. Confocal microscopy of double immunolabeling for tyrosine phosphorylated proteins ((b), PY20 antibody, green) and A kinase anchoring protein 3 (AKAP3) ((d), anti-AKAP3 antibody, red) reveals positivity for both antibodies in sperm tails. Simultaneous analysis of dual fluorescence confirms that tyrosine phosphorylation corresponds to AKAP3 in the tail ((f), double fluorescence, yellow). (a), (c), (e), negative controls without primary antibody. From reference 9, with permission. See also Color plate 2 on page xxvi

acids secreted by the epithelium[76]. Conversely, upon ejaculation, spermatozoa are subjected to the relatively hyposmotic environment of the female genital tract (osmotic pressure falls from 420 to 300 mmol/kg, from the epididymal cauda to the uterus[76,77]), and in order to prevent swelling, spermatozoa lose water and osmolytes acquired in the epididymis. Defects in such a delicate mechanism of volume regulation can cause an abnormal increase in sperm head volume and angulation of the sperm tail[76], resulting in defects of sperm motility and fertility.

A similar hairpin shape in the sperm tail and its detrimental consequence on motility has been demonstrated in both c-*ros* knock-out mice and following sperm treatment with the ion-channel blocker quinine[78]. Interestingly, seminal plasma osmolarity (intermediate between epididymis and uterus) is significantly higher in asthenozoospermic patients, irrespective of the cause of asthenozoospermia, than in normozoospermic men[79]. Moreover, seminal osmolarity correlates negatively with sperm progressive motility and kinetic characteristics[80], suggesting a potential pathological role for seminal hyperosmolarity in the reduction of sperm motility in asthenozoospermic subjects. Sperm exposure to low-osmolarity media such as oviductal and uterine fluids activates an influx of Ca^{2+} through osmolarity-sensitive calcium channels[79].

The role of fluid resorption in sperm maturation in the apical region of the epididymis has been extensively investigated[81]. Estrogens control differential expression of Na^+/H^+ exchangers[82] and aquaporin channels[83] through estrogen receptor α in the initial segment and caput of the epididymis. Aquaporin channels (e.g. AQ7) are also expressed in sperm tails and seem to be important for the control of cell volume, motility and fertility[84]. Therefore, it is conceivable that sperm maturation in the epididymis may be modulated by active water transport at two levels: the non-ciliated epidydimal epithelium and the sperm plasma membrane. L-carnitine, which is one of the main osmolytes captured by sperm during their transit through the epididymis, is essential for acyl transport in the mitochondrial β-oxidation of long-chain fatty acids, and may also prevent sperm DNA and membrane damage induced by reactive oxygen species. Indeed, a positive effect of oral administration of carnitine in increasing semen quality, in particular sperm forward motility, in oligoasthenoteratozoospermic and asthenozoospermic patients has been demonstrated in clinical trials[85,86].

Reactive oxygen species

Reactive oxygen species (ROS), in particular hydrogen peroxide, produced either by spermatozoa or seminal leukocytes, have been described to affect different sperm functions including motility[87]. Their effects appear to depend on the concentration of ROS; low levels can induce the cAMP–PKA signaling cascade leading to an increase in sperm motility and tyrosine phosphorylation of proteins associated with capacitation, while high levels exert an inhibitory effect[88,89]. The detrimental action of ROS on sperm motility has been associated with increased lipid peroxidation of the plasma membrane[90].

High production of ROS as well as low antioxidant capacity may account for certain types of sperm pathology, in particular asthenozoospermia[91]. In such cases, the use of antioxidants may be indicated[92,93]. However, levels of glutathione-dependent seleno-enzymes in human spermatozoa, which are responsible for more general protection against ROS, have been reported to be similar in spermatozoa isolated from both normozoospermic and asthenozoospermic subjects[94].

HYPERACTIVATED MOTILITY

Hyperactivation is a special type of sperm motility developed in association with the process of capacitation in the female genital tract. It can also be achieved *in vitro* by seminal plasma removal and incubation of sperm in capacitating media[95]. It is characterized by a more energetic and less symmetric flagellar beat, which helps sperm to progress through the cervical mucus, the oviduct and, finally, the cumulus oophorus and zona pellucida surrounding the oocyte[96–98]. Furthermore, in species in which the oviductal isthmus represents a reservoir for spermatozoa, this particular swimming pattern seems to be important for the release of sperm entrapped in the folds and crypts of the oviductal epithelium[98]. In these cases, ovulation appears to induce a modification in the carbohydrate moieties of the oviductal epithelium, resulting in the release of fully activated sperm which have developed hyperactivation. This phenomenon ensures appropriate timing for the acquisition of sperm fertilization potential[99]. The development of hyperactivation, especially at the oviducts, may be orchestrated by ovulation, since follicular fluid has been demonstrated to have a dose-dependent stimulatory effect on sperm hyperactivation[100,101]. The specific component capable of directly affecting sperm motility, however, has not yet been isolated[102,103].

The importance of adequate timing for hyperactivation has been demonstrated by the infertile *t*-haplotype mice, whose spermatozoa undergo premature hyperactivation in the female reproductive tract[104]. Interestingly, forward progressive motility and hyperactivation appear to be discontinuous and reversible processes, allowing sperm to switch alternately from one pattern to the other[105].

Capacitation and hyperactivation are two complementary aspects of sperm activation and develop simultaneously under physiological conditions. If capacitation is conceptualized as the complex of physiological changes enabling sperm to fertilize[95], hyperactivation should be considered as part of such a process. However, they occur as independent pheomonena. In *t*-haplotype mice, spermatozoa show premature hyperactivation, but normal timing of capacitation *in vitro*. Although sharing similar signaling pathways, capacitation and hyperactivation are distinct processes that show different thresholds for activating factors. Indeed, the calcium and bicarbonate concentrations required for hyperactivation are far higher than those needed for capacitation[16,97].

The molecular bases underlying hyperactivation have been studied by different investigators, especially using a demembranated sperm model in which both plasma and mitochondrial membranes were removed by Triton X 100, leaving the axonemal structure intact and functional[97]. The development of hyperactivated and activated motility share the same signaling pathways and molecular players; however, different activation thresholds are involved. In particular, although ATP and cAMP are able to stimulate motility of demembranated spermatozoa, it is only following the addition of calcium that hyperactivation begins[106], suggesting that this ion is a key regulator of the process[97].

Both external sources and intracellular stores are important for the increase in intracellular calcium levels associated with hyperactivation. Intracellular calcium stores showing inositol 1,4,5-trisphosphate receptors (IP3R) have been demonstrated not only in the acrosome[15], but also in the neck of the sperm[16]. In the distal region of the sperm neck, the axoneme associates with mitochondria and is surrounded by a redundant nuclear envelope, whose enlarged cisternae represent the flagellum intracellular calcium stores[16]. The release of calcium from this structure through IP3-gated channels seems to initiate sperm hyperactivation directly[97,107], perhaps through the activation of calmodulin-dependent kinases. Calmodulin kinase II is one of the few discovered calcium targets in spermatozoa. Upon its activation by the calcium/calmodulin complex, it specifically stimulates hyperactivation[20].

Hyperactivation is also modulated by calcium entry through plasma membrane-specific channels such as voltage-gated, receptor-associated, store-operated and cyclic nucleotide-gated channels (for reviews see references 11 and 12). A recently discovered family of sperm-specific voltage-operated calcium channels, the CatSper family, plays a pivotal role in the development and maintenance of sperm motility. The four members of the family are differentially expressed along the tail. While CatSper1 seems to regulate sperm-activated motility[14], CatSper2 is important for hyperactivation. CatSper2 knock-out mice are infertile due to their inability to develop hyperactivation and penetrate the zona pellucida; however, capacitation, motility and the acrosome reaction are normal[108]. Interestingly, male infertility in a mutant CatSper2 family has recently been described[109].

Similar to activated motility, hyperactivation is regulated by a complex balance between kinase and phosphatase activity. Increased tyrosine phosphorylation of several sperm proteins in the tail

has been described to be associated with physiological[59,66,69,110] and temperature-induced hyperactivation[111]. Inhibition of tyrosine and cAMP-dependent kinases decreases hyperactivated motility[55,69,112], whereas an increase in intracellular cAMP enhances this type of motility[55,69,113].

CHEMOTAXIS AND SPERM MOTILITY

Spermatozoa from invertebrates and mammals demonstrate attraction to chemoattractants secreted by the egg. This mechanism plays a pivotal role in guiding sperm towards the oocyte, which is particularly important for those species characterized by external fertilization. By binding to sperm-specific receptors, these molecules affect sperm motility, inducing a directed movement towards the chemical gradient of the chemoattractant (chemotaxis). In the sea urchin, speract secreted by the eggs induces, in a species-specific manner, a sperm chemotactic response by stimulating a transmembrane guanylate cyclase receptor complex associated with K+ channels preferentially localized along the flagellum, which results in an increase in intracellular cAMP and calcium[114,115].

In vitro induction of chemotaxis by follicular fluid (FF) has been extensively demonstrated in human sperm[116]. Progesterone[117] and chemokines such as RANTES (T)[118] have been suggested to be the active components of FF involved in sperm chemotaxis, even when the major effect of the steroid appears to be on sperm hyperactivation rather than on chemotaxis[119]. Furthermore, odorant-like molecules, through their specific olfactory receptors expressed on human spermatozoa, induce a membrane adenylate cyclase-dependent increase in intracellular calcium, resulting in redirection of sperm along the ascending gradient of the odorant[120,121]. Sperm chemoattractants are secreted by the preovulatory follicle as well as the mature oocyte and its surrounding cumulus[122], contributing to guiding sperm to the site of fertilization. However, the physiological role of chemotaxis in human spermatozoa is still controversial. Rather than being important in guiding sperm toward the oocyte, chemotaxis in humans seems more likely to be involved in recruiting a selected, activated subpopulation of spermatozoa[123,124].

COMPUTER-ASSISTED ASSESSMENT OF SPERM MOTILITY

Classically, sperm motility has been assessed using phase-contrast microscopy, subjectively classifying sperm trajectories as forward progression (a and b), *in situ* (c) and immotile (d) according to the World Health Organization (WHO) *Manual for the Examination of Human Semen and Sperm–Cervical Mucus Interaction* (1999)[125]. The definition of asthenozoospermia is based on this classification, using 50% of forward-motile sperm as the normal cut-off. Computer-assisted analysis of sperm movement has significantly increased the objectivity of this assessment, providing a series of measurements such as sperm velocity, amplitude of head displacement and flagellar beat frequency, which otherwise could not be obtained with classical subjective microscopic evaluation. Furthermore, computer-assisted sperm analysis (CASA) systems are capable of sorting sperm subpopulations according to established threshold values, allowing for the quick and accurate determination of the percentage of spermatozoa displaying hyperactivated motility (for review see Mortimer 1997)[126].

The sensitivity and confidence of these instruments have greatly improved in the past few years, and they can now be referred to as potent research and clinical tools to measure both basic and hyperactivation parameters[1]. Essentially, CASA allows for the simultaneous evaluation of kinematic parameters in a high number of spermatozoa in a short period. All parameters are measured by CASA using the sperm head (centroid-derived movement) instead of the tail, as head movement passively reflects the flagellar beat and can be more easily followed due to its lower frequency of move-

ment. Velocity values are based on curvilinear velocity (VCL), straight-line velocity (VSL) and average path velocity (VAP). The VCL is referred to as the real distance that the sperm head covers during the observation time; the VAP is the distance that the sperm covers in the average direction of movement; and the VSL is the straight-line distance between the starting and the ending points of the sperm trajectory (Figure 2.4). More strictly associated with sperm head characteristics, lateral head displacement (ALH) and beat cross frequency (BCF) measure, respectively, the width of lateral movement and the number of times that the sperm head crosses the direction of movement.

As indicated above, CASA systems can also derive from the obtained data in terms of a sort fraction, which represents the percentage of spermatozoa showing hyperactivation. The criteria for sorting hyperactivated sperm at 60 Hz can be manually set, and have been defined as VCL $> 150\,\mu m/s$, $ALH_{max} > 7.0\,\mu m$, linearity LIN $< 50\%$[127]. Modern CASA instruments capture 60 images per second, which is ideal for properly characterizing sperm hyperactivated motility. To allow for unimpeded tridimensional sperm movement, motility should be analyzed in > 30-μm chambers, prewarmed to $37°C$[128].

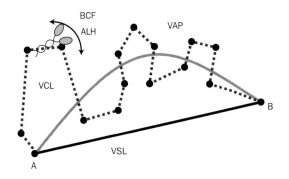

Figure 2.4 Schematic representation of a digitized sperm trajectory analyzed by a computer-assisted sperm analysis (CASA) system. VCL, curvilinear velocity; VSL, straight-line velocity; VAP, average path velocity; BCF, beat cross frequency; ALH, lateral head displacement; LIN, linearity = VSL/VSL; STR, straightness = VSL/VAP. From reference 9, with permission

Besides its undisputed utility for research studies, CASA has also been widely adopted in the clinic. Several studies have correlated CASA parameters with assisted reproductive technologies (ART) outcomes[129–131]. Although no single parameter has shown good predictive value, some are valuable contributors to a multiparameter equation that predicts fertilization potential.

ETIOLOGY AND PATHOPHYSIOLOGY OF ASTHENOZOOSPERMIA

Alterations in the previously described external and internal factors regulating sperm motion and metabolism in the flagellar structure may result in defects in sperm motility and infertility. A recent study reported that out of 1085 sperm samples analyzed from infertile subjects, 81% had defective motility, 20% of which presented pure asthenozoospermia[132]. Thus, asthenozoospermia is one of the main seminal pathologies underlying male infertility.

Severe asthenozoospermia is frequently caused by flagellar alterations[133]. Ultrastructural studies of men with severe asthenozoospermia revealed two types of tail abnormalities: non-specific flagellar anomalies, which are random secondary alterations that affect variable numbers of spermatozoa in different samples, and dysplasia of the fibrous sheath (DFS), which is a systemic primary anomaly that affects most spermatozoa and is associated with respiratory pathology and familial incidence[134,135].

Non-specific flagellar anomalies constitute the most frequent flagellar pathology underlying asthenozoospermia. Its structural phenotype of random microtubular alterations is characteristically heterogeneous, and is sometimes associated with other andrological disorders (e.g. varicocele). Some of these patients respond to conservative treatment, while others require ART[136].

Dysplasia of the fibrous sheath is a different condition associated with extreme asthenozoospermia or total sperm immobility. It has a homogeneous and distinctive phenotype characterized by distortions of the fibrous sheath and other axonemal and periaxonemal structures[135,136]. It has been postulated to be a variant of the immotile cilia syndrome, also known as primary ciliary dyskinesia, a congenital anomaly presenting with respiratory disease and male infertility. The axonemes of the respiratory cilia and sperm flagella show missing dynein arms, radial spokes and central microtubules, and general microtubular translocations[137]. In the Kartagener's syndrome presentation, the ciliary/flagellar immotility is accompanied by dextrocardia. The familial clustering of these syndromes strongly suggests a genetic origin of the disease[134]. Intracytoplasmic sperm injection is the treatment of choice, but genetic counseling is required[138].

Not all cases of asthenozoospermia, especially those that are not severe in nature, are associated with structural anomalies of the flagellum, however. Our studies demonstrate that spermatozoa from less severe asthenozoospermic patients show a clear impairment in motility and their capacity to develop hyperactivation, which is associated with low membrane fluidity and a concomitant inability to undergo protein tyrosine phosphorylation[59,60]. This is particularly evident when spermatozoa are challenged with a capacitating incubation (e.g. 6 hours at 37°C, 5% CO_2, in protein-supplemented medium) (Figure 2.5).

Changes in membrane dynamics have been associated with tyrosine phosphorylation, as well as sperm function and fertilizing ability[139,140]. Spermatozoa from asthenozoospermic patients reveal significantly less fluid membranes before and after capacitation, in comparison with normozoospermic patients and proven-fertile donors[60]. Such a difference in membrane fluidity could be due to the increased susceptibility of these spermatozoa to suffer peroxidative damage[91], as the generation of membrane lipid hydroperoxides has been associated with membrane fluidity reduction[141,142]. This susceptibility of asthenozoospermic sperm could be explained, in part, by their membrane composition, which is

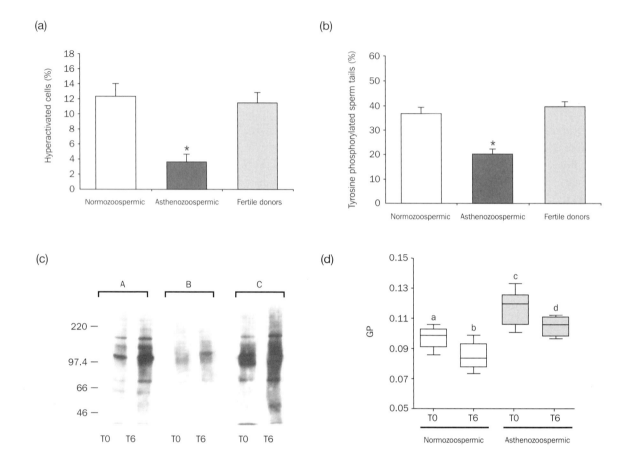

Figure 2.5 Tyrosine phosphorylation, hyperactivation and membrane fluidity deficiencies in asthenozoospermic samples in comparison with samples from normozoospermic and proven-fertile men. Spermatozoa were incubated for 0 (T0, baseline) or 6 h under capacitating conditions and the incidence of hyperactivated motility (a), the incidence (immunofluorescence) and intensity (Western blot) of tyrosine phosphorylation (b) and (c) and the sperm membrane fluidity (fluorometry) (d) were determined. Asterisks (*) and letters (a vs. b, c vs. d, a vs. c and b vs. d) above bars indicate statistical significance. In the Western blot image (c), A = normozoospermic, B = asthenozoospermic, C = proven-fertile. In the membrane fluidity plot (d) GP is Laurdan's general polarization. From reference 60, with permission

responsible for their reported higher oxidation coefficient[91]. Sperm membranes of asthenozoospermic samples contain high levels of polyunsaturated fatty acids, making them more prone to attack by reactive oxygen species. Since oxidizing conditions are normal during sperm capacitation and have been linked to signal transduction and tyrosine phosphorylation[87,143], the predisposition of the asthenozoospermic samples to oxidative damage may be the origin of their membrane dysfunction, resulting in tyrosine phosphorylation deficiency and alteration of motility.

TREATMENT OF ASTHENOZOOSPERMIA

Systemic modalities

Before considering any treatment, a correct diagnosis has to be established. Hence, the evaluation of subfertile men begins with a detailed history and physical examination. The history should identify the duration of attempted conception, intercourse timing and frequency, erectile function, ejaculation, life-style factors (alcohol, smoking, etc.) and any medications[144]. Other pertinent details include previous mumps orchitis, chemotherapy and/or radiation for cancer, cryptorchidism, previous reproductive tract infections, prior illnesses and any systemic disease. Physical examination should seek any sign of hypogonadism (virilization, body proportions, gynecomastia, etc.); a careful genitourinary examination should be performed to evaluate testicular size and consistency and the presence of masses and eventual penile pathology (hypospadias, etc.), and to identify the presence of the most common condition associated with male infertility – varicocele[145,146]. Severe ultrastructural sperm anomalies such as dysplasia of the fibrous sheath should also be ruled out.

If a treatable condition responsible for male factor infertility, such as hypogonadism, varicocele, infections, immunologic infertility, obstructions and cryptorchidism, is found, then it should be corrected using current medical and/or surgical therapies[147]. Conversely, if a diagnosis of idiopathic asthenozoospermia is made, there are a few treatment options that have some degree of evidence-based support.

Placebo-controlled double-blind randomized trials of men with idiopathic asthenozoospermia have demonstrated that L-carnitine and its analogs, especially L-acetyl-carnitine, after daily oral administration, increase sperm motility and kinematic parameters[85,148,149]. Although these studies do not have enough statistical power in themselves to draw unequivocal conclusions, they all show clear trends toward improvement of motility. This was especially notable in patients who started with the lower values of motility and motion parameters.

Although the etiopathogenic mechanisms being modified by the oral administration of carnitines are not clearly established, increases in mitochondrial energy production and total antioxidant capacity have been suggested[85,86,149,150]. Glutathione and coenzyme Q10 administration may also have beneficial effects in the treatment of idiopathic asthenozoospermia[151,152].

Another systemic treatment that has been tested in ART patients presenting with oligozoospermia or combined oligoasthenoteratozoospermia is pure follicle stimulating hormone (FSH). Although results are still controversial, several studies show an improvement of in vitro fertilization (IVF) outcome[153–157].

Assisted reproductive modalities

To date, albeit not curative, the most efficient treatment for asthenozoospermia is ART. Improving sperm motility in vitro before insemination is a common practice for moderate asthenozoospermic samples.

Certain molecules have been demonstrated to be capable of improving sperm motility in vitro. Among them are inhibitors of phosphodiesterases such as pentoxifylline (PF), analogs of cAMP and a plasma membrane phospholipid, platelet-activating factor (PAF), which is physiologically produced and released by sperm[158]. PF is often used in ART to improve the fertilization rate and outcome in couples with male factor infertility[159,160], since this compound not only stimulates motility in sperm obtained from asthenozoospermic subjects, but also positively affects sperm capacitation, binding to the zona pellucida and the acrosome reaction[161]. Sperm treatment with PF before IVF has been demonstrated not to be teratogenic for the developing embryo[160]; however, potential toxic effects cannot be definitively ruled out[162]. Furthermore, the presence of non-responder subjects decreases the overall efficacy of the treatment[163]. The most striking negative side-effect exerted by the majority of these compounds, including PF, is their ability also to stimulate the acrosome reaction[102]. Unfortunately, acrosome-reacted spermatozoa are unable to bind the oocyte's zona pellucida, thus decreasing their efficacy in conventional IVF.

In this regard, during the past few years, our research has been focused on two molecules which seem very good candidates for potential adjuvant *in vitro* treatment of asthenozoospermia. LY294002 is a pharmacological inhibitor of phosphatidylinositol 3-kinase (PI3K), a kinase which phosphorylates in the 3-OH position, the inositol ring of the plasma membrane phosphoinositides[164]. This enzyme has been demonstrated to play a negative role in the control of sperm motility[68,165–167], and its inhibition by LY294002 stimulates a significant increase in forward and rapid motility in both ejaculated and selected human spermatozoa, independently from the technique used for selection[10,68,166]. This stimulatory effect was more evident on samples from oligoasthenozoospermic compared with normozoospermic subjects[10,165,166]. In particular, direct addition of LY294002 to seminal samples of severe asthenozoospermic subjects increases the number of sperm showing forward motility recovered after a swim-up selection for ART[166]. PI3K inhibition by LY294002 stimulates tyrosine phosphorylation of AKAP3 in the fibrous sheath of sperm tails, allowing local recruitment and activation of PKA by increased binding of PKA regulatory subunit RIIβ to the phosphorylated form of AKAP3[10,68,167]. PKA activation finally results in stimulation of sperm motility and hyperactivation[68]. Interestingly, in contrast to the above-mentioned molecules, LY294002 effects on sperm motility are not associated with an increase in the acrosome reaction[165]. Moreover, no toxic effect on embryo development has been demonstrated following sperm, oocyte or embryo treatment with LY294002 in a mouse model[168]. All these findings support the possible use of this drug as well as other PI3K inhibitors as potential tools to improve sperm motility in ART.

In addition to the use of this pharmacological tool, our group (University of Florence) has also focused its attention on a physiological stimulus of sperm motility, the bicarbonate ion (HCO_3^-). We have recently demonstrated that in swim-up-selected human spermatozoa, physiological concentrations of bicarbonate (15 and 75 mmol/l) rapidly stimulate an increase in intracellular cAMP levels and tyrosine phosphorylation of AKAP3, the latter phenomenon resulting in an increased amount of PKA bound to this scaffolding protein, in a manner resembling LY294002 effects[68,69]. The stimulatory effects of bicarbonate on both sperm motility and AKAP3 phosphorylation seem to involve entry of the ion into the cell and activation of sAC, since they are inhibited by 4,4′-diisothiocyanostilbene-2,2′-disulfonic acid, a specific blocker of bicarbonate transporter, and by 2OH-estradiol, a selective inhibitor of sAC[69]. Thus, our findings strongly suggest that both HCO_3^- and LY294002 increase sperm motility by converging on the same signaling pathway involving stimulation of cAMP production by sAC and tyrosine phosphorylation of AKAP3 in the sperm tail. Redundancy of the signaling pathways leading to AKAP3 phosphorylation further highlights the importance of this process in regulating sperm motility. Molecules acting in promoting phosphorylation could potentially be used for increasing the number of motile spermatozoa selected for ART, offering infertile couples better chances for less invasive and expensive techniques.

CONCLUSIONS AND FUTURE DIRECTIONS

Although progress has been significant, much remains to be elucidated concerning the biochemical pathways that regulate and maintain sperm motility. In particular, it is still unclear how spermatozoa begin to move following their release from the testis and their transit through the epididymis, and which signals are necessary for such activation. The identification of molecules involved in controlling sperm motility appears difficult, however. Genetic studies in mice show that many genes are involved in the development and maintenance of sperm motility. Some of them are testis-specific genes belonging to the fibrous sheath of the principal piece. Clarifying the molecular mechanisms involved in the onset of sperm motility will be of great benefit for the development of possible therapeutic strategies. Indeed, although some systemic therapies (such as oral administration of carnitine and antioxidants) have proved to be relatively efficacious, at present *in vitro* treatments remain the best option for the treatment of asthenozoospermia.

ACKNOWLEDGMENTS

GF Doncel wishes to thank CONRAD and the US Agency for International Development for supporting his work on sperm motility and immobilizing agents. The views expressed in this manuscript do not necessarily represent those of the funding agencies or their programs. The authors also wish to express gratitude to Ms Charlotte Neumann for her editorial assistance.

REFERENCES

1. Mortimer, S.T. CASA – practical aspects, J. Androl 21; 515: 2000
2. Fawcett DW. The mammalian spermatozoon. Dev Biol 1975; 44: 394
3. Baltz JM, Williams PO, Cone RA. Dense fibers protect mammalian sperm against damage. Biol Reprod 1990; 43: 485
4. Vernon GG, Woolley DM. Basal sliding and the mechanics of oscillation in a mammalian sperm flagellum. Biophys J 2004; 87: 3934
5. Woolley DM, Neesen J, Vernon GG. Further studies on knockout mice lacking a functional dynein heavy chain (MDHC7). A developmental explanation for the asthenozoospermia. Cell Motil Cytoskeleton 2005; 61: 74
6. Narisawa S, et al. Testis-specific cytochrome c-null mice produce functional sperm but undergo early testicular atrophy. Mol Cell Biol 2002; 22: 5554
7. Miki K, et al. Glyceraldehyde 3-phosphate dehydrogenase-S, a sperm-specific glycolytic enzyme, is required for sperm motility and male fertility. Proc Natl Acad Sci USA 2004; 101: 16501
8. Visconti PE, et al. Properties and localization of a tyrosine phosphorylated form of hexokinase in mouse sperm. Mol Reprod Dev 1996; 43: 82
9. Luconi M, Forti G, Baldi E. Pathophysiology of sperm motility. Front Biosci 2006; in press
10. Luconi M, Baldi E. How do sperm swim? Molecular mechanisms underlying sperm motility. Cell Mol Biol (Noisy-le-grand) 2003; 49: 357
11. Darszon A, et al. Ion transport in sperm signalling. Dev Biol 2001; 240: 1
12. Darszon A, et al. Calcium channels and Ca2+ fluctuations in sperm physiology. Int Rev Cytol 2005; 243: 79
13. Castellano LE, et al. Transient receptor potential (TRPC) channels in human sperm: expression, cellular localization and involvement in the regulation of flagellar motility. FEBS Lett 2003; 541: 69
14. Ren D, et al. A sperm ion channel required for sperm motility and male fertility. Nature 2001; 413: 603
15. Walensky LD, Snyder SH. Inositol 1,4,5-trisphosphate receptors selectively localized to the acrosomes of mammalian sperm. J Cell Biol 1995; 130: 857
16. Ho HC, Suarez SS. An inositol 1,4,5-trisphosphate receptor-gated intracellular Ca(2+) store is involved in regulating sperm hyperactivated motility. Biol Reprod 2001; 65: 1606
17. Gross MK, Toscano DG, Toscano WA Jr. Calmodulin-mediated adenylate cyclase from mammalian sperm. J Biol Chem 1987; 262: 8672
18. Jaiswal BS, Conti M. Calcium regulation of the soluble adenylyl cyclase expressed in mammalian spermatozoa. Proc Natl Acad Sci USA 2003; 100: 10676
19. Marin-Briggiler CI, et al. Evidence of the presence of calcium/calmodulin-dependent protein kinase IV in human sperm and its involvement in motility regulation. J Cell Sci 2005; 118: 2013
20. Ignotz GG, Suarez SS. Calcium/calmodulin and calmodulin kinase II stimulate hyperactivation in demembranated bovine sperm. Biol Reprod 2005; 73: 519
21. Rusnak F, Mertz P. Calcineurin: form and function. Physiol Rev 2000; 80: 1483
22. Wasco WM, Orr GA. Function of calmodulin in mammalian sperm: presence of a calmodulin-dependent cyclic nucleotide phosphodiesterase associated with demembranated rat caudal epididymal sperm. Biochem Biophys Res Commun 1984; 118: 636

23. Lindemann CB, et al. The calcium-induced curvature reversal of rat sperm is potentiated by cAMP and inhibited by anti-calmodulin. Cell Motil Cytoskeleton 1991; 20: 316

24. Reyes A, et al. Concentrations of calmodulin in sperm in relation to their motility in fertile euspermic and infertile asthenozoospermic men. Int J Androl 1987; 10: 507

25. Aitken RJ, et al. Analysis of calmodulin acceptor proteins and the influence of calmodulin antagonists on human spermatozoa. Gamete Res 1988; 21: 93

26. Luconi M, et al. Extracellular calcium negatively modulates tyrosine phosphorylation and tyrosine kinase activity during capacitation of human spermatozoa. Biol Reprod 1996; 55: 207

27. Carrera A, et al. Regulation of protein tyrosine phosphorylation in human sperm by a calcium/calmodulin-dependent mechanism: identification of A kinase anchor proteins as major substrates for tyrosine phosphorylation. Dev Biol 1996; 180: 284

28. Lewis B, Aitken RJ. Impact of epididymal maturation on the tyrosine phosphorylation patterns exhibited by rat spermatozoa. Biol Reprod 2001; 64: 1545

29. Vijayaraghavan S, Hoskins DD. Changes in the mitochondrial calcium influx and efflux properties are responsible for the decline in sperm calcium during epididymal maturation. Mol Reprod Dev 1990; 25: 186

30. Williams KM, Ford WC. The motility of demembranated human spermatozoa is inhibited by free calcium ion activities of 500 nmol/L or more. Int J Androl 2001; 24: 216

31. McLaughlin EA, Ford WC. Effects of cryopreservation on the intracellular calcium concentration of human spermatozoa and its response to progesterone. Mol Reprod Dev 1994; 37: 241

32. Schuh K, et al. Plasma membrane Ca2+ ATPase 4 is required for sperm motility and male fertility. J Biol Chem 2004; 279: 28220

33. Tash JS, et al. Identification, characterization, and functional correlation of calmodulin-dependent protein phosphatase in sperm. J Cell Biol 1988; 106: 1625

34. Baker MA, et al. Analysis of the mechanism by which calcium negatively regulates the tyrosine phosphorylation cascade associated with sperm capacitation. J Cell Sci 2004; 117: 211

35. Holt WV, Harrison RA. Bicarbonate stimulation of boar sperm motility via a protein kinase A-dependent pathway: between-cell and between-ejaculate differences are not due to deficiencies in protein kinase A activation. J Androl 2002; 23: 557

36. Osheroff JE, et al. Regulation of human sperm capacitation by a cholesterol efflux-stimulated signal transduction pathway leading to protein kinase A-mediated up-regulation of protein tyrosine phosphorylation. Mol Hum Reprod 1999; 5: 1017

37. Rathi R, et al. Evaluation of in vitro capacitation of stallion spermatozoa. Biol Reprod 2001; 65: 462

38. Visconti PE, et al. Roles of bicarbonate, cAMP, and protein tyrosine phosphorylation on capacitation and the spontaneous acrosome reaction of hamster sperm. Biol Reprod 1999; 61: 76

39. Okamura N, et al. Lowered levels of bicarbonate in seminal plasma cause the poor sperm motility in human infertile patients. Fertil Steril 1986; 45: 265

40. David A, Frenkel G, Kraicer PF. Chemical composition of rabbit follicular fluid. Fertil Steril 1973; 24: 227

41. Okamura N, et al. Sodium bicarbonate in seminal plasma stimulates the motility of mammalian spermatozoa through direct activation of adenylate cyclase. J Biol Chem 1985; 260: 9699

42. Chen Y, et al. Soluble adenylyl cyclase as an evolutionarily conserved bicarbonate sensor. Science 2000; 289: 625

43. Sinclair ML, et al. Specific expression of soluble adenylyl cyclase in male germ cells. Mol Reprod Dev 2000; 56: 6

44. Litvin TN, et al. Synergism between calcium and bicarbonate. J Biol Chem 2003; 278: 15922

45. Leclerc P, Kopf GS. Mouse sperm adenylyl cyclase: general properties and regulation by the zona pellucida. Biol Reprod 1995; 52: 1227

46. Baxendale RW, Fraser LR. Evidence for multiple distinctly localized adenylyl cyclase isoforms in mammalian spermatozoa. Mol Reprod Dev 2003; 66: 181

47. Harrison RA. Cyclic AMP signalling during mammalian sperm capacitation – still largely terra incognita. Reprod Domest Anim 2003; 38: 102

48. Zippin JH, et al. Compartmentalization of bicarbonate-sensitive adenylyl cyclase in distinct signaling microdomains. FASEB J 2003; 17: 82

49. Zippin JH, et al. Bicarbonate-responsive 'soluble' adenylyl cyclase defines a nuclear cAMP microdomain. J Cell Biol 2004; 164: 527

50. Lefievre L, et al. Activation of protein kinase A during human sperm capacitation and acrosome reaction. J Androl 2002; 23: 709

51. Braun T, Dods RF. Development of a Mn-2+-sensitive, 'soluble' adenylate cyclase in rat testis. Proc Natl Acad Sci USA 1975; 72: 1097

52. Esposito G, et al. Mice deficient for soluble adenylyl cyclase are infertile because of a severe sperm-motility defect. Proc Natl Acad Sci USA 2004; 101: 2993

53. Hess KC, et al. The 'soluble' adenylyl cyclase in sperm mediates multiple signaling events required for fertilization. Dev Cell 2005; 9: 249

54. Livera G, et al. Inactivation of the mouse adenylyl cyclase 3 gene disrupts male fertility and spermatozoon function. Mol Endocrinol 2005; 19: 12770

55. Bajpai M, Doncel GF. Involvement of tyrosine kinase and cAMP-dependent kinase cross-talk in the regulation of human sperm motility. Reproduction 2003; 126: 183

56. Ficarro S, et al. Phosphoproteome analysis of capacitated human sperm. Evidence of tyrosine phosphorylation of a kinase-anchoring protein 3 and valosin-containing protein/p97 during capacitation. J Biol Chem 2003; 278: 11579

57. Mandal A, et al. FSP95, a testis-specific 95-kilodalton fibrous sheath antigen that undergoes tyrosine phosphorylation in capacitated human spermatozoa. Biol Reprod 1999; 61: 1184

58. Petrunkina AM, et al. Specific order in the appearance of protein tyrosine phosphorylation patterns is functionally coordinated with dog sperm hyperactivation and capacitation. J Androl 2003; 24: 423

59. Yunes R, Doncel GF, Acosta AA. Incidence of sperm-tail tyrosine phosphorylation and hyperactivated motility in normozoospermic and asthenozoospermic human sperm samples. Biocell 2003; 27: 29

60. Buffone MG, et al. Capacitation-associated protein tyrosine phosphorylation and membrane fluidity changes are impaired in the spermatozoa of asthenozoospermic patients. Reproduction 2005; 129: 697

61. Buffone MG, et al. Decreased protein tyrosine phosphorylation and membrane fluidity in spermatozoa from infertile men with varicocele. Mol Reprod Dev 2006; in press 6 [review]

62. Buffone MG, et al. Human sperm subpopulations: relationship between functional quality and protein tyrosine phosphorylation. Hum Reprod 2004; 19: 139

63. Vijayaraghavan S, et al. A tyrosine-phosphorylated 55-kilodalton motility-associated bovine sperm protein is regulated by cyclic adenosine 3',5'-monophosphates and calcium. Biol Reprod 1997; 56: 1450

64. Leclerc P, de Lamirande E, Gagnon C. Cyclic adenosine 3',5'monophosphate-dependent regulation of protein tyrosine phosphorylation in relation to human sperm capacitation and motility. Biol Reprod 1996; 55: 684

65. Patil SB, et al. Reactivation of motility of demembranated hamster spermatozoa: role of protein tyrosine kinase and protein phosphatases. Andrologia 2002; 34: 74

66. Si Y, Okuno M. Role of tyrosine phosphorylation of flagellar proteins in hamster sperm hyperactivation. Biol Reprod 1999; 61: 240

67. Visconti PE. Regulation, localization, and anchoring of protein kinase A subunits during mouse sperm capacitation. Dev Biol 1997; 192: 351

68. Luconi M, et al. Increased phosphorylation of AKAP by inhibition of phosphatidylinositol 3-kinase enhances human sperm motility through tail recruitment of protein kinase A. J Cell Sci 2004; 117: 1235

69. Luconi M, et al. Tyrosine phosphorylation of the A kinase anchoring protein 3 (AKAP3) and soluble adenylate cyclase are involved in the increase of human sperm motility by bicarbonate. Biol Reprod 2005; 72: 22

70. Galantino-Homer HL, Visconti PE, Kopf GS. Regulation of protein tyrosine phosphorylation during bovine sperm capacitation by a cyclic adenosine 3'5'-monophosphate-dependent pathway. Biol Reprod 1997; 56: 707

71. Visconti PE, et al. Capacitation of mouse spermatozoa. II. Protein tyrosine phosphorylation and capacitation are regulated by a cAMP-dependent pathway. Development 1995; 121: 1139

72. O'Flaherty C, de Lamirande E, Gagnon C. Phosphorylation of the arginine-X-X-(serine/threonine) motif in human sperm proteins during capacitation modulation and protein kinase A dependency. Mol Hum Reprod 2004; 10: 355

73. Miki K, et al. Targeted disruption of the Akap4 gene causes defects in sperm flagellum and motility. Dev Biol 2002; 248: 331

74. Turner RM, et al. Molecular genetic analysis of two human sperm fibrous sheath proteins, AKAP4 and AKAP3, in men with dysplasia of the fibrous sheath. J Androl 2001; 22: 3025

75. Baccetti B, et al. Gene deletions in an infertile man with sperm fibrous sheath dysplasia. Hum Reprod 2005; 20: 2790

76. Yeung CH, Sonnenberg-Riethmacher E, Cooper TG. Infertile spermatozoa of c-ros tyrosine kinase receptor knockout mice show flagellar angulation and maturational defects in cell volume regulatory mechanisms. Biol Reprod 1999; 61: 1062

77. Yeung CH, et al. The cause of infertility of male c-ros tyrosine kinase receptor knockout mice. Biol Reprod 2000; 63: 612

78. Yeung CH, et al. Sperm volume regulation: maturational changes in fertile and infertile transgenic mice and association with kinematics and tail angulation. Biol Reprod 2002; 67: 269

79. Rossato M, et al. Role of seminal osmolarity in the reduction of human sperm motility. Int J Androl 2002; 25: 230

80. Rossato M, Di Virgilio F, Foresta C. Involvement of osmo-sensitive calcium influx in human sperm activation. Mol Hum Reprod 1996; 903

81. O'Donnell L, et al. Estrogen and spermatogenesis. Endocr Rev 2001; 22: 289

82. Zhou Q, et al. Estrogen action and male fertility: roles of the sodium/hydrogen exchanger-3 and fluid reabsorption in reproductive tract function. Proc Natl Acad Sci USA 2001; 98: 14132

83. Oliveira CA, et al. Aquaporin-1 and -9 are differentially regulated by oestrogen in the efferent ductule epithelium and initial segment of the epididymis. Biol Cell 2005; 97: 385

84. Saito K, et al. Localization of aquaporin-7 in human testis and ejaculated sperm: possible involvement in maintenance of sperm quality. J Urol 2004; 172: 2073

85. Lenzi A, et al. Use of carnitine therapy in selected cases of male factor infertility: a double-blind crossover trial. Fertil Steril 2003; 79: 292

86. Garolla A, et al. Oral carnitine supplementation increases sperm motility in asthenozoospermic men with normal sperm phospholipid hydroperoxide, glutathione peroxidase levels. Fertil Steril 2005; 83: 355

87. Aitken RJ, et al. A novel signal transduction cascade in capacitating human spermatozoa characterised by a redox-regulated, cAMP-mediated induction of tyrosine phosphorylation. J Cell Sci 1998; 111: 645

88. Aitken RJ, Sawyer D. The human spermatozoon – not waving but drowning. Adv Exp Med Biol 2003; 518: 85

89. Ford WC. Regulation of sperm function by reactive oxygen species. Hum Reprod Update 2004; 10: 387

90. Williams AC, Ford WC. Relationship between reactive oxygen species production and lipid peroxidation in human sperm suspensions and their association with sperm function. Fertil Steril 2005; 83: 929

91. Calamera J, et al. Superoxide dismutase content and fatty acid composition in subsets of human spermatozoa from normozoospermic, asthenozoospermic, and polyzoospermic semen samples. Mol Reprod Dev 2003; 66: 422

92. Martin-Du Pan RC, Sakkas D. Is antioxidant therapy a promising strategy to improve human reproduction? Are anti-oxidants useful in the treatment of male infertility? Hum Reprod 1998; 13: 2984

93. Lenzi A, Gandini L, Picardo M. A rationale for glutathione therapy. Hum Reprod 1998; 13: 1419

94. Tramer F, et al. Native specific activity of glutathione peroxidase (GPx-1), phospholipid hydroperoxide glutathione peroxidase (PHGPx) and glutathione reductase (GR) does not differ between normo- and hypomotile human sperm samples. Int J Androl 2004; 27: 88

95. Yanagimachi R. Mammalian fertilization. In Knobil E, Neill JD, eds. The Physiology of Reproduction. New York: Raven Press, 1994: 189

96. Suarez SS, Dai X. Hyperactivation enhances mouse sperm capacity for penetrating viscoelastic media. Biol Reprod 1992; 46: 686

97. Ho HC, Suarezs SS. Hyperactivation of mammalian spermatozoa: function and regulation. Reproduction 2001; 122: 519

98. Demott RP, Suarez SS. Hyperactivated sperm progress in the mouse oviduct. Biol Reprod 1992; 46: 779

99. Gualtieri R, Talevi R. Selection of highly fertilization-competent bovine spermatozoa through adhesion to the Fallopian tube epithelium in vitro. Reproduction 2003; 125: 251

100. Fabbri R, et al. Follicular fluid and human granulosa cell cultures: influence on sperm kinetic parameters, hyperactivation, and acrosome reaction. Fertil Steril 1998; 69: 112

101. Yao Y, Ho P, Yeung WS. Human oviductal cells produce a factor(s) that maintains the motility of human spermatozoa in vitro. Fertil Steril 2000; 73: 479

102. Kay VJ, Coutts JR, Robertson L. Effects of pentoxifylline and progesterone on human sperm capacitation and acrosome reaction. Hum Reprod 1994; 9: 2318

103. Sueldo CE et al. Effect of progesterone on human zona pellucida sperm binding and oocyte penetrating capacity. Fertil Steril 1993; 60: 137

104. Olds-Clarke P, Johnson LR. t haplotypes in the mouse compromise sperm flagellar function. Dev Biol 1993; 155: 14

105. Tessler S, Olds-Clarke P. Linear and nonlinear mouse sperm motility patterns. A quantitative classification. J Androl 1985; 6: 35

106. Lindemann CB, Goltz JS. Calcium regulation of flagellar curvature and swimming pattern in triton X-100-extracted rat sperm. Cell Motil Cytoskeleton 1988; 10: 420

107. Ho HC, Suarez SS. Characterization of the intracellular calcium store at the base of the sperm flagellum that regulates hyperactivated motility. Biol Reprod 2003; 68: 1590

108. Quill TA, et al. A voltage-gated ion channel expressed specifically in spermatozoa. Proc Natl Acad Sci USA 2001; 98: 12527

109. Avidan N, et al. CATSPER2, a human autosomal nonsyndromic male infertility gene. Eur J Hum Genet 2003; 11: 497

110. Nassar A, et al. Modulation of sperm tail protein tyrosine phosphorylation by pentoxifylline and its correlation with hyperactivated motility. Fertil Steril 1999; 71: 919

111. Si Y. Hyperactivation of hamster sperm motility by temperature-dependent tyrosine phosphorylation of an 80-kDa protein. Biol Reprod 1999; 61: 247

112. Bajpai M, Asin S, Doncel GF. Effect of tyrosine kinase inhibitors on tyrosine phosphorylation and motility parameters in human sperm. Arch Androl 2003; 49: 229

113. Yunes R, et al. Cyclic nucleotide phosphodiesterase inhibition increases tyrosine phosphorylation and hypermotility in normal and pathological human spermatozoa. Biocell 2005; 29: 287

114. Cook SP, et al. Sperm chemotaxis: egg peptides control cytosolic calcium to regulate flagellar responses. Dev Biol 1994; 165: 10

115. Wood CD, et al. Real-time analysis of the role of Ca(2+) in flagellar movement and motility in single sea urchin sperm. J Cell Biol 2005; 169: 725

116. Villanueva-Diaz C, et al. Evidence that human follicular fluid contains a chemoattractant for spermatozoa. Fertil Steril 1990; 54: 1180

117. Villanueva-Diaz C, et al. Progesterone induces human sperm chemotaxis. Fertil Steril 1995; 64: 1183

118. Isobe T, et al. The effect of RANTES on human sperm chemotaxis. Hum Reprod 2002; 17: 1441

119. Jaiswal BS, et al. Human sperm chemotaxis: is progesterone a chemoattractant? Biol Reprod 1999; 60: 1314

120. Spehr M, et al. Identification of a testicular odorant receptor mediating human sperm chemotaxis. Science 2003; 299: 2054

121. Spehr M, et al. Particulate adenylate cyclase plays a key role in human sperm olfactory receptor-mediated chemotaxis. J Biol Chem 2004; 279: 40194

122. Sun F, et al. Human sperm chemotaxis: both the oocyte and its surrounding cumulus cells secrete sperm chemoattractants. Hum Reprod 2005; 20: 761

123. Eisenbach M, Ralt D. Precontact mammalian sperm–egg communication and role in fertilization. Am J Physiol 1992; 262: C1095

124. Cohen-Dayag A, et al. Sperm capacitation in humans is transient and correlates with chemotactic responsiveness to follicular factors. Proc Natl Acad Sci USA 1995; 92: 11039

125. World Health Organization. WHO Laboratory Manual for the Examination of Human Semen and Sperm–Cervical Mucus Interaction. Cambridge: Cambridge University Press, 1999

126. Mortimer ST. A critical review of the physiological importance and analysis of sperm movement in mammals. Hum Reprod Update 1997; 3: 403

127. Mortimer ST, Swan MA, Mortimer D. Effect of seminal plasma on capacitation and hyperactivation in human spermatozoa. Hum Reprod 1998; 13: 2139

128. Mortimer ST, Swan MA. Variable kinematics of capacitating human spermatozoa. Hum Reprod 1995; 10: 3178

129. Paston MJ, et al. Computer-aided semen analysis variables as predictors of male fertility potential. Arch Androl 1994; 33: 93

130. Hirano Y, et al. Relationships between sperm motility characteristics assessed by the computer-aided sperm analysis (CASA) and fertilization rates in vitro. J Assist Reprod Genet 2001; 18: 213

131. Shibahara H, et al. Prediction of pregnancy by intrauterine insemination using CASA estimates and strict criteria in patients with male factor infertility. Int J Androl 2004; 27: 63

132. Curi SM, et al. Asthenozoospermia: analysis of a large population. Arch Androl 2003; 49: 343

133. Chemes H. The significance of flagellar pathology in the evaluation of asthenozoospermia. In Baccetti B, ed. Comparative Spermatology 20 years later. Serono Symposia Publications. New York: Raven Press, 1991; 75: 815

134. Chemes HE, et al. Ultrastructural pathology of the sperm flagellum: association between flagellar

pathology and fertility prognosis in severely astheno-zoospermic men. Hum Reprod 1998; 13: 2521

135. Chemes HE, et al. Dysplasia of the fibrous sheath: an ultrastructural defect of human spermatozoa associated with sperm immotility and primary sterility. Fertil Steril 1987; 48: 664

136. Chemes HE. Phenotypes of sperm pathology: genetic and acquired forms in infertile men. J Androl 2000; 21: 799

137. Afzelius BA, et al. Lack of dynein arms in immotile human spermatozoa. J Cell Biol 1975; 66: 2252

138. Olmedo SB, et al. Pregnancies established through intracytoplasmic sperm injection (ICSI) using spermatozoa with dysplasia of fibrous sheath. Asian J Androl 2000; 2: 1252

139. Gadella BM, et al. Dynamics in the membrane organization of the mammalian sperm cell and functionality in fertilization. Vet Q 1999; 21: 142

140. Flesch FM, et al. Bicarbonate stimulated phospholipid scrambling induces cholesterol redistribution and enables cholesterol depletion in the sperm plasma membrane. J Cell Sci 2001; 114: 3543

141. Aitken RJ, et al. Analysis of the responses of human spermatozoa to A23187 employing a novel technique for assessing the acrosome reaction. J Androl 1993; 14: 132

142. Windsor DP, White IG. Assessment of ram sperm mitochondrial function by quantitative determination of sperm rhodamine 123 accumulation. Mol Reprod Dev 1993; 36: 354

143. Aitken J, Fisher H. Reactive oxygen species generation and human spermatozoa: the balance of benefit and risk. Bioessays 1994; 16: 259

144. Isidori A, Latini M, Romanelli F. Treatment of male infertility. Contraception 2005; 72: 314

145. Redmon JB, Carey P, Pryor JL. Varicocele – the most common cause of male factor infertility? Hum Reprod Update 2002; 8: 53

146. Fretz PC, Sandlow JI. Varicocele: current concepts in pathophysiology, diagnosis, and treatment. Urol Clin North Am 2002; 29: 921

147. Liu PY, Handelsman DJ. The present and future state of hormonal treatment for male infertility. Hum Reprod Update 2003; 9: 9

148. Lenzi A, Gandini L. Characterization of human sperm. Hum Reprod 2002; 17: 842

149. Balercia G, et al. Placebo-controlled double-blind randomized trial on the use of L-carnitine, L-acetylcarnitine, or combined L-carnitine and L-acetylcarnitine in men with idiopathic asthenozoospermia. Fertil Steril 2005; 84: 662

150. Costa M, et al. L-carnitine in idiopathic asthenozoospermia: a multicenter study. Italian Study Group on Carnitine and Male Infertility. Andrologia 1994; 26: 155

151. Lenzi A, et al. Placebo-controlled, double-blind, cross-over trial of glutathione therapy in male infertility. Hum Reprod 1993; 8: 1657

152. Balercia G, et al. Coenzyme Q(10) supplementation in infertile men with idiopathic asthenozoospermia: an open, uncontrolled pilot study. Fertil Steril 2004; 81: 93

153. Acosta AA, Khalifa E, Oehninger S. Pure human follicle stimulating hormone has a role in the treatment of severe male infertility by assisted reproduction: Norfolk's total experience. Hum Reprod 1992; 7: 1067

154. Ashkenazi J, et al. The role of purified follicle stimulating hormone therapy in the male partner before intracytoplasmic sperm injection. Fertil Steril 1999; 72: 670

155. Dirnfeld M, et al. Pure follicle-stimulating hormone as an adjuvant therapy for selected cases in male infertility during in-vitro fertilization is beneficial. Eur J Obstet Gynecol Reprod Biol 2000; 93: 105

156. Caroppo E, et al. Recombinant human follicle-stimulating hormone as a pretreatment for idiopathic oligoasthenoteratozoospermic patients undergoing intracytoplasmic sperm injection. Fertil Steril 2003; 80: 1398

157. Foresta C, et al. Treatment of male idiopathic infertility with recombinant human follicle-stimulating hormone: a prospective, controlled, randomized clinical study. Fertil Steril 2005; 84: 654

158. Krausz C, et al. Effect of platelet-activating factor on motility and acrosome reaction of human spermatozoa. Hum Reprod 1994; 9: 471

159. Yovich JL. Pentoxifylline: actions and applications in assisted reproduction. Hum Reprod 1993; 8: 1786

160. Rizk B, et al. Successful use of pentoxifylline in male-factor infertility and previous failure of in vitro fertilization: a prospective randomized study. J Assist Reprod Genet 1995; 12: 710

161. Paul M, Sumpter JP, Lindsay KS. The paradoxical effects of pentoxifylline on the binding of spermatozoa to the human zona pellucida. Hum Reprod 1996; 11: 814

162. Centola GM, Cartie RJ, Cox C. Differential responses of human sperm to varying concentrations of pentoxyfylline with demonstration of toxicity. J Androl 1995; 16: 136

163. Tournaye H, et al. Use of pentoxifylline in assisted reproductive technology. Hum Reprod 1995; 10 (Suppl 1): 72

164. Wymann MP, Pirola L. Structure and function of phosphoinositide 3-kinases. Biochim Biophys Acta 1998; 1436: 127

165. du Plessis SS, et al. Phosphatidylinositol 3-kinase inhibition enhances human sperm motility and sperm–zona pellucida binding. Int J Androl 2004; 27: 19

166. Luconi M, et al. Phosphatidylinositol 3-kinase inhibition enhances human sperm motility. Hum Reprod 2001; 16: 1931

167. Aparicio IM, et al. Inhibition of phosphatidylinositol 3-kinase modifies boar sperm motion parameters. Reproduction 2005; 129: 283

168. Luconi M, et al. Enhancement of mouse sperm motility by the PI3-kinase inhibitor LY294002 does not result in toxic effects on preimplantation embryo development. Hum Reprod 2005; 20: 3500

3

The pathophysiology and genetics of human male reproduction

Christaan F Hoogendijk, Ralf Henkel

INTRODUCTION

The male germ cells, the spermatozoa, are produced in a unique process named spermatogenesis. During this process, spermatogenic stem cells undergo reduction of the genome from diploid cells to haploid cells, as well as unequaled morphological and functional changes. In this respect, spermatozoa are not only the smallest (length of sperm head: 4–5 μm) and most polarized cells (sperm head in front, flagellum at rear) in the body, but also the only cells that fulfill their function outside the body, even in a different individual, the female reproductive tract. Therefore, spermatozoa are highly specialized cells, simply a 'means of transportation', that transfer the genetic information from the male to the female, the oocyte for which specific physiological functions of these cells are required. For the sperm cells to acquire these functions, morphological and physiological development of the spermatozoa has to take place. In addition, proper chromosomal and genetic constitution is mandatory, i.e. chromosomal and DNA integrity must be given.

During spermatogenesis, spermatozoa acquire the morphological and physiological foundations, which eventually have to mature during epididymal maturation, for normal sperm function. This means that if the processes taking place in the course of spermatogenesis are defective, this will result in malformed, dysfunctional male germ cells. Therefore, to understand the physiology of fertilization, the understanding of spermatogenesis and its morphological and genetic processes is of paramount importance.

GENETIC CONTROL OF SPERMATOGENESIS

The relationship between structurally abnormal and genetically defective spermatozoa poses a crucial unknown. The long sequence of events involved in spermatogenesis, from germ cell differentiation to functionally mature spermatozoa, is fraught with the possibility of both structural and genetic damage. Spermatogenesis consists of three distinct phases: (1) proliferation and differentiation of diploid spermatogonial stem cells, (2) meiosis where chromosome pairing and genetic recombination occurs and (3) spermiogenesis, a unique series of events in which the rather commonplace-appearing, albeit haploid, round spermatids differentiate into species-specific-shaped spermatozoa. Collectively, these intervals consist of many developmental events, which offer numerous opportunities for the introduction of damage into the genome of the male gamete. These concerns are exacerbated by the ability of scientists and embryologists to use differentiating male germ cells, prior to the completion of spermatogenesis, for fertilization. This raises the question: are we not introducing 'incomplete' male gametes into oocytes?

Spermatogonial differentiation

The intricate mechanisms whereby stem cells maintain a population of proliferating and differentiating cells are only beginning to be unraveled[1]. In the mammalian testis, spermatogonial type A stem cells proliferate, producing three classes of spermatogonia: (1) a group of presumably identical spermatogonial stem cells, (2) a population of differentiating spermatogonia and (3) a large number of cells that undergo cell death by apoptosis[2]. The originators of this developmental cascade, type A spermatogonia, represent a mixed population of cell types designated type A_0, A_1, A_2, A_3 or A_4 spermatogonia. Among these cells, the identity of 'true' stem cells is yet to be definitively established. Although multiple stem-cell renewal models have been put forward, one commonly accepted model proposes that type A_0 spermatogonia represents a reserve population of stem cells, which divide slowly and can repopulate the testis after damage[3]. Thus, types A_1–A_4 spermatogonia are believed to be the renewing stem-cell spermatogonia, and these cells maintain the fertility of a man.

Type A spermatogonia differentiate into intermediate and type B spermatogonia, which in turn divide and enter the differentiating pathway leading to spermatozoa. These cellular programming events appear to be irreversible, because once committed to differentiation, the spermatogonia appear incapable of re-entering the pathway that produces stem cells. The implications of genetically defective spermatogonia are substantial, since it is these cells that will function as the precursors of spermatozoa throughout the life of the individual. The large number of spermatogonial stem cells that undergo apoptosis suggests that a sophisticated monitoring system has evolved in which 'defective' stem cells are removed. Currently,

much effort is being directed towards studies defining mechanisms of apoptosis in somatic cells. Research efforts need to be extended to define the mechanisms by which specific populations of stem cells are selected to be targets for cell death. Specifically in the testis, an understanding of how the differentiating germ cells are continually being assessed, presumably by a self-monitoring system, will help greatly to minimize the production of genetically defective germ cells.

Meiosis

Meiosis represents a fascinating interval of spermatogenesis in which genetic alterations, including genetic damage, are intentionally introduced into the genome, which in turn contributes to the evolutionary change of species. In addition to its essential role in producing haploid gametes from diploid stem cells, the extended interval of meiotic prophase has evolved to provide the critical cellular milieu for precise genetic recombination[4].

Meiotic prophase commences with preleptotene primary spermatocytes, the cell type in which the last semiconservative DNA replication of the male germ cell occurs. All subsequent DNA synthesis in differentiating male germ cells represents DNA repair synthesis. Chromosome condensation initiates concomitantly with the movement of leptotene and zygotene spermatocytes to the adluminal compartment of the seminiferous tubule from the basal membrane region. Alignment and complete pairing of the chromosomal homologs are completed in pachytene spermatocytes. As the chromosomes condense, axial elements appear between the two sister chromatids of each chromosomal homolog. The addition of a visible central element to the chromosomes produces the synaptonemal complex, a highly conserved structure in the meiotic cells of organisms ranging from water mold to the human, that is needed for effective synapsis. Because synapsis of chromosomes represents an event unique and critical to genetic recombination, meiotic cells contain many novel structural proteins and enzymes needed for chromosome and DNA alignment, DNA breakage, recombination and DNA repair.

Among the proteins recently shown to be important in the genetic recombination process are Rad 51, a human homolog of a bacterial recombination protein[5]; BRCA1, a tumor-suppressor gene implicated in familial breast and ovarian cancers[5]; ATM-related genes, members of a gene family proposed to prevent DNA damage[6–8]; a ubiquitin-conjugating repair enzyme believed to be involved in protein turnover[9,10]; a mammalian homolog to a meiosis-specific DNA double-strand breaking enzyme[11]; DNA recombination genes[12,13]; and a meiotic-specific heat shock protein[14]. Since meiosis is crucial for the survival of a species, an elaborate series of safeguards has evolved to pair, break and repair chromosomal DNA. Despite such regulatory mechanisms, it is well known that translocations and aneuploidy are regularly introduced during the meiotic divisions. Moreover, in a sizeable population of infertile men, germ cell differentiation arrests during meiosis[15]. Anomalies in pairing and chromosome segregation are likely to contribute to this population of infertile men. Moreover, the many specific molecular processes essential for meiosis provide many targets for both genetic damage and for the introduction of structural defects, leading to the arrest of germ cell development. Our rapidly advancing knowledge of the mechanisms of meiosis in both males and females will provide substantial insights into a significant cause of male infertility.

Spermiogenesis

Spermiogenesis represents an interval of spermatogenesis that appears exceptionally susceptible to the introduction of both genetic and structural defects in the maturing male gamete, as the round spermatid is transformed into the highly elongated and polarized (sperm head in front, flagellum at rear) spermatozoon at a time of reduced repair capabilities. Moreover, during spermiogenesis, a major reorganization of the cell occurs. The nucleus elongates and an acrosome containing a group of proteolytic enzymes develops. At the chromosomal level, the histones, the predominant chromatin proteins of somatic cells, are replaced by the highly basic transition proteins, which in turn are replaced by the protamines, producing a tightly compacted nucleus with extensive disulfide bridge crosslinking. In fact, sperm chromatin condensation during spermiogenesis results in DNA taking up about 90% of the total volume of the sperm nucleus. In contrast, in normal somatic cells, the DNA takes up only 5% of the nucleus volume, while in mitotic chromosomes DNA takes up about 15% of the nuclear volume[16].

Displacement of the histones from the nucleosomes during spermiogenesis may leave the DNA of the haploid genome especially susceptible to damage at a time of limited repair capabilities. Although unscheduled DNA repair has been demonstrated to occur in early stages of spermatid development[17], as spermiogenesis proceeds, unscheduled DNA synthesis diminishes, and it is not known whether any of the sophisticated DNA repair mechanisms that function during meiosis are still operational. In addition to the major nuclear restructuring taking place during spermiogenesis, the axoneme and tail of the developing male germ cell are produced, requiring synthesis of many structural proteins, including those of the fibrous sheath[18] and the outer dense fiber proteins[19]. These cellular changes require extensive gene expression from the actively transcribed haploid genome before it matures into a genetically quiescent nucleus. In fact, transcription of RNA ceases during mid-spermiogenesis[20], and translational regulation plays a prominent regulatory role in the extensive protein synthesis throughout the latter half of spermiogenesis that is required to produce spermatozoa[21–23].

The major reorganizational events of the differentiating spermatid are accompanied by significant alterations in the energy suppliers of the cell, the mitochondria. Mitochondria exhibit several distinct morphologies as germ cell differentiation proceeds[24]. Spermatogonia and somatic testicular cells contain the 'cigar-shaped' mitochondria found in most somatic tissues. During meiosis, mitochondria with diffuse and vacuolated matrices start replacing the 'somatic' mitochondria. By the beginning of spermiogenesis, the 'somatic' mitochondria have been totally replaced by 'germ cell' mitochondria, which in turn are replaced by the crescent-shaped mitochondria of spermatozoa. These structural changes in mitochondria are accompanied by major changes in protein composition[25,26]. Although spermatocytes and spermatids are estimated to contain over 103 mitochondria, each spermatozoa midpiece contains only approximately 75 uniquely helically shaped mitochondria. This requires the reduction or possibly selection of mitochondria as the germ cells differentiate[27]. At the conclusion of spermiogenesis, most of the cytoplasm of the elongated spermatid is removed as the residual body is pinched off, leaving spermatozoa with little cytoplasm, and no cytoplasmic ribosomes. Although cytoplasmic protein synthesis does not occur in spermatozoa, cytoplasmic mitochondrial protein synthesis continues[28].

Considering the massive changes that occur during spermiogenesis, it is not surprising that many cases of germ cell blockage during spermiogenesis lead to infertility in men. Defects in the synthesis of the midpiece, axoneme, mitochondria or tail assembly would result in structurally abnormal spermatozoa often with poor motility, while mutations in proteins needed for the compaction of sperm nuclei or sperm head shaping would lead to spermatozoa with abnormal heads. Despite the presence of aberrant-appearing spermatozoa, it is premature to equate morphological aberrations with genetic aberrations. More disquieting, minor base-pair substitutions in critical genes that would not alter spermatozoon morphology would lead to genetically defective but normal-appearing spermatozoa!

Our inability to detect genetically defective male gametes is of great concern when round spermatid nucleus injections (ROSNI) and round spermatid injections (ROSI) are used to overcome the sterility of men incapable of completing spermatogenesis[29,30]. The success of ROSNI and ROSI has demonstrated that although spermiogenesis is essential for reorganization of the male germ cell to become a motile cell, it is not needed for fertilization. Thus, the normal physiological selection processes leading to fertilization can be bypassed in mice and men. Unfortunately, morphological examination of the spermatids tells little of any underlying genetic defects in the spermatid chosen for injection. A major research effort must be undertaken with a mammalian model system such as the mouse in which a large population of progeny produced by ROSNI and ROSI are produced and evaluated. Among the concerns raised by these procedures is whether we are circumventing gene imprinting in the male genome. The detection of DNA methylation of spermatozoa in the epididymis also raises questions[31]. Without a detailed analysis of this approach in an animal system, we could be facing major genetic dangers introduced by the ROSNI and ROSI technologies.

GENETICS OF THE SPERMATOZOON

During the past few years, many exciting discoveries, previously unsuspected by scientists, have been made about the structure and function of sperm DNA. For example, the paternal genome has been shown to contain endogenous nicks, probably as a normal part of spermiogenesis[32]. In patients in whom these nicks are left unrepaired during the final stages of spermiogenesis, fertility is decreased[33]. Topoisomerases, the enzymes thought to be responsible for these nicks, are present throughout spermatogenesis; nonetheless, they are not present in spermatozoa[34,35]. Evenson and colleagues[36–38] developed the sperm chromatin structure assay (SCSA) that assesses the potential of sperm DNA to denature under certain conditions. This potential also correlates with reduced fertility[39]. Perhaps most surprising of all, evidence published by Spadafora and colleagues[40,41] shows that fully mature mouse spermatozoa have the potential to incorporate exogenous DNA sequences into the paternal genome. Finally, since a sheep has been cloned from an adult cell[42], and this technique has also been successful in several other mammalian species such as cattle, the mouse, goat, pig, cat and rabbit and even a primate, the rhesus monkey, this has raised the question of the importance of the paternal genome and its unique structure in embryogenesis.

The above-mentioned discoveries have forced us to rethink the idea of sperm DNA structure in which we visualize the paternal genome as being so tightly packaged into an almost crystalline state that it is virtually inert until it is unfolded during fertilization. The sperm chromosome structure is, in fact, very complex – some attributes are similar to somatic cell DNA organization, and others are unique to spermatogenic cells.

When discussing sperm chromatin packaging, several different aspects of structure need to be addressed. These can be divided into different levels of complexity based on the length of DNA being discussed. Each chromosome consists of one double-stranded DNA molecule, containing telomeric repeats at both ends, and centromeric repeats somewhere along its length. Chromosomes are in the order of several million base pairs in length, and, when fully decondensed, are each many times longer than the sperm nucleus itself. At the other end of the spectrum are sperm-specific protamines, each of which bind to only a few base pairs of DNA.

Sperm DNA packaging can be subdivided into four levels. In the following paragraphs, we discuss the structural relationship between the different levels of DNA packaging in the mature sperm nucleus.

Level I: chromosomal anchoring by the nuclear annulus

In the first step of the assembly of sperm chromatin, the two strands of naked DNA that make up the chromosomes are attached to a sperm-specific structure, the nuclear annulus. This represents a novel type of DNA organization, termed chromosomal anchoring, that is found only in spermatogenic cells. Spermatozoa that are washed with non-ionic detergents such as NP-40, and then treated with high salt and reducing agents to extract the protamines, will decondense completely, leaving no trace of nuclear structure. The DNA, however, remains anchored to the base of the tail, so that the sperm chromatin resembles a broom, with the tail acting as the handle[43]. Since this chromosomal anchoring is maintained in sperm nuclei from which protamines have been extracted, it is independent of protamine binding. Ward and Coffey[43] have isolated a small structure that is located at the implantation fossa in hamster spermatozoa, which they have termed the nuclear annulus, to which the DNA is attached in these decondensed nuclei. The nuclear annulus is shaped like a bent ring, and is about 2 μm in length. It is found only in sperm nuclei, although it is currently unknown at what stage of spermiogenesis it is first formed. Thus, so far, no evidence for a nuclear annulus-like structure in any somatic cell type has been found. In contrast, there is evidence of its existence in hamster[43], human[44], mouse and Xenopus sperm nuclei. Its existence in a wide variety of species suggests a fundamental role in sperm function.

Unique DNA sequences were found to be associated with the nuclear annulus. Ward and Coffey[43] termed these sequences NA-DNA. The existence of these unique sequences suggests that the nuclear annulus anchors chromosomes according to particular sequences and not by random DNA binding. They also hypothesized that NA-DNAs on different chromosomes become associated early during spermiogenesis, to initiate chromatin condensation by aggregating specific sites of each chromosome to one point.

This hypothesis is supported by the work of Zalensky et al.[45], who suggested that sperm chromosomes are packaged as extended fibers along the length of the nucleus. Each chromosome so far examined has only one site at the base of the nucleus, where the nuclear annulus is located. By organizing the chromosomes so that the NA-DNA sites of each chromosome are aggregated onto one structure, the nuclear annulus may also affect the determination of sperm nuclear shape. For example, in the hamster spermatozoon the longer chromosomes may extend into the thinner hook of the nucleus, while a portion of every chromosome is located at the nuclear annulus. This is supported by image analysis of the distribution of DNA throughout the hamster sperm nucleus, which demonstrates that the highest concentration of DNA in the packaged sperm nucleus is at the base, where the nuclear annulus is located; in contrast, the lowest concentration of DNA is in the hooked portion[46].

The hypothesis is further supported by electron microscopic evidence that chromatin near the implantation fossa is one of the first areas to condense during spermiogenesis[47]. Thus, the nuclear annulus may represent the only known aspect of sperm chromatin condensation that is specific for individual chromosome sites.

Level II: sperm DNA loop domain organization

DNA loop domain organization

At this level, anchored chromosomes are organized into DNA loop domains. Parts of the nuclear matrix, protein structural fibers, attach to the DNA every 30–50 kb by specific sequences termed matrix attachment regions (MARs). This arranges the chromosome strands into a series of loops. This type of organization can be visualized experimentally in preparations, and is known as a nuclear halo. A nuclear halo comprises the nuclear matrix with a halo of DNA surrounding it. This halo consists of loops of naked DNA, 25–100 kb in length, attached at their bases to the matrix. Each loop domain visible in the nuclear halo consists of a structural unit of chromatin that exists *in vivo* in a condensed form.

As with chromosomal anchoring, DNA loop domain formation is independent of protamine binding. The organization of DNA into loop domains is the only type of structural organization resolved thus far that is present in both somatic and sperm cells. In somatic cells, DNA is coiled into nucleosomes, then further coiled into a 30-nm solenoid-like fiber and then organized into DNA loop domains. The corresponding structures in sperm chromatin have a very different appearance. Protamine binding causes a different type of coiling, and DNA is folded into densely packed toroids, but still organized into loop domains. Mammalian sperm nuclei contain a small amount of histones, which are presumably organized into nucleosomes[48,49], but most of the DNA is reorganized by protamines. This means that with the evolutionary pressure to condense sperm DNA, all aspects of chromatin structure are sacrificed other than the organization of DNA into loop domains. This suggests that DNA loop domains play a crucial role in sperm DNA function.

DNA loop domain function

In somatic cells, DNA loop domain organization has been implicated in both the control of gene expression and in DNA replication. Each DNA loop domain replicates at a fixed site on the nuclear matrix, by being reeled through the enzymatic machinery located at the base of the loop[50,51]. DNA replication origins have been localized to the nuclear matrix in mammals[52], and the varying sizes of replicons in different species have been correlated with the sizes of loop domains[53]. A replicon can be thought of as the distance between two regions of replication. The attachment sites of individual genes to the nuclear matrix vary between cell types, and are also involved in transcription. Active genes are tightly associated with the nuclear matrix, but inactive genes are usually located within the extended part of the DNA loop[54–58]. In this manner, the three-dimensional organization of DNA plays an important role in DNA function.

Possible function of sperm DNA loop domains

It has been demonstrated that the specific configurations of DNA loop domains are markedly different in sperm and somatic cells[44,59]. In somatic cells, DNA replication and transcription are the major functions in which DNA loop domain structures are involved[48–53,56–58]. However, since mature sperm nuclei perform neither process[60], it is not clear what is the function of sperm DNA loop domain organization. Two possibilities exist. First, the DNA loop domain structures in spermatozoa may be residual structures that were required for transcription or DNA replication that occurred during spermatogenesis. Second, they may be involved in regulating these functions during embryonic development, if the embryo inherits them. If, for example, paternal genes in the male pronucleus of a newly fertilized egg were organized into the same DNA loop configurations that they have in sperm nuclei, it would suggest that this organization might help to regulate transcription and DNA replication in early embryonic development. This would have the exciting implication that the sperm nucleus provides the embryo with a specific chromosomal architecture that may be functional during embryogenesis.

Level III: protamine decondensation

In the third step of assembly of the sperm chromatin structure, the binding of protamines condenses the DNA loops into tightly packaged chromatin. Hud *et al.*[61] have demonstrated that when protamines bind DNA, they form toroidal, or doughnut-shaped, structures in which the DNA is very concentrated. During spermiogenesis, histones, the DNA-binding proteins of somatic spermatogenic precursor cells, are replaced by protamines. Since histone-bound DNA requires much more volume than the same amount of DNA bound to protamines[16], this change in chromatin structure probably accounts for some of the

nuclear condensation that occurs during spermiogenesis. Histones package DNA by organizing it into nucleosomes, in which the DNA is wrapped around an octamer of histone proteins. Protamines, on the other hand, bind DNA in a markedly different manner. These positively charged proteins bind DNA along the major groove, completely neutralizing the DNA so that neighboring DNA strands bind to each other by van der Waals forces. Protamines are believed to coil the DNA into doughnut-like structures in which the DNA exists in an almost crystalline-like state[61]. If each toroid is a single DNA loop domain[62], protamine binding will lead to condensation and preservation of the DNA loop domain organization present in the round spermatid.

Level IV: chromosome organization

The next level of sperm chromatin packaging is the spatial arrangement of the condensed chromosomes within the mature sperm nucleus. This has been investigated in several different ways. First, Zalensky and co-workers[45] demonstrated that, in human sperm nuclei, the centromeres of all chromosomes are aggregated in the center of the nucleus, while the telomeres are located at the periphery. In a second approach, Haaf and Ward[63] analyzed whole chromosomes and found similar results. Finally, Ward and co-workers[64] mapped the three-dimensional location of three genes in the hamster sperm nucleus and found that while each one tended to be located in the outer third of the nucleus, there was otherwise little specificity to the positioning of the genes. These data led to the proposal of a model[65] in which there are limited constraints on the actual position of chromosomes in the sperm nucleus. The NA-DNA sequences are located at the base of the nucleus, centromeres are located centrally and the telomeres are located peripherally. Outside these three constraints, the folding of the chromosomal p and q arms is flexible. Interestingly, this type of organization does not seem to be present in montreme mammal spermatozoa. In these species, chromosomes are aligned end-to-end[66]. In most eutherian mammals examined, however, the centromeres are organized in a central location, making such an end-to-end arrangement impossible.

ROLE OF SPERMATOZOA IN EMBRYOGENESIS

For many years, male fertility has been defined *in vitro* as the possibility of sperm to fertilize the oocyte, and to obtain early cleavage-stage embryos. In human *in vitro* fertilization (IVF), the gold-standard/test for sperm fertility potential was the ability of a fertilized egg to develop into a 2–4-cell embryo. It was assumed that all embryos obtained had the same developmental potential, independent of the quality of sperm. Thereafter, several authors[67–69] observed that poor morphological embryonic quality and poor embryonic developmental ability are associated with severe sperm morphological defects and oligoasthenozoospermia. In addition, Janny and Ménézo[70] observed a negative relationship between sperm quality and the ability to reach the blastocyst stage. We now know that differences in sperm fertility are not simply related to sperm penetration failure. The following is an analysis of the chronology of the steps involved in these embryonic failures.

Early defects at the time of fertilization

The centrosome

The first epigenetic contribution of the spermatozoon is the centrosome, the microtubule-organizing center of the cell. Correct assembly and function of microtubules is fundamental for the separation of chromosomes at meiosis and migration of the male and female pronuclei. Maternal inheritance of the centrosome observed

in mice brought about confusion until the work of Schatten[71] and Simerly *et al.*[72]. Considering the semiconservative form of this organelle and its critical role in mitosis, it seems obvious that a functionally imperfect centrosome borne by a subnormal spermatozoon induces problems in early embryogenesis, i.e. the formation of cytoplasmic fragments and abnormal distribution of chromosomes[72,73]. Asch *et al.*[74] reported that up to 25% of non-segmented eggs are in fact fertilized but submitted to cell division defects. Centrin and γ-tubulin could be involved in this pathology of the centrosome[75]. In bovine oocytes, Navara *et al.*[76] observed a positive relationship between size and quality of the sperm aster and reproductive performance in bulls.

Oocyte activation factor(s)

The process of meiosis reinitiation is probably completed through an exit from the M phase due to cyclin B degradation and re-phosphorylation of $p34^{cdc2}$ following a decrease in cytostatic factor (CSF)[77]. It is generally accepted that intracellular Ca^{2+} is the universal signal for triggering oocytes into metabolic activity. It is still not clear how the spermatozoon causes this calcium oscillation. A heat-sensitive[78] and soluble protein called oscillin, acting through the inositol phosphate pathway, could be at the origin of these calcium oscillations[79].

Defects in oscillin (or other soluble activating factors) could account for delays in zygote formation, as described by Ron-El *et al.*[68]. However, for Eid *et al.*[80], based on their observations in bovine zygotes, this hypothesis might not be the only one. In a group of embryos sired by low-fertility bulls, they did not observe any delay in pronuclear formation, but a delayed initiation and reduced length of zygotic S-phase correlated with reduced embryonic development *in vitro*. A longer S-phase was correlated with higher fertility *in vivo*.

Poor chromatin packaging and/or anomalies in DNA packaging could contribute to the failure of sperm decondensation, independently of any activation problems[81].

Developmental arrests between fertilization and the beginning of genomic activation

It is quite surprising to expect a paternal-derived influence between fertilization and genomic activation, i.e. before the appearance of the first products resulting from the first massive transcriptions involving the paternal genome. It is now well documented that the longest cleavage stage is linked to embryonic genome activation[82]. There is obviously a race against the clock between, first, the ineluctable turnover of the maternal mRNA and, on the other hand, the first massive synthesis of the embryonic transcripts. The cumulative delays observed, cycle after cycle, due to epigenetic defects brought about by suboptimal spermatozoa lead to developmental arrests, the maternal stores being exhausted before the beginning of transcription. Under *in vitro* conditions, one-third of human IVF embryos block around the time of genomic activation[70].

Antisperm antibodies may also have a deleterious effect on early preimplantation development. Naz[83] observed that antibodies against very special epitopes might block embryos, especially if cleavage signal proteins (CS-1) or regulatory products of the OCT-3 gene are immunoneutralized.

Developmental arrests between genomic activation and implantation

After genomic activation, the very sensitive transition between morula and blastocyst follows. Complex remodeling within the embryo occurs with the first differentiation. Janny and Ménézo[70] observed a loss of blastocysts at this point, which was significantly increased in men with poor sperm quality (31% vs. 22% for the control group). They concluded that poor-quality sperm has a negative influence on preimplantation development even after genomic activation.

The lesson from ICSI

One of the most exciting breakthroughs in the treatment of male infertility is intracytoplasmic sperm injection (ICSI). The success that we observe in ICSI, considering the poor quality of the sperm, can partially be ascribed to the following. In human IVF with poor-quality sperm, delay in the fertilization process[68] and delays associated with epigenetic problems, the cumulative effect may be prolonged cell cycles and late divisions (2-cell embryos on day 2, 4-cell on day 3), leading to developmental arrest around genomic activation, in relation to depletion of the mRNA maternal store. In contrast, the fertilization process in ICSI is shorter, since the sperm is introduced into the cytoplasm.

Van Landuyt and co-workers[84] showed that the blastocyst formation rate after ICSI compares to the rate after regular IVF. An in-depth analysis, however, demonstrates that more patients have embryos which are unable to reach the blastocyst stage. Interestingly, there seems to be an 'all or nothing' trend regarding blastocyst development. If one blastocyst is obtained, then all embryos from the patient in question normally develop into blastocysts, whilst if no blastocysts are seen at day 5, it is highly unlikely that any embryos will go on to develop into blastocysts.

ICSI is of no use if performed 24 hours after failed fertilization: the maternal mRNA reserves are already at this point too depleted to allow development from fertilization to genomic activation. It is very likely that major sperm defects cannot be corrected by the application of ICSI.

The ICSI process itself carries other genetic-related problems such as the genetic link between oligoasthenoteratozoospermia and sperm genetic disorders. Some of these features include microdeletions of the Y chromosome[85]. The negative influence of suboptimal spermatozoa is linked to the integrity and quality of the paternal DNA. In 1985, Bourrouillou and co-workers[86] observed an increase in chromosomal abnormalities as a function of sperm count; in 1995, Moosani and co-workers[87] clearly demonstrated increased chromosomal disorders in the sperm population of infertile men with idiopathic infertility.

In this context, it is also important to mention the consequences of fertilization of oocytes with sperm deriving from an ejaculate containing a high incidence of disturbed DNA integrity in IVF and, especially, in ICSI patients. According to present knowledge, sperm DNA fragmentation might cause not only impaired embryonic development and early embryonic death[74,88,89], but also an increased risk of childhood cancer in the offspring[90,91]. The latter is due to the vulnerability of human sperm DNA during late stages of spermatogenesis and epididymal maturation. At this stage, DNA repair mechanisms have been switched off, resulting in a genetic instability of the male germ cells[92], especially on the Y chromosome, resulting in male-specific cancers[93]. However, this DNA damage is not only caused by these intrinsic factors, but can also be triggered by extrinsic factors such as excess amounts of oxidants producing leukocytes in the ejaculate[94]. The influence of the spermatozoon-carried mitochondria during ICSI, on early or late embryogenesis, is, however, still a matter of debate.

Genomic imprinting

Experimental manipulations of mouse zygotes have clearly proved the necessary complementary relationship between the maternal and the paternal genome to ensure normal embryonic development. Even if implantation and late development can be observed in the rabbit and mouse, parthenogenesis never leads to live births. Surani *et al.*[95] observed that hypertrophy of the inner cell mass and hypotrophy of the extraembryonic tissue is related to gynogenesis. In contrast, androgenesis performed by removal of the female pronucleus followed by duplication of the paternal genome leads to hypertrophy of extraembryonic tissues. This is due to genomic imprinting, which occurs as early as the pronuclear stage. Genomic imprinting seems to be directly related to variations in the methylation pattern of some genes. One of the most important systems in genomic imprinting is IGF2/IGF2-R[96]. The ligand is contributed by the paternal genome and the receptor by the maternal one. The maternal and paternal X chromosomes are submitted to differential inactivation, related to different methylation patterns of the Xist locus, in the preimplantation period. Xist is the initiator of methylation carried by the X chromosome.

The H19 gene, a tumor suppressor, is expressed in the placenta but not in the mole. The potential invasiveness of the placenta and/or placental tumors is directly related to the paternal genome qualitatively and quantitatively[97]. Disorganized imprinting may have harmful effects on early-preimplantation and late-postimplantation development.

CONCLUSIONS

As discussed, it is clear that paternal factors have major effects on early embryogenesis. In the past decade, major advances have been made in assisted reproductive technologies. ICSI has been proposed as a tool for overcoming sperm deficiencies observed at the time of fertilization. This technology can assist in overcoming some of the defects affecting early-preimplantation development. Time gained by direct sperm insertion into the cytoplasm may help in avoiding delays that impair early-preimplantation development.

However, it is unlikely that ICSI can universally compensate for male-factor defects. Moreover, it raises questions regarding the genetic basis of some of the defects observed, and on some other hidden genetic links. The growing number of children that have followed the application of ICSI is beginning to provide us with a good base to evaluate the transmission of genetic defects. To date, there is evidence showing that infertility in fathers due to microdeletions in the Y chromosome is transmitted from one male generation to the next[98,99]. These examples of male infertility are believed to be due to deletion of genes such as the DAZ (deleted in azoospermia) and RBM (RNA-binding motif) genes. These genes show mapping to Y chromosome-linked microdeletions[100–103].

REFERENCES

1. Morrison SJ, Shah NM, Anderson DJ. Regulatory mechanisms in stem cell biology. Cell 1997; 88: 287
2. Dym M. Spermatogonial stem cells of the testis. Proc Natl Acad Sci USA 1994; 91: 11287
3. Dym M, Clermont Y. Role of spermatogonia in the repair of the seminiferous epithelium following X radiation of the rat testis. Am J Anat 1970; 128: 265
4. Stern H. The process of meiosis. In Ewing L, Desjardin C, eds. Cell and Molecular Biology of the Testis. New York: Oxford University Press, 1993: 296
5. Scully R, et al. Association of BRCA1 with Rad 51 in mitotic and meiotic cells. Cell 1997; 88: 256
6. Zakian VA. ATM-related genes: what do they tell us about functions of the human gene? Cell 1995; 82: 685
7. Barlow C, et al. A paradigm of ataxia telangiectasia. Cell 1996; 86: 159
8. Keegan KS, et al. The Atr and Atm protein kinases associate with different sites along meiotically pairing chromosomes. Genes Dev 1996; 10: 2423
9. Roest HP, et al. Inactivation of the HR6B ubiquitin-conjugating DNA repair enzyme in mice causes male sterility associated with chromatin modification. Cell 1996; 86: 799
10. Kovalenko OV, et al. Mammalian ubiquitin-conjugating enzyme Ubc9 interacts with Rad51 recombination protein and localizes in synaptonemal complexes. Proc Natl Acad Sci USA 1996; 93: 2958
11. Keeney S, Giroux CN, Kleckner N. Meiosis-specific DNA double-strand breaks are catalyzed by Spo11, a member of a widely conserved protein family. Cell 1997; 88: 375
12. Edelmann W, Kucherlapati R. Role of recombination enzymes in mammalian cell survival. Proc Natl Acad Sci USA 1996; 93: 6225
13. Edelmann W, et al. Meiotic pachytene arrest in MLH1-deficient mice. Cell 1996; 85: 1125
14. Dix DJ, et al. Targeted gene disruption of Hsp 70-2 results in failed meiosis, germ cell apoptosis, and male infertility. Proc Natl Acad Sci USA 1996; 93: 3264
15. Reijo R, et al. Diverse spermatogenic defects in humans caused by Y chromosome deletions encompassing a novel RNA-binding protein gene. Nat Genet 1995; 10: 383
16. Ward WS, Coffey DS. DNA packaging and organization in mammalian spermatozoa: comparison with somatic cells [Review]. Biol Reprod 1991; 44: 569
17. Sega GA. Unscheduled DNA synthesis (DNA repair) in germ cells of male mice – its role in the study of mammalian mutagenesis. Genetics 1979; 92: 49
18. Morales CR, Oko R, Clermont Y. Molecular cloning and developmental expression of an mRNA encoding the 27 kDa outer dense fiber protein of rat spermatozoa. Mol Reprod Dev 1994; 37: 229
19. Carrera A, Gerton GL, Moss B. The major fibrous sheath polypeptide of mouse sperm: structural and functional similarities to the A-kinase anchoring proteins. Dev Biol 1994; 165: 272
20. Kierszenbaum AL. Mammalian spermatogenesis in vivo and in vitro: a partnership of spermatogenic and somatic cell lineages. Endocr Rev 1994; 15: 116
21. Hecht NB. The making of a spermatozoon: a molecular perspective. Dev Genet 1995; 16: 95
22. Spirin AS. Storage of messenger RNA in eukaryotes: envelopment with protein, translocation barrier at 5′ side, or conformational masking by 3′ side? Mol Reprod Dev 1994; 38: 107
23. Schäfer M, et al. Translocational control in spermatogenesis. Dev Biol 1995; 172: 344
24. De Martino C, et al. Morphological, histochemical, and biochemical studies on germ cell mitochondria of normal rats. Cell Tissue Res 1979; 196: 1
25. Hecht NB, Bradley FM. Changes in mitochondrial protein composition during testicular differentiation in mouse and bull. Gamete Res 1981; 4: 433
26. Hake LE, Alcivar AA, Hecht NB. Changes in length accompany translocational regulation of the somatic and testis-specific cytochrome c genes during spermatogenesis in the mouse. Development 1990; 110: 249
27. Hecht NB, Liem H. Mitochondrial DNA is synthesized during meiosis and spermiogenesis in the mouse. Exp Cell Res 1984; 154: 293
28. Alcivar AA, et al. Mitochondrial gene expression in male germ cells of the mouse. Dev Biol 1989; 135: 263
29. Ogura A, Matsuda J, Yanagimachi R. Birth of normal young after electrofusion of mouse oocytes with round spermatids. Proc Natl Acad Sci USA 1994; 91: 7460
30. Fishel S, Aslam I, Tesarik J. Spermatid conception: a stage too early, or a time too soon? Hum Reprod 1996; 11: 1371
31. Ariel M, Cedar H, McCarrey J. Developmental changes in methylation of spermatogenesis-specific genes include reprogramming in the epididymis. Nat Genet 1994; 7: 59
32. Bianchi PG, et al. Effect of DNA protamination on fluorochrome staining and in situ nick-translation of

murine and human mature spermatozoa. Biol Reprod 1993; 49: 1083

33. Sakkas D, et al. Sperm chromatin anomalies can influence decondensation after intracytoplasmic sperm injection. Hum Reprod 1996; 11: 837

34. Morse-Gaudio M, Risley MS. Topoisomerase II expression and VM-26 induction of DNA breaks during spermatogenesis in Xenopus laevis. J Cell Sci 1994; 107: 2887

35. Chen JL, Longo FJ. Expression and localisation of DNA topoisomerase II during rat spermatogenesis. Mol Reprod Dev 1996; 45: 61

36. Evenson DP, et al. Relation of mammalian sperm chromatin heterogeneity to fertility. Science 1980; 210: 1131

37. Evenson DP, Melamed MR. Rapid analysis of normal and abnormal cell types in human semen and testis biopsies by flow cytometry. J Histochem Cytochem 1983; 31: 248

38. Evenson DP, Jost LK. Sperm chromatin structure assay: DNA denaturability. In Darzynkiewicz Z, Robinson JP, Crissman HA, eds. Methods in Cell Biology. Flow Cytometry, 2nd edn. Orlando: Academic Press, 1994; 42: 159

39. Sailer BL, Jost LK, Evenson DP. Bull sperm head morphometry related to abnormal chromatin structure and fertility. Cytometry 1996; 24: 167

40. Lavitrano M, et al. Sperm cells as vectors for introducing foreign DNA into eggs; genetic transformation of mice. Cell 1989; 57: 717

41. Zoraqi G, Spadafora C. Integration of foreign DNA sequences into mouse sperm genome. DNA Cell Biol 1997; 16: 291

42. Wilmut I, et al. Viable off-spring derived from fetal and adult mammalian cells. Nature 1997; 385: 810

43. Ward WS, Coffey DS. Identification of a sperm nuclear annulus: a sperm DNA anchor. Biol Reprod 1989; 41: 361

44. Barone JG, et al. DNA organization in human spermatozoa. J Androl 1994; 15: 139

45. Zalensky AO, et al. Well-defined genome architecture in the human sperm nucleus. Chromosoma 1995; 103: 577

46. Ward WS, et al. Localization of the three genes in the assymetric hamster sperm nucleus by fluorescent in situ hybridization. Biol Reprod 1996; 54: 1271

47. Loir M, Courtens JL. Nuclear reorganization in ram spermatids. J Ultrastruct Res 1979; 67: 309

48. Tanphaichitr N, et al. Basic nuclear proteins in testicular cells and ejaculated spermatozoa in man. Exp Cell Res 1978; 117: 347

49. Choudhary SK, et al. A haploid expressed gene cluster exists as a single chromatin domain in human sperm. J Biol Chem 1995; 270: 8755

50. Vogelstein B, Pardoll DM, Coffey DS. Supercoiled loops and eucaryotic DNA replication. Cell 1980; 22: 79

51. Jackson DA, Dickinson P, Cook PR. The size of chromatin loops in HeLa cells. EMBO J 1990; 9: 567

52. Vaughn JP, et al. Replication forks are associated with the nuclear matrix. Nucleic Acids Res 1990; 18: 1965

53. Buongiorno-Nardelli M, et al. A relationship between size and supercoiled loop domains in the eukaryotic genome. Nature 1982; 298: 100

54. Robinson SI, Nelkin BD, Vogelstein B. The Ovalbumin gene is associated with the nuclear matrix of chicken oviduct cells. Cell 1982; 28: 99

55. Cockerill PN, Garrard WT. Chromosomal loop anchorage of the kappa immunoglobulin gene occurs next to the enhancer in a region containing topoisomerase II sites. Cell 1986; 44: 273

56. Gasser SM, Laemmli UK. Cohabitation of scaffold binding regions with upstream-enhancer elements of three developmentally regulated genes of D. melanogaster. Cell 1986; 46: 521

57. Mirkovitch J, Gasser SM, Laemmli UK. Relation of chromosome structure and gene expression. Philos Trans R Soc Lond Biol 1987; 317: 563

58. Gerdes MG, et al. Dynamic changes in the higher-level chromatin organization of specific sequences revealed by in situ hybridization to nuclear halos. J Cell Biol 1994; 126: 289

59. Nadel B, et al. Cell specific organization of the 5S rRNA gene cluster DNA loop domains in spermatozoa and somatic cells. Biol Reprod 1995; 53: 1222

60. Stewart TA, Bellvé AR, Leder P. Transcription and promoter usage of the myc gene in normal somatic and spermatogenic cells. Science 1984; 226: 707

61. Hud NV, Downing KH, Balhorn R. A constant radius of curvature model for the organization of DNA in toroidal condensates. Proc Natl Acad Sci USA 1995; 92: 3581

62. Ward WS. DNA loop domain tertiary structure in mammalian spermatozoa. Biol Reprod 1993; 48: 1193

63. Haaf T, Ward DC. Higher order nuclear structure in mammalian sperm revealed by in situ hybridization and extended chromatin fibers. Exp Cell Res 1995; 219: 604

64. Ward WS, et al. Localization of three genes in the hook-shaped hamster sperm nucleus by fluorescent in situ hybridisation. Biol Reprod 1996; 54: 1271

65. Ward WS, Zalensky A. The unique, complex organization of the transcriptionally silent sperm chromatin. Crit Rev Eukaryot Gene Expr 1996; 6: 139

66. Watson JM, Meyne J, Graves JA. Ordered tandem arrangement of chromosomes in the sperm heads of monotreme mammals. Proc Natl Acad Sci USA 1996; 93: 10200

67. Yovitch JL, Stanger JD. The limitations of in vitro fertilization from males with severe oligospermia and abnormal sperm morphology. J In Vitro Fert Embryo Transf 1984; 1: 172

68. Ron-El R, et al. Delayed fertilization and poor embryonic development associated with impaired semen quality. Fertil Steril 1991; 55: 338

69. Parinaud J, et al. Influence of sperm parameters on embryo quality. Fertil Steril 1993; 60: 888

70. Janny L, Ménézó YJR. Evidence for a strong paternal effect on human preimplantation embryo development and blastocyst formation. Mol Reprod Develop 1994; 38: 36

71. Schatten G. The centrosome and its mode of inheritance: the reduction of the centrosome during gametogenesis and its restoration during fertilization. Dev Biol 1994; 165: 299

72. Simerly C, et al. The paternal inheritance of the centrosome, the cell's microtubule-organizing center, in humans, and the implications for infertility. Nat Med 1995; 1: 47

73. Palermo G, Munné S, Cohen J. The human zygote inherits its mitotic potential from the male gamete. Hum Reprod 1994; 9: 1220

74. Asch R, et al. The stages at which human fertilization arrests: microtubule and chromosome configurations in inseminated oocytes which failed to complete fertilization and development in humans. Hum Reprod 1995; 10: 1897

75. Navara CS, et al. The implications of a paternally derived centrosome during human fertilization: consequences for reproduction and treatment of male factor infertility. Am J Reprod Immunol 1997; 37: 39

76. Navara CS, First N, Schatten G. Individual bulls affect sperm aster size and quality: relationship between the sperm centrosome and development. Mol Biol Cell 1993; 4: 828

77. Murray A. Creative blocks: cell cycle checkpoints and feed-back controls. Nature 1996; 359: 599

78. Dozortsev D, et al. Human oocyte activation following intracytoplasmic injection: the role of the sperm cell. Hum Reprod 1995; 10: 399

79. Swann K. The soluble sperm oscillogen hypothesis. Zygote 1993; 1: 273

80. Eid LN, Lorton SP, Parrish JJ. Paternal influence on S-phase in the first cell cycle of the bovine embryo. Biol Reprod 1994; 51: 1232

81. Sakkas D, et al. Sperm chromatin anomalies can influence decondensation after intracytoplasmic sperm injection. Hum Reprod 1996; 11: 837

82. Sakkas D, Batt PA, Cameron AWN. Development of pre-implantation goat (Capra hircus) embryos in vivo and in vitro. J Reprod Fertil 1989; 87: 359

83. Naz RK. Effect of antisperm antibodies on early cleavage of fertilized ova. Biol Reprod 1992; 46: 130

84. Van Landuyt L, et al. Blastocyst formation in in vitro fertilization versus intracytoplasmic sperm injection cycles: influence of the fertilization procedure. Fertil Steril 2005; 83: 1397

85. Kremer JAM, et al. Microdeletions of Y chromosome and intracytoplasmic sperm injection: from gene to clinic. Hum Reprod 1997; 12: 687

86. Bourrouillou G, Dastugue N, Colobies P. Chromosome studies in 952 infertile males with sperm count below 10 million/ml. Hum Genet 1985; 71: 366

87. Moosani N, et al. Chromosomal analysis of sperm from men with idiopathic infertility using sperm karyotyping and fluoresence in situ hybridisation. Fertil Steril 1995; 64: 811

88. Jurisicova A, et al. Embryonic human leukocyte antigen-G expression: possible implications for human preimplantation development. Fertil Steril 1996; 65: 997

89. Simerly C, et al. The inheritance, molecular dissection and reconstitution of the human centrosome during fertilization: consequences for infertility. In Barratt C, De Jonge C, Mortimer D, Parinaud J, eds. Genetics of Human Male Fertility. Paris: EDK Press, 1997: 258

90. Ji BT, et al. Paternal cigarette smoking and the risk of childhood cancer among offspring of nonsmoking mothers. J Natl Cancer Inst 1997; 89: 238

91. Aitken RJ, et al. Relative impact of oxidative stress on the functional competence and genomic integrity of human spermatozoa. Biol Reprod 1998; 59: 1037

92. Aitken RJ, Krausz C. Oxidative stress, DNA damage and the Y chromosome. Reproduction 2001; 122: 497

93. McElreavey K, Quintana-Murci L. Male reproductive function and the human Y chromosome: is selection acting on the Y? Reprod Biomed Online 2003; 7: 17

94. Henkel R, et al. Effect of reactive oxygen species produced by spermatozoa and leukocytes on sperm functions in non-leukocytospermic patients. Fertil Steril 2005; 83: 635

95. Surani MAH, Barton SC, Norris ML. Experimental reconstruction of mouse eggs and embryos: an analysis of mammalian development. Biol Reprod 1987; 36: 1

96. De Groot N, Hochberg A. Gene imprinting during placental and embryonic development. Mol Reprod Dev 1993; 36: 390

97. Goshen R, et al. The role of genomic imprinting in implantation. Fertil Steril 1994; 62: 903

98. Chandley AC, et al. Deleted Yq in the sterile son of a man with a sattelite Y chromosome (Yqs). J Med Genet 1989; 26: 145

99. Kent-First MG, et al. Infertility in intracytoplasmic-sperm-injection-derived sons. Lancet 1996; 348: 332

100. Reijo R, et al. Diverse spermatogenic defects in humans caused by Y chromosome deletions encompassing a novel RNA-binding protein gene. Nat Genet 1995; 10: 383

101. Najmabadi H, et al. Substantial prevalence of microdeletions of the Y chromosome in infertile men with idiopathic azoospermia and oligozoospermia detected using a sequence-tagged site-based mapping strategy. J Clin Endocrinol Metab 1996; 81: 1347

102. Reijo R, et al. Severe oligozoospermia resulting from deletions of azoospermia factor gene on Y chromosome. Lancet 1996; 347: 1290

103. Pryor JL, et al. Microdeletions in the Y chromosome of infertile men. N Engl J Med 1997; 336: 534

4

Contribution of the male gamete to fertilization and embryogenesis

Gerardo Barroso, Sergio Oehninger

INTRODUCTION

The normal progression of fertilization of mammalian oocytes followed by cleavage, blastocyst formation and implantation is dependent upon the successful activation of specific genetic and developmental programs. Successful interaction of the paternal and maternal gametes is required for normal embryonic development. The oocyte controls several important aspects of meiosis, fertilization and early cleavage, and modulates the epigenetic development of the embryonic genome that manifests later in embryogenesis[1].

The contributing role of the spermatozoon has remained largely ignored. However, a large body of evidence is accumulating demonstrating that (1) the fertilizing spermatozoon plays a significant part in bringing about the development of the zygote, with its contributions being well beyond the delivery of the paternal DNA; and (2) infertile men with or without altered 'classic' semen parameters may have associated sperm dysfunction(s) at different levels, including nuclear[2], organelle-cytoplasmic[3] and cytoskeletal systems[4], that can result in aberrant embryogenesis.

The mechanism(s) underlying these phenomena is/are not completely understood. This review focuses on examination of the paternal effects that become manifest before and after the major activation of embryonic gene expression.

BIOLOGY OF FERTILIZATION

Sperm–oocyte fusion

The sperm equatorial region plays a pivotal role in gamete fusion. The inner and outer acrosomal membranes and the plasma membrane of the equatorial region remain intact after completion of the acrosome reaction and zona penetration[5]. Electron microscopic studies have shown convincingly that sperm–oocyte membrane fusion takes place at the sperm equatorial region, whereas the posterior acrosome itself is engulfed by the oocyte microvilli in a phagocytic manner.

Acrosome-reacted sperm bind to and fuse with eggs by using the plasma membrane at the postacrosomal region of the sperm; this region is capable of fusion only after acrosomal exocytosis has taken place[6]. Binding of the sperm to the egg plasma membrane appears to be mediated by a member of the ADAM (a disintegrin and metalloprotease) family of transmembrane proteins on the sperm and integrin $\alpha6\beta1$ receptors on the egg[7]. Fertilin is a heterodimeric ADAM glycoprotein that was first identified in the guinea-pig using monoclonal antibodies to sperm surface antigens that could inhibit sperm–egg fusion[8]. The protein is composed of an α and a β subunit with similar domain structures[9,10], and is proteolytically processed during sperm development by removal of the prodomain and metalloprotease domain. Processing of fertilin is crucial for exposing the disintegrin domain that mediates sperm–egg binding, and for allowing proper localization of fertilin in the head of the mature sperm[11,12]. More recently, a member of the immunoglobulin superfamily (the membrane protein Izumo) has been found to be critically involved in murine sperm–oocyte fusion[13].

Equatorin is a sperm-head equatorial protein, the antigenic molecule of the monoclonal antibody mMN9[14]. In mice, after sperm–egg fusion, equatorin dissociates from the sperm-head equatorial region and remains at the vicinity of the decondensing male pronucleus. The equatorial segment containing equatorin is maintained away from the nuclei, possibly due to chromatin swelling and nuclear membrane reconstruction. It remains at the vicinity of the sperm head for a considerable length of time during the first cell cycle, and, after that, it is inherited by one of the proembryonic cells. After intracytoplasmic sperm injection (ICSI), the equatorial segment is directly exposed to the oocyte cytoplasm without prior interaction with the cortical membrane system, but displays similar cellular events of equatorin degeneration to the oocyte after *in vitro* fertilization (IVF). These observations argue in favor of membrane interaction not being a prerequisite for shedding the equatorial posterior acrosome, equatorin, and their subsequent disintegration after ICSI[15].

The persistence of equatorin through early-proembryonic cleavage is comparable with that of sperm-tail microtubules and the midpiece mitochondrial sheath. The residual tail microtubules are retained up to the 8-cell or blastocyst stage. However, the residual equatorin seems to degenerate a little early, before the 4-cell stage[15].

Oocyte activation

The oocyte and spermatozoon are metabolically quiescent; sperm–oocyte binding and fusion initiate a cascade of events that transform the dormant oocyte into the dynamic, animated zygote. These processes include metabolic oocyte activation and resumption of meiosis. Although there are still diverse opinions as to the precise manner in which the spermatozoon activates this cascade, it is clear in all fertilization systems that an elevation of intracellular calcium ion concentration is the central messenger in communicating the activating signal.

The signaling mechanism(s) utilized by the spermatozoon to initiate and perpetuate these responses is unclear. Two theories have been proposed: the fusion and the receptor theories (reviewed in reference 16). The fusion theory suggests the presence of active calcium-releasing components in the sperm head. It has experimental support in that injections of sperm-derived cytosolic fractions elicit calcium oscillations, and also in that ICSI results in activation without sperm interaction with the membrane.

It was recently reported that a cytosolic sperm factor containing a 33-kDa protein called oscillin, which is related to a prokaryote glucosamine phosphate deaminase, appeared to be responsible for causing the calcium oscillations that trigger egg activation at fertilization in mammals[17]. Oscillin is located in the equatorial segment of the spermatozoon, the region where the spermatozoon is fused with the oocyte in mammals. However, multiple pieces of experimental evidence have now shown that oscillin is not the mammalian sperm calcium oscillogen (reviewed in reference 16).

In eggs of all animal species, sperm-triggered inositol (1,4,5)-triphosphate (IP3) production regulates the vast array of calcium wave-patterns observed. Present evidence supports the concept that an IP3 receptor system is the main mediator of calcium oscillations in oocytes (reviewed in reference 16). The spatial organization of calcium waves is driven either by intracellular distribution of the calcium-release machinery or by localized and dynamic production of calcium-releasing second messengers.

In the highly polarized egg cell, cortical endoplasmic reticulum-rich clusters act as pacemaker sites dedicated to the initiation of global calcium waves. The polarized nature of the calcium signals may in itself influence embryonic patterning by regulating early embryonic cleavage. Finding out whether calcium wave-patterns play a role in later development will require studies that interfere with the normal spatial–temporal pattern of calcium waves without perturbing mitosis and cleavage. The rather simple ascidian embryo, which displays two different meiotic calcium-wave pacemakers and develops into a swimming tadpole within a day, is particularly suited to studies of the relationship between meiotic calcium waves and development[18]. It should be possible in the future to relate patterns of calcium waves and phenotypic differences in embryos.

In recent years, mitochondria have been shown to be major regulators of intracellular calcium homeostasis[19,20]. In cells such as sea urchin[21] and ascidian eggs[22], mitochondria sequester calcium during the fertilization calcium transients. Calcium sequestration by mitochondria has two main consequences. First, mitochondria act as passive calcium buffers that can regulate intracellular calcium release[19,20]. The second consequence is that calcium in the mitochondrial matrix is a 'multisite' activator of oxidative phosphorylation (or mitochondrial adenosine triphosphate (ATP) synthesis); it activates the dehydrogenases of the Krebs cycle and the electron transport chain[23,24] and has a direct action on the F_0/F_1 ATP synthase[25].

In somatic cells and in ascidian eggs, mitochondrial calcium uptake has been shown to stimulate mitochondrial respiration by promoting the reduction of mitochondrial nicotinamide–adenine dinucleotide (NAD^+) to NADH[22,26–28]. Furthermore, mitochondrial ATP production may directly regulate intracellular calcium release: ATP sensitizes the IP3 receptor to activation by calcium[29,30], while magnesium-complexed ATP is consumed to refill the endoplasmic reticulum calcium stores. The tight coupling of ATP supply and demand therefore provides a major advantage for early mammalian development. The maternal inheritance of mitochondria requires that mitochondria be protected from potentially damaging reactive oxygen species (ROS).

The maintenance of a low level of oxidative phosphorylation that can be stimulated upon increased ATP demand provides a means of lowering the exposure of mitochondria to damaging oxidative stress. Data suggest that calcium is the functional link that provides a mechanism for coupling ATP supply and demand. As maternal aging is associated with increased oxidative stress in human eggs[31], it will be interesting to define whether mitochondrial physiology and the coupling of ATP supply and demand are impaired in eggs from aged women.

It has recently been shown that the soluble sperm factor that triggers calcium oscillations and egg activation (oocyte activating factor, OAF) in mammals is a novel form of phospholipase C (PLC) referred to as PLCζ[32]. This has been demonstrated by injection into eggs of both cRNA encoding PLCζ and a recombinant PLCζ[32,33]. According to a present hypothesis, after fusion of the sperm and egg plasma membrane, the sperm-derived PLCζ protein (possibly a sperm cytosolic factor) diffuses into the egg cytoplasm. This results in hydrolysis of phosphatidylinositol-4,5-bisphosphate (PIP2) from an unknown source to generate IP3 (reviewed in reference 34).

The earliest indicators of the transition to embryos in mammalian eggs, or egg activation, are cortical granule extrusion by exocytosis (CGE) and resumption of meiosis. Although these events are triggered by calcium oscillations as described above, the pathways within the egg leading to intracellular calcium release and to downstream cellular events are not completely understood. The calcium transients actuate resumption of the cell cycle by decreasing the activity of both the M phase-promoting factor and the cytostatic factor (reviewed in reference 35). The calcium transients and/or activation of PLCζ lead to CGE by an, as yet, undefined mechanism[36].

Src family kinases (SFKs) have been suggested as possible inducers of some aspects of egg activation (reviewed in reference 37). A present model claims that sperm fusion with the egg membrane results in hydrolysis of PIP2 to form IP3 and diacylglycerol (DAG). IP3 triggers calcium release from the endoplasmic reticulum via the IP3 receptor while DAG activates protein kinase C (PKC). Both an intracellular calcium rise and DAG contribute to egg activation, CGE and resumption of meiosis. The existence of SFK activity is associated with the resumption of meiosis in response to the fertilization signal, whereas the occurrence of CGE is independent of SFK activity. Also, a role for SFKs upstream of calcium release remains plausible (reviewed in reference 37).

Sperm mitochondrial DNA and its role during fertilization

Mitochondria have a profound role to play in mammalian-tissue bioenergetics during the processes of growth, aging and apoptosis, and yet they descend from an asexually reproducing independent life form. Most cells in the body contain between 103 and 104 copies of mitochondrial (mt)DNA. There are slightly higher copy numbers (about 105) in mature oocytes. This may be in preparation for the energetic demands of embryogenesis[38], but an alternative explanation is that replication does not occur during early embryogenesis and that high copy numbers are needed to give a sufficient reservoir. The DNA exists mainly as a circular molecule of approximately 16.6 kb, encoding 13 proteins that are transcribed and translated in the mitochondrion. These are essential subunits of the electron transport complexes on the inner mitochondrial membrane. The mitochondrial genome also encodes the RNA molecules that are necessary for translation of these proteins[39,40].

Spermatozoa are metabolically flexible and, in some species, can switch between aerobic and anaerobic metabolism. This perhaps reflects the great range of oxygen tensions that they experience, from near anoxia in the testis and epididymis to ambient tensions in the vagina and in vitro[3,41,42]. Like somatic mtDNA, that of

spermatozoa is highly vulnerable to mutation, and a significant number of mtDNA deletions are found in the semen of at least 50% of normospermic men[43].

Given the lengthy process of spermiogenesis and epididymal maturation, during which the sperm mitochondria have to survive the likelihood that they will be exposed to mutagenic agents, this is perhaps not surprising. Indeed, the need to exclude defective sperm mtDNA from contributing to the embryo is possibly one of the major selection pressures against survival of paternal mtDNA. Indeed, Short[44] has suggested that this asymmetric inheritance of mtDNA, through the oocyte but not the spermatozoon, may be the fundamental driving force behind amphimixis and anisogamy. This is because of the need to conserve a healthy stock of mtDNA for embryo development through a long period of quiescence in meiosis[43].

It is well established that the mitochondria from spermatozoa are targeted for destruction by endogenous proteolytic activity during early embryogenesis. Uniparental (generally maternal) inheritance of cytoplasmic organelles such as mitochondria is accomplished by a wide variety of strategies, and thus is clearly of profound importance to long-term fitness. Most evidence indicating the possibility of paternal transmission of mtDNA derives from interspecific crosses, which by definition are uncommon in nature[45]. In a previous study, Kaneda et al.[45] proposed that the zygote cytoplasm has a species-specific mechanism that recognizes and eliminates sperm mitochondria, on the basis of nuclear DNA-encoded proteins in the sperm midpiece, and neither on the mtDNA itself, nor on the proteins it encodes.

The ubiquitination–proteasome pathway

The fate of various accessory structures of the penetrating spermatozoon came under scrutiny recently, as it became obvious that in addition to the sperm-borne chromosomes, other structures of the fertilizing spermatozoon make important contributions to the mammalian zygote. Yet other sperm accessory structures are degraded in an orderly fashion so as to not interfere with normal embryo development. These include the sperm proximal centriole, perinuclear theca, sperm mitochondria and axonemal fibrous sheath and outer dense fibers.

In most mammals, except rodents, the spermatozoon contains a reduced, inactive form of the centrosome, within which one of the two centrioles as well as the entourage of pericentriolar material are degraded during the final stages of spermiogenesis. Such an incomplete centrosome, consisting of a proximal centriole embedded in the dense mass of sperm-tail capitulum, must be released into the oocyte cytoplasm at fertilization in order to attract microtubule-nucleating pericentriolar proteins from the surrounding oocyte cytoplasm. Failure to convert the reduced sperm centriole into such an active zygotic centrosome may be a reason for postfertilization developmental arrests affecting couples treated at IVF clinics.

The strictly maternal inheritance of mtDNA in mammals is a developmental paradox, because the fertilizing spermatozoon introduces up to 100 functional mitochondria into the oocyte cytoplasm at fertilization. However, the mandatory destruction of sperm mitochondria appears to be an evolutionary and developmental advantage[46], because the paternal mitochondria and their DNA may be compromised by the deleterious action of reactive oxygen species encountered by the sperm during spermatogenesis, storage, migration and fertilization[47].

Although a number of studies have supported the notion that sperm mitochondria are actively destroyed by the egg, the actual mechanism of this process is not known[48–50]. Earlier claims that the sperm mitochondria disperse evenly throughout embryonic cytoplasm[51] and the misconception about sperm mitochondria not entering the egg were overturned by new research. The dilution of paternal mtDNA in the maternal cytoplasm genome[52] and the oxidative damage of sperm mitochondria during fertilization[53] were also implicated in this process, but were not adequately supported by experimental data.

Ubiquitination of the sperm mitochondria during spermatogenesis has been implicated in the targeted degradation of paternal mitochondria after fertilization, a mechanism proposed to promote the predominantly maternal inheritance of mitochondria DNA in humans. Recent studies[54,55] have shown that some unknown proteins in mammalian sperm mitochondria are tagged with a proteolytic peptide, ubiquitin, which may target sperm mitochondria for destruction in the egg cytoplasm after fertilization. Both lysosomal and proteasomal proteolysis have been implicated in such targeted degradation of sperm mitochondria inside the fertilized oocyte[55].

This mechanism seems to be feasible for the selective degradation of paternal mitochondria at fertilization, sometimes described as the 'ultimate war of the sexes', and is consistent with the prevailing view that the inheritance of mtDNA in mammals is predominantly maternal[56]. Such a scenario is also supported by studies of mitochondrial inheritance in inter- and intraspecies murine crosses as well as in their back-crossed progeny, in which the mitochondrial membrane proteins, rather than mtDNA, seemed to determine whether the sperm mitochondria and mtDNA were passed on or degraded[45].

Ubiquitination is the major means in eukaryotic cells for targeted protein proteolysis. By the covalent addition of polyubiquitin to specific proteins, the ubiquitination system regulates protein levels and thereby influences diverse cellular processes. There are three well-established types of enzymes involved in ubiquitination, termed E1, E2 and E3. E1 is the ubiquitin-activating enzyme, which forms a thiol-ester linkage with ubiquitin through its active site cysteine. Ubiquitin is subsequently transferred to an E2 ubiquitin-conjugating enzyme; the E3 enzyme is the ubiquitin protein ligase, which transfers ubiquitin from the E2 enzyme to lysines of a specific protein, targeting the protein for degradation by the proteasome.

More recently, E4 enzymes have been described that appear to function in ubiquitin chain polymerization.

Pronuclear formation and nuclear fusion

The fertilizing spermatozoon is essential for contributing three critical components: (1) the paternal haploid genome, (2) the signal to initiate the metabolic–maturational activation of the oocyte and (3) the centrosome, which directs microtubule assembly within the penetrated oocyte leading to oocyte–sperm activation as well as formation of the mitotic spindles during initial zygote development (Figure 4.1). Fertilization is completed once the parental genomes unite (syngamy), and requires migration of the egg nucleus to the sperm nucleus (female and male pronuclei) on microtubules within the penetrated oocyte.

The male pronucleus is tightly associated with the centrosome, which nucleates microtubules to form the sperm aster. The growth of the sperm aster drives the centrosome and associated male pronucleus from the cell cortex towards the center of the oocyte. In contrast to the male pronucleus, the female pronucleus has neither an associated centrosome nor microtubule-nucleating activity. Nevertheless, the female pronucleus moves along microtubules from the cell cortex towards the centrosome located in the center of the sperm aster. The current model for movement of the female pronucleus involves its translocation along the microtubule lattice using the minus-end-directed motor dynein[53,57,58], in a manner analogous to organelle motility.

Mammalian fertilization requires dynein and dynactin to mediate genomic union, and that dynein concentrates exclusively around the female pronucleus. Dynactin, by contrast, localizes around both pronuclei and associates with nucleoporins and vimentin in addition to dynein. The findings that a sperm aster is required for dynein to localize to the female pronucleus and the microtubules are necessary to retain dynein,

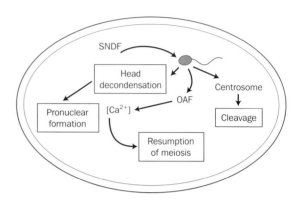

Figure 4.1   Critical sperm components during fertilization. OAF, oocyte activating factor; SNDF, sperm nuclear decondensing factor

but not dynactin, at its surface, suggest that nucleoporins, vimentin and dynactin might associate upon pronuclear formation, and that subsequent sperm aster contact with the female pronuclear surface allows dynein to interact with these proteins[59].

EVIDENCE FOR PATERNAL CONTRIBUTIONS TO ABNORMAL EMBRYOGENESIS

Clinical evidence: lessons from the IVF/ICSI setting

Several lines of clinical evidence resulting from the use of assisted reproductive technologies have provided additional support for the concept of paternal contribution to faulty fertilization and abnormal embryogenesis:

• Abnormal sperm parameters, particularly teratozoospermia ('poor prognosis pattern' as defined by strict criteria), are associated with fertilization disorders in IVF, including failure (partial or complete) and delayed fertilization[60,61].

- Results of standard (conventional) IVF in men with severe teratozoospermia and other seminal abnormalities showed not only decreased fertilization but also lower implantation rates compared with normozoospermic samples[62–65].

- The application of corrective measures in conventional IVF (such as increasing sperm insemination concentration) resulted in an enhanced fertilization rate but implantation rates remained lower than anticipated[66].

- Poor sperm quality was associated with a decreased ability to reach the blastocyst stage *in vitro*[67].

- A comparative analysis of embryo implantation potential in patients with severe teratozoospermia undergoing IVF with a high insemination concentration or ICSI revealed that ICSI produced a significant proportion of embryos with superior morphology and implantation competence[68].

- Although multiple studies have shown that the outcome of clinical pregnancies following ICSI is not affected by semen quality[69–72], patients with total teratozoospermia demonstrated a very low implantation rate[73].

- Spermatozoa of infertile men have also been shown to contain various nuclear alterations. They include an abnormal chromatin structure, aneuploidy, chromosomal microdeletions and DNA strand breaks[74–81].

Different theories have been proposed to explain the origin of DNA damage in spermatozoa (reviewed in references 2, 80 and 82). Damage could occur at the time of, or be the result of, DNA packing during the transition of histone to the protamine complex during spermiogenesis. DNA fragmentation could also be the consequence of direct oxidative damage (free radical-induced DNA damage has been associated with antioxidant depletion, smoking, xenobiotics, heat exposure, leukocyte contamination of semen and the presence of ions in sperm culture media).

Alternatively, DNA damage could be the consequence of apoptosis.

- Numerous studies have demonstrated associations between poor sperm quality and increased sperm aneuploidy, DNA damage, fragmentation and instability and single-stranded DNA, with poor pregnancy potential documented in such cases undergoing intrauterine insemination (IUI) or ICSI therapies[83–89].

- Although the major congenital malformation rate and developmental potential of children conceived after IVF or ICSI and naturally are similar, ICSI is associated with a slight increase in *de novo* chromosomal abnormalities. Moreover, recent publications mention that diseases caused by imprinting disorders affect a few ICSI children, and sperm from men with severely impaired semen quality may carry microdeletions of the Y chromosome and other genetic disorders (reviewed in references 90 and 91). Consequently, spermatozoa from infertile men may carry chromosomal and/or genetic abnormalities that can be potentially transmitted to the offspring[92].

In addition, findings in animals and in the human have provided evidence of paternal transmission of genetic damage, including data on paternally mediated behavioral effects, male-mediated teratogenicity and tumor induction and susceptibility in the offspring. The available evidence indicates that preconception paternal exposure to certain mutagens can, under certain conditions, have adverse effects on the offspring. Two principal mechanisms proposed are the induction of germ-line genomic instability or the suppression of germ cell apoptosis (reviewed in reference 93).

It is well established that the presence of sperm abnormalities can lead to failure of fertilization. A high proportion of infertile men possess sperm functional deficiencies that result in poor interaction with the zona pellucida, including a diminished capacity to achieve tight binding and/or to undergo acrosomal exocytosis. Moreover, a deficient interaction with the oolema can lead to binding or fusion abnormalities[94–97]. Obviously, failure of the spermatozoon to penetrate the oocyte's investments or to arrive at the cytoplasm negates fertilization and embryogenesis.

Other sperm abnormalities have been associated with failed fertilization and aberrant or arrested embryo development. Such instances include delayed fertilization, abnormal oocyte activation, deficient sperm-head decondensation, defective pronuclear formation and poor embryo cleavage (reviewed in references 96, 98 and 99). Once the spermatozoon penetrates the oocyte, several events must take place to ensure fertilization, including incorporation of the entire spermatozoon into the oocyte, completion of oocyte meiotic maturation with extrusion of the second polar body, metabolic activation of the previously quiescent oocyte, decondensation of the sperm nucleus and the maternal chromosomes into the male and female pronuclei, respectively, and cytoplasmic migrations of the pronuclei, which bring them into apposition. Defects in any of these events can be lethal to the zygote and can be causes of infertility.

As mentioned earlier, it is generally accepted that the contributions of the fertilizing spermatozoon to the oocyte include delivery of the DNA/chromatin, a putative oocyte-activating factor (OAF) and a centriole. The DNA/chromatin complex is obviously the most significant contribution to originating a new diploid individual. Nevertheless, the OAF and centriole play a critical part in bringing about oocyte activation, cortical granule extrusion and the first mitotic division, and without these contributions embryogenesis would also be neglected or proceed abnormally.

The fate of sperm components in primate models (human and subhuman) during fertilization is being unraveled. The centrosome, introduced by the sperm at fertilization, organizes a microtubule array that is responsible for bringing the parental genomes together at first mitosis. Structural a*bnormalities* or *incomplete functioning*

of the centrosome have been identified as a novel form of infertility[100]. Moreover, the paternal sperm-borne mitochondria also enter the cytoplasm and are specifically targeted for degradation by the resident oocyte ubiquitin system[101]. This phenomenon allows for maternal inheritance of mitochondrial DNA. *Defects of paternal mitochondrial degradation* could result in heteroplasmy.

New evidence has challenged the traditional view of the transcriptional dormancy of terminally differentiated spermatozoa. Several reports have indicated the presence of mRNAs in ejaculated human spermatozoa (reviewed in reference 102). It has been hypothesized that these templates could be critically involved in late spermiogenesis, including a function to equilibrate imbalances in spermatozoal phenotypes brought about by meiotic recombination and segregation, and furthermore, that they could also be involved in early postfertilization events such as establishing imprints during the transition from maternal to embryonic genes.

Cell divisions in the human embryo can be compromised by deficiencies in the sperm nuclear genome or sperm-derived cytoplasmic factors, including the OAF and centriole. The newly formed zygote undergoes early cleavage divisions depending upon the oocyte's endogenous machinery, and at the 4–8-cell stage initiates transcription of the embryonic genome[103]. Consequently, sperm nuclear deficiencies are usually not dctcctcd before the 8-cell stage, when a major expression of sperm-derived genes has begun. On the other hand, sperm cytoplasm deficiencies can be detected as early as the 1-cell zygote and then throughout the preimplantation development[104,105].

The terms 'late' and 'early' paternal effect have been suggested to denote these two pathological conditions[106]. The diagnosis of an *early paternal effect* is based upon poor zygote and early embryo morphology and low cleavage speed, and is not associated with sperm DNA fragmentation. The *late paternal effect*, on the other hand, is manifested by poor developmental competence leading to failure of implantation, and is associated with an increased incidence of sperm DNA fragmentation in the absence of zygote and early cleavage-stage morphological abnormalities. It has been suggested that ICSI with testicular sperm can be an efficient treatment for the late paternal effect[107].

It can be speculated that the *early paternal effect* probably includes dysfunctions related to oocyte activation and the centrosome and cytoskeletal apparatus, as well as possible abnormal mRNA delivery. Conversely, the *late paternal effect* is associated with dysfunctions/abnormalities of the DNA/chromatin (including sperm chromosomal–genetic aberrations, retention of histones and/or DNA damage), and perhaps mitochondrial dysfunctions. Alterations due to genomic imprinting anomalies probably result in both early and late paternal effects.

Disorders of oocyte activation, centrosome and cytoskeletal apparatus dysfunction and mitochondria elimination

PLCζ offers the molecular basis for an explanation of how calcium release is triggered during mammalian fertilization. There are clinical situations that can be explained by the absence or dysfunction of the OAF. For example, it has been suggested that up to 40% of failed fertilization cases after ICSI could be due to *failure of the egg to activate*[99]. In these cases the sperm is within the cytoplasm, but a stimulus for activation is apparently missing. Certainly, there may be cases where the spermatozoon provides the OAF, but any of the multiple elements of the oocyte-responsive system (SFKs, PIP2, IP3 receptor or PKC) is aberrant, resulting in failure to resume meiosis or to undergo CGE.

During fertilization the zygotic centrosome organizes a large sperm aster critical for uniting the pronuclei before the first mitosis. Dysfunctional microtubule organization in failed

fertilization during human IVF suggests that *centrosomal dysfunction* might be a cause of fertilization arrest. In a study by Asch et al.[98] microtubules and DNA were imaged in inseminated human oocytes that had been discarded as unfertilized. The presence and number of incorporated sperm tails were also documented using a monoclonal antibody specific for the post-translationally modified, acetylated α-tubulin found in the tail, but not oocyte, microtubules. Results showed that fertilization arrested at various levels: (1) metaphase II arrest; (2) arrest after successful incorporation of the spermatozoon; (3) arrest after formation of the sperm aster; (4) arrest during mitotic cell cycle progression; and (5) arrest during meiotic cell cycle progression.

Rawe et al.[99] analyzed the distribution of β-tubulins to detect spindle and cytoplasmic microtubules, α-acetylated tubulins for sperm microtubules and chromatin configuration in oocytes showing fertilization failure after conventional IVF or ICSI. Immunofluorescence analysis showed that the main reason for fertilization failure after IVF was no sperm penetration (55.5%). The remaining oocytes showed different abnormal patterns, e.g. oocyte activation failure (15.1%) and defects in pronuclei apposition (19.2%). On the other hand, fertilization failure after ICSI was mainly associated with incomplete oocyte activation (39.9%), and to a lesser extent with defects in pronuclei apposition (22.6%) and failure of sperm penetration (13.3%). A further 13.3% of the ICSI oocytes arrested their development at the metaphase of the first mitotic division.

Fluorescent imaging scanning has shown that centrosomal defects may result in abnormal microtubule nucleation, preventing genomic union. In a primate model, ICSI (using apparently normal gametes) resulted in abnormal nuclear remodeling during sperm decondensation due to the presence of the sperm acrosome and perinuclear theca, structures normally removed at the oolema during IVF; this in turn caused a delay of DNA synthesis[108]. Such unusual modifications raised concerns about the 'normalcy' of the fertilization process and cell-cycle checkpoints during ICSI (reviewed in references 108 and 109).

During the ICSI procedure, a spermatozoon is deposited into the ooplasm with both the acrosomal and plasma membranes intact, in addition to the other sperm components that are naturally eliminated in fertilized oocytes. The sperm acrosome contains a variety of hydrolytic enzymes, the release of which into the ooplasm might be harmful[110]. It is unclear how an oocyte that has been injected with an acrosome-intact spermatozoon will cope with the sperm acrosome. It is believed that an acrosome introduced into the ooplasm by ICSI seems physically to disturb sperm chromatin decondensation. Synthesis of DNA is delayed in both pronuclei when the paternal pronucleus is still undergoing decondensation in the apical region under the acrosomal cap, identifying a unique G_1/S cell-cycle checkpoint[111]. Katayama et al.[112] showed morphological characteristics in detail of the acrosome of boar sperm through ICSI, showing that the lectin-binding properties of sperm-head components introduced into the cytoplasm were different from those after IVF. Resumption of meiosis and cortical-granules exocytosis were achieved after micromanipulation techniques.

Terada et al.[113] assessed centrosomal function of human sperm using heterologous ICSI with rabbit eggs. They demonstrated that the sperm-aster formation rate was lower in infertile men compared with controls. Moreover, the sperm-aster formation rate correlated with the embryonic cleavage rate following human IVF. The data suggested that reproductive success during the first cell cycle requires a functional sperm centrosome and that dysfunctions of this organelle could be present in cases of unexplained infertility.

Kovacic and Vlaisavljevic[114] studied the microtubules and chromosomes of human oocytes failing to fertilize after ICSI, to establish how sperm chromatin and sperm-astral microtubule configuration is related to the phases of the oocyte cell cycle, and to find the defects in these structures causing fertilization arrest. A high proportion of

oocytes were arrested at metaphase II. Damage of the second meiotic spindle was noted in some oocytes. Intact sperm were found in some cases, and a swollen sperm head and prematurely condensed sperm chromosomes were apparent in others. Many monopronucleate oocytes contained sperm, with delay in the process of sperm nucleus decondensation. It was concluded that sperm that do not activate the oocyte may continue decondensing the chromatin, but the oocyte prevents male pronucleus formation before the female one, mostly by causing premature chromatin condensation in the sperm and by duplicating the sperm centrosome.

The functional role of the sperm tail (either attached or dissected) in early human embryonic growth is not known. In microinjection experiments, it was demonstrated that the injection of isolated sperm segments (heads or flagella) could permit oocyte activation and bipronuclear formation. However, a high rate of mosaicism was observed in the embryos with disrupted sperm, suggesting that the structural integrity of the intact fertilizing spermatozoon appears to contribute to normal human embryogenesis[115]. In addition, oocytes injected with mechanically dissected spermatozoa, although capable of pronuclear formation, did not undergo normal mitotic division. The lack of a bipolar spindle, in combination with mosaicism, suggested abnormalities of the mitotic apparatus when sperm integrity is impaired following dissection[116].

Fertilization is completed once the parental genomes unite, and requires migration of the egg nucleus to the sperm nucleus (female and male pronuclei, respectively) on microtubules within the inseminated egg. The failure of zygotic development in some patients suggests that abnormalities of this step may contribute to infertility. Recently, Payne et al.[59] showed that preferentially localized dynein and perinuclear dynactin associate with the nuclear pore complex and vimentin, and are required to mediate genomic union. The data suggest a model in which dynein accumulates and binds to the female pronucleus on sperm-aster microtubules, where it acts with dynactin, nucleoporins and vimentin.

Mutations in the human gene ubiquitin-specific protease-9 Y chromosome (USP9Y), which encodes a protein with a C-terminal ubiquitin hydrolase domain, result in azoospermia and male infertility[117]. Knock-out mice lacking the E3 ubiquitin protein ligase SIAH1A or the E2 ubiquitin-conjugating enzyme HR6B demonstrated defects in meiosis, postmeiotic germ cell development and male infertility[118]. Ubiquitin-mediated proteolysis is also critical for other aspects of reproduction, including the elimination of defective sperm in the epididymis, clearance of paternal mitochondria and progression of embryonic development in mammals[119].

Sutovsky et al.[101] showed that increased sperm ubiquitin (measured through a flow cytometric sperm–ubiquitin tag immunoassay) was inversely correlated with sperm quality. Conversely, Muratori et al.[120] observed a positive correlation between sperm ubiquitination and sperm quality. More studies are therefore needed to establish whether sperm ubiquitination can be used as a biomarker of sperm functional capacity and whether anomalies of fertilization result from anomalies of ubiquitin sperm marking.

Ubiquitin-mediated degradation targets cell-cycle regulators for proteolysis. Cullins are core components of E3 ubiquitin ligases, and CUL-4A has a possible role in cell cycle control. In experiments with CUL-4A deletion mutations in mice, it was observed that homozygous mutants generated no viable pups or recovery of homozygous embryos after 7.5 days postcoitum[119]. Results indicated that appropriate CUL-4A expression appears to be critical for early embryonic development.

The true identity of ubiquitinated substrates in the sperm mitochondria is not known. Nevertheless, it was recently shown that prohibitin, a mitochondrial membrane protein, is one of the ubiquitinated substrates that makes the sperm mitochondria responsible for the egg's ubiquitin–proteasome-dependent proteolytic machinery after fertilization[121]. Abnormalities of this recognition system might be involved in the dysregulation of mitochondrial inheritance and sperm quality control.

Occasional occurrence of paternal inheritance of mtDNA has been suggested in mammals, including humans. While most such evidence has been widely disputed, of particular concern is the documented heteroplasmic or mixed mtDNA inheritance after ooplasmic transfusion[122]. Indeed, there is evidence that heteroplasmy is a direct consequence of ooplasm transfer, a technique that was used to 'rescue' oocytes from older women by injecting ooplasm from young oocytes. ICSI has an inherent potential for delaying the degradation of sperm mitochondria. However, paternal mtDNA inheritance after ICSI has not been documented (reviewed in reference 101).

Putative dysfunctions resulting from aberrant delivery of mRNA

Recently, mRNA has been discovered in human ejaculated sperm. A non-exhaustive list of transcripts, including c-myc, human leukocyte antigen (HLA) class 1, protamines 1 and 2, heat shock proteins 70 and 90, β-integrins, transition protein-1, β-actin, variants of phosphodiesterase, progesterone receptor and aromatase, reveals a wide range of transcripts in mammalian sperm[123–126].

In mammals, round spermatids contain a number of transcripts that are produced either throughout early spermatogenesis[127] or during spermiogenesis from the haploid gene encoding sperm-specific proteins such as transition proteins and protamines[128], or sperm-tail cytoskeletal proteins implied in the molecular make-up of the outer dense fibers[129] and fibrous sheath[130]. The arrest of transcription that is concomitant with major changes in chromatin organization occurs during mid-spermiogenesis[131]. However, the presence of extremely varied transcripts in mature sperm cells has been described in both rodent[132,133] and human spermatozoa[134–138].

Most investigations into RNA identification in mature spermatozoa have been performed with techniques based on the detection of specific or particular sets of RNA by means of polymerase chain reaction (PCR) after reverse transcription (RT-PCR). Indeed, nested RT-PCR of RNA from a single spermatozoon has shown apparently aberrant transcripts in human sperm cells, such as those encoding synapsin I, immunoglobulins or Y-cell receptor α[139]. Such a phenomenon, named illegitimated transcription, has been defined as a very low-level transcription of any gene in any cell type[140].

Different mRNA species were found in human ejaculated spermatozoa by carrying out a step-by-step analysis with macroarray hybridization, RT-PCR and *in situ* hybridization. An extended pattern of several transcripts encoding factors (NFκB, HOX2A, ICSBP, JNK2, HBEGF, RXRβ and ErbB3) essential for cellular functioning (including signal transduction and cell proliferation) were demonstrated in human sperm nuclei. The presence of residual DNA and RNA polymerase activity within the sperm chromatin was also formerly reported[141–143].

Complementary investigations have indicated that, in spite of a high degree of DNA packaging within the human sperm head, chromatin retains some features of active chromatin, mainly acetylated histones[144] and the arrangement of certain chromatin domains into nucleosomes[145,146]. The existence of transcriptional and translational activities in human sperm during capacitation and the acrosome reaction has been described, which could also explain the presence of mRNA in mature sperm[147]. Lambard *et al.*[124] showed a significant decrease of aromatase mRNA level in sperm with low motility, compared with highly motile sperm from the same sample of normospermic patients; these data suggest that the establishment of sperm mRNA profiles could be used as a genetic fingerprint of normal fertile men.

The data therefore suggest that spermatozoa are a repository of information regarding meiotic and postmeiotic gene expression in the human,

and are likely to contain transcripts for genes playing an essential role during spermiogenesis (Figure 4.2). Use of the whole ejaculate as a wholly noninvasive biopsy of the spermatid should therefore be evaluated[123].

Different mRNA-encoding proteins are probably implicated in cell–cell and cell–substratum interactions, enhancement of fertility rate, lipid transportation, membrane recycling and stabilization of stress proteins, and promotion or inhibition of the death cell mechanism[148].

It is possible that if the mRNA accumulated in the sperm nucleus is not residual non-functional material, it might be viewed as the male gamete's contribution to early embryogenesis[149]. Delivering spermatozoon RNA to the oocyte has been demonstrated in mice[150] and humans[148]. Some sperm transcripts encoding proteins known to participate in fertilization and embryonic development have been specifically detected in early embryos after *in vitro* fertilization failure, while they have not been found in the oocyte[138]. Thus, human spermatozoa could act not only as genome carriers but also as providers of specific transcripts necessary for zygote viability and development before activation of the embryonic genome.

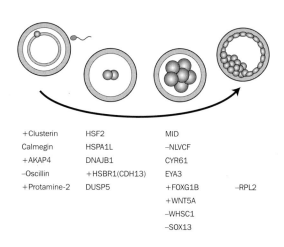

+Clusterin	HSF2	MID	
Calmegin	HSPA1L	−NLVCF	
+AKAP4	DNAJB1	CYR61	
−Oscillin	+HSBR1(CDH13)	EYA3	
+Protamine-2	DUSP5	+FOXG1B	−RPL2
		+WNT5A	
		−WHSC1	
		−SOX13	

Figure 4.2 Spermatozoa mRNA transcripts and putative temporal expression during embryo development (+ refers to mRNA transcripts that are possibly involved in development as reported in reference 148)

Ostermeier et al.[102] recently reported a suite of novel human spermatozoal mRNAs. The authors identified a group of RNAs previously defined as micro-RNAs, and others that were antisense mRNAs of in silico predicted transcripts (or silencing mRNAs). The authors speculated that the delivery of these antisense RNAs upon fertilization could enable their participation in early post-fertilization processes. They could be involved in regulation of the transition from maternal to embryonic genome, and could even be related to imprinting. Fukagawa et al.[151] and Morris et al.[152] have shown that this class of mRNA could confer transcriptional silencing by methylation.

Aberrant embryogenesis secondary to nuclear/chromatin anomalies

As mentioned above, spermatozoa of infertile men have been shown to contain various nuclear alterations, including an abnormal chromatin structure, aneuploidy, chromosomal microdeletions and DNA strand breaks (reviewed in reference 2). Since meiosis is crucial for the survival of a species, an elaborate series of safeguards have evolved to pair, break and repair the chromosomal DNA. Despite such regulatory mechanisms, it is well known that translocations and aneuploidy are regularly introduced during the meiotic divisions.

Esterhuizen et al.[153] evaluated the role of chromatin packaging (CMA3 staining), sperm morphology during sperm–zona binding, sperm decondensation and the presence of polar bodies in oocytes that failed IVF. Odds ratio analyses indicated that being in the $\geq 60\%$ CMA3 staining group resulted in a 15.6-fold increase in the risk of decondensation failure, relative to CMA3 staining of $< 44\%$. Using CMA3 fluorescence to discriminate, 51% of oocytes in the group with elevated CMA3 fluorescence had no sperm in the ooplasm, compared with 32% and 16% penetration failure in the CMA3 staining groups $\geq 44–59\%$ and $< 44\%$, respectively. Sperm chromatin packaging quality and sperm morphology assessments were demonstrated as useful clinical indicators of human fertilization failure.

Ectopic expression and inactivation of apoptosis-related genes have been shown to cause abnormalities in spermatogenesis. During spermatogenesis, the process of germ cell proliferation and maturation causes diploid spermatogonia to develop into mature haploid sperm. A number of the developing germ cells die by apoptosis before reaching maturity, even under normal conditions[154]. In addition to the physiological germ-cell apoptosis that occurs continuously throughout life, increased germ-cell apoptosis results from such external disturbances as irradiation or exposure to toxicants[155]. Evidence suggests that within the cellular component of the testicular tissue, caspases play a central role in the apoptotic process that leads to DNA fragmentation of Sertoli cells[104].

The presence of apoptosis in ejaculated spermatozoa could be the result of various types of injuries[156,157]. In vivo, apoptosis could be triggered at the testicular (hormonal depletion, irradiation, toxic agents, chemicals and heat have been shown to induce apoptosis), epididymal (the result of signals released by abnormal and/or senescent spermatozoa or by leukocytes – such as ROS and other mediators of inflammation/infection) or seminal (ROS, lack of antioxidants or other causes) levels. Also, apoptosis could be triggered by factors present in the female tract. In vitro, apoptosis could be triggered upon incubation with inappropriate culture media or other manipulation procedures. Irrespective of the stimulus, spermatozoa undergoing apoptosis and unrecognized by currently used methodologies may be dysfunctional (resulting in failure of fertilization) or, more dramatically, they may pose the risk of carrying a damaged genome into the egg resulting in poor embryo development, miscarriage or childhood anomalies[158,159].

We have published compelling evidence indicative of the presence of somatic cell apoptosis markers, including key constituents of the apoptotic machinery and activation upon defined stimuli, in human ejaculated spermatozoa. It can be summarized as follows:

- Human spermatozoa exhibit somatic cell apoptosis markers. Spermatozoa from fertile and infertile men demonstrated variable levels of phosphatidylserine (PS) externalization (by Annexin V-FITC (fluorescein isothiocyanate) binding using indirect immunofluorescence) and DNA fragmentation (by immuno-fluorescence using TUNEL (terminal deoxy nucleotide transferase-mediated dUTP nick-end labeling) and also the monoclonal antibody (mAb) F7-26) upon ejaculation and incubation under capacitating conditions[2,160,161].

- The apoptosis markers PS externalization and DNA fragmentation are expressed with a higher frequency in fractions of sperm with low motility (where dysmorphic and dysfunc-tional sperm are found), when compared with high-motility fractions[2,161].

- Apoptosis markers are expressed with a sig-nificantly higher frequency in sperm of infertile men when compared with fertile controls[156,161].

- Human sperm contain caspase-3, the major executioner caspase, in both inactive and active forms. We have unequivocally demonstrated the presence of inactive caspase-3 (32 kDa) and also caspase-3 activation (17-kDa proteolytic fragment) in ejaculated sperm by immunoblot-ting, and have also confirmed caspase activa-tion by immunofluorescent and enzymatic techniques[161]. Using immunofluorescence with a FITC-labeled antibody that specifically recognizes the active form, active caspase-3 was exclusively detected to the midpiece, where mitochondria and residual cytoplasm are present.

- Human sperm exhibit other members of the caspase family, caspase-7 and -9. By immuno-blotting, we have demonstrated the presence of inactive caspase-7 (35 kDa) and caspase-9 (45 kDa) in many samples, as well as active cas-pase-7 (32 kDa) and caspase-9 (37 kDa) in samples of infertile men[162].

- Human sperm possess apoptosis-inducing fac-tor (AIF). By immunoblotting, we have demonstrated that human sperm express AIF (67 kDa) (although further studies are needed to establish its cellular location) and possibly a unique PARP (poly [ADP-ribose] polymerase), a specific caspase substrate of 66 kDa, with a different molecular weight from that of the 116–85-kDa analog and proteolytic fragment found in somatic cells[162,163].

- Human sperm appear not to express Bid pro-tein (neither the 24-kDa intact nor the 15-kDa proapoptotic fragment) as measured by immunoblotting (unpublished observations).

- Caspase activation can be triggered in ejacu-lated human sperm by the mitochondrial dis-rupter staurosporine. Staurosporine at 10 μmol/l (apoptosis-inducing dose in somatic cells) significantly enhanced caspase activation (by DEVD assay (Asp-Glu-Val-Asp) that measures caspase-3, -6 and -7) and DNA frag-mentation, suggesting a mitochondria-dependent pathway of caspase activation[162]. We analyzed the dose-dependent effect of stau-rosporine on sperm viability, and found no deleterious effects in the range 1–15 μmol/l. Preincubation with the pan-caspase inhibitor zVAD (benzoxy-Val-Ala-Asp) (50 μmol/l, 30 min) inhibited staurosporine-induced DNA fragmentation by 50% (unpublished observations).

- Human sperm did not exhibit a response to Fas ligand. Fas ligand did not trigger caspase activation, PS translocation or DNA fragmen-tation. The Fas ligand (anti-Fas monoclonal antibody) was tested at 1 μg/ml (apoptosis-inducing dose in somatic cells) with and with-out G-protein as a linker (at 2 μg/ml), and did not elicit caspase activation, PS translocation or DNA fragmentation[162]. These data are in agreement with recent studies that failed to demonstrate Fas receptors in ejaculated human sperm[164].

- Hydrogen peroxide, the most damaging ROS in sperm, induces expression of apoptosis markers. We demonstrated that H_2O_2 increased PS translocation and DNA fragmentation[165]. H_2O_2 produced a dose-dependent effect on PS translocation, with a significant increase at 200 μmol/l, a dose that we previously reported initiated impairment of motility and other sperm functions without affecting viability *in vitro*[166]. In addition, H_2O_2 resulted in a moderate increase in caspase activation.

- Ejaculated human sperm show a strong correlation between ROS production and DNA fragmentation, linking mitochondrial dysfunction and expression of apoptosis markers. We have shown a positive, significant correlation between the endogenous generation of ROS (measured by chemiluminescence) and DNA strand breaks in ejaculated sperm[2].

- Ejaculated sperm show a strong correlation between disruption of mitochondrial transmembrane potential and PS translocation, again linking mitochondrial dysfunction and expression of apoptosis markers. We have documented that samples with live cells presenting PS externalization demonstrated changes in mitochondrial transmembrane potential using a mitochondrial membrane sensor kit[167]. The test uses a cationic dye, which fluoresces differently in apoptotic and healthy cells. Results showed alterations of the mitochondrial membrane potential that were three times higher in sperm fractions with low motility, compared with high-motility fractions.

The oocyte has the capability to repair DNA damage, as oocytes fertilized by DNA-damaged spermatozoa did not develop further *in vitro* when they were cultured in the presence of inhibitors to DNA repair[168–171]. The capacity of the oocyte to repair is limited, and is related to the degree of sperm DNA damage. The fertilization capacity of apoptotic sperm has been observed to be at the same rate as that of intact spermatozoa; however, embryo development to the blastocyst stage is closely related to the integrity of the DNA[171].

During spermatogenesis, a complex and dynamic process of proliferation and differentiation occurs as spermatogonia are transformed into mature spermatozoa. This unique process involves a series of meioses and mitoses, changes in cytoplasmic architecture, replacement of somatic cell-like histones with transition proteins and the final addition of protamines, leading to highly packaged chromatin[172]. The human is of particular interest, as a single ejaculate normally contains a heterogeneous population of spermatozoa. It has been known for many years that the chromatin of the mature sperm nucleus can be abnormally packaged[173]. In addition, abnormal chromatin packaging and nuclear DNA damage appear to be linked[174], and there is a strong association between the presence of nuclear DNA damage in the mature spermatozoa of men and poor semen parameters[77,175].

It is postulated that an endogenous nuclease, topoisomerase II, creates and ligates nicks to provide relief of torsional stress and to aid chromatin rearrangement during protamination[176]. The DNA damage in ejaculated human sperm consists of both single- and double-stranded DNA breaks. Endogenous nicks in DNA are normally expressed at specific stages of spermiogenesis in different animal models; these endogenous nicks are evident during spermiogenesis, but are not observed once chromatin packaging is completed. It is possible that endogenous nuclease topoisomerase II may play a role in both creating and ligating nicks during spermiogenesis, that these nicks may provide relief of torsional stress and that they aid chromatin rearrangement during the displacement of histones by protamines[177–179].

Several studies have shown that sperm DNA quality has robust power to predict fertilization *in vitro*[175,180–182]. Tomlinson *et al.*[183] have reported that the only parameter showing a significant difference between pregnant and non-pregnant groups in IVF was the percentage of DNA fragmentation assessed by *in situ* nick translation. Sperm-derived effects, particularly the degree of DNA fragmentation, have been suggested to affect human embryo development[104].

The sperm chromatin structure assay (SCSA) has been proposed as a diagnostic tool to predict fertilization by evaluating sperm DNA stability[79]. The SCSA measures susceptibility to DNA denaturation *in situ* in sperm exposed to acid for 30 s, followed by acridine orange staining. The use of flow cytometry in the SCSA increases its dependability.

Duran *et al.*[84] studied a large infertility population undergoing IUI therapy in a prospective cohort fashion. A total of 119 patients underwent 154 cycles of IUI. DNA fragmentation evaluated by TUNEL and acridine orange staining were measured. The authors reported that sperm DNA quality played a major role as a predictor of pregnancy under such *in vivo* conditions.

Epigenetic factors

'Epigenetics' refers to a process that regulates gene activity without affecting the genetic (DNA) code and is heritable through cell division. Germ cell development and early embryogenesis are crucial windows in the erasure, acquisition and maintenance of genomic imprints. Moreover, a number of genes regulated by imprinting have been shown to be essential to fetal growth and placental function. Increasing attention has recently focused on potential epigenetic disturbances resulting from embryo culture, somatic cell nuclear cloning and assisted reproductive technologies[184,185], indicating that a better understanding of genomic imprinting or parent-of-origin effects on gene expression is highly significant to the current study of reproduction and development.

Imprinting is an epigenetically controlled phenomenon, because something other than DNA sequence must distinguish the parental alleles and determine sex-specific gene expression. The role of DNA methylation in genomic imprinting has been extensively investigated. It is estimated that the total number of imprinted genes in the mouse and human genomes may range between 100 and 200. Of those that have been identified to date, a significant number appear to have important roles in fetal development. It has been argued that imprinted genes play essential roles in controlling the placental supply of maternal nutrients to the fetus, by regulating the growth of the placenta and/or the activity of transplacental transport systems.

Methylation is important for somatic cell maintenance of imprinting after the global wave of demethylation in the blastocyst[186]. However, the question arises of how maternal and paternal alleles can be distinguished after global demethylation arises[187,188]. It has been found that different methylation sites within imprinted genes may demonstrate significant temporal differences in methylation pattern, and that establishment of the final methylation pattern is a dynamic process[189].

Epigenetic modifications serve as an extension of the information content by which the underlying genetic code may be interpreted. These modifications mark genomic regions and act as heritable and stable instructions for the specification of chromatin organization and structure that dictate transcriptional states. In mammals, DNA methylation and the modification of histones account for the major epigenetic alterations. Two cycles of DNA methylation reprogramming have been characterized (reviewed in reference 190). During germ cell development, epigenetic reprogramming of DNA methylation resets parent-of-origin-based genomic imprints and restores totipotency to gametes.

During fertilization, the second cycle is triggered, resulting in an asymmetric difference between parental genomes. Further epigenetic asymmetry is evident in the establishment of the first two lineages at the blastocyst stage. This differentiative event sets the epigenetic characteristics of the lineages as derivatives of the inner cell mass (somatic) and trophectoderm (extraembryonic).

The erasure and subsequent retracing of the epigenetic checkpoints pose the most serious obstacles to somatic nuclear transfer. Elaboration of the mechanisms of these interactions will be invaluable in our fundamental understanding of biological processes and in achieving substantial therapeutic advances[190].

Recent studies have suggested a possible link between human assisted reproductive technologies and genomic imprinting disorders (reviewed in reference 191). The presence of Angelman syndrome (caused by a loss of function of the maternal allele or duplication of the paternal allele within a region that spans *UBE3A*) and Beckwith–Wiedemann syndrome (another disease that exhibits parent-of-origin effects in its inheritance) has been observed following the use of ICSI.

Assisted reproductive technologies include the isolation, handling and culture of gametes and early embryos at times when imprinted genes are likely to be particularly vulnerable to external influences. Evidence of sex-specific differences in imprint acquisition suggests that male and female germ cells may be susceptible to perturbations in imprinted genes at specific prenatal and postnatal stages. Imprints acquired first during gametogenesis must be maintained during preimplantation development when reprogramming of the overall genome occurs. The identification of the mechanisms and timing of imprint erasure, acquisition and maintenance during germ cell development and early embryogenesis, as well as their implications for future epigenetic studies in assisted reproductive technologies, should constitute research priorities[191].

CONCLUSIONS

The fertilizing spermatozoon has a very dynamic and critical participation in embryogenesis during and after the fertilization process. A defective spermatozoon that penetrates the oocyte may cause arrest of development at multiple levels during embryo preimplantational development.

Moreover, sublethal and lethal effects can be 'carried over' following implantation, resulting in human disease.

The contributions of the fertilizing spermatozoon to the oocyte during normal development include delivery of the DNA/chromatin, the oocyte-activating factor (OAF) and a centriole. The DNA/chromatin complex is obviously the most significant contribution to originating a new diploid individual. Nevertheless, the OAF and centriole play a critical part in bringing about oocyte activation and the first mitotic division, and without their contributions embryogenesis would also be neglected. In addition, recent data have indicated that spermatozoa provide the zygote with a unique suite of paternal mRNAs. Such transcripts might be crucial for early and late embryonic development, and deficient delivery or aberrant transcription might contribute to abnormal development and arrest.

A large body of evidence is accumulating demonstrating that abnormal oocyte activation and embryonic development might be the consequence of aberrant paternal contribution(s). An early paternal effect results in failure to complete the fertilization process, syngamy or early cleavage. It can be demonstrated by morphological abnormalities observed at the pronuclear and 2–4-cell stage. It is speculated that these defects are mediated by sperm deficiencies, including an abnormal release of OAF and by dysfunctions of the centrosome and cytoskeletal apparatus. A late paternal effect is characterized by failure to achieve implantation competence, but could also be associated with pregnancy loss and postnatal developmental abnormalities. It is associated with sperm nuclear/chromatin defects, including the presence of aneuploidy, genetic anomalies, DNA damage and possible other causes.

The strictly maternal inheritance of mitochondrial DNA (mtDNA) in mammals is a developmental paradox promoted by an unknown mechanism responsible for the destruction of sperm mitochondria shortly after fertilization. It has been shown that sperm mitochondria are tagged and later subjected to directed proteolysis during preimplantation development. Abnormalities of this process could lead to aberrant embryogenesis.

In addition, recent data have indicated that spermatozoa provide the zygote with a unique suite of paternal mRNAs. Such transcripts might be crucial for early and late embryonic development, and deficient delivery or aberrant transcription might lead to abnormal embryogenesis. Furthermore, limited RNA synthesis can be detected in human pronuclei and failure of this early transcription is associated with abnormal pronuclear development and arrest. Finally, gene-imprinting abnormalities, either of gamete origin or taking place during early embryogenesis, may be responsible for severe human disease. Such a problem has a potential impact when using certain forms of assisted reproductive technologies.

REFERENCES

1. Latham KE, Sapienza C. Localization of genes encoding egg modifiers of paternal genome function to mouse chromosomes one and two. Development 1998; 125: 929
2. Barroso G, Morshedi M, Oehninger S. Analysis of DNA fragmentation, plasma membrane translocation of phosphatidylserine and oxidative stress in human spermatozoa. Hum Reprod 2000; 15: 1338
3. Cummins JM, Jequier AM, Kan R. Molecular biology of human male infertility links with aging, mitochondrial genetics, and oxidative stress? Mol Reprod Dev 1994; 37: 345
4. Simerly C, Wu GJ, Zoran S. The paternal inheritance of the centrosome, the cell's microtubule organizing center, in humans, and the implications for infertility. Nat Med 1995; 1: 47
5. Bedford JM. Ultrastructural changes in the sperm head during fertilization in the rabbit. Am J Anat 1968; 123: 329
6. Yanagimachi R. Mammalian fertilization In Knobil E, Neill JO, eds. The Physiology of Reproduction. New York: Raven 1994: 189
7. Snell WJ, White JM. The molecules of mammalian fertilization. Cell 1996; 85: 175
8. Primakoff P, Hyatt H, Tredick-Kline J. Identification and purification of a sperm surface protein

9. with a potential role in sperm–egg membrane fusion. J Cell Biol 1987; 104: 141
9. Blobel CP, White JM. Structure, function and evolutionary relationship of proteins containing a disintegrin domain. Curr Opin Cell Biol 1992; 4: 760
10. Blobel CP, et al. A potential fusion peptide and an integrin ligand domain in a protein active in sperm–egg fusion. Nature 1992; 356: 248
11. Cowan AE, et al. Guinea pig fertilin exhibits restricted lateral mobility in epididymal sperm and becomes freely diffusing during capacitation. Dev Biol 2001; 236: 502
12. Primakoff P, Myles DG. The ADAM gene family: surface proteins with adhesion and protease activity. Trends Genet 2000; 16: 83
13. Inoue N, et al. The immunoglobulin superfamily protein Izumo is required for sperm to fuse with eggs. Nature 2005; 434: 234
14. Toshimori K, et al. An MN9 antigenic molecule, equatorin, is required for successful sperm–oocyte fusion in mice. Biol Reprod 1998; 59: 22
15. Manandhar G, Toshimori K. Exposure of sperm head equatorin after acrosome reaction and its fate after fertilization in mice. Biol Reprod 2001; 65: 1425
16. Fissore RA, Reis MM, Palermo GD. Isolation of the Ca2+ releasing component(s) of mammalian sperm extracts: the search continues. Mol Hum Reprod 1999; 5: 189
17. Parrington J, et al. Calcium oscillations in mammalian eggs triggered by a soluble sperm protein. Nature 1996; 379: 364
18. Dumollard R, Sardet C. Three different calcium wave pacemakers in ascidian eggs. J Cell Sci 2001; 1: 2471
19. Duchen M. Mitochondria and calcium: from cell signalling to cell death. J Physiol 2000; 529: 57
20. Rizzuto R, Bernardi P, Pozzan T. Mitochondria as all-round players of the calcium game. J Physiol 2000; 529: 37
21. Eisen A, Reynolds GT. Source and sinks for the calcium released during fertilization of single sea urchin eggs. J Cell Biol 1985; 100: 1522
22. Dumollard R, et al. Mitochondrial respiration and Ca2+ waves are linked during fertilisation and meiosis completion. Development 2003; 130: 683
23. McCormick JG, Denton RM. Mitochondrial Ca2+ transport and the role of intramitochondrial Ca2+ in the regulation of energy metabolism. Dev Neurosci 1993; 15: 3

24. Hansford RG. Physiological role of mitochondrial Ca2+ transport. J Bioenerg Biomembr 1994; 26: 495

25. Territo PR, et al. Ca(2+) activation of heart mitochondrial oxidative phosphorylation: role of the F(0)/F(1)-ATPase. Am J Physiol Cell Physiol 2000; 278: C423

26. Duchen MR, Biscoe TJ. Mitochondrial function in type I cells isolated from rabbit arterial chemoreceptors. J Physiol 1992; 450: 13

27. Pralong WF, Spat A, Wollheim CB. Dynamic pacing of cell metabolism by intracellular Ca2+ transients. J Biol Chem 1994; 269: 27310

28. Hajnoczky G, et al. Decoding of cytosolic calcium oscillations in the mitochondria. Cell 1995; 11: 415

29. Mak DO, McBride S, Foskett JK. ATP regulation of type 1 inositol 1,4,5-trisphosphate receptor channel gating by allosteric tuning of Ca(2+) activation. J Biol Chem 1999; 274: 22231

30. Mak DO, McBride S, Foskett JK. ATP regulation of recombinant type 3 inositol 1,4,5-trisphosphate receptor gating. J Gen Physiol 2001; 117: 447

31. Tarin JJ. Potential effects of age-associated oxidative stress on mammalian oocytes/embryos. Mol Hum Reprod 1996; 2: 717

32. Saunders CM, et al. PLC zeta: a sperm-specific trigger of Ca(2+) oscillations in eggs and embryo development. Development 2002; 129: 3533

33. Kouchi Z, et al. Recombinant phospholipase Czeta has high Ca2+ sensitivity and induces Ca2+ oscillations in mouse eggs. J Biol Chem 2004; 279: 10408

34. Swann K, et al. The cytosolic sperm factor that triggers Ca2+ oscillations and egg activation in mammals is a novel phospholipase C: PLCzeta. Reproduction 2004; 127: 431

35. Dupont G. Theoretical insights into the mechanism of spiral Ca2+ wave initiation in Xenopus oocytes. Am J Physiol 1998; 275: C317

36. Eliyahu E, Shalgi R. A role for protein kinase C during rat egg activation. Biol Reprod 2002; 67: 189

37. Talmor-Cohen A, et al. Are Src family kinases involved in cell cycle resumption in rat eggs? Reproduction 2004; 127: 455

38. Piko L, Matsumoto L. Number of mitochondria and some properties of mitochondrial DNA in the mouse egg. Dev Biol 1976; 49: 1

39. Lodish H, et al. Molecular Cell Biology, 3rd edn. New York: WH Freeman and Co., 1995

40. Shadel GS, Clayton DA. Mitochondrial DNA maintenance in vertebrates. Ann Rev Biochem 1997; 66: 409

41. Ford WCL, Rees JM. The bioenergetics of mammalian sperm motility. In Gagnon C, ed. Controls of Sperm Motility: Biological and Clinical Aspects. Boca Raton, FL: CRC Press, 1990: 175

42. Max B. This and that: hair pigments, the hypoxic basis of life and the Virgilian journey of the spermatozoon. Trends Pharmacol Sci 1992; 13: 272

43. Cummins J. Mitochondrial DNA in mammalian reproduction. Rev Reprod 1998; 3: 172

44. Short RV. The difference between a testis and an ovary. J Exp Zool 1998; 281: 359

45. Kaneda H, et al. Elimination of paternal mitochondrial DNA in intraspecific crosses during early mouse embryogenesis. Proc Natl Acad Sci USA 1995; 92: 4542

46. Ankel-Simons F, Cummins JM. Misconceptions about mitochondria and mammalian fertilization – implications for theories on human evolution. Proc Nat Acad Sci USA 1996; 93: 13859

47. Aitken RJ. Free radicals, lipid peroxidation and sperm function. Reprod Fertil Dev 1995; 7: 659

48. Shalgi R, et al. Fate of sperm organelles during early embryogenesis in the rat. Mol Reprod Dev 1994; 37: 264

49. Sutovsky P, Navara C, Schatten G. Fate of the sperm mitochondria, and the incorporation, conversion, and disassembly of the sperm tail structures during bovine fertilization. Biol Reprod 1996; 55: 1195

50. Smith LC, Alcívar AA. Cytoplasmic inheritance and its effects on development and performance. J Reprod Fertil 1993; 48 (Suppl): 31

51. Gresson RAR. Presence of the sperm middle-piece in the fertilized egg of the mouse (Mus musculus). Nature 1940; 145: 425

52. Smith LC, et al. Sea urchin genes expressed in activated coelomocytes are identified by expressed sequence tags. Complement homologues and other putative immune response genes suggest immune system homology within the deuterostomes. J Immunol 1996; 15: 593

53. Allen V. Role of motor proteins in organizing the endoplasmic reticulum and Golgi apparatus. Semin Cell Dev Biol 1996; 7: 335

54. Sutovsky P, et al. Ubiquitin tag for sperm mitochondria. Nature 1999; 402: 371

55. Sutovsky P, et al. Ubiquitinated sperm mitochondria selective proteolysis and the regulation of mitochondrial inheritance in mammalian embryos. Biol Reprod 2000; 63: 582

56. Ingman M, et al. Mitochondrial genome variation and the origin of modern humans. Nature 2000; 408: 708

57. Schatten G. The centrosome and its mode of inheritance: the reduction of the centrosome during gametogenesis and its restoration during fertilization. Dev Biol 1994; 165: 299

58. Reinsch S, Karsenti E. Movement of nuclei along microtubules in Xenopus egg extracts. Curr Biol 1997; 7: 211

59. Payne C, et al. Preferentially localized dynein and perinuclear dynactin associate with nuclear pore complex proteins to mediate genomic union during mammalian fertilization. J Cell Sci 2003; 116: 4727

60. Oehninger S, et al. Failure of fertilization in in vitro fertilization: the 'occult' male factor. J In Vitro Fert Embryo Transf 1988; 5: 181

61. Oehninger S, et al. Delayed fertilization during in vitro fertilization and embryo transfer cycles: analysis of causes and impact on overall results. Fertil Steril 1989; 52: 991

62. Kruger TF, et al. Predictive value of abnormal sperm morphology in in vitro fertilization. Fertil Steril 1988; 49: 112

63. Ron-el R, et al. Delayed fertilization and poor embryonic development associated with impaired semen quality. Fertil Steril 1991; 55: 338

64. Parinaud J, et al. Influence of sperm parameters on embryo quality. Fertil Steril 1993; 60: 888

65. Grow DR, et al. Sperm morphology as diagnosed by strict criteria: probing the impact of teratozoospermia on fertilization rate and pregnancy outcome in a large in vitro fertilization population. Fertil Steril 1994; 62: 559

66. Oehninger S, et al. Corrective measures and pregnancy outcome in in vitro fertilization in patients with severe sperm morphology abnormalities. Fertil Steril 1988; 50: 283

67. Janny L, Menezo YJ. Evidence for a strong paternal effect on human preimplantation embryo development and blastocyst formation. Mol Reprod Dev 1994; 38: 36

68. Oehninger S, et al. A comparative analysis of embryo implantation potential in patients with severe teratozoospermia undergoing in-vitro fertilization with a high insemination concentration or intracytoplasmic sperm injection. Hum Reprod 1996; 11: 1086

69. Nagy ZP, et al. The result of intracytoplasmic sperm injection is not related to any of the three basic sperm parameters. Hum Reprod 1995; 10: 1123

70. Oehninger S, et al. Intracytoplasmic sperm injection: achievement of high pregnancy rates in couples with severe male factor infertility is dependent primarily upon female and not male factors. Fertil Steril 1995; 64: 977

71. Mansour RT, et al. The effect of sperm parameters on the outcome of intracytoplasmic sperm injection. Fertil Steril 1995; 64: 982

72. Mercan R, et al. The outcome of clinical pregnancies following intracytoplasmic sperm injection is not affected by semen quality. Andrologia 1998; 30: 91

73. Tasdemir I, et al. Effect of abnormal sperm head morphology on the outcome of intracytoplasmic sperm injection in humans. Hum Reprod 1997; 12: 1214

74. Gorczyca W, et al. Presence of strand breaks and increased sensitivity of DNA in situ to denaturation in abnormal human sperm: analogy to apoptosis of somatic cells. Exp Cell Res 1993; 207: 202

75. Manicardi GC, et al. Presence of endogenous nicks in DNA of ejaculated human spermatozoa and its relationship to chromomycin A3 accessibility. Biol Reprod 1995; 52: 864

76. Hughes CM, et al. A comparison of baseline and induced DNA damage in human spermatozoa from fertile and infertile men, using a modified comet assay. Mol Hum Reprod 1996; 2: 613

77. Lopes S, et al. Sperm deoxyribonucleic acid fragmentation is increased in poor-quality semen samples and correlates with failed fertilization in intracytoplasmic sperm injection. Fertil Steril 1998; 69: 528

78. Aitken RJ, et al. Relative impact of oxidative stress on the functional competence and genomic integrity of human spermatozoa. Biol Reprod 1998; 59: 1037

79. Evenson DP, et al. Utility of the sperm chromatin structure assay as a diagnostic and prognostic tool in the human fertility clinic. Hum Reprod 1999; 14: 1039

80. Sakkas D, et al. Origin of DNA damage in ejaculated human spermatozoa. Rev Reprod 1999; 4: 31

81. Pfeffer J, et al. Aneuploidy frequencies in semen fractions from ten oligoasthenoteratozoospermic patients donating sperm for intracytoplasmic sperm injection. Fertil Steril 1999; 72: 472

82. Sakkas D, et al. Sperm nuclear DNA damage and altered chromatin structure: effect on fertilization and embryo development. Hum Reprod 1998; 13 (Suppl 4): 11

83. Rubio C, et al. Incidence of sperm chromosomal abnormalities in a risk population: relationship with sperm quality and ICSI outcome. Hum Reprod 2001; 16: 2084

84. Duran EH, et al. Sperm DNA quality predicts intrauterine insemination outcome: a prospective cohort study. Hum Reprod 2002; 17: 3122

85. Virant-Klun I, Tomazevic T, Meden-Vrtovec H. Sperm single-stranded DNA, detected by acridine orange staining, reduces fertilization and quality of ICSI-derived embryos. J Assist Reprod Genet 2002; 19: 319

86. Burrello N, et al. Lower sperm aneuploidy frequency is associated with high pregnancy rates in ICSI programmes. Hum Reprod 2002; 18: 1371

87. Liu CH, et al. DNA fragmentation, mitochondrial dysfunction and chromosomal aneuploidy in the spermatozoa of oligoasthenoteratozoospermic males. J Assist Reprod Genet 2004; 21: 119

88. Virro MR, Larson-Cook KL, Evenson DP. Sperm chromatin structure assay (SCSA) parameters are related to fertilization, blastocyst development, and ongoing pregnancy in in vitro fertilization and intracytoplasmic sperm injection cycles. Fertil Steril 2004; 81: 1289

89. Petit FM, et al. Could sperm aneuploidy rate determination be used as a predictive test before intracytoplasmic sperm injection? J Androl 2005; 26: 235

90. Devroey P, Van Steirteghem A. A review of ten years experience of ICSI. Hum Reprod Update 2004; 10: 19

91. Foresta C, et al. Genetic abnormalities among severely oligospermic men who are candidates for intracytoplasmic sperm injection. J Clin Endocrinol Metab 2005; 90: 152

92. St John JC. Incorporating molecular screening techniques into the modern andrology laboratory. J Androl 1999; 20: 692

93. Brinkworth MH. Paternal transmission of genetic damage: findings in animals and humans. Int J Androl 2000; 23: 123

94. Lanzendorf SE, et al. Penetration of human spermatozoa through the zona pellucida of nonviable human oocytes. J Soc Gynecol Invest 1994; 1: 69

95. Oehninger S, et al. Clinical significance of human sperm–zona pellucida binding. Fertil Steril 1997; 67: 1121

96. Oehninger S. Normal fertilization. In El-Shafie M, et al., eds. An Atlas of the Ultrastructure of Human Oocytes – A Guide for Assisted Reproduction. London: Parthenon Publishing, 2000: 23

97. Liu de Y, Garrett C, Baker HW. Clinical application of sperm–oocyte interaction tests in in vitro fertilization–embryo transfer and intracytoplasmic sperm injection programs. Fertil Steril 2004; 82: 1251

98. Asch R, et al. The stages at which human fertilization arrests: microtubule and chromosome configurations in inseminated oocytes which failed to complete fertilization and development in humans. Hum Reprod 1995; 10: 1897

99. Rawe VY, et al. Cytoskeletal organization defects and abortive activation in human oocytes after IVF and ICSI failure. Mol Hum Reprod 2000; 6: 510

100. Hewitson L, Simerly CR, Schatten G. Fate of sperm components during assisted reproduction: implications for infertility. Hum Fertil (Camb) 2002; 5: 110

101. Sutovsky P, Hauser R, Sutovsky M. Increased levels of sperm ubiquitin correlate with semen quality in men from an andrology laboratory clinic population. Hum Reprod 2004; 19: 628

102. Ostermeier GC, et al. A suite of novel human spermatozoal RNAs. J Androl 2005; 26: 70

103. Braude P, Bolton V, Moore S. Human gene expression first occurs between the four- and eight-cell stages of preimplantation development. Nature 1988; 332: 459

104. Tesarik J, et al. In-vitro effects of FSH and testosterone withdrawal on caspase activation and DNA fragmentation in different cell types of human seminiferous epithelium. Hum Reprod 2002; 17: 1811

105. Tesarik J. The paternal effects on cell division in the human preimplantation embryo. Reprod Biomed Online 2005; 10: 370

106. Tesarik J, Greco E, Mendoza C. Late, but not early, paternal effect on human embryo development is related to sperm DNA fragmentation. Hum Reprod 2004; 19: 611

107. Greco E, et al. Efficient treatment of infertility due to sperm DNA damage by ICSI with testicular spermatozoa. Hum Reprod 2005; 20: 226

108. Hewitson L, Simerly CR, Schatten G. Cytoskeletal aspects of assisted fertilization. Semin Reprod Med 2000; 18: 151

109. Hewitson L, Simerly CR, Schatten G. ICSI, male pronuclear remodeling and cell cycle checkpoints. Adv Exp Med Biol 2003; 518: 199

110. Tesarik J, Mendoza C. In vitro fertilization by intracytoplasmic sperm injection. BioEssays 1999; 21: 791

111. Ramalho-Santos J, et al. SNAREs in mammalian sperm: possible implications for fertilization. Dev Biol 2000; 223: 54

112. Katayama M, Koshida M, Miyake M. Fate of the acrosome in ooplasm in pigs after IVF and ICSI. Hum Reprod 2002; 17: 2657

113. Terada Y, et al. Centrosomal function assessment in human sperm using heterologous ICSI with rabbit eggs: a new male factor infertility assay. Mol Reprod Dev 2004; 67: 360

114. Kovacic B, Vlaisavljevic V. Configuration of maternal and paternal chromatin and pertaining microtubules in human oocytes failing to fertilize after intracytoplasmic sperm injection. Mol Reprod Dev 2000; 55: 197

115. Colombero LT, et al. The role of structural integrity of the fertilising spermatozoon in early human embryogenesis. Zygote 1999; 7: 157

116. Moomjy M, et al. Sperm integrity is critical for normal mitotic division and early embryonic development. Mol Hum Reprod 1999; 5: 836

117. Sun C, et al. An azoospermic man with a de novo point mutation in the Y-chromosomal gene USP9Y. Nat Genet 1999; 23: 429

118. Dickins RA, et al. The ubiquitin ligase component Siah1a is required for completion of meiosis I in male mice. Mol Cell Biol 2002; 22: 2294

119. Li B, Ruiz JC, Chun KT. CUL-4A is critical for early embryonic development. Mol Cell Biol 2002; 22: 4997

120. Muratori M, et al. Sperm ubiquitination positively correlates to normal morphology in human semen. Hum Reprod 2005; 20: 1035–43

121. Thompson WE, Ramalho-Santos J, Sutovsky P. Ubiquitination of prohibitin in mammalian sperm mitochondria: possible roles in the regulation of mitochondrial inheritance and sperm quality control. Biol Reprod 2003; 69: 254

122. Brenner CA, Kubisch HM, Pierce KE. Role of the mitochondrial genome in assisted reproductive technologies and embryonic stem cell-based therapeutic cloning. Reprod Fertil Dev 2004; 16: 743

123. Miller D. RNA in the ejaculate spermatozoon: a window into molecular events in spermatogenesis and a record of the unusual requirements of haploid gene expression and post-meiotic equilibration. Mol Hum Reprod 1997; 3: 669

124. Lambard S, et al. Expression of aromatase in human ejaculated spermatozoa: a putative marker of motility. Mol Hum Reprod 2003; 9: 117

125. Wykes SM, Miller D, Krawetz SA. Mammalian spermatozoal mRNAs: tools for the functional analysis of male gametes. J Submicrosc Cytol Pathol 2000; 32: 77

126. Dadoune JP, et al. Identification of transcripts by macroarrays, RT–PCR and in situ hybridization in human ejaculate spermatozoa. Mol Hum Reprod 2005; 11: 133

127. Eddy EM. Male germ cell gene expression. Recent Prog Horm Res 2002; 57: 103

128. Steger K. Transcriptional and translational regulation of gene expression in haploid spermatids. Anat Embryol (Berl) 1999; 199: 471

129. Petersen C, Fuzesi L, Hoyer-Fender S. Outer dense fibre proteins from human sperm tail: molecular cloning and expression analyses of two cDNA transcripts encoding proteins of approximately 70 kDa. Mol Hum Reprod 1999; 5: 627

130. Eddy EM, Toshimori K, O'Brien DA. Fibrous sheath of mammalian spermatozoa. Microsc Res Tech 2003; 61: 103

131. Dadoune JP. Expression of mammalian spermatozoal nucleoproteins. Microsc Res Tech 2003; 61: 56

132. Pessot CA, et al. Presence of RNA in the sperm nucleus. Biochem Biophys Res Commun 1989; 158: 272

133. Passananti C, et al. The product of Zfp59 (Mfg2), a mouse gene expressed at the spermatid stage of spermatogenesis, accumulates in spermatozoa nuclei. Cell Growth Differ 1995; 6: 1037

134. Kumar G, Patel D, Naz RK. c-myc mRNA is present in human sperm cells. Cell Mol Biol Res 1993; 39: 111

135. Miller D, et al. Differential RNA fingerprinting as a tool in the analysis of spermatozoal gene expression. Hum Reprod 1994; 9: 864

136. Goodwin LO, Karabinus DS, Pergolizzi RG. Presence of N-cadherin transcripts in mature spermatozoa. Mol Hum Reprod 2000; 6: 487

137. Carreau S, et al. Aromatase expression in male germ cells. J Steroid Biochem Mol Biol 2001; 79: 203

138. Ostermeier GC, et al. Spermatozoal RNA profiles of normal fertile men. Lancet 2002; 360: 772

139. Kimoto Y. A single human cell expresses all messenger ribonucleic acids: the arrow of time in a cell. Mol Gen Genet 1998; 258: 233

140. Chelly J et al. Illegitimate transcription: transcription of any gene in any cell type. Proc Natl Acad Sci USA 1989; 86: 2617

141. Hecht NB. A DNA polymerase isolated from bovine spermatozoa. J Reprod Fertil 1974; 41: 345

142. Witkin SS, Korngold GC, Bendich A. Ribonuclease-sensitive DNA-synthesizing complex in human sperm heads and seminal fluid. Proc Natl Acad Sci USA 1975; 72: 3295

143. Miteva K, Valkov N, Goncharova-Peinoval J. Electron microscopic data for the presence of post-meiotic gene expression in isolated ram sperm chromatin. Cytobios 1995; 83: 85

144. Gatewood JM, et al. Isolation of four core histones from human sperm chromatin representing a minor subset of somatic histones. J Biol Chem 1990; 265: 20662

145. Gineitis AA, et al. Human sperm telomere-binding complex involves histone H2B and secures telomere membrane attachment. J Cell Biol 2000; 151: 1591

146. Zalenskaya IA, Bradbury EM, Zalensky AO. Chromatin structure of telomere domain in human sperm. Biochem Biophys Res Commun 2000; 279: 213

147. Naz RK. Effect of actinomycine D and cycloheximide on human sperm function. Arch Androl 1998; 41: 135

148. Ostermeier GC, et al. Reproductive biology: delivering spermatozoan RNA to the oocyte. Nature 2004; 429: 154

149. Dadoune JP, Siffroi JP, Alfonsi MF. Transcription in haploid male germ cells. Int Rev Cytol 2004; 237: 1

150. Hayashi S, et al. Mouse preimplantation embryos developed from oocytes injected with round spermatids or spermatozoa have similar but distinct patterns of early messenger RNA expression. Biol Reprod 2003; 69: 1170

151. Fukagawa T, et al. Dicer is essential for formation of the heterochromatin structure in vertebrate cells. Nat Cell Biol 2004; 6: 784

152. Morris KV, et al. Small interfering RNA-induced transcriptional gene silencing in human cells. Science 2004; 305: 1289

153. Esterhuizen AD, et al. Defective sperm decondensation: a cause for fertilization failure. Andrologia 2002; 34: 1

154. Billig H, et al. Apoptosis in testis germ cells: developmental changes in gonadotropin dependence and localization to selective tubule stages. Endocrinology 1995; 136: 5

155. Pentikainen V, Erkkila K, Dunkel L. Fas regulates germ cell apoptosis in the human testis in vitro. Am J Physiol 1999; 276: E310

156. Oehninger S, et al. Presence and significance of somatic cell apoptosis markers in human ejaculated spermatozoa. Reprod Biomed Online 2003; 7: 469

157. Oehninger S. Biochemical and functional characterization of the human zona pellucida. Reprod Biomed Online 2003; 7: 641

158. Bowen JR, et al. Medical and developmental outcome at 1 year for children conceived by intracytoplasmic sperm injection. Lancet 1998; 351: 1529

159. Bonduelle M, et al. Seven years of intracytoplasmic sperm injection and follow-up of 1987 subsequent children. Hum Reprod 1999; 14: 243

160. Schuffner A, et al. Effect of different incubation conditions on phosphatidylserine externalization and motion parameters of purified fractions of highly motile human spermatozoa. J Androl 2002; 23: 194

161. Weng S, et al. Caspase activity and apoptotic markers in ejaculated human sperm. Mol Hum Reprod 2002; 8: 984

162. Taylor SL, et al. Somatic cell apoptosis markers and pathways in human ejaculated sperm: potential utility as indicators of sperm quality. Mol Hum Reprod 2004; 10: 825

163. Benchoua A, et al. Active caspase-8 translocates into the nucleus of apoptotic cells to inactivate poly(ADP-ribose) polymerase-2. J Biol Chem 2002; 277: 34217

164. Castro A, et al. Absence of Fas protein detection by flow cytometry in human spermatozoa. Fertil Steril 2004; 81: 1019

165. Duru NK, et al. Cryopreservation–thawing of fractionated human spermatozoa is associated with membrane phosphatidylserine externalization and not DNA fragmentation. J Androl 2001; 22: 646

166. Oehninger S, et al. Effects of hydrogen peroxide on human spermatozoa. J Assist Reprod Genet 1995; 12: 41

167. Barroso G, et al. Mitochondrial membrane potential integrity and plasma membrane translocation of phosphatidylserine: a comparison of subpopulations of sperm with high and low motility from men consulting for infertility. Fertil Steril 2006; 85: 149

168. Ahmadi A, Ng SC. Destruction of protamine in human sperm inhibits sperm binding and penetration in the zona-free hamster penetration test but increases sperm head decondensation and male pronuclear formation in the hamster-ICSI assay. J Assist Reprod Genet 1999; 16: 128

169. Ahmadi A, Ng SC. Developmental capacity of damaged spermatozoa. Hum Reprod 1999; 14: 2279

170. Ahmadi A, Ng SC. Influence of sperm plasma membrane destruction on human sperm head

decondensation and pronuclear formation. Arch Androl 1999; 42: 1

171. Ahmadi A, Ng SC. Fertilizing ability of DNA-damaged spermatozoa. J Exp Zool 1999; 284: 696

172. Poccia D. Remodeling of nucleoproteins during gametogenesis, fertilization, and early development. Int Rev Cytol 1986; 105: 1

173. Evenson DP, Darzynkiewicz Z, Relamed MR. Relation of mammalian sperm chromatin heterogeneity to fertility. Science 1980; 210: 1131

174. Bianchi PG, et al. Effect of deoxyribonucleic acid protamination on fluorochrome staining and in situ nick-translation of murine and human mature spermatozoa. Biol Reprod 1993; 49: 1083

175. Sun JG, Jurisicova A, Casper RF. Detection of deoxyribonucleic acid fragmentation in human sperm: correlation with fertilization in vitro. Biol Reprod 1997; 56: 602

176. McPherson SM, Longo FJ. Nicking of rat spermatid and spermatozoa DNA: possible involvement of DNA topoisomerase II. Dev Biol 1993; 158: 122

177. McPherson S, Longo FJ. Chromatin structure–function alterations during mammalian spermatogenesis: DNA nicking and repair in elongating spermatids. Eur J Histochem 1993; 37: 109

178. Sakkas D, et al. Relationship between the presence of endogenous nicks and sperm chromatin packaging in maturing and fertilizing mouse spermatozoa. Biol Reprod 1995; 52: 1149

179. Chen JL, Longo FJ. Expression and localization of DNA topoisomerase II during rat spermatogenesis. Mol Reprod Dev 1996; 45: 61

180. Duran EH, et al. A logistic regression model including DNA status and morphology of spermatozoa for prediction of fertilization in vitro. Hum Reprod 1998; 13: 1235

181. Larson KL, et al. Sperm chromatin structure assay parameters as predictors of failed pregnancy following assisted reproductive techniques. Hum Reprod 2000; 15: 1717

182. Chan PJ, et al. A simple comet assay for archived sperm correlates DNA fragmentation to reduced hyperactivation and penetration of zona-free hamster oocytes. Fertil Steril 2001; 75: 186

183. Tomlinson MJ, et al. Interrelationships between seminal parameters and sperm nuclear DNA damage before and after density gradient centrifugation: implications for assisted conception. Hum Reprod 2001; 16: 2160

184. De Rycke M, Liebaers I, Van Steirteghem A. Epigenetic risks related to assisted reproductive technologies: risk analysis and epigenetic inheritance. Hum Reprod 2002; 17: 2487

185. Gosden R, et al. Rare congenital disorders, imprinted genes, and assisted reproductive technology. Lancet 2003; 361: 1975

186. Bartolomei MS, Tilghman SM. Genomic imprinting in mammals. Annu Rev Genet 1997; 31: 493

187. Barlow DP. Gametics imprinting in mammals. Science 1995; 270: 1610

188. Jaenisch R. DNA methylation and imprinting: why bother? Trends Genet 1997; 13: 323

189. Shemer R, et al. Dynamic methylation adjustment and counting as part of imprinting mechanisms. Proc Natl Acad Sci USA 1996; 93: 6371

190. Santos F, Dean W. Epigenetic reprogramming during early development in mammals. Reproduction 2004; 127: 643

191. Lucifero D, Chaillet JR, Trasler JM. Potential significance of genomic imprinting defects for reproduction and assisted reproductive technology. Hum Reprod Update 2004; 10: 3

5

Genome architecture in human sperm cells: possible implications for male infertility and prediction of pregnancy outcome

Olga Mudrak, Andrei Zalensky

INTRODUCTION

Infertility and birth defects are often the result of chromosomal abnormalities in gametes[1–3], with more than 80% of cases being paternally derived[4]. The development of multicolor fluorescence *in situ* hybridization (FISH) has allowed detection and analysis of several types of chromosomal defects in sperm, such as aneuploidies, partial chromosomal duplications, deletions and inversions, translocations and chromosomal breaks[2,5–7].

While there is consensus concerning a strong correlation between sperm chromosomal abnormalities and male infertility, the analysis of such abnormalities does not guarantee the selection of a 'good spermatozoon' without chromosomal defects, especially if intracytoplasmic sperm injection (ICSI) is performed for male factor infertility. There is no doubt that ICSI can enable men with severely impaired sperm to overcome naturally existing barriers to fertilization, yet in doing so it increases the possibility of transmitting genetic defects to the offspring. For example, it was demonstrated that oligozoospermic men carry a higher burden of transmissible chromosome damage[8]. A common attitude is emerging that detailed molecular cytogenetic tests should be performed on sperm samples from men with abnormal fertility before the execution of ICSI[9–11]. Here, we put forward a hypothesis that yet another previously unattended class of sperm chromosome abnormalities may have an impact on fertilization and early development. These aberrations are connected with chromosome packaging and the higher-order chromosome architecture in sperm nuclei.

GENOME ARCHITECTURE

More than a century ago, Rabl and Boveri proposed the existence of spatial order within the cell nucleus, which is manifested in the preservation of distinct individuality chromosomes in interphase[12,13]. Nevertheless, until recently, the view prevailed that interphase chromosomes were chromatin 'spaghetti' floating randomly in the nucleoplasm[14]. According to the modern assumption, the ordered and dynamic global architecture of interphase chromosomes exists, and is involved in a variety of nuclear functions (for recent reviews see references 15 and 16).

This view resulted from a major breakthrough in the elucidation of chromosome organization that became possible because of FISH techniques, the development of instrumentation for microscopy and completion of the Human Genome Project. The central postulate of this concept is chromosome territorial organization. Interphase chromosomes occupy distinct non-overlapping intranuclear volumes called chromosome territories (CTs)[16,17]. We refer here to the higher-order spatial arrangement of CTs within the nuclear volume as genome architecture (GA).

Two major characteristics of GA may be distinguished[18]: chromosome positioning (spatial localization of chromosomes relative to each other or to defined nuclear structures), and chromosome path (chromosome trajectory within nuclei). It appears that intranuclear positioning of CTs in interphase is non-random[19]. The spatial positioning of a chromosome relative to the center of the nucleus is defined as radial positioning[20–22]. A number of studies indicate that gene-rich chromosomes are located closer to the nuclear center, while gene-poor chromosomes are preferentially found at the nuclear periphery[23,24]. In addition to the radial positioning, chromosomes may be localized non-randomly with respect to each other[21,25]. For example, some authors declare fixed, deliberate chromosome positioning in the prometaphase ring[26,27], while another study did not establish such an order in relative chromosome position[28]. Therefore, this issue is controversial.

While dynamic changes in the relative spatial grouping of chromosome domains have been observed during cell-cycle progression, differentiation and malignant transformation[29–31], the internal organization of CTs is still largely unknown. Recent studies indicate a relationship between the nuclear arrangement of CTs and the G–R-banding patterns of mitotic chromosomes[32]. In interphase nuclei, the R-band sequences, which are enriched in constitutively expressed housekeeping genes, are directed towards the nuclear interior. Current studies are focused on elucidation of the higher-order chromatin structures/ chromosome paths within CTs[33] and relative spatial arrangement of individual CTs[34].

Chromosome territories and chromosome architecture in sperm cells

The sperm cell is a highly differentiated cell type, which results from the specialized genetic and morphological process of spermatogenesis. During postmeiotic stages (spermiogenesis), the somatic histones are gradually replaced with protamines[35,36]. Consequently, the chromatin structure is reorganized, DNA becomes supercondensed and genetic activity is completely shut down[37,38]. For a long time, biological functions of this remodeling have been considered limited to the creation of a compact hydrodynamically efficient nuclear shape, with inert DNA fairly well protected from the environment. Therefore, the spermatozoon nucleus has been perceived as a 'sac' of genes that are to be transferred to an egg.

Contrary to this point of view, specific and non-random chromosome architecture has recently been demonstrated for human sperm cells. In these studies, selected DNA sequences and chromosomal proteins were localized by FISH and immunocytochemistry followed by epifluorescent or laser scanning confocal microscopy. Several elements of GA in human sperm have been established:

- Similar to somatic cells, individual chromosomes occupy distinct territories[39–41] (Figure 5.1a).

- Each chromosome has a preferred intranuclear localization (position), and the relative positioning of chromosomes is non-random[42–46].

- Centromeres (CEN) belonging to non-homologous chromosomes are collected into a compact chromocenter buried within a nuclear volume[41,47,48] (Figure 5.1b).

- Telomeres (TEL) are localized at the nuclear periphery where they interact in the form of dimers and tetramers[44,49,50] (Figure 5.1c).

- Telomere dimers correspond to the contacts between two ends of one chromosome rather than random association between chromosomal ends, and therefore chromosomes in sperm are looped[51,52] (Figure 5.1d and e).

Based on the acquired data, a general model for GA in human sperm has been proposed (Figure 5.1f).

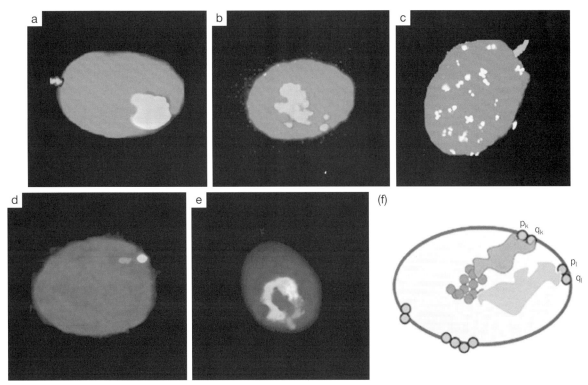

Figure 5.1   Chromosome organization in human sperm. (a) Chromosome territory: chromosome 6 (CHR6) (green) was localized using a painting probe. Total DNA counterstained with propidium iodide (PI) (red). (b) Centromeres (green) were visualized using immunofluorescence with antibodies against CENP-A (centromere protein A). Total DNA counterstained with PI (red). (c) Fluorescence *in situ* hybridization (FISH) using TTAGGG probe (yellow/green) shows that the majority of telomeres are joined as dimers and tetramers. Total DNA counterstained with PI (red). (d) Subtelomeric sequences located at the p and q arms of chromosome 3 (subTEL3q, pink; subTEL3p, emerald) are spatially close. Total DNA counterstained with diamidino-2-phenylindole (DAPI) (blue). (e) FISH using arm-specific probes microdissected from CHR1 (1q, green; 1p, red) indicates looping of this chromosome. Total DNA counterstained with DAPI (blue). (f) Schematic model of sperm nuclear architecture. Selected chromosome territories (pink and ocher), telomeres (TEL) (green circles) and centromeres (CEN) (red circles) are shown within a section through the nucleus. Non-homologous CEN are clustered into a chromocenter, while TEL interact at the nuclear periphery. Modified from Ward and Zalensky 1996 (reference 38). See also Color plate 1 on page xxv

SPERM NUCLEAR STATUS AND MALE INFERTILITY

Annually in the USA, more than 2 million conceptions are lost before the 20th week of gestation, and approximately half of these carry chromosomal defects such as numerical abnormalities, breaks/rearrangements and mutations[1,53]. Biochemical and FISH-based diagnostic procedures for detection of these chromosomal defects in germ-line cells and early embryos are either currently set up or being developed[54–58].

Defective fertilization and/or early development may also be a consequence of abnormal DNA packaging in gamete nuclei. While structural organization of DNA in oocytes is poorly studied, it is generally accepted that a significant fraction of infertile males produce sperm with malformations in spermatozoa nuclei or chromatin defects. Among these are deficiencies in basic chromosomal proteins[59,60], or broadly instituted chromatin condensation defects[61–64]. The latter defects have been determined using cytochemical and electron microscopy methods, while the molecular basis of flawed nuclear organization has remained unidentified. Male-factor infertility is a heterogeneous disorder, and the abnormalities in sperm chromatin/nuclear organization are most probably complex and diverse. In the following sections, we provide a few examples of nuclear aberrations that are connected with sperm genome architecture. We use for illustration sperm samples obtained from patients undergoing treatment in the fertility clinic. Comprehensive semen analysis indicated normal sperm count and motility but significantly abnormal sperm morphology (e.g. presence of round or torpedoid cells). Physical examination of the patients failed to reveal any abnormalities, including varicocele.

COMPACTNESS OF CHROMOSOME TERRITORY

In 95% of sperm cells of fertile donors, FISH signals obtained using whole-chromosome painting probes (Figure 5.2a) or a combination of p and q arm-specific painting probes (Figure 5.2b) were confined to relatively small areas, and had sharp chromosome territory (CT) contours. Thus, FISH detects tightly packed, compact CTs formed by closely located p and q arms. The CT in normal sperm is approximately four times more condensed than the metaphase chromosome, and therefore is much more condensed than the interphase CT.

In sperm of some patients with idiopathic infertility (three of the ten studied), abnormal hybridization patterns were observed (Figure 5.2c). In more detail, 42% of cells in sample P44 and 36% in P09 had large and diffuse signals; 27% of cells in sample P12 had multiple signals. The hybridization picture indicates that sperm in samples P44 and P09 may have had lesions in the formation of chromosome higher-order structures. Sperm of patient P12 may have had aneuploidy of chromosome 1 and/or large-scale rearrangement in its DNA (Figure 5.2 right hand panels.

CHROMOSOME POSITIONING

Determination of the intranuclear chromosome position in human sperm is possible because these cells have a non-symmetrical elongated shape, and the site of tail attachment may easily be used as a spatial reference point[46]. Nevertheless, only a few studies in this direction have been performed so far. FISH using painting probes indicated that chromosome X[43,44,46] and chromosome 6[46] were preferentially located in the anterior part of sperm nuclei, chromosome 18, near the sperm tail[43], while chromosome 13 seemed to be randomly positioned[44]. In recent work, we found that in 90% of cells, chromosome 1 was located in the apical half of the nucleus, and 80% of chromosome 2 and 85% of chromosome 5 were preferentially located in the basal half[52]. Using another approach, FISH with chromosome-specific centromere probes, preferential intranuclear positioning was shown for chromosomes 2, 6, 7, 16, 17, X and Y[46].

In the examples provided in Figure 5.2d–f, we traced the positioning of chromosomes by localization of FISH signals resulting from hybridization with DNA chromosomepainting probes. For each nucleus the position of chromosomes was assigned to a particular nuclear sector, I–IV, as illustrated in Figure 5.2d. About 100 nuclei from each sperm sample were analyzed, and the location of CTs is presented using diagrams of spatial distribution (Figure 5.2e and f). Figure 5.2e demonstrates that in sperm from fertile donors, chromosome 6 had a tendency towards more anterior localization compared with chromosome 1, and both were rarely found in the posterior half of the nucleus.

We also compared the position of chromosome 1 within nuclei of normal sperm and sperm of infertile patient P44. Figure 5.2f shows that the nuclear position of this chromosome in the infertile sperm sample was less confined. This might be a result of improper packaging, as noted above, and/or of an aberration in unknown mechanism(s) governing non-random chromosome localization.

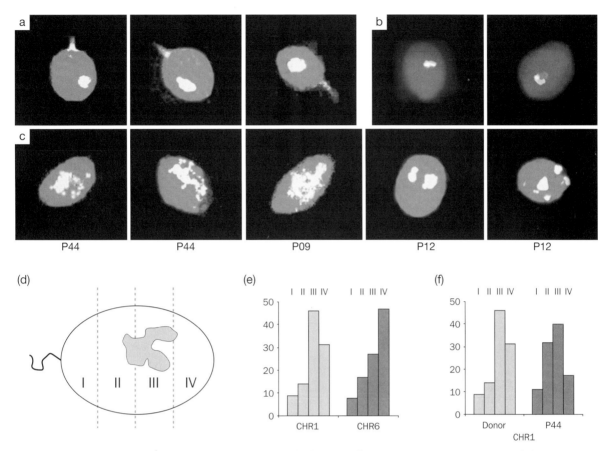

Figure 5.2 Determination of chromosome intranuclear localization using fluorescence *in situ* hybridization (FISH) with painting probes. (a) Typical patterns of chromosome 1 (CHR1) painting probe hybridization (yellow) in normal sperm. (b) Typical patterns of CHR1 arm-specific probe hybridization (1p, green; 1q, red) in normal sperm. (c) Patterns of CHR1 hybridization in three samples of abnormal sperm. (d) Schematic example of CHR territory position in a sectioned sperm nucleus. (e) Charts showing distribution of CHR1 and CHR6 localization within sectors I–IV (percentage of hits to a sector from total FISH signals analyzed). (f) Comparison of nuclear positioning of CHR1 in normal and abnormal sperm cells. See also Color plate 3 on page xxvi

TELOMERE LOCALIZATION

Localization of telomere repeat sequences $(TTAGGG)_N$ in human sperm reveals that most, if not all, telomeres are joined in dimers and tetramers (Figures 5.1c and 5.3a)[49]. As a result, on a frequency distribution plot (Figure 5.3c), the majority of nuclei fall into two peaks: the first corresponds to 12 hybridization loci (TEL tetramers), and the second to 24 loci (TEL dimers). In the absence of telomere–telomere interactions in human sperm, 46 hybridization signals (2 telomeres×23 chromosomes) should be observed.

We compared the localization of telomeres in sperm between donors and patients (total 20 patients) (Figure 5.3). Three sperm samples obtained from infertile males showed strikingly different telomere localizations. In the majority of cells, hybridization was in numerous small dots dispersed over the nucleus (Figure 5.3b). As a result, no telomere grouping was seen in the frequency distribution plot (Figure 5.3c). Such localization reflects the absence of telomere–telomere interactions, which are characteristic of normal human sperm. The molecular basis of this phenotype is unknown. Atypical sperm telomere-binding

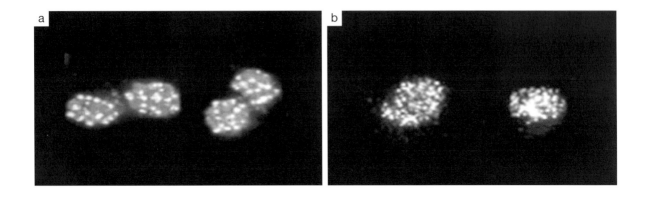

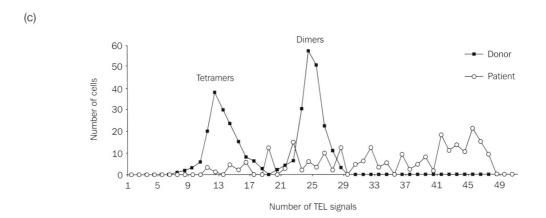

Figure 5.3   Comparison of nuclear localization of telomeres in normal and abnormal cells. (a) Telomeres are joined as dimers and tetramers in normal sperm. (b) Telomere hybridization appears as numerous small dots dispersed over the nucleus in abnormal sperm cells. (c) Frequency of telomere (TEL) hybridization signal distribution in sperm cells determined by fluorescence *in situ* hybridization (FISH). In the majority of normal sperm cells, the number of TEL hybridization signals peaks at 24 (TEL dimers) and 12 (TEL tetramers)

proteins[65] or aberrant telomere DNA may be involved.

GENOME ARCHITECTURE AND UNPACKING OF SPERM GENOME DURING FERTILIZATION

Data above were obtained using small, random selections of patients with idiopathic male infertility. Nevertheless, they clearly illustrate the existence of three categories of deviations from the standard genome architecture characteristic of sperm cells: (1) atypical packing of chromosome territories, (2) unstable or aberrant nuclear positioning of chromosomes and (3) disturbed telomere interactions. What are the possible effects of such faults on successful fertilization and early development?

Normal mammalian embryogenesis requires the participation of both a maternal and a paternal genome[66]. Genetically inert chromatin of the spermatozoa is remodeled into the decondensed and transcriptionally competent chromatin of the male pronucleus upon entry into the ooplasm; this remodeling is controlled by an oocyte activity that appears during meiotic maturation[67]. Reorganization of the sperm genome after fertilization is a complex process that involves chromosome withdrawal from the nucleus, their decoration with histones (decondensation), formation of the male pronucleus and its movement towards the female pronucleus[68,69]. Exchange of the basic chromosomal proteins involves chaperones of the nucleoplasmin family[70]. Overall, the molecular characterization of participants responsible for pronucleus development is at an early stage. While the activity of sperm chromosome remodeling is of maternal origin, the structural organization and biochemical composition of sperm nuclei are equally important. Improperly packed and spatially unorganized sperm chromosomes will have a high probability of being inadequately processed by egg cytoplasm.

Transcription is influenced by the underlying chromatin structure, including the organization of chromosome territories[71], and therefore activation of the male genome will depend on the specific sperm GA. Recent data show that in mammals, transcription begins earlier than in zygotes from other classes of organisms, starting several hours after fertilization in male pronuclei and continuing in embryonic nuclei[72–74]. Hence, it is highly probable that *abnormal genome architecture in sperm (or undeveloped GA in immature gametes) may cause irregularities in early development.* In addition, since paternal and maternal genomes are spatially separated up to the 4-cell embryo stage, chromatin remodeling after fertilization occurs in separate nuclear compartments and consequently may be regulated in a parent-specific manner[75].

The data overviewed above indicate that each chromosome in human sperm has a preferential intranuclear position. Since, during normal fertilization, sperm penetration begins with the acrosome, there is a sequential order of exposure of sperm chromosomes to the egg cytoplasm during sperm entry. Therefore, a predetermined order of chromosome activation induced by chromatin remodeling by egg factors may exist. We propose that *deviation from regular sperm chromosome localization may be deleterious for proper fertilization and development.*

It is noteworthy that, in all mammals, sex chromosomes are located in the region nearest to the acrosome, and are presumably the first chromosomes to enter the egg on fertilization[76]. Such a position has been preserved between monotreme and marsupial mammals, which diverged from eutherian mammals 170 and 130 million years ago, respectively[77]. This strongly supports the hypothesis of a functional significance of the intranuclear localization of sperm chromosomes.

While modern clinical assisted reproductive technologies broadly use intracytoplasmic injection using sperm and occasionally even immature gametes, the molecular/cellular mechanisms of fertilization after ISCI have been poorly studied[78]. Some publications have reported an increased rate of *de novo* chromosomal anomalies in human babies following ICSI[79]. Importantly, in several species, delayed decondensation of the apical region of the sperm nucleus and postponed replication of the male genome after ICSI were observed[43,80–82]. Immunofluorescent analysis showed that the perinuclear theca of sperm persisted around the condensed apical portion following ICSI, whereas it was removed completely from the sperm nucleus after *in vitro* insemination[80]. The presence of sex chromosomes in the condensed apical region of the sperm nucleus might lead to sex chromosomal anomalies, introducing the delay of S-phase entry.

In particular, this atypical decondensation may unbalance normal remodeling of sex chromosomes (e.g. introducing delay of their entry to the S-phase, or gene activation), which are located in this region of the nucleus. Therefore, an ICSI procedure itself may lead to birth defects because of improper processing of a well-defined GA characteristic of normal sperm.

Examples provided above (Figure 5.3) show disturbed localization of telomeres and telomere–telomere interactions in sperm from patients with idiopathic infertility. In human sperm, the telomere chromosomal domain is characterized by elongated DNA (in comparison with somatic cells) and sperm-specific telomeric proteins[49,83,84]. The elongation of telomere DNA during spermatogenesis is characteristic of all mammals[85], and is provided by telomerase, a specific reverse transcriptase, which is highly active in germline cells[86,87]. In the mouse, the fertilization of oocytes with sperm obtained from telomerase knock-out males resulted in aberrant cleavage and development[88]. These results suggest that the state of telomere DNA in sperm contributes to defective fertilization and cleavage. Currently there are no equivalent data obtained in humans. Nevertheless, we propose a general hypothesis that telomeres in human spermatozoa have unique molecular and structural features critical for function during fertilization and early embryonic development. Experiments to characterize telomeres in infertile patients are under way in our laboratory.

ACKNOWLEDGMENTS

This work was supported by a National Institutes of Health (NIH) grant HD-042748 to one of the authors (AZ).

REFERENCES

1. McFadden DE, Friedman JM. Chromosome abnormalities in human beings. Mutat Res 1997; 396: 129
2. Sloter E, et al. Effects of male age on the frequencies of germinal and heritable chromosomal abnormalities in humans and rodents. Fertil Steril 2004; 81: 925
3. Perreault SD, et al. Integrating new tests of sperm genetic integrity into semen analysis: breakout group discussion. Adv Exp Med Biol 2003; 518: 253
4. Chandley AC. On the parental origin of de novo mutation in man. J Med Gene 1991; 28: 217
5. Shi Q, Martin RH. Aneuploidy in human spermatozoa: FISH analysis in men with constitutional chromosomal abnormalities, and in infertile men. Reproduction 2001; 121: 655
6. Egozcue J, et al. Genetic analysis of sperm and implications of severe male infertility. Placenta 2003; 24: 62
7. Tempest HG, Griffin DK. The relationship between male infertility and increased levels of sperm disomy. Cytogenet Genome Res 2004; 107: 83
8. Schmidt E, et al. Detection of structural and numerical chromosomal abnormalities by ACM-FISH analysis in sperm of oligozoospermic infertility patients. Hum Reprod 2004; 19: 1395
9. Petit FM, et al. Could sperm aneuploidy rate determination be used as a predictive test before intracytoplasmic sperm injection? J Androl 2005; 26: 235
10. Foresta C, et al. Genetic abnormalities among severely oligospermic men who are candidates for intracytoplasmic sperm injection. J Clin Endocrinol Metab 2005; 90: 152
11. Pang MG, et al. The high incidence of meiotic errors increases with decreased sperm count in severe male factor infertilities. Mol Vis 2005; 11: 152
12. Rabl C. Ueber Zelltheilung [On cell division]. Morphol Jahrbuch 1895; 10: 214
13. Boveri T. Die blastomerenkerne von Ascaris megalocephala und die Theorie der Chromosomenindividualitat [The blastomere nucleus of Ascaris megalocephala and the theory of chromosome individuality on cell division]. Arch Zellforsch 1909; 3: 181
14. Marshall WF. Order and disorder in the nucleus. Curr Biol 2002; 12: 185
15. Taddei A, et al. The function of nuclear architecture: a genetic approach. Annu Rev Genet 2004; 38: 305
16. Cremer T, et al. Higher order chromatin architecture in the cell nucleus: on the way from structure to function. Biol Cell 2004; 96: 555
17. Cremer T, Cremer C. Chromosome territories, nuclear architecture and gene regulation in mammalian cells. Nat Rev Genet 2001; 2: 292
18. Zalensky AO. Genome architecture. In Verma RS, ed. Advances in Genome Biology. Greenwich, London: JAI Press, 1998: 179
19. Cremer M, et al. Inheritance of gene density-related higher order chromatin arrangements in normal and tumor cell nuclei. J Cell Biol 2003; 162: 809
20. Cremer M, et al. Non-random radial higher-order chromatin arrangements in nuclei of diploid human cells. Chromosome Res 2001; 9: 541
21. Parada L, Misteli T. Chromosome positioning in the interphase nucleus. Trends Cell Biol 2002; 12: 425
22. Kozubek S, et al. 3D structure of the human genome: order in randomness. Chromosoma 2002; 111: 321
23. Boyle S, et al. The spatial organization of human chromosomes within the nuclei of normal and emerin-mutant cells. Hum Mol Genet 2001; 10: 211
24. Croft JA, et al. Differences in the localization and morphology of chromosomes in the human nucleus. J Cell Biol 1999; 145: 1119

25. Parada LA, et al. Conservation of relative chromosome positioning in normal and cancer cells. Curr Biol 2002; 12: 1692

26. Leitch A, et al. The spatial localization of homologous chromosomes in human fibroblasts at mitosis. Hum Genet 1994; 93: 275

27. Nagele R, et al. Precise spatial positioning of chromosomes during prometaphase: evidence for chromosome order. Science 1995; 270: 1831

28. Allison DC, Nestor AL. Evidence for a relatively random array of human chromosomes on the mitotic ring. J Cell Biol 1999; 145: 1

29. Manuelidis L. Indications of centromere movement during interphase and differentiation. Ann NY Acad Sci 1985; 450: 205

30. Neves H, et al. The nuclear topography of ABL, BCR, PML, and RAR alpha genes: evidence for gene proximity in specific phases of the cell cycle and stages of hematopoietic differentiation. Blood 1999; 93: 1197

31. Bridger JM, et al. Re-modelling of nuclear architecture in quiescent and senescent human fibroblasts. Curr Biol 2000; 10: 149

32. Sadoni N, et al. Nuclear organization of mammalian genomes. Polar chromosome territories build up functionally distinct higher order compartments. J Cell Biol 1999; 146: 1211

33. Stadler S, et al. The architecture of chicken chromosome territories changes during differentiation. BMC Cell Biol 2004; 5: 44

34. Parada LA, et al. Tissue-specific spatial organization of genomes. Genome Biol 2004; 5: R44

35. Meistrich M. Histone and basic nuclear protein transitions in mammalian spermatogenesis. In Hnilica LS, Stein GS, Stein JL, eds. Histones and Other Basic Nuclear Proteins. Boca Raton, FL: CRC Press, 1989: 165

36. Churikov D, et al. Male germline-specific histones in mouse and man. Cytogenet Genome Res 2004; 105: 203

37. Balhorn R. A model for the structure of chromatin in mammalian sperm. J Cell Biol 1982; 93: 298

38. Ward WS, Zalensky AO. The unique, complex organization of the transcriptionally silent sperm chromatin. Crit Rev Eukaryot Gene Expr 1996; 6: 139

39. Brandriff BF, Gordon LA. Spatial distribution of sperm-derived chromatin in zygotes determined by fluorescence in situ hybridization. Mutat Res 1992; 296: 33

40. Haaf T, Ward DC. Higher order nuclear structure in mammalian sperm revealed by in situ hybridization

and extended chromatin fibers. Exp Cell Res 1995; 219: 604

41. Zalensky AO, et al. Well-defined genome architecture in the human sperm nucleus. Chromosoma 1995; 103: 577

42. Geraedts JP, Pearson PL. Spatial distribution of chromosomes 1 and Y in human spermatozoa. J Reprod Fertil 1975; 45: 515

43. Luetjens CM, et al. Non-random chromosome positioning in human sperm and sex chromosome anomalies following intracytoplasmic sperm injection. Lancet 1999; 353: 1240

44. Hazzouri M, et al. Genome organization in the human sperm nucleus studied by FISH and confocal microscopy. Mol Reprod Dev 2000; 55: 307

45. Tilgen N, et al. Heterochromatin is not an adequate explanation for close proximity of interphase chromosomes 1-Y, 9-Y, and 16-Y in human spermatozoa. Exp Cell Res 2001; 265: 283

46. Zalenskaya IA, Zalensky AO. Non-random positioning of chromosomes in human sperm nuclei. Chromosome Res 2004; 12: 163

47. Zalensky AO, et al. Organization of centromeres in the decondensed nuclei of mature human sperm. Chromosoma 1993; 102: 509

48. Hoyer-Fender S, et al. The murine heterochromatin protein M31 is associated with the chromocenter in round spermatids and is a component of mature spermatozoa. Exp Cell Res 2000; 254: 72

49. Zalensky AO, et al. Telomere–telomere interactions and candidate telomere binding protein(s) in mammalian sperm cells. Exp Cell Res 1997; 232: 29

50. Meyer-Ficca M, et al. Clustering of pericentromeres initiates in step 9 of spermiogenesis of the rat (Rattus norvegicus) and contributes to a well defined genome architecture in the sperm nucleus. J Cell Sci 1998; 111: 1363

51. Solov'eva L, et al. Nature of telomere dimers and chromosome looping in human spermatozoa. Chromosome Res 2004; 12: 817

52. Mudrak OS, et al. Chromosome architecture in the human sperm nucleus. J Cell Sci 2005; 118: 4541

53. Wyrobek AJ. Methods and concepts in detecting abnormal reproductive outcomes of paternal origin. Reprod Toxicol 1993; 7: 3

54. Sloter ED, et al. Multicolor FISH analysis of chromosomal breaks, duplications, deletions, and numerical abnormalities in the sperm of healthy men. Am J Hum Genet 2000; 67: 862

55. Fung J, et al. Detection of structural and numerical chromosome abnormalities in interphase cells using

spectral imaging. J Histochem Cytochem 2001; 49: 797

56. Plachot M. Genetic analysis of the oocyte – a review. Placenta 2003; 24: 66

57. Evenson DP, et al. Sperm chromatin structure assay: its clinical use for detecting sperm DNA fragmentation in male infertility and comparisons with other techniques. J Androl 2002; 23: 25

58. Virro MR, et al. Sperm chromatin structure assay (SCSA) parameters are related to fertilization, blastocyst development, and ongoing pregnancy in in vitro fertilization and intracytoplasmic sperm injection cycles. Fertil Steril 2004; 81: 1289

59. Bench G, et al. Protein and DNA contents in sperm from an infertile human male possessing protamine defects that vary over time. Mol Reprod Dev 1998; 50: 345

60. De Yebra L, et al. Complete selective absence of protamine P2 in humans. J Biol Chem 1993; 268: 10553

61. Francavilla S, et al. Chromatin defects in normal and malformed human ejaculated and epididymal spermatozoa: a cytochemical ultrastructural study. J Reprod Fertil 1996; 106: 259

62. Francavilla S, et al. Ultrastructural analysis of chromatin defects in testicular spermatids in azoospermic men submitted to TESE–ICSI. Hum Reprod 2001; 16: 1440

63. Sakkas D, et al. Sperm nuclear DNA damage and altered chromatin structure: effect on fertilization and embryo development. Hum Reprod 1998; 13: 11

64. Bianchi PG, et al. Chromatin packaging and morphology in ejaculated human spermatozoa: evidence of hidden anomalies in normal spermatozoa. Mol Hum Reprod 1996; 2: 139

65. Gineitis AA, et al. Histone H2B variant is a part of the telomere-binding complex that secures telomere membrane attachment in human sperm. J Cell Biol 2000; 151: 1591

66. Hall JG. Genomic imprinting: nature and clinical relevance. Annu Rev Med 1997; 48: 35

67. McLay DW, Clarke HJ. Remodelling the paternal chromatin at fertilization in mammals. Reproduction 2003; 125: 625

68. Wright SJ. Sperm nuclear activation during fertilization. Curr Top Dev Biol 1999; 46: 133

69. Sutovsky P, Schatten G. Paternal contributions to the mammalian zygote: fertilization after sperm–egg fusion. Int Rev Cytol 2000; 5: 1

70. Burns KH, et al. Roles of NPM2 in chromatin and nucleolar organization in oocytes and embryos. Science 2003; 300: 633

71. Gilbert N, et al. Chromatin organization in the mammalian nucleus. Int Rev Cytol 2005; 242: 283

72. Bouniol-Baly C, et al. Dynamic organization of DNA replication in one-cell mouse embryos: relationship to transcriptional activation. Exp Cell Res 1997; 236: 201

73. Aoki F, et al. Regulation of transcriptional activity during the first and second cell cycles in the preimplantation mouse embryo. Dev Biol 1997; 181: 296

74. Capco DG. Molecular and biochemical regulation of early mammalian development. Int Rev Cytol 2001; 207: 195

75. Mayer W, et al. Spatial separation of parental genomes in preimplantation mouse embryos. J Cell Biol 2000; 148: 629

76. Greaves IK, et al. Conservation of chromosome arrangement and position of the X in mammalian sperm suggests functional significance. Chromosome Res 2003; 11: 503

77. Kirsch JAW, et al. DNA-hybridisation studies of marsupials and their implications for metatherian classification. Aust J Zool 1997; 45: 211

78. Schatten G, et al. Cell and molecular biological challenges of ICSI: ART before science? J Law Med Ethics 1998; 26: 29

79. Bonduelle M, et al. Seven years of intracytoplasmic sperm injection and follow-up of 1987 subsequent children. Hum Reprod 1999; 14: 243

80. Sutovsky P, et al. Intracytoplasmic sperm injection for rhesus monkey fertilization results in unusual chromatin, cytoskeletal, and membrane events, but eventually leads to pronuclear development and sperm aster assembly. Hum Reprod 1996; 11: 1703

81. Hewitson L, et al. Unique checkpoints during the first cell cycle of fertilization after intracytoplasmic sperm injection in rhesus monkeys. Nat Med 1999; 5: 431

82. Terada Y, et al. Atypical decondensation of the sperm nucleus, delayed replication of the male genome, and sex chromosome positioning following intracytoplasmic human sperm injection (ICSI) into golden hamster eggs: does ICSI itself introduce chromosomal anomalies? Fertil Steril 2000; 74: 454

83. Zalenskaya IA, Bradbury EM, Zalensky AO. Chromatin structure of telomere domain in human sperm. Biochem Biophys Res Commun 2000; 279: 213

84. Bekaert S, et al. Telomere biology in mammalian germ cells and during development. Dev Biol 2004; 274: 15

85. Kozik A, et al. Identification and characterization of a bovine sperm protein that binds specifically to

single-stranded telomeric deoxyribonucleic acid. Biol Reprod 2000; 62: 340

86. Kim NW, et al. Specific association of human telomerase activity with immortal cells and cancer. Science 1994; 266: 2011

87. Achi MV, et al. Telomere length in male germ cells is inversely correlated with telomerase activity. Biol Reprod 2000; 63: 591

88. Liu L, et al. An essential role for functional telomeres in mouse germ cells during fertilization and early development. Dev Biol 2002; 249: 74

6

Sperm pathology: pathogenic mechanisms and fertility potential in assisted reproduction

Hector E Chemes, Vanesa Y Rawe

INTRODUCTION

Teratozoospermia, asthenozoospermia and necro-zoospermia are frequently responsible for infertility in men, and have a negative influence on the fertility prognosis when assisted reproductive technologies (ART), including *in vitro* fertilization (IVF), are attempted. The introduction of intra-cytoplasmic sperm injection (ICSI) allowed examination of the motility and morphology of the very same spermatozoon that was to be micro-injected. It then became clear that abnormal and immotile spermatozoa could successfully fertilize oocytes, and the issue of the convenience of using them in ART procedures was raised. Some androl-ogists have stressed the importance of using different tools to characterize sperm pathologies and establish a diagnosis; still others have been more inclined to use spermatozoa in ICSI without paying much attention to the nature of the pathologies involved.

Sperm morphology, the subject of numerous studies, has been subjectively assessed or charac-terized by manual or computer-assisted objective methods[1–3]. Strict criteria for sperm classification have been introduced, and a correlation between sperm morphology and prognosis in ART has received general acceptance[4,5]. In all of these methods, the morphometric parameters of the sperm head, middle piece and flagellum have been analyzed in detail with the light microscope, which allows detailed observation of the external profile of the spermatozoon but does not give information on its internal structure. The combi-nation of high-resolution light and electron microscopy, immunocytochemistry and molecular studies has provided new insights into the struc-ture of normal and abnormal spermatozoa, and defined the subcellular basis of sperm aberrations.

Furthermore, correlation of these data with rel-evant clinical and fertility information has shed new light on this field. This approach goes beyond descriptive morphology of *the appearance* of sper-matozoa. Several important questions remain. What is it that impairs sperm function in mor-phologically abnormal sperm? *What is wrong with a wrong sperm shape? What hides behind the head-shape change in amorphous or tapering spermatozoa?* Is it just the abnormal shape, or is there something wrong with specific sperm components? *Sperm pathology is the discipline of characterizing struc-tural and functional deficiencies in abnormal sper-matozoa.* This is significant because it helps to explain the mechanisms of sperm inefficiency, identifies genetic phenotypes, suggests strategies to improve fertilization and opens a door to molecular genetic studies that will probably lead to the design of therapeutic tools of the future.

Two main examples of sperm alterations can be distinguished. The most frequent is characterized by a heterogeneous array of sperm anomalies that do not follow a uniform pattern, and demonstrate different combinations in each individual and among different patients. These are non-specific anomalies that are potentially reversible and usually secondary to diverse conditions affecting the reproductive system. The second type is characterized by a well-defined, uniform pattern of anomalies that affect the vast majority of spermatozoa, and present a similar configuration in different patients suffering from the same condition. These alterations are stable in time, do not respond to therapeutic interventions, may display family clustering and have a recognized or presumed genetic origin. Because of these characteristics, these alterations are known as systematic sperm defects.

PATHOLOGICAL SPERM PHENOTYPES ASSOCIATED WITH MOTILITY DISORDERS

To understand fully the physiopathology of asthenozoospermia, it is first necessary to summarize briefly the ultrastructure of the sperm tail. The human sperm flagellum is a long structure, approximately 50 μm in length and 0.4–0.5 μm in diameter. It is composed of a central element, the axoneme, which is a cylinder comprising a circumferential array of nine peripheral microtubular doublets surrounding a central pair of microtubules, the so-called 9 + 2 configuration (Figure 6.1a). Each peripheral doublet is composed of two apposed subunits, microtubules A and B, consisting of protofilaments of tubulin heterodimers. Extending from subunit A, two arms project toward the B subunit of the next doublet. These arms are composed of dynein, a structural protein with adenosine triphosphatase (ATPase) activity that utilizes ATP as an energy source to generate axonemal movement[6,7]. The axoneme is surrounded by the outer dense fibers (ODFs) and the fibrous sheath. The ODFs are nine slender cylindrical structures associated with the corresponding peripheral doublet. The fibrous sheath is a sort of flagellar exoskeleton, present only at the main piece, and organized into two longitudinal columns that run along the length of the principal piece and insert into microtubular pairs 3 and 8. These columns are joined regularly by transverse semicircular ribs.

Asthenozoospermia is a frequent cause of male infertility. Both non-specific and systematic sperm phenotypes can be responsible for alterations in sperm motility.

Non-specific flagellar anomalies (NSFAs) are the underlying cause in most men with severe asthenozoospermia[8–12]. In NSFAs, the normal 9 + 2 organization of the sperm tail is replaced by a combination of modifications in the number, topography and organization of microtubular pairs and periaxonemal structures of the flagellum (Figure 6.1b). Affected flagella appear normal under light microscopy, and are only identified by ultrastructural examination, because their outer diameter and profile are not modified. NSFAs are either idiopathic or secondary to various andrological conditions such as varicocele, infections, immune factor, orchitis and other endogenous or environmental factors. Since these same kinds of anomalies are found in lower numbers in most fertile men, their incidence should be determined in each particular asthenozoospermic patient by means of careful quantification of no less than 100 transverse sections of the sperm tail. We have set the upper normal limit of NSFAs to 40% of the sperm population; values in the 40–60% range are borderline; and above the 60% threshold they are certainly pathological. There is no genetic background in NSFAs which are potentially responsive to etiological or empirical therapeutic interventions. Their prevalence fluctuates during clinical evolution and among different asthenozoospermic men[12–16].

Genetically determined sperm phenotypes causing asthenozoospermia have been the subject of numerous studies since the mid 1970s, when the lack of dynein arms was identified as the main underlying cause of ciliar and flagellar paralysis in men suffering from extreme asthenozoospermia

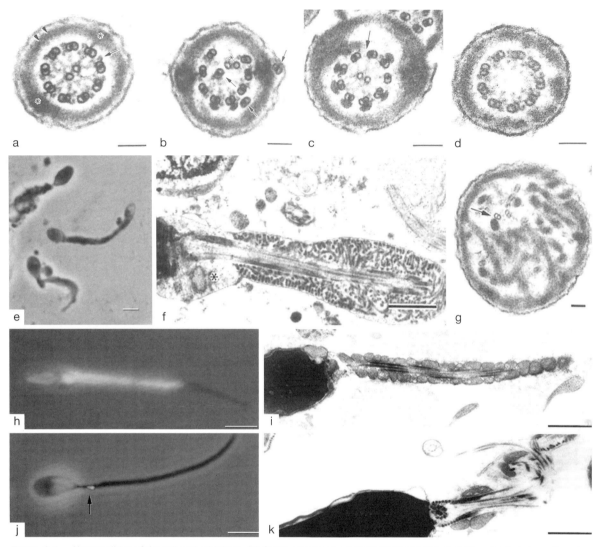

Figure 6.1 Abnormalities of the tail and midpiece. (a) Cross-section of a normal sperm flagellum at the principal piece. The nine peripheral doublets of the axoneme, central pair, dynein arms (arrow) and radial spokes are clearly seen. The fibrous sheath is composed of two lateral columns inserted in doublets 3 and 8 (asterisks) and semicircumferential ribs (arrowheads). (b) Sperm tail with non-specific flagellar anomalies. The central pair is displaced (asterisk) and there is microtubular translocation to the center and the periphery of the axoneme or outside the fibrous sheath (arrows). (c, d) Spermatozoa from two patients with primary ciliary dyskinesia. There is a lack of dynein arms (arrow, c) or absence of the central pair (d). Bars (a–d) = 0.1 μm. (e–g) Light and transmission electron microscopy (TEM) of spermatozoa with dysplasia of the fibrous sheath (DFS). (e) Very short, thick and irregular tails are seen (phase-contrast microscopy). (f) Longitudinal section of a DFS sperm. Note absence of the mitochondrial sheath (asterisk) and redundant elements of the fibrous sheath. (g) Cross-section of flagellum with disorganized and hyperplastic fibrous sheath. The axoneme is almost completely obliterated with few remaining microtubular doublets and missing dynein arms (arrow). Bars = 5 μm (e), 1 μm (f), 0.1 μm (g). (h–k) Alterations of the mitochondrial sheath (MS). (h) Under epifluorescence, this spermatozoon displays intense and uniform labeling of the MS that covers a length > 15 μm (normal length 3–5 μm). (i) Abnormally long and distorted MS observed in TEM. (j) Absence of MS (very small labeling in the midpiece corresponding to isolated mitochondrion, arrow). (k) Under TEM, the midpiece is not formed and mitochondria are either absent or abnormal in location and/or arrangement. Bars = 5 μm (h, j), 1 μm (i, k). Panels (f) and (g) were originally published in reference 12. Copyrights European Society of Human Reproduction and Embryology. Reproduced by permission of Oxford University Press/*Human Reproduction*

and chronic respiratory disease in the so-called immotile cilia syndrome (ICS)[17–19]. ICS was more recently renamed as primary ciliary dyskinesia (PCD), because various degrees of reduced or qualitatively abnormal motility were reported in some of these patients[20–22]. PCD patients are infertile owing to sperm immotility or severe asthenozoospermia, suffer from rhinosinusitis and chronic pneumopathy caused by infections secondary to faulty mucociliary clearance, and have alterations in the visceral situs, with dextrocardia in 50% of patients[23]. Familial incidence of PCD, most possibly due to autosomal recessive mutation(s), has been reported. There is extensive locus heterogeneity, with a number of mutations in dynein genes found in families with members carrying the PCD phenotype[24–29].

Spermatozoa in PCD patients have immotile or dyskinetic flagella of normal appearance under the light microscope. The underlying alteration consists of the lack of one or both dynein arms, absence of the central pair, microtubular transposition or a number of less frequent abnormal configurations of the sperm axoneme (Figures 6.1c and d)[17,18,20,24,30–35]. The possibility also exists of isolated immotility in either cilia or flagella.

Another systematic sperm phenotype responsible for severe asthenozoospermia/sperm immotility is dysplasia of the fibrous sheath (DFS). Patients are young males with primary sterility and immotile spermatozoa. Sperm flagella are typically short, thick and of very irregular profile (Figure 6.1e). This appearance prompted the denomination 'stump tails' or 'short tails', a descriptive name that does not give any clues as to the nature and subcellular basis of this pathology. We have proposed DFS, which recognizes the main alterations in the sperm fibrous sheath and identifies its testicular origin as a consequence of a dysplastic development of the tail during spermiogenesis[12,16,36–38]. Other authors[39,40] have previously indicated that this anomaly involves various components of the tail cytoskeleton, the fibrous sheath being the most visibly affected. DFS sperm should not be confused with other alterations secondary to necrozoospermia, or sperm aging in men with partial obstruction of the seminal pathway, that lead to flagellar disintegration and thickening. Familial and geographical clustering of DFS has been reported[12,39–41]. A striking contrast between the high incidence of DFS and low incidence of PCD has been noted in a population of multiethnic origin[16], which may indicate the interaction between genetic and environmental influences in the generation of this phenotype.

The subcellular basis of DFS is a serious disarray of the sperm-tail cytoskeletal components. The fibrous sheath appears hyperplastic and completely disorganized, and the axoneme may be disrupted. There is also frequent absence of the central pair, missing dynein arms and lack or minimal development of the mitochondrial sheath of the midpiece (Figure 6.1f and g). These abnormalities are very stable during evolution, do not respond to any therapeutic measures, have familial incidence and may be associated with a lack of dynein in the respiratory cilia (see below). These alterations point to a genetic origin of DFS, possibly an autosomic recessive trait[12,42–45]. About 20% of patients also suffer from chronic respiratory disease due to a lack of dynein in the respiratory cilia. This subgroup of DFS patients constitutes a variety of primary ciliary dyskinesia in which a lack of dynein in the respiratory cilia is associated with the DFS phenotype in spermatozoa[35,41].

In recent years, extensive work has been carried out on the protein composition of the fibrous sheath. A kinase anchoring protein 3 (AKAP3) and AKAP4 have been recognized as the most abundant structural proteins of the fibrous sheath. They bind to one another and provide the structural framework for docking of protein kinase A to the fibrous sheath[46]. To analyze the possible role of these proteins in generation of the DFS phenotype, sequence analysis of the AKAP3 and AKAP4 binding sites in DFS patients was carried out, but did not reveal mutations[47]. However, targeted disruption of the AKAP4 gene in mice resulted in sperm immotility and abnormally short flagella with localized aggregations of fibrous sheath material, somewhat reminiscent of the DFS phenotype[48] (Eddy, personal communication). Very recently, Baccetti et al.[49] have reported deletion of the AKAP4/AKAP3 binding regions and absence of the AKAP4 protein in spermatozoa of one of five patients with DFS. This report suggests that lack of AKAP4 could be pathogenically responsible for the DFS phenotype. It is possible that DFS is a multigenic disease caused by alterations in several different gene products. Intensive research into this field is currently being carried out.

Other more rare forms of axonemal pathologies of genetic origin include deficient respiratory cilia and sperm axonemes in patients with retinitis pigmentosa[14,50] or albinism (unpublished personal observation). Mitochondrial anomalies in the sperm midpiece such as an abnormally long extension or absence of the mitochondrial sheath are very infrequent sperm anomalies that are also associated with asthenozoospermia (Figures 6.1h–k)[51]. Recent investigations have identified various mutations/deletions in mitochondrial genes of immotile spermatozoa whose products are involved in oxidative phosphorylation and generation of ATP necessary for sperm motility[52,53]. No structural correlates of these anomalies have been described so far.

ABNORMAL HEAD–NECK ATTACHMENT AND ACEPHALIC SPERMATOZOA

The region of head–neck attachment or the connecting piece derives from interaction of the centrioles with the spermatid nucleus (Figure 6.2c). Early in spermiogenesis, the sperm flagellum grows from the centriolar complex, while this approaches the nucleus and attaches to its caudal pole, ensuring linear alignment of the tail with the longitudinal axis of the head.

Spermatozoa without heads ('acephalic', 'decapitated', 'pin heads'; Figure 6.2b) or with an abnormal head–midpiece relationship ('abaxial implantation'; Figure 6.2a) can be detected in very small numbers in the semen of fertile men, and

can rise up to 10–20% in subfertile patients[36,54]. Its significance for fertility is not clear in these situations. There are infertile patients in whom 80–100% of the sperm population is composed of acephalic forms and loose heads, or spermatozoa with heads and tails not aligned along the same axis. Each of these two forms can predominate or combine in different proportions. This sperm defect is of rare occurrence albeit underdiagnosed, since these patients are usually considered to suffer from 'severe teratozoospermia', without the specificity of this sperm defect being recognized. Several authors[55–57] reported individual patients with headless flagella in the semen, and more recently, other authors[36,58–60] reported 15 more cases, including familial incidence. The term 'pin heads' has been used in reference to this peculiar appearance, but this denomination adds confusion, since there is no nuclear material in these minute 'heads'. Acephalic forms appear as headless flagella ending cranially in a small cytoplasmic droplet that, when bigger, simulates a head, but has no DNA content (Figure 6.2b and e)[36]. When a head is present, it attaches either to the tip or to the sides of the midpiece, without linear alignment with the sperm axis (Figure 6.2a and d). This misalignment ranges from complete lack of connection to lateral positioning of the nucleus at a 90–180° angle. All forms of this defect result from failure of the sperm centriole to attach normally to the caudal pole of the maturing spermatid nucleus, reported on the few occasions on which testicular biopsies from these patients have been studied (Figure 6.2f)[61,62]. These variants express different degrees of abnormality of the head–neck junction, with acephalic forms representing the most extreme situation, and hence the more inclusive denomination of *alterations* of the head–neck attachment[59,62,63]. When the relationship between the head and midpiece is looser, increased fragility of this junction determines the generation of acephalic forms and loose heads[59,64]. The latter are frequently phagocytosed within the testis, and their frequency in semen is lower than that of headless flagella.

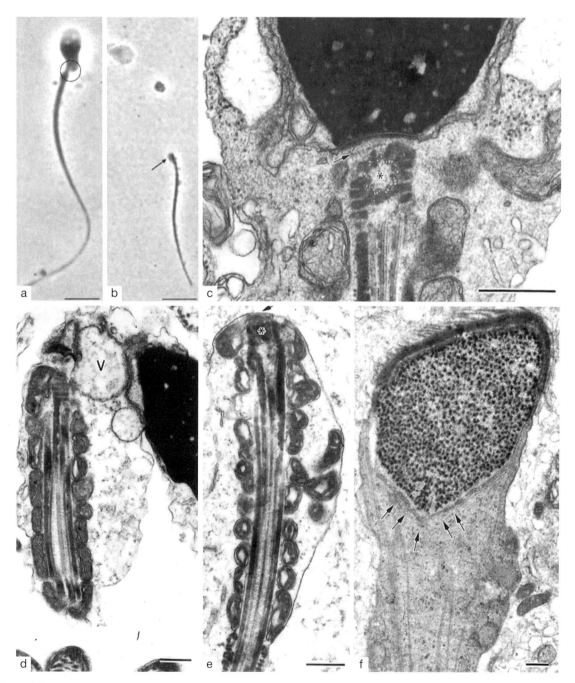

Figure 6.2 Abnormalities of the connecting piece (head–tail junction). In (a) the head and the tail are not aligned along the same axis (abaxial implantation of the tail). (b) Acephalic spermatozoon with minute thickening (arrow). (c) Normal configuration of the connecting piece. The tail is lodged in the concave implantation fossa (arrow). Note the triplets of the proximal centriole (asterisk) and beginning of the axoneme. (d) The head and midpiece are not properly attached and a vesicular structure (V) separates them. (e) Acephalic spermatozoon. The plasma membrane (arrow) covers the connecting piece (asterisk). The midpiece is well formed. (f) Elongating spermatid in testicular biopsy. Note lack of attachment of the tail anlagen to the caudal pole of the nucleus (arrows). Bars = 5 μm (a, b), 0.5 μm (c–f). Panels (a) and (b) were originally published in reference 62 and panels (c–f) in reference 59. Copyrights European Society of Human Reproduction and Embryology. Reproduced by permission of Oxford University Press/*Human Reproduction*

The uniform pathological phenotype, its origin as a consequence of a systematic alteration during spermiogenesis, the fact that seminal characteristics remain constant along clinical evolution even when a pharmacological germ cell depletion–repopulation has been induced, and the familial incidence indicate that this condition is very likely of genetic origin[59,60].

The need for normal migration of the spermatid centriole to generate a normal head–midpiece attachment, and the abnormalities that have been observed in sperm aster formation, syngamy and embryo cleavage when these spermatozoa have been microinjected in bovine and human oocytes, point to a sperm centriolar dysfunction, the nature of which remains to be elucidated. Proteins such as centrin, pericentrin, γ-tubulin and MPM-2 have been localized to the sperm connecting piece and zygote centrosome, but no studies are available that show their (possible) significance in the pathogenesis of this syndrome[63,65]. Sequencing across the exons of the gene for speriolin (another protein localized to the sperm neck region) has failed to demonstrate any abnormality in two patients with the syndrome (Eddy, personal communication).

The release of the sperm centriole after fertilization probably involves the action of sperm proteasomes recently localized to the neck region of human spermatozoa[66,67]. Experimental neutralization of proteasomes in the zygote has also resulted in defective sperm-aster and pronuclear formation[67]. Defective enzymatic activity of sperm proteasomes in patients with defects of the head–midpiece attachment has recently been reported[68]. We are currently conducting research in this exciting area of sperm pathology.

PATHOLOGY OF THE SPERM HEAD: ACROSOME AND CHROMATIN ANOMALIES

The sperm acrosome is an organelle derived from the Golgi complex of spermatids. It consists of a flattened sac covering the anterior two-thirds of the sperm head and is formed by two membranes (the internal and external acrosomal membranes), delimiting a space with a dense content rich in hydrolytic enzymes.

The lack or insufficient development of the acrosome are specific sperm defects causing infertility, characterizing two well-defined syndromes: acrosomeless spermatozoa and acrosomal hypoplasia.

Spermatozoa lacking acrosomes usually display spherical heads, which has prompted the denominations 'globozoospermia' or 'round-headed acrosomeless spermatozoa'. They can be found in small numbers (approximately 0.5%) in the semen of fertile individuals, and may increase up to 2–3% in cases of infertility[69]. The denomination globozoospermia applies when they predominate in the vast majority of spermatozoa (up to 100% of ejaculated spermatozoa). Affected spermatozoa have an absence of or detached acrosomes, or very small perinuclear densities that may be abortive attempts at acrosome formation (Figure 6.3a and c).

The generation of spermatozoa with absence of an acrosome corresponds to more than one mechanism. Most reports indicate that the Golgi complex fails to join the nucleus and develops a detached acrosome with irregular secretory activity. This structure remains free in the cytoplasm of maturing spermatids, to be eliminated with the residual cytoplasm at spermiation. In this situation, acrosomes are formed but do not attach to the nucleus[70–73]. In some other patients there is a real lack of or serious deficiency in acrosome formation. In these cases, a rudimentary acrosome may be found on the anterior pole of the spermatozoon[71]. One characteristic finding is delayed maturation of the chromatin; it appears granular, with incomplete compaction frequently in the form of hypodense areas. These changes are due to failure of the histone–protamine transition and increased rates of DNA fragmentation.

Lack of the acrosome is associated with absence of the perinuclear theca, a subacrosomal structure of the sperm nuclear–perinuclear skeletal

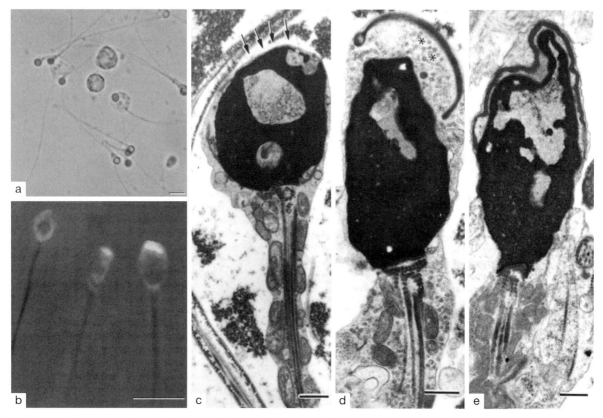

Figure 6.3   Acrosome and chromatin anomalies. (a) Light microscopy of spermatozoa from a patient with globozoospermia. Heads are characteristically spherical. (b) Detailed visualization of sperm heads with pathological acrosomes. Immunolabeling using antiacrosin antibody shows fluorescence on the acrosome. Lack (left) or variable hypoplasia (two right spermatozoa) are clearly observed. (c) A round-headed spermatozoon lacks the acrosome (arrows). There is also a marked lacunar defect of the chromatin. (d) Acrosomal hypoplasia: small and detached acrosome (asterisks). (e) Severe lacunar defect of the chromatin in a grossly distorted amorphous head. Bars = 5 μm (a, b), 0.5 μm (c–e).

complex involved in modeling the shape of sperm heads, attachment of the acrosome to the nucleus and also oocyte activation after sperm penetration[74–77]. These abnormalities of the perinuclear theca are probably the molecular basis responsible for spherical sperm heads, detached acrosomes and insufficient oocyte activation in acrosomeless spermatozoa.

Familial incidence has been reported in men suffering from globozoospermia, and a mono- or polygenic origin has been suggested but not proven[43,72,78]. Various animal models with similar characteristics have recently been described.

Acrosomal hypoplasia is a poorly understood and frequently underdiagnosed sperm pathology that, according to Zamboni[79], is frequent in severe teratozoospermia. Acrosomes are very small, and often lack contact with the amorphous nucleus (Figure 6.3b and d). Chemes[16] reported a series of 35 patients with acrosomal anomalies in whom lack of the acrosome or acrosomal hypoplasia was present as a predominant form or in combination. Sperm heads are mostly round, but may also be amorphous or oval. Acrosomal hypoplasia should be investigated in cases of severe teratozoospermia, and can be readily recognized under the electron microscope[80], with the use of various antibodies that react against the acrosome or by lectin binding to intact spermatozoa. In the classification of spermatozoa by strict criteria, these abnormalities are included among the severe amorphous varieties that have poor fertility prognosis[5].

Other forms of acrosomal defects have been reported in infertile males. Premature occurrence of and/or failure to undergo the acrosome reaction have been recognized[81]. More rare and not well-characterized defects of the acrosome include the 'crater defect'[82] and acrosomal inclusions[80]. In both cases, fertility is compromised by the inability of these spermatozoa to penetrate oocytes normally.

The chromatin of maturing spermatids suffers a complex series of chemical and macromolecular changes that are reflected in the structure of the nucleus. Early round spermatids have euchromatic nuclei with dispersed chromatin. During maturation, the chromatin condenses progressively in the form of discrete granules that enlarge as they approach each other and condense to acquire finally a dense, homogeneous structure in which only small ($0.1–0.2\,\mu m$) hypodense, clear areas can be discerned. This process of progressive maturation and compaction is due to the replacement of nuclear histones that associate with the DNA in a supercoiled structure, similar to that found in somatic cells. Histones are interchanged first by transition proteins and later by protamines that organize in a side-to-side configuration along the groove of the DNA helix, so that chromatin fibers can compact tightly to determine the typical condensed structure of mature spermatids and spermatozoa[83–85]. In this compacted state, individual chromatin granules cannot be discerned.

When the process of chromatin maturation and compaction is altered, the heads of the spermatozoa display large lacunar defects ($2–3\,\mu m$ in diameter), where the compact arrangement of the chromatin is replaced by granulofibrillar or 'empty' areas that occupy as much as 20–50% of the nucleus (Figure 6.3c–e)[79,86]. They originate in the testis as a consequence of abnormal spermiogenesis, as confirmed by their presence in immature spermatids found in testicular biopsies and semen. Spermatozoa with chromatin abnormalities frequently demonstrate abnormal head shapes, have diminished fertility potential or are

associated with first-trimester abortions[16]. Single-stranded DNA, DNA breaks, abnormal histone–protamine transition or apoptotic changes have been reported, as well as insufficient chromatin condensation, immaturity and intranuclear lacunae that are their ultrastructural correlates. There is not much information about the genetic constitution of morphologically abnormal spermatozoa. A positive correlation between sperm aneuploidy and teratozoospermia has been reported, but in other studies no increased numerical chromosomal aberrations have been found in abnormal spermatozoa[87–89]. Recent fluorescence in situ hybridization (FISH) studies of infertile men with poor semen quality have shown increased aneuploidy in spermatozoa, despite a normal blood karyotype[90,91], which suggests that the same factor(s) causing aneuploidy may also induce teratozoospermia.

The question of the acquired versus the genetic etiology of chromatin anomalies has received attention, but is not solved to date. Men who suffer from infectious bowel disease and are treated with sulfasalazine may present with this type of abnormality in the spermatozoa. The question remains whether they are caused by the pathological process itself or the treatment instituted. The same alterations can also be found in men with varicocele, fever, seminal infections and even testicular tumors[92–95]. In these last cases they are found mixed with other types of non-specific sperm anomalies. Accounts of genetic etiology in patients with chromatin anomalies are not frequent. There are reports of abnormal removal of histones and transition proteins from sperm nuclei, selective absence of protamine P2 or altered ratios of nucleoproteins in spermatozoa from infertile individuals, but no or only occasional mutations in protamine genes have been documented[93,95–99].

Other nuclear abnormalities include macronuclear/multinuclear polyploid spermatozoa derived from meiotic alterations in nuclear cleavage. A familial pedigree with this anomaly has been reported[100–102].

ACQUIRED SPERM ABNORMALITIES SECONDARY TO ANDROLOGICAL CONDITIONS AND ENDOGENOUS OR ENVIRONMENTAL FACTORS

Non-specific anomalies are the most frequent finding in astheno- and teratozoospermic patients. Non-specific flagellar anomalies are dealt with in the section on pathology of asthenozoospermia (see above). With regard to non-specific head anomalies, these constitute a heterogeneous condition in which various anomalies in the acrosome, chromatin, head cytoskeleton and the neck region coexist in different proportions. Their individualization in clinical andrology is based on the abnormal appearance of the spermatozoa. They constitute the foundation of all current classifications of sperm morphology, including those based on strict criteria. These classifications undoubtedly have an important application in predicting the fertility potential of a given semen sample. However, with the exception of acrosome anomalies that are taken into consideration in the classification presented by Kruger[4,5], most head alterations are classified according to their external appearance, without any indication of the nature of the pathologies involved or the morphogenetic mechanisms that originate them. Alterations in chromatin maturation and compaction and insufficient development or vacuolization of the acrosome are frequent findings in amorphous sperm heads. They have been noted to be associated with inflammatory bowel disease[80], varicocele[103], contact with alkylated imino sugars or pesticides[104,105], exposure to fuels, oils, organic solvents, exhaust fumes and hydrocarbons[106], cigarette-smoking[107], ionizing radiation[108,109] or temperatures higher than physiological[110].

Even though there have been attempts to associate certain types of alterations with specific etiologies (e.g. tapered forms with varicocele[1]), this has not been confirmed and their non-specific nature is currently accepted.

SPERM PATHOLOGY AND FERTILITY PROGNOSIS: THE SIGNIFICANCE OF SPERM PATHOLOGY IN THE STUDY OF INFERTILE MALES

It has been asserted that the results of ICSI are independent of most sperm parameters, but recent evidence indicates otherwise. Teratozoospermia should be understood not solely as a morphological abnormality but also as the corresponding impairment in sperm function. A higher pregnancy rate has been reported in coincidence with morphology values above the 4% threshold[5], and various reports have stressed the importance of normal acrosome and chromatin structure, head–neck junction and centrosomes for adequate fertilization and pregnancy[16,62,111–114]. It has been claimed[115,116] that abnormal morphology does not influence ICSI results, but in 10 of their 15 patients with total fertilization failure, strict morphology was ≤2%, and also failed fertilization was documented by these authors in six patients with acrosomeless spermatozoa[115,116]. In conclusion, many studies have shown that, depending on the nature of the pathologies involved, the outcome of ART can change dramatically. The recent introduction of ICSI provides access to the structural and functional features of spermatozoa that are being used for fertilization. This information can be applied to evaluate the relationship between sperm quality and fertility outcome, and hence a more objective picture is emerging of the differential roles played by specific sperm components in fertilization, early embryonic development and implantation.

Asthenozoospermia: flagellar pathologies and fertility prognosis

As previously noted when discussing the subcellular basis of asthenozoospermia, increased rates of non-specific flagellar anomalies (NSFAs) were the underlying cause in 70% of 201 men with severe motility disorders (mean fast forward progression

3.6%)[10]. In patients with asthenozoospermia of genetic origin (fast forward progression 0.2%), specific sperm phenotypes such as primary ciliary dyskinesia and dysplasia of the fibrous sheath (PCD and DFS) were present in all spermatozoa[12]. Longitudinal studies in these men have shown that 33% of patients with NSFAs, but 0% of those with DFS, obtained fertilizations/pregnancies within 2–6 years of diagnosis, either spontaneously or with the use of ART, including IVF (but not ICSI). These findings indicate that one-third of cases of NSFA are reversible and can obtain fair fertility results, while DFS does not respond to conventional fertility treatments or IVF, as confirmed by the lack of other positive results in the literature. One publication by Kay and Irvine[117] has documented a live birth after IVF using sperm with no progressive motility from a patient with primary ciliary dyskinesia. When there are 100% immotile sperm, a misleading tendency exists to equate complete asthenozoospermia with total necrozoospermia. This creates unnecessary confusion in view of the very different natures and fertility potentials of immotile (but live) and dead spermatozoa. Others have reported poor ICSI results with the use of 'immotile spermatozoa', but careful examination of the data indicates that, in their 'immotile' population, viability was always lower than 10%, which makes it very likely, as also noted by the authors, that their poor results were due to injection of dead spermatozoa (rather than live, immotile)[115,116]. ICSI has been of great help in cases of men with genetic asthenozoospermia. Indeed, there are now several publications reporting fertilizations/pregnancies with the use of immotile but live spermatozoa[118–121]. The difficulty in distinguishing between dead and completely immotile but live spermatozoa has been circumvented by various methods, including the hypo-osmotic swelling test, stimulation of motility with pentoxifylline or retrieving testicular spermatozoa[122–125].

We have recently reviewed numerous reports of ICSI results in 11 patients with PCD and 12 with DFS[126]. Fertilization was in the 55–70% range, and there were numerous pregnancies and 21 live births. The abortion rate was 20% (three of 15 pregnancies). The encouraging results indicate that this subpopulation of severe male-factor patients can expect good outcomes with microinjection of *in situ* motile or live, immotile spermatozoa. Therefore, flagellar pathologies causing sperm immotility do not compromise ICSI outcome if sperm viability is not affected.

As stated before, DFS and PCD are genetic conditions, and there are concerns about the (possible) transmission of these anomalies to the next generation. Even though the number of cases is limited, there have been no reports of respiratory disease (a common finding in PCD and some DFS) in newborns. The question of fertility potential will have to remain unresolved for some years until the offspring attain reproductive age. Prospective parents should be made aware of the risks involved, but comprehensive genetic counseling will not be possible until the genes involved and the mechanism of inheritance are identified. Informed consent should always be obtained. Affected men tend to accept the risks if transmission of reproductive failure is the only concern, as is the case for individuals carrying Y-chromosome microdeletions that surely will pass to their male descendants.

Fertility potential in abnormalities of the connecting piece

We have previously stated that, depending on the sperm anomalies involved, fertility outcomes change dramatically. This is illustrated by anomalies of the connecting piece, which, in contrast to the relatively good results attained in cases of flagellar pathology, are associated with a poor fertility prognosis in ICSI.

Anomalies of the connecting piece have a heterogeneous phenotypic manifestation. In some of these patients, acephalic spermatozoa are the only form observed in semen, which makes impossible any attempt at fertilization. Other patients have acephalic forms in lower numbers, and spermatozoa with abnormal head–midpiece alignment predominate. Various recent ICSI procedures have been reported in these last patients. Chemes *et al.*[59] documented the first ICSI failure using spermatozoa with a faulty alignment of the head–midpiece junction. Four metaphase II oocytes were fertilized by ICSI but remained at the pronuclear stage, and degenerated after failure to undergo syngamy and cleavage. Shortly after this there were two other failed attempts, with similar characteristics (Saias-Magnan *et al.*[127], one patient, 1 cycle; Rawe *et al.*[62], one patient, 5 cycles) and a further two with pregnancies and live deliveries (Porcu *et al.*[63], two patients, five cycles, two pregnancies; Kamal *et al.*[64], 16 patients, three pregnancies) as well as another successful attempt in one of our patients (personal unreported communication). In summary, from five reports available, four live births resulted from 26 cycles with numerous arrested or degenerated embryos. The question can be asked whether these different evolutions were connected with selection of the 'right' spermatozoon for injection. This seemed to be the case in one of our patients (five failed ICSI attempts), since two chemical pregnancies were obtained when the sperm selection criteria were very strict and the 'best' spermatozoa were microinjected. However, the two pregnancies reported by Porcu *et al.*[63] seem to indicate otherwise, because the published morphology of the spermatozoa used for ICSI indicated a serious abnormality with severe misalignment at the head–midpiece junction.

Fertility outcome in men with acrosome and chromatin abnormalities

Patients with acrosomeless spermatozoa are infertile because their spermatozoa are unable to penetrate oocytes due to the lack of acrosomes, physiologically involved in penetration of the cumulus oophorus that surrounds the oocyte and also in binding and penetration of the zona pellucida[128]. When ICSI was introduced, it was soon hypothesized that, since microinjection bypasses all the penetration steps previous to fertilization, it may be an ideal solution for globozoospermia. The practice of ICSI with acrosomeless spermatozoa indicated that this was not exactly the case. While fertilization took place in a good number of instances, it failed in others, suggesting that besides penetration problems these spermatozoa may carry other deficiencies. Unsuccessful ICSI attempts in nine cases of acrosomeless spermatozoa were reported by Bourne *et al.*[129], Liu *et al.*[116], Battaglia *et al.*[130] and Edirishinge *et al.*[131]. It was soon realized that the abnormality in cases of failure was probably due to insufficient activation of the oocyte, a function recently attributed to the perinuclear theca of spermatozoa. Indeed, acrosomeless spermatozoa have alterations of the perinuclear theca, and also lack various proteins associated with this structure (see above). Rybouchkin *et al.*[132] and Kim *et al.*[133] obtained successful pregnancies with acrosomeless spermatozoa by means of Ca^{2+} ionophore activation of the oocytes. However, artificially induced oocyte activation is not always followed by pregnancy[130]. Since chromatin anomalies are frequently associated with a lack of acrosome, their negative influence on fertilization should be taken into consideration. Besides these failures, there are also various reports of ICSI successes after microinjection of acrosomeless spermatozoa, but fertilization rates were low (10–50%)[134–139]. These results indicate that even though human acrosomeless spermatozoa are able to fertilize human or hamster oocytes and achieve pregnancies in numerous couples, they bear abnormalities responsible for unsuccessful or low fertilization rates or the need for artificial activation.

The maturational changes that chromatin undergoes during spermiogenesis are an essential component of its fertilizing capacity. Spermatozoa with amorphous, elongated or round heads have been shown to have a four-fold increase in chromosomal abnormalities[87]. Large, intranuclear, hypodense regions (incorrectly called 'nuclear vacuoles') represent areas in which the DNA itself or the associated proteins have structural abnormalities. DNA breaks, single-stranded DNA, deletions of variable magnitude and other alterations significantly affect sperm quality, fertilization, embryo development and implantation. Infertility or abortions during the first trimester have been reported in these patients[16,79,80,140]. Similar results were reported by Francavilla *et al.*[141] when comparing the results of 21 testicular sperm extraction (TESE)–ICSI cycles in azoospermic men with or without chromatin abnormalities. While the fertilization rate was similar in both groups, the delivery rate per cycle was significantly diminished in men with chromatin abnormalities. Others have also reported normal fertilization rates and low pregnancy rates in a study of 17 males with megalohead multitailed spermatozoa that have been shown to be polyploid[142]. Careful selection of motile spermatozoa for ICSI by means of very high-resolution light microscopy yields dramatic differences in implantation and pregnancy rates between normal spermatozoa and those with 'nuclear vacuoles' (indicative of abnormal chromatin constitution)[143]. The negative influence of DNA fragmentation on ICSI outcome was reported by Greco *et al.*[144] in men with high rates of DNA fragmentation, by comparing ICSI with testicular spermatozoa (low DNA damage) versus ejaculated spermatozoa (found to have high DNA damage).

CONCLUDING REMARKS

Sperm pathology is the discipline that characterizes structural and functional deficiencies in spermatozoa. It is not just another denomination for abnormal sperm morphology; it is rather a new concept in which a multidisciplinary approach is applied to the precise description of sperm abnormalities and the understanding of the pathogenic mechanisms that underlie abnormal sperm appearance. Used jointly with classical sperm morphology (in particular the strict criteria), it allows a clear appreciation of what is wrong with abnormal sperm shapes and facilitates a rational approach to the use of abnormal spermatozoa in assisted reproduction. The distinction between non-specific anomalies and systematic defects of genetic origin is an important one, and couples undergoing ICSI have the right to be informed not only of their diminished chances when this is the case, but also of the possible risk of transmission to their offspring. Whenever possible, genetic counseling is important and follow-up of newborns desirable. However, in view of our present uncertainties, care should be taken to protect patients from excessive information, particularly when no unambiguous conclusions are available.

Another important issue refers to the use of appropriate nomenclature, previously addressed by Chemes and Rawe[126]. We have attempted to highlight each pathological phenotype with a denomination that identifies the organelles involved and the pathogenic mechanisms. The problem of nomenclature is not a trivial one: the way we speak and write conditions the way we think. If descriptive terms are used, thoughts will not go beyond appearances. It is essential to distinguish a dead (immotile) from an immotile (live) spermatozoon, and to use denominations that give us the basic understanding of each pathology. A 'stump tail' can either belong to a DFS spermatozoon or be the result of tail disintegration in aging spermatozoa; an 'amorphous' head can correspond to a lack of acrosome or to abnormal chromatin maturation and compaction.

The introduction of innovative therapeutic approaches such as ICSI has revolutionized the field of reproductive medicine. Besides its obvious advantages for men with severe male factor infertility, it has created new concerns about the ethical and social role of therapeutic interventions. The possibility of *inherited sterility* is certainly one of the most perplexing paradoxes of our times.

ACKNOWLEDGMENTS

The present chapter including most of its information is based on our previous publication:

Chemes HE, Rawe VY. Sperm pathology: a step beyond descriptive morphology. Origin, characterization and fertility potential of abnormal sperm phenotypes in infertile men. *Hum Reprod Update* 2003; 9: 405. Figures 6.1a–d and 6.3c–e in the present chapter are taken from the same paper. Copyrights European Society of Human Reproduction and Embryology. Reproduced by permission of Oxford University Press/*Human Reproduction*.

This work was supported by grants from the National Research Council (PIP 0900 and 4584), ANPCyT (PICT 9591) and CEGyR Foundation.

REFERENCES

1. MacLeod J. The significance of deviations in human sperm morphology. In Rosenberg E, Paulsen AC, eds. The Human Testis. New York: Plenum Press, 1970: 481
2. Kruger TF, et al. Sperm morphology: assessing the agreement between the manual method (strict criteria) and the sperm morphology analyzer IVOS. Fertil Steril 1995; 63: 134
3. Hofman GE, et al. Intraobserver, interobserver variation of sperm critical morphology: comparison of examiner and computer assisted analysis. Fertil Steril 1996; 65: 1021
4. Kruger TF, et al. Sperm morphologic features as a prognostic factor in in vitro fertilization. Fertil Steril 1986; 46: 1118
5. Kruger TF, et al. Predictive value of abnormal sperm morphology in in vitro fertilization. Fertil Steril 1988; 49: 112
6. Gibbons IR. Structure and function of flagellar microtubules. In Brinkley BR, Porter KR, eds. International Cell Biology. New York: Rockefeller University Press, 1977: 348
7. Baccetti B, et al. Human dynein and sperm pathology. J Cell Biol 1981; 88: 102
8. Williamson RA, et al. Ultrastructural sperm tail defects associated with sperm immotility. Fertil Steril 1984; 41: 103
9. Ryder TA, et al. A survey of ultrastructural defects associated with absent or impaired human sperm motility. Fertil Steril 1990; 53: 556
10. Chemes H. The significance of flagellar pathology in the evaluation of asthenozoospermia. In Baccetti

B, ed. Comparative Spermatology 20 years Later. Serono Symposia Publications 75. New York: Raven Press, 1991: 815
11. Wilton LJ, Temple-Smith PD, de Kretser DM. Quantitative ultrastructural analysis of sperm tails reveals flagellar defects associated with persistent asthenozoospermia. Hum Reprod 1992; 7: 510
12. Chemes H, et al. Ultrastructural pathology of the sperm flagellum. Association between flagellar pathology and fertility prognosis in severely asthenozoospermic men. Hum Reprod 1998; 13: 2521
13. Wilton LJ, et al. Structural heterogeneity of the axonemes of respiratory cilia and sperm flagella in normal men. J Clin Invest 1985; 75: 825
14. Hunter DG, Fishman GA, de Kretser FL. Abnormal axonemes in X-linked retinitis pigmentosa. Arch Ophtalmol 1988; 106: 362
15. Afzelius BA. Immotile cilia syndrome and ciliary abnormalities induced by infection and injury. Annu Rev Respir Dis 1981; 124: 107
16. Chemes H. Phenotypes of sperm pathology: genetic and acquired forms in infertile men. J Androl 2000; 21: 799
17. Afzelius BA, et al. Lack of dynein arms in immotile human spermatozoa. J Cell Biol 1975; 66: 225
18. Pedersen H, Rebbe H. Absence of arms in the axoneme of immotile human spermatozoa. Biol Reprod 1975; 12: 541
19. Afzelius BA. A human syndrome caused by immotile cilia. Science 1976; 193: 317
20. Afzelius BA, Eliasson R. Flagellar mutants in man: on the heterogeneity of the immotile cilia syndrome. J Ultrastr Res 1979; 69: 43
21. Camner P, et al. Relation between abnormalities of human sperm flagella and respiratory tract diseases. Int J Androl 1979; 2: 211
22. Rossman CM, et al. The dyskinetic cilia syndrome: abnormal ciliary motility in association with abnormal ciliary ultrastructure. Chest 1981; 80: 860
23. Kartagener MI. Mitteilung: Bronchiektasien bei situs viscerum inversus. Beitr Klin Tuberk 1935; 83: 489
24. Schneeberger EE, et al. Heterogeneity of ciliary morphology in the immotile cilia syndrome in man. J Ultrastruct Res 1980; 73: 34
25. Afzelius BA. Genetical and ultrastructural aspects of the immotile-cilia syndrome. Am J Hum Genet 1981; 33: 852
26. Pennarun G, et al. Loss-of-function mutations in a human gene related to Chlamydomonas reinhardtii

dynein IC78 result in primary ciliary dyskinesia. Am J Hum Genet 1999; 65: 1508

27. Blouin JL, et al. Primary ciliary dyskinesia: a genome-wide linkage analysis reveals extensive locus heterogeneity. Eur J Hum Genet 2000; 8: 109

28. Guichard C, et al. Axonemal dynein intermediate-chain gene (DNAI1) mutations result in situs inversus and primary ciliary dyskinesia (Kartagener syndrome). Am J Hum Genet 2001; 68: 1030

29. Bartoloni L, et al. Mutations in the DNAH11 (axonemal heavy chain dynein type 11) gene cause one form of situs inversus totalis and most likely primary ciliary dyskinesia. Proc Natl Acad Sci USA 2002; 99: 10282

30. Baccetti B. '9+0' immotile spermatozoa in an infertile man. Andrologia 1979; 11: 437

31. Baccetti B, Burrini AG, Pallini V. Spermatozoa and cilia lacking axoneme in an infertile man. Andrologia 1980; 12: 525

32. Sturges JM, et al. Cilia with defective radial spokes. A cause of human respiratory disease. N Engl J Med 1979; 300: 53

33. Sturges JM, Chao J, Turner JAP. Transposition of ciliary microtubules: another cause of impaired ciliary motility. N Engl J Med 1980; 303: 318

34. Walt H, et al. Mosaicism of dynein in spermatozoa and cilia and fibrous sheath aberrations in an infertile man. Andrologia 1983; 15: 295

35. Chemes H, Morero JL, Lavieri JC. Extreme asthenozoospermia and chronic respiratory disease. A new variant of the immotile cilia syndrome. Int J Androl 1990; 13: 216

36. Chemes HE, et al. Lack of a head in human spermatozoa from sterile patients: a syndrome associated with impaired fertilization. Fertil Steril 1987; 47: 310

37. Rawe VY, et al. Incidence of tail structure distortions associated with dysplasia of the fibrous sheath in human spermatozoa. Hum Reprod 2001; 16: 879

38. Rawe VY, et al. Sperm ubiquitination in patients with dysplasia of the fibrous sheath. Hum Reprod 2002; 17: 2119

39. Bisson JP, David G. Anomalies morphologiques du spermatozoide humain. 2) Étude ultrastructurale. J Gynecol Obstet Biol Reprod 1975; 4: 37

40. Escalier D, David G. Pathology of the cytoskeleton of the human sperm flagellum: axonemal and peri-axonemal anomalies. Biol Cell 1984; 50: 37

41. Chemes H, et al. Dysplasia of the fibrous sheath. An ultrastructural defect of human spermatozoa

associated with sperm immotility and primary sterility. Fertil Steril 1987; 48: 664

42. Baccetti B, et al. The short-tailed human spermatozoa, ultrastructural alterations and dynein absence. J Submicrosc Cytol 1975; 7: 349

43. Baccetti B, et al. Genetic sperm defects and consanguinity. Hum Reprod 2001; 16: 1365

44. Alexandre C, Bisson JP, David G. Asthenospermie totale avec anomalie ultrastructurale du flagelle chez deux frères stériles. J Gynecol Obstet Biol Reprod 1978; 7: 31

45. Bisson JP, Leonard C, David G. Caractère familial de certaines perturbations morphologiques des spermatozoides. Arch Anat Cytol Pathol 1979; 27: 230

46. Carrera A, Gerton GL, Moss SB. The major fibrous sheath polypeptide of mouse sperm: structural and functional similarities to the A-kinase anchoring proteins. Dev Biol 1994; 165: 272

47. Turner RMO, et al. Molecular genetic analysis of two human sperm fibrous sheath proteins, AKAP4 and AKAP3, in men with dysplasia of the fibrous sheath. J Androl 2001; 22: 302

48. Miki K, et al. Targeted disruption of the Akap4 gene causes defects in sperm flagellum and motility. Dev Biol 2002; 248: 331

49. Baccetti B, et al. Gene deletions in an infertile man with sperm fibrous sheath dysplasia. Hum Reprod 2005; 20: 2790

50. Bonneau D, et al. Usher syndrome type I associated with bronchiectasis and immotile nasal cilia in two brothers. J Med Genet 1993; 30: 253

51. Rawe VY, et al. Abnormal organization of mitochondrial sheaths in two cases of severe asthenozoospermia. Int J Androl 2005; 28 (Suppl 1): 88

52. Holyoake AJ, et al. High incidence of single nucleotide substitutions in the mitochondrial genome is associated with poor semen parameters in men. Int J Androl 2001; 243: 175

53. Thangaraj K, et al. Sperm mitochondrial mutations as a cause of low sperm motility. J Androl 2003; 24: 388

54. Panidis D, et al. Headless spermatozoa in semen specimens from fertile and subfertile men. J Reprod Med 2001; 46: 947

55. Le Lannou D. Teratozoospermie consistant en l'absence de tete spermatique par defaut de connexion. J Gynecol Obstet Biol Reprod (Paris) 1979; 8: 43

56. Perotti ME, Gioria M. Fine structure and morphogenesis of 'headless' human spermatozoa associated with infertility. Cell Biol Int Rep 1981; 5: 113

57. Baccetti B, Selmi MG, Soldani P. Morphogenesis of 'decapitated spermatozoa' in a man. J Reprod Fertil 1984; 70: 395

58. Holstein AF, Schill WB, Breucker H. Dissociated centriole development as a cause of spermatid malformation in a man. J Reprod Fertil 1986; 78: 719

59. Chemes HE, et al. Acephalic spermatozoa and abnormal development of the head–neck attachment. A human syndrome of genetic origin. Hum Reprod 1999; 14: 1811

60. Baccetti B, et al. Morphogenesis of the decapitated and decaudated sperm defect in two brothers. Gamete Res 1989; 23: 181

61. Perotti ME, Giarola A, Gioria M. Ultrastructural study of the decapitated sperm defect in an infertile man. J Reprod Fertil 1981; 63: 543

62. Rawe VY, et al. A pathology of the sperm centriole responsible for defective sperm aster formation, syngamy and cleavage. Hum Reprod 2002; 17: 2344

63. Porcu G, et al. Pregnancies after ICSI using sperm with abnormal head–tail junction from two brothers: case report. Hum Reprod 2003; 18: 562

64. Kamal A, et al. Easily decapitated spermatozoa defect: a possible cause of unexplained infertility. Hum Reprod 1999; 14: 2791

65. Manandhar G, Schatten G. Centrosome reduction during rhesus spermiogenesis: gamma-tubulin, centrin, and centriole degeneration. Mol Reprod Dev 2000; 56: 502

66. Wojcik C, et al. Proteasomes in human spermatozoa. Int J Androl 2000; 23: 169

67. Rawe VY. Proteasome function in mammalian fertilization: implications ferilization faileur in humans. Int J Androl 2005; 28 (Suppl 1): 13

68. Morales P, et al. Decreased proteasome enzymatic activity in sperm from patients with genetic abnormalities of the head–tail junction and acephalic spermatozoa. J Androl 2004; 25 (March–April Suppl): 41

69. Kalahanis J, et al. Round-headed spermatozoa in semen specimens from fertile and subfertile men. J Reprod Med 2002; 47: 489

70. Baccetti B, et al. Further observations on the morphogenesis of the round-headed human spermatozoa. Andrologia 1977; 9: 255

71. Holstein AF, Schirren C. Classification of abnormalities in human spermatids based on recent advances in ultrastructure research on spermatid differentiation. In Fawcett DW, Bedford JM, eds. The Spermatozoon: Maturation, Motility, Surface Properties and Comparative Aspects. Baltimore: Urban and Schwarzenberg, 1979: 341

72. Florke-Gerloff S, et al. Biochemical and genetic investigation of round-headed spermatozoa in infertile men including two brothers and their father. Andrologia 1984; 16: 187

73. Florke-Gerloff S, et al. On the teratogenesis of round-headed spermatozoa: investigations with antibodies against acrosin, an intraacrosomally located acrosin-inhibitor, and the outer acrosomal membrane. Andrologia 1985; 17: 126

74. Longo FJ, Krohne G, Franke WW. Basic proteins of the perinuclear theca of mammalian spermatozoa and spermatids: a novel class of cytoskeletal elements. J Cell Biol 1987; 105: 1105

75. Sutovsky P, et al. The removal of the sperm perinuclear theca and its association with the bovine oocyte surface during fertilization. Dev Biol 1997; 188: 75

76. Sutovsky P, et al. Interactions of sperm perinuclear theca with the oocyte: implications for oocyte activation, anti-polyspermy defense, and assisted reproduction Microsc Res Tech 2003; 61: 362

77. Oko R, et al. The sperm head cytoskeleton. In Robaire B, Chemes H, Morales C, eds. Andrology in the 21st Century. Englewood: Medimond Publishing Company, 2001: 37

78. Nistal M, Herruzo A, Sanchez Corral F. Teratozoospermia absoluta de presentación familiar: espermatozoides microcéfalos irregulares sin acrosoma. Andrologia 1978; 10: 234

79. Zamboni L. The ultrastructural pathology of the spermatozoon as a cause of infertility: the role of electron microscopy in the evaluation of semen quality. Fertil Steril 1987; 48: 711

80. Zamboni L. Sperm structure and its relevance to infertility. An electron microscopic study. Arch Pathol Lab Med 1992; 116: 325

81. Liu DY, Baker HW. Disordered acrosome reaction of spermatozoa bound to the zona pellucida: a newly discovered sperm defect causing infertility with reduced sperm-zona pellucida penetration and reduced fertilization in vitro. Hum Reprod 1994; 9: 1694

82. Baccetti B. et al. Crater defect in human spermatozoa. Gamete Res 1989; 22: 249

83. Balhorn R. A model for the structure of chromatin in mammalian sperm. J Cell. Biol 1982; 93: 298

84. Ward WS, Coffey DS. DNA packaging and organization in mammalian spermatozoa: comparison with somatic cells. Biol Reprod 1991; 44: 569

85. Brewer L, Corzett M, Balhorn R. Condensation of DNA by spermatid basic nuclear proteins. J Biol Chem 2002; 277: 38895

86. Holstein AF. Morphologische Studien an abnormen Spermatiden und Spermatozoen des Menschen. Virchows Arch 1975; 367: 93

87. Lee JD, Kamiguchi Y, Yanagimachi R. Analysis of chromosome constitution of human spermatozoa with normal and aberrant head morphologies after injection into mouse oocytes. Hum Reprod 1996; 11: 1942

88. Calogero AE, et al. Aneuploidy rate in spermatozoa of selected men with abnormal semen parameters. Hum Reprod 2001; 16: 1172

89. Kovanci E, et al. FISH assessment of aneuploidy frequencies in mature and immature human spermatozoa classified by the absence or presence of cytoplasmic retention. Hum Reprod 2001; 16: 1209

90. Lewis-Jones I, et al. Sperm chromosomal abnormalities are linked to sperm morphologic deformities. Fertil Steril 2003; 1: 212

91. Vicari E, et al. Absolute polymorphic teratozoospermia in patients with oligo-asthenozoospermia is associated with an elevated sperm aneuploidy rate. J Androl 2003; 4: 598

92. Hrudka F, Singh A. Sperm nucleomalacia in men with inflammatory bowel disease. Arch Androl 1984; 13: 37

93. Schlicker M, et al. Disturbances of nuclear condensation in human spermatozoa: search for mutations in the genes for protamine 1, protamine 2 and transition protein 1. Hum Reprod 1994; 9: 2313

94. Evenson DP, et al. Characteristics of human sperm chromatin structure following an episode of influenza and high fever: a case study. J Androl 2000; 21: 739

95. Tanaka H, et al. Single-nucleotide polymorphisms in the protamine-1 and -2 genes of fertile and infertile human male populations. Mol Hum Reprod 2003; 9: 69

96. Balhorn R, Reed S, Tanphaichitr N. Aberrant protamine 1/protamine 2 ratios in sperm of infertile human males. Experientia 1988; 44: 52

97. Blanchard Y, Lescoat D, Le Lannou D. Anomalous distribution of nuclear basic proteins in round-headed human spermatozoa. Andrologia 1990; 22: 549

98. de Yebra L, et al. Complete selective absence of protamine P2 in humans. J Biol Chem 1993; 268: 10553

99. de Yebra L, et al. Detection of P2 precursors in the sperm cells of infertile patients who have reduced protamine P2 levels. Fertil Steril 1998; 69: 755

100. Escalier D. Human spermatozoa with large heads and multiple flagella: a quantitative ultrastructural study of 6 cases. Biol Cell 1983; 48: 65

101. Benzacken B, et al. Familial sperm polyploidy induced by genetic spermatogenesis failure. Hum Reprod 2001; 16: 2646

102. Devillard F, et al. Polyploidy in large-headed sperm: FISH study of three cases. Hum Reprod 2002; 17: 1292

103. Muratori M, et al. Functional and structural features of DNA-fragmented human sperm. J Androl 2000; 21: 903

104. ElJack AH, Hrudka F. Patterns and dynamics of teratospermia induced in rams by parenteral treatment with ethylene dibromide. J Ultrastruct Res 1979; 67: 124

105. Bustos-Obregon E, Diaz O, Sobarzo C. Parathion induces mouse germ cells apoptosis. Ital J Embryol 2001; 2: 199

106. Harrison KL. Semen parameter defects and toxin contact related occupation in infertility patients. Middle East Fertil Soc J 1998; 3: 3

107. Banerjee A, et al. Semen characteristics of tobacco users in India. Arch Androl 1993; 30: 35

108. Sailer BL, et al. Effects of X-irradiation on mouse testicular cells and sperm chromatin structure. Environ Mol Mutagen 1995; 25: 23

109. Schevchenko VA, et al. Genetic effects of 131I in reproductive cells of male mice. Mutat Res 1989; 226: 87

110. Mieusset R. Influence of lifestyle on male infertility: potential testicular heating factors. Middle East Fertil Soc J 1998; 3 (Suppl 1): 40

111. Tasdemir I, et al. Effect of abnormal sperm head morphology on the outcome of intracytoplasmic sperm injection in humans. Hum Reprod 1997; 12: 1214

112. Oehninger S, et al. Failure of fertilization in in vitro fertilization: the 'occult' male factor. J In Vitro Fert Embryo Transf 1988; 5: 181

113. Nikolettos N, et al. Fertilization potential of spermatozoa with abnormal morphology. Hum Reprod 1999; 14: 47

114. Bartoov B, et al. Real-time fine morphology of motile human sperm cells is associated with IVF–ICSI outcome. J Androl 2002; 23: 1

115. Nagy ZP, et al. The result of intracytoplasmic sperm injection is not related to any of the three basic sperm parameters. Hum Reprod 1995; 10: 1123

116. Liu J, et al. Analysis of 76 total fertilization failure cycles out of 2732 intracytoplasmic sperm injection cycles. Hum Reprod 1995; 10: 2630

117. Kay VJ, Irvine DS. Successful in-vitro fertilization pregnancy with spermatozoa from a patient with Kartagener's syndrome: case report. Hum Reprod 2000; 15: 135

118. Nijs M, et al. Fertilizing ability of immotile spermatozoa after intracytoplasmic sperm injection. Hum Reprod 1996; 11: 2180

119. Barros A, et al. Pregnancy and birth after intracytoplasmic sperm injection with totally immotile sperm recovered from the ejaculate. Fertil Steril 1997; 67: 1091

120. Kahraman S, et al. A healthy birth after intracytoplasmic sperm injection by using immotile testicular spermatozoa in a case with totally immotile ejaculated spermatozoa before and after Percoll gradients. Hum Reprod 1997; 12: 292

121. von Zumbusch A, et al. Birth of healthy children after intracytoplasmic sperm injection in two couples with male Kartagener's syndrome. Fertil Steril 1998; 70: 643

122. Kahraman S, et al. Pregnancies achieved with testicular and ejaculated spermatozoa in combination with intracytoplasmic sperm injection in men with totally or initially immotile spermatozoa in the ejaculate. Hum Reprod 1996; 11: 1343

123. Ved S, et al. Pregnancy following intracytoplasmic sperm injection of immotile spermatozoa selected by the hypo-osmotic swelling-test: a case report. Andrologia 1997; 29: 241

124. Wang CW, et al. Pregnancy after intracytoplasmic injection of immotile sperm. A case report. J Reprod Med 1997; 42: 448

125. Terriou P, et al. Pentoxifylline initiates motility in spontaneously immotile epididymal and testicular spermatozoa and allows normal fertilization, pregnancy, and birth after intracytoplasmic sperm injection. J Assist Reprod Genet 2000; 17: 194

126. Chemes HE, Rawe VY. Sperm pathology: a step beyond descriptive morphology. Origin, characterization and fertility potential of abnormal sperm phenotypes in infertile men. Hum Reprod Update 2003; 9: 405

127. Saias-Magnan J, et al. Failure of pregnancy after intracytoplasmic sperm injection with decapitated spermatozoa: case report. Hum Reprod 1999; 14: 1989

128. Schmiady H, Radke E, Kentenich H. Round-headed spermatozoa – contraindication for IVF. Geburtshilfe Frauenheilkd 1992; 52: 301

129. Bourne H, et al. Normal fertilization and embryo development by intracytoplasmic sperm injection of round-headed acrosomeless sperm. Fertil Steril 1995; 63: 1329

130. Battaglia DE, et al. Failure of oocyte activation after intracytoplasmic sperm injection using round-headed sperm. Fertil Steril 1997; 68: 118

131. Edirisinghe WR, et al. Cytogenetic analysis of unfertilized oocytes following intracytoplasmic sperm injection using spermatozoa from globozoospermic man. Hum Reprod 1998; 13: 3094

132. Rybouchkin A, et al. Disintegration of chromosomes in dead sperm cells as revealed by injection into mouse oocytes. Hum Reprod 1997; 12: 1693

133. Kim ST, et al. Successful pregnancy and delivery from frozen–thawed embryos after intracytoplasmic sperm injection using round-headed spermatozoa and assisted oocyte activation in a globozoosperic patient with mosaic Down syndrome. Fertil Steril 2001; 75: 445

134. Lunding K, et al. Fertilization and pregnancy after intracytoplasmic microinjection of acrosomeless spermatozoa. Fertil Steril 1994; 62: 1266

135. Liu J, et al. Successful fertilization and establishment of pregnancies after intracytoplasmic sperm injection in patients with globozoospermia. Hum Reprod 1995; 10: 626

136. Trokoudes KM, et al. Pregnancy with spermatozoa from a globozoospermic man after intracytoplasmic sperm injection. Hum Reprod 1995; 10: 880

137. Stone S, et al. A normal livebirth after intracytoplasmic sperm injection for globozoospermia without assisted oocyte activation: case report. Hum Reprod 2000; 15: 139

138. Nardo LG, et al. Ultrastructural features and ICSI treatment of severe teratozoospermia: report of two human cases of globozoospermia. Eur J Obstet Gynecol Reprod Biol 2002; 104: 40

139. Zeyneloglu HB, et al. Achievement of pregnancy in globozoospermia with Y chromosome microdeletion after ICSI. Hum Reprod 2002; 17: 1833

140. Francavilla S, et al. Chromatin defects in normal and malformed human ejaculated and epididymal spermatozoa: a cytochemical ultrastructural study. J Reprod Fertil 1996; 106: 259

141. Francavilla S, et al. Ultrastructural analysis of chromatin defects in testicular spermatids in azoospermic men submitted to TESE–ICSI. Hum Reprod 2001; 16: 1440

142. Kahraman S, et al. Fertility of ejaculated and testicular megalohead spermatozoa with intracytoplasmic sperm injection. Hum Reprod 1999; 14: 726

143. Bartoov B, et al. High power light microscope morphological examination as a tool for single sperm selection pryor IVF–ICSI. Int J Androl 2005; 28 (Suppl 1): 8

144. Greco E, et al. Efficient treatment of infertility due to sperm DNA damage by ICSI with testicular spermatozoa. Hum Reprod 2005; 20: 226

7

Testicular dysgenesis syndrome: biological and clinical significance

Niels Jørgensen, Camilla Asklund, Katrine Bay, Niels E Skakkebæk

INTRODUCTION

A few years ago it was suggested that testicular cancer, hypospadias, cryptorchidism and low sperm counts were all symptoms of a disease complex, the testicular dysgenesis syndrome (TDS), with a common origin in fetal life[1] (Figure 7.1). Knowledge of the etiology of TDS is still rather limited, but environmental and life-style factors are suggested as contributing agents. However, genetic polymorphisms or aberrations may render some individuals particularly susceptible to these exogenous factors. The most severe cases of TDS may include all four symptoms, whereas the least

affected may show only reduced spermatogenesis which is fully compatible with fertility[1]. Consequently, a person diagnosed with one of the TDS symptoms must be considered at increased risk of harboring one or more of the other symptoms as well.

PRENATAL ORIGIN OF TESTICULAR DYSGENESIS SYNDROME

The prenatal origin of hypospadias and cryptorchidism is evident, owing to their congenital nature. However, testicular cancers that do not

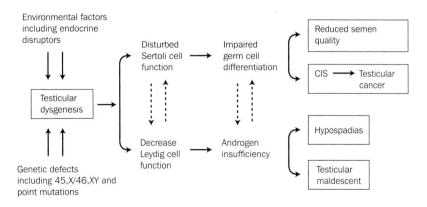

Figure 7.1 Schematic presentation of the components and clinical manifestations of testicular dysgenesis syndrome. CIS, carcinoma *in situ*. Adapted with permission from reference 1

manifest until later in life are most probably also of fetal origin. Likewise, the potential of a man's semen quality may also be determined prenatally.

Spermatogenesis

At the beginning of the fourth week of fetal development, germ cells begin to migrate via the yolk sac through the gut and into the mesentery, ending in the celomic epithelium of the gonadal ridges[2]. The indifferent gonad is composed of three cell types: germ cells, supporting cells, which in the male fetus give rise to Sertoli cells, and stromal (interstitial) cells. The first sign of gonadal differentiation is development of the Sertoli cells and their aggregation into primitive seminiferous cords during the eighth week of development[3]. Differentiation of the gonad into a testis rather than an ovary is genetically dependent on the SRY gene (the gene of the sex-determining region of the Y chromosome), which is expressed by testicular (Sertoli) cells[4]. The majority of the Sertoli cell multiplication occurs during fetal life, and only to a lesser extent later[5]. The final number of Sertoli cells reached during development has consequences in adult life, as these cells can only support a limited number of germ cells[6,7]. Thus,

factors affecting Sertoli cell development and function during fetal life will have important consequences for a man's future spermatogenic capacity, as the number of Sertoli cells essentially determines the maximal achievable sperm output. The final sperm output may, however, be adversely influenced by postnatal factors such as irradiation, medical treatment, pesticides, organic solvents, metals and physical agents.

Testicular cancer

Testicular germ-cell cancers occurring from puberty and onwards originate from preinvasive carcinoma *in situ* of the testis (CIS) cells, which are considered to be gonocyte-like transformed germ cells that failed to differentiate during the fetal period[8,9]. CIS cells have stem-cell properties, as evident from the expression of a number of genes also expressed by gonocytes and embryonic stem cells, for example alkaline phosphatase, c-*kit*, Oct-4, SSEA-3 (stage-specific embryonic antigen 3) and others[8,10–13] (Figure 7.2). Furthermore, CIS cells and gonocytes lack expression of other genes that are specific for postmeiotic germ cells[14]. Clinical data also indicate that CIS cells arise before adult life[15], and CIS cells have been detected even

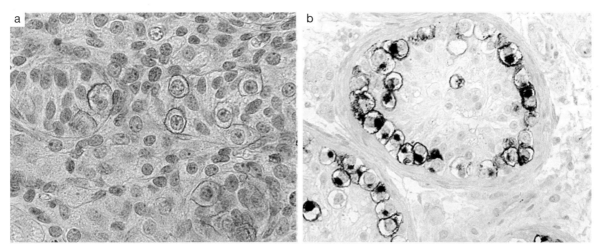

Figure 7.2 Immunohistochemical staining with placental-like alkaline phosphatase (PLAP). (a) Expression in normal, immature germ cells of 9-week-old fetal testis, and (b) expression in an adult testis with carcinoma *in situ* cells. Note in both images that the immunohistochemical reaction is not seen in Sertoli cells or interstitial cells

in the neonatal period[16]. Epidemiologically, it has been shown that Danish and other Scandinavian men born during the Second World War have a lower risk in all age groups of developing germ-cell tumors than expected from the overall trend in incidences, indicating that important etiological events take place during prenatal life[17,18].

Hypospadias and cryptorchidism

The secondary sex characteristics are dependent on hormones produced by the newly formed testicles. Testosterone is secreted by the fetal Leydig cells, and is responsible for differentiation of the Wolffian duct into the epididymis, vas deferens and seminal vesicle[19]. Testosterone is converted to 5α-dihydrotestosterone at the bipotential external genitalia, and stimulates formation of the penile urethra, the penis and the scrotum. Decreased testosterone secretion may lead to formation disturbances, resulting in hypospadias[20], for example.

Testicular descent appears in two phases. The intra-abdominal descent is quite complex, and its regulation is not fully understood; however, it occurs in the second trimester and is largely dependent on the Leydig cell hormone insulin-like factor 3 (INSL3)[21]. The following descent through the inguinal canal and into the scrotum is dependent on adequate testosterone secretion[22]. Thus, impaired INSL3 and/or testosterone may lead to cryptorchidism.

RISK FACTORS FOR TESTICULAR DYSGENESIS SYNDROME

Many investigators have found that the TDS symptoms are to be regarded as risk factors for each other, and frequently, patients present with more than one of the symptoms. The association between testicular cancer and low semen quality is firmly established. CIS cells were first detected in infertile men[23], and later Berthelsen showed reduced spermatogenesis in testicles contralateral to testicular cancer already before treatment of the

cancer[24,25]. More recently, men with unilateral testicular cancer have been shown to have poorer semen quality than expected from a man with only one functioning testicle[26]. Epidemiologically, the link between testicular cancer and low semen quality has indirectly been confirmed by the detection of reduced fertility in men who later developed testicular cancer[27]. At the histological level, the non-tumor-bearing testicles in men with testicular cancer often show carcinoma *in situ* (5–8%), Sertoli-cell-only tubules (13.8%), microcalcifications (6.0%) and undifferentiated Sertoli cells (4.6%). All in all, signs of histological testicular dysgenesis were detected in 25.2% of the examined contralateral testes[28].

Cryptorchidism is a well-known risk factor for both testicular cancer and poor semen quality[29–31], and the association between cryptorchidism and hypospadias is well documented[31,32].

The associations between the four TDS symptoms point to abnormal germ-cell and/or Sertoli-cell development during fetal life, and are all coupled to the intrauterine milieu, such as low birth weight, premature birth and low parity[33–35]. Genetic factors seem to contribute, as indicated by the fact that African-Americans have significantly lower incidence than Caucasians living in the same areas of the USA[36,37]. Additionally, patients with genetic disorders such as 45,X/46,XY mosaicism or androgen insensitivity syndrome often show testicular dysgenesis due to impaired androgen production or function already in fetal life, increased risk of cryptorchidism, testicular cancer and impaired spermatogenesis. The genetic mechanism(s) behind this is still unresolved; however, genes on the Y chromosome seem to be important for proper testicular function[38,39].

REGIONAL AND TEMPORAL TRENDS IN TESTICULAR DYSGENESIS SYNDROME SYMPTOMS

For many years, the incidence of testicular germ-cell cancer has increased in numerous European countries[40]. In particular, the situation in the two Nordic countries Denmark and Finland is remarkable. Danish men have one of the highest incidences of testicular cancer, and Finnish men one of the lowest incidences (11.1 per 10[5] and 2.8 per 10[5], respectively)[41]. The sharp increase in incidence among Danish men shows a birth cohort-dependency, as men born recently have a higher lifetime risk than men born in previous decades[17,42].

In line with the geographical trends observed for testicular cancer, the prevalence of cryptorchidism and hypospadias in Finnish newborn boys is considerably lower than in Danish boys (2.4% vs. 9.0% and 0.27% vs. 1.03%, respectively)[43,44].

Semen quality also shows a regional difference, with a better situation among Finnish than among Danish men. Young, normal men from the Danish general population have a median sperm concentration of 41×10^6/ml in contrast to Finnish men having 54×10^6/ml[45], and overall an East–West gradient in sperm concentration exists in the Nordic–Baltic area[45–48], with a better situation in the eastern than in the western part (Figure 7.3).

There are, however, indications that the otherwise good reproductive health of Finnish men is also following a worsening tendency. Despite being low, the testicular cancer incidence is increasing[40], while the sperm count may be decreasing[45].

In 1992, Carlsen and co-workers[49] reported the results of a meta-analysis of previously published semen quality data, and indicated that sperm concentration among men in Europe and North America had decreased. Following this, reports from several other research groups were published. Some did not find any change over time[50–53], whereas others suggested that sperm counts had declined significantly[54–57], and thereby also indicated the presence of geographical differences in the adverse male reproductive-health trends.

Associations between the individual TDS symptoms are seen not only in Danish and Finnish populations. Norwegian men have a high frequency of testicular cancer and low sperm

(a)

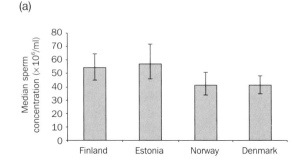

(b)

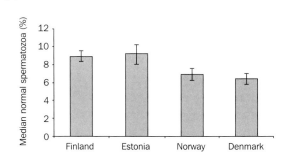

Figure 7.3   Illustration of the regional difference in (a) sperm concentration (adjusted for period of abstinence and interlaboratory variation) and (b) frequency of morphologically normal spermatozoa of young men from the Nordic–Baltic area. Bars indicate median values and 95% confidence level of the estimates (from linear regression models taking confounders into account). See text for further explanation. Adapted from reference 45. Results from references 47 and 48 are not included as the presentations in these publications do not provide sufficient information to draw similar bars

counts, whereas the opposite is true for Estonian and Lithuanian men[45,46]. Unfortunately, very limited information exists from countries outside the Nordic–Baltic area to elucidate the occurrence of TDS. Japanese fertile men seem to have semen quality at the same level as that of comparable Danish fertile men, but at the same time Japanese men have a risk of testicular cancer at or below the level in Finnish men[40,58]. This finding is compatible with Japanese (or Asian) men having a lower sperm quality, without being at increased risk for the other symptoms of TDS. However, a more thorough analysis is needed before any firm conclusions can be reached.

Studies have revealed the existence of regional differences in semen quality among fertile US men[59], whereas other studies have shown African-Americans having significantly lower incidences of testicular cancer than Caucasians living in the same areas[37]. These results are compatible with both an environmental and a genetic influence on male reproductive health, but the studies cannot provide any firm information about associations between the different TDS symptoms among US men. Likewise, data from other countries outside Northern Europe are lacking.

TESTICULAR DYSGENESIS SYNDROME AND FECUNDITY

It is of concern that the birth rate in many industrialized countries has declined to below replacement level of the populations. The social structure in these countries acts against a high birth rate, but it is becoming clearer that reduced biological fecundity may also be considered an important contributing factor. The World Health Organization (WHO) states that the reference value for sperm concentration is 20×10^6 spermatozoa/ml[60]. Whether this is a relevant 'threshold' can be questioned) owing to the findings of a prospective study of fecundity. Decreasing waiting time to pregnancy (TTP) with increasing sperm concentrations up to approximately 40×10^6 spermatozoa/ml was shown[61]. Additionally, a recent cross-sectional study of European fertile men demonstrated a reduced TTP with increasing sperm concentration up to 55×10^6 spermatozoa/ml[62]. Thus, a large fraction of normal young Danish and Norwegian men may already have a semen quality with sperm concentrations below these levels; 20% of the investigated Danish and Norwegian men had a sperm concentration below the WHO reference level, and approximately 40% of the men had fewer than 40×10^6 spermatozoa/ml. Sperm concentration is only one of the parameters having an impact on fecundity. A recent publication by Guzick *et al.* has indicated

that men with fewer than 9% morphologically normal spermatozoa belong to a group of subfertile men, and that men ought to have more than 12% normal forms to be regarded as fertile[63]. The Danish and Norwegian young, normal men had only a few more than 6% (median) normal forms[45]. The majority of these young men were 19 years of age; however, a follow-up study of these men indicated that their low semen quality is unlikely to be a result of immaturity[64].

POSSIBLE LIFE-STYLE OR ENVIRONMENTAL FACTORS CAUSING IMPAIRED MALE REPRODUCTIVE HEALTH

It is possible that genetic predisposition may play a partial role in the observed trends in male reproductive health, at least for some populations. For example, impaired spermatogenesis has in some studies been associated with polymorphisms in the androgen receptor gene or in the Y chromosome[39,65]. The speed of the observed increase in testicular cancer indicates that life-style or environmental factors may also be contributing agents. Furthermore, poor semen quality, cryptorchidism or hypospadias – at least in some areas – have become more frequent[40,43,45], and thus exogenous etiological factors are likely.

Three recent studies detected that men exposed to smoking *in utero* (via maternal smoking during pregnancy) had decreased sperm concentrations: a 20% reduction compared with men not exposed at all[66], a 48% reduction among sons exposed to maternal smoking of more than ten cigarettes per day[67] and a dose-dependent association between fetal tobacco exposure, lower semen quality and higher risk of oligozoospermia[68]. The men's own history of tobacco-smoking was shown to be only of minor importance when taking into account mothers smoking while pregnant.

Obesity has increased in the Western world, and a body mass index (BMI) above $25 \, \text{kg/m}^2$ has been associated with reductions in sperm concentration, total sperm count and morphologically normal spermatozoa[69]. Any causal relationship between semen quality and BMI has yet to be resolved.

Generally, TDS is suggested to result from disruption of fetal gonadal development caused by endocrine-disrupting compounds. During recent years, focus has been on the possible disruption of the androgen–estrogen balance and impaired androgen action[33,70].

Recent experimental evidence comes from a possible animal model for TDS, in which rats exposed *in utero* to the antiandrogen dibutyl phthalate developed cryptorchidism, hypospadias, infertility and testis abnormalities[71,72]. The finding that phthalates can induce TDS-like symptoms is of concern, as neonates can be exposed to considerable daily doses of phthalates via breast-milk[73,74]. Moreover, many of the so-called 'environmental estrogens', including a number of pesticides, have also appeared to possess antiandrogenic properties[75].

In the absence of possibilities to provide evidence of a causal relationship between human exposure to harmful chemicals and male reproductive health, rising concern has led to a number of epidemiological studies dealing with associations between parental exposure to substances with endocrine-disrupting properties and congenital abnormalities in the reproductive organs of their sons[34,76–80]. Interestingly, an American group has recently published a report using shortening of the anogenital distance (AGD) as a new and more sensitive marker for demasculinization in humans. In 134 boys aged 2–30 months they found a significant inverse correlation between AGD and urinary concentrations of a number of phthalate metabolites[81].

CONCLUSIONS

Testicular dysgenesis syndrome (TDS) encompasses the disease entities cryptorchidism, hypospadias, testicular cancer and poor semen quality. Exogenous factors exhibiting antiandrogenic properties or reducing androgen/estrogen functions are suspected to affect the developing fetal gonad, leading to the TDS symptoms. However, a genetic susceptibility to these exposures may contribute to the development. In its most severe form, a man may suffer from all the TDS symptoms, whereas the least affected may only have a slightly reduced semen quality, compatible with fertility. Most likely, all cases of testicular germ-cell cancers are due to TDS. The three other symptoms may also be due to TDS; however, alternative contributing factors may be relevant. A man's potential semen quality may already be determined prenatally, but may be adversely affected by factors acting postnatally. Nevertheless, diagnosis of one of the TDS symptoms should alert physicians to look for manifestations of the other symptoms, especially the occurrence of preinvasive carcinoma *in situ* germ cells. Eradication of these cells will prevent the development of overt testicular cancer[82].

REFERENCES

1. Skakkebaek NE, Rajpert-De ME, Main KM. Testicular dysgenesis syndrome: an increasingly common developmental disorder with environmental aspects. Hum Reprod 2001; 16: 972
2. Witschi E. Migration of the germ cells of human embryos from the yolk sac to the primitive gonadal folds. Contributions to Embryology, No. 209. Washington, DC: Carnegie Institute of Washington, 1948: 69
3. Jirasek JE. Principles of reproductive embryology. In Simpson JL, ed. Disorders of Sexual Differentiation. New York: Academic Press, 1976: 51
4. Gubbay J, et al. A gene mapping to the sex-determining region of the mouse Y chromosome is a member of a novel family of embryonically expressed genes. Nature 1990; 346: 245
5. Cortes D, Muller J, Skakkebaek NE. Proliferation of Sertoli cells during development of the human testis assessed by stereological methods. Int J Androl 1987; 10: 589
6. Russell LD, Peterson RN. Determination of the elongate spermatid–Sertoli cell ratio in various mammals. J Reprod Fertil 1984; 70: 635

7. Orth JM, Gunsalus GL, Lamperti AA. Evidence from Sertoli cell-depleted rats indicates that spermatid number in adults depends on numbers of Sertoli cells produced during perinatal development. Endocrinology 1988; 122: 787

8. Skakkebaek NE, et al. Carcinoma-in-situ of the testis: possible origin from gonocytes and precursor of all types of germ cell tumours except spermatocytoma. Int J Androl 1987; 10: 19

9. Rajpert-De Meyts E, et al. Developmental arrest of germ cells in the pathogenesis of germ cell neoplasia. APMIS 1998; 106: 198

10. Jacobsen GK, Nørgaard-Pedersen B. Placental alkaline phosphatase in testicular germ cell tumours and in carcinoma-in-situ of the testis. APMIS 1984; 92: 323

11. Jørgensen N, et al. Expression of immunohistochemical markers for testicular carcinoma in situ by normal human fetal germ cells. Lab Invest 1995; 72: 223

12. Looijenga LH, et al. POU5F1 (OCT3/4) identifies cells with pluripotent potential in human germ cell tumors. Cancer Res 2003; 63: 2244

13. Damjanov I, et al. Immunohistochemical localization of murine stage-specific embryonic antigens in human testicular germ cell tumors. Am J Pathol 1982; 108: 225

14. Rapley EA, et al. Localisation of susceptibility genes for familial testicular germ cell tumour. APMIS 2003; 111: 128

15. Giwercman A, von der Maase H, Skakkebaek NE. Epidemiological and clinical aspects of carcinoma in situ of the testis. Eur Urol 1993; 23: 104

16. Müller J, Skakkebaek NE. Testicular carcinoma in situ in children with androgen insensitivity (testicular feminisation) syndrome. Br Med J 1984; 288: 1419

17. Møller H. Clues to the aetiology of testicular germ cell tumours from descriptive epidemiology. Eur Urol 1993; 23: 8

18. Adami HO, et al. Testicular cancer in nine northern European countries. Int J Cancer 1994; 59: 33

19. Wilson JD, Lasnitzki I. Dihydrotestosterone formation in fetal tissues of the rabbit and rat. Endocrinology 1971; 89: 659

20. Baskin LS. Hypospadias and urethral development. J Urol 2000; 163: 951

21. Toppari J, Kaleva M. Maldescendus testis. Horm Res 1999; 51: 261

22. Wilson JD, George FW, Renfree MB. The endocrine role in mammalian sexual differentiation. Recent Prog Horm Res 1995; 50: 349

23. Skakkebaek NE. Possible carcinoma-in-situ of the testis. Lancet 1972; 2: 516

24. Berthelsen JG, Skakkebaek NE. Gonadal function in men with testis cancer. Fertil Steril 1983; 39: 68

25. Berthelsen JG. Andrological aspects of testicular cancer. Int J Androl 1984; 7: 451

26. Petersen PM, et al. Gonadal function in men with testicular cancer. Semin Oncol 1998; 25: 224

27. Møller H, Skakkebaek NE. Risk of testicular cancer in subfertile men: case–control study. Br Med J 1999; 318: 559

28. Hoei-Hansen CE, et al. Histological evidence of testicular dysgenesis in contralateral biopsies from 218 patients with testicular germ cell cancer. J Pathol 2003; 200: 370

29. Sohval AR. Testicular dysgenesis as an etiologic factor in cryptorchidism. J Urol 1954; 72: 693

30. Huff DS, et al. Histologic maldevelopment of unilaterally cryptorchid testes and their descended partners. Eur J Pediatr 1993; 152 (Suppl 2): S11

31. Khuri FJ, Hardy BE, Churchill BM. Urologic anomalies associated with hypospadias. Urol Clin North Am 1981; 8: 565

32. Weidner IS, et al. Risk factors for cryptorchidism and hypospadias. J Urol 1999; 161: 1606

33. Sharpe RM. The 'oestrogen hypothesis' – where do we stand now? Int J Androl 2003; 26: 2

34. Pierik FH, et al. Maternal and paternal risk factors for cryptorchidism and hypospadias: a case–control study in newborn boys. Environ Health Perspect 2004; 112: 1570

35. Berkowitz GS, et al. Maternal and neonatal risk factors for cryptorchidism. Epidemiology 1995; 6: 127

36. Spitz MR, et al. Incidence and descriptive features of testicular cancer among United States whites, blacks, and Hispanics, 1973–1982. Cancer 1986; 58: 1785

37. McGlynn KA, et al. Increasing incidence of testicular germ cell tumors among black men in the United States. J Clin Oncol 2005; 23: 5757

38. Krausz C, Forti G, McElreavey K. The Y chromosome and male fertility and infertility. Int J Androl 2003; 26: 70

39. McElreavey K, Quintana-Murci L. Y chromosome haplogroups: a correlation with testicular dysgenesis syndrome? APMIS 2003; 111: 106

40. Richiardi L, et al. Testicular cancer incidence in eight northern European countries: secular and recent trends. Cancer Epidemiol Biomarkers Prev 2004; 13: 2157

41. Bray F, et al. Estimates of cancer incidence and mortality in Europe in 1995. Eur J Cancer 2002; 38: 99

42. Møller H. Trends in incidence of testicular cancer and prostate cancer in Denmark. Hum Reprod 2001; 16: 1007

43. Boisen KA, et al. Difference in prevalence of congenital cryptorchidism in infants between two Nordic countries. Lancet 2004; 363: 1264

44. Boisen KA, et al. Hypospadias in a cohort of 1072 Danish newborn boys: prevalence and relationship to placental weight, anthropometrical measurements at birth, and reproductive hormone levels at three months of age. J Clin Endocrinol Metab 2005; 90: 4041

45. Jørgensen N, et al. East–West gradient in semen quality in the Nordic–Baltic area: a study of men from the general population in Denmark, Norway, Estonia and Finland. Hum Reprod 2002; 17: 2199

46. Punab M, et al. Regional differences in semen qualities in the Baltic region. Int J Androl 2002; 25: 243

47. Richthoff J, et al. Higher sperm counts in Southern Sweden compared with Denmark. Hum Reprod 2002; 17: 2468

48. Tsarev I, et al. Sperm concentration in Latvian military conscripts as compared with other countries in the Nordic–Baltic area. Int J Androl 2005; 28: 208

49. Carlsen E, et al. Evidence for decreasing quality of semen during past 50 years. Br Med J 1992; 305: 609

50. Vierula M, et al. High and unchanged sperm counts of Finnish men. Int J Androl 1996; 19: 11

51. Fisch H, et al. Semen analyses in 1,283 men from the United States over a 25-year period: no decline in quality. Fertil Steril 1996; 65: 1009

52. Paulsen CA, Berman NG, Wang C. Data from men in greater Seattle area reveals no downward trend in semen quality: further evidence that deterioration of semen quality is not geographically uniform. Fertil Steril 1996; 65: 1015

53. Handelsman DJ. Sperm output of healthy men in Australia: magnitude of bias due to self-selected volunteers. Hum Reprod 1997; 12: 2701

54. Swan SH, Elkin EP, Fenster L. The question of declining sperm density revisited: an analysis of 101 studies published 1934–1996. Environ Health Perspect 2000; 108: 961

55. Auger J, et al. Decline in semen quality among fertile men in Paris during the past 20 years. N Engl J Med 1995; 332: 281

56. Irvine S, et al. Evidence of deteriorating semen quality in the United Kingdom: birth cohort study in 577 men in Scotland over 11 years. Br Med J 1996; 312: 467

57. Van Waeleghem K, et al. Deterioration of sperm quality in young healthy Belgian men. Hum Reprod 1996; 11: 325

58. Iwamoto T, et al. Semen quality of 324 fertile Japanese men. Hum Reprod 2006; 21: 760

59. Swan SH, et al. Semen quality in relation to biomarkers of pesticide exposure. Environ Health Perspect 2003; 111: 1478

60. World Health Organization. WHO Laboratory Manual for the Examination of Human Semen and Sperm–Cervical Mucus Interaction, 4th edn. Cambridge: Cambridge University Press, 1999

61. Bonde JP, et al. Relation between semen quality and fertility: a population-based study of 430 first-pregnancy planners. Lancet 1998; 352: 1172

62. Slama R, et al. Time to pregnancy and semen parameters: a cross-sectional study among fertile couples from four European cities. Hum Reprod 2002; 17: 503

63. Guzick DS, et al. Sperm morphology, motility, and concentration in fertile and infertile men. N Engl J Med 2001; 345: 1388

64. Carlsen E, et al. Longitudinal changes in semen parameters in young Danish men from the Copenhagen area. Hum Reprod 2005; 20: 942

65. Ochsenkuhn R, De Kretser DM. The contributions of deficient androgen action in spermatogenic disorders. Int J Androl 2003; 26: 195

66. Jensen TK, et al. Association of in utero exposure to maternal smoking with reduced semen quality and testis size in adulthood: a cross-sectional study of 1,770 young men from the general population in five European countries. Am J Epidemiol 2004; 159: 49

67. Storgaard L, et al. Does smoking during pregnancy affect sons' sperm counts? Epidemiology 2003; 14: 278

68. Jensen MS, et al. Lower sperm counts following prenatal tobacco exposure. Hum Reprod 2005; 20: 2559

69. Jensen TK, et al. Body mass index in relation to semen quality and reproductive hormones among 1,558 Danish men. Fertil Steril 2004; 82: 863

70. Rivas A, et al. Induction of reproductive tract developmental abnormalities in the male rat by lowering androgen production or action in combination with a low dose of diethylstilbestrol: evidence for importance of the androgen–estrogen balance. Endocrinology 2002; 143: 4797

71. Fisher JS, et al. Human 'testicular dysgenesis syndrome': a possible model using in-utero exposure of the rat to dibutyl phthalate. Hum Reprod 2003; 18: 1383

72. Mahood I K, et al. Abnormal Leydig cell aggregation in the fetal testis of rats exposed to di (n-butyl) phthalate and its possible role in testicular dysgenesis. Endocrinology 2005; 146: 613

73. Calafat AM, et al. Automated solid phase extraction and quantitative analysis of human milk for 13 phthalate metabolites. J Chromatogr B Analyt Technol Biomed Life Sci 2004; 805: 49

74. Mortensen GK, et al. Determination of phthalate monoesters in human milk, consumer milk, and infant formula by tandem mass spectrometry (LC-MS-MS). Anal Bioanal Chem 2005; 382: 1084

75. Sohoni P, Sumpter JP. Several environmental oestrogens are also anti-androgens. J Endocrinol 1998; 158: 327

76. Dolk H, et al. Risk of congenital anomalies near hazardous-waste landfill sites in Europe: the EUROHAZCON study. Lancet 1998; 352: 423

77. Garcia-Rodriguez J, et al. Exposure to pesticides and cryptorchidism: geographical evidence of a possible association. Environ Health Perspect 1996; 104: 1090

78. Weidner IS, et al. Cryptorchidism and hypospadias in sons of gardeners and farmers. Environ Health Perspect 2004; 106: 793

79. Hardell L, et al. Concentrations of polychlorinated biphenyls in blood and the risk for testicular cancer. Int J Androl 2004; 27: 282

80. Hauser R, et al. The relationship between human semen parameters and environmental exposure to polychlorinated biphenyls and p,p′-DDE. Environ Health Perspect 2003; 111: 1505

81. Swan SH, et al. Decrease in anogenital distance among male infants with prenatal phthalate exposure. Environ Health Perspect 2005; 113: 1056

82. Rorth M, et al. Carcinoma in situ in the testis. Scand J Urol Nephrol Suppl 2000: 166

Section 2

Diagnosis of male infertility

8

Evaluation of the subfertile male

Agnaldo P Cedenho

INTRODUCTION

Based on the literature, it can be expected that 15–20% of couples within reproductive age will encounter difficulties in achieving a pregnancy, and medical attention will be required in order to start a family. Around 30% of these couples are infertile due to a significant isolated male factor, and associated male and female factors are present in an additional 20% of cases[1]. Therefore, an abnormal male factor is involved in about half of the couples seeking infertility treatment.

Although male factor infertility plays such a dramatic role in a couple's infertility, it has been left aside for decades. In fact, for a long time the man was examined solely using conventional semen analysis, without even an interview or a physical examination. Since the advent of intracytoplasmic sperm injection (ICSI) in 1992[2], this situation has become even worse. ICSI is without doubt a breakthrough in male infertility treatment, but since this technique overcomes virtually all natural barriers to fertilization, research on male factor infertility has lost its momentum, and both physicians and patients have shifted their focus from seeking and treating the cause of male infertility to achieving pregnancy only. Fortunately, as usually occurs in medicine, time and evidence puts everything back in its place. Perhaps more now than ever before, the subfertile man

needs to be studied with extreme care in search of the true cause of infertility, for once it is found, the physician will be able to decide what is the best treatment plan (with the best possible cost/benefit ratio) for the couple. Evidence-based andrology will thus ultimately allow childless couples to be spared the enormous stress associated with infertility.

For many decades it has been conventional to define infertility as 1 year of failed attempts to conceive, and a couple should be investigated for infertility only after 1 year of regular sexual activity without the use of any contraceptives. This period of time was selected from epidemiological studies suggesting that around 85% of couples are able to achieve pregnancy within 1 year[3]. Therefore, after 1 year only 15% of couples will need infertility work-up. Even though the logic behind this rationale is evident, concessions need to be made considering the current situation and history of each partner in the infertile couple.

If, for example, a woman is over 35 years old, or one of the partners has a clinical history that could lower his/her ability to conceive, this period of time may be shortened. On the other hand, since evaluation of the male partner in an infertile couple is simple, fast, inexpensive and usually non-invasive, it may be performed as soon as the infertile couple seeks medical assistance, or whenever the male partner decides to evaluate his fertility status[4]. Evaluation of the male partner should be carried out following basic medical guidelines, which are: the patient's history, physical examination, as well as all the laboratory and imaging resources available at the time. While the patient's history and physical examination are of fundamental importance to all patients, imaging and laboratory techniques should be used as required. Many patients will require only two separate standard semen analyses, while others will need to go through many tests in order to find the cause of infertility. Each patient must be evaluated according to the individual situation.

PATIENT HISTORY

Patient history and a careful physical examination may be of great help in evaluating the male partner of an infertile couple (Table 8.1) Although this chapter focuses on the infertile man, information regarding the female partner is not only useful, but also extremely relevant in deciding a treatment plan. We should not forget that as far as reproduction is concerned the couple must be seen as one functional unit, not as two separate individuals. It is therefore important to know the female history concerning menstrual cycle regularity, previous infections, pregnancies, abortions, abdominal surgery and possible risks related to sexually transmitted diseases (STDs).

In many cases, coupling seminal analysis with the female partner's examinations, such as pelvic ultrasound and hysterosalpingography, will allow the examiner to assess whether the couple can still achieve pregnancy through natural conception. On the other hand, the reproductive history is one of the most important areas to investigate in the infertile couple. It is very important to know how long the couple has been trying to achieve pregnancy without success, mainly because the longer is this period (> 7 years), the lower are the chances of natural conception and the graver are the factors involved. This is especially true when the female partner has normal menstrual cycles,

Table 8.1 Work-up sheet addressing anamnesis in a chronological fashion

Conception	Natural conception or ART was needed
Prenatal	Drugs, pharmaceutical, environmental agents and endocrine disruptors
Childhood	Cryptorchidism, inguinal herniorrhaphy, bladder neck, pelvic or retroperitoneal surgery, testicular torsion
Puberty onset	Precocious or late, testicular trauma or torsion
Adolescence or young adult	Sexual behavior and STDs, viral or bacterial orchitis, recreational drugs, anabolic steroids, inguinal herniorrhaphy
Adult	Tricyclic antidepressives, antihypertensives, sulfasalazine, nitrofurantoin, cimetidine, chemotherapy, radiotherapy, retroperitoneal lymphadenectomy, inguinal herniorrhaphy, diabetes, multiple sclerosis, chronic respiratory diseases
Reproductive issues (female)	Menstrual cycle, infections, pregnancies, abortions, STDs, previous investigation and treatments
Reproductive issues (male)	Previous paternity, investigation, treatments, potency
Reproductive issues (couple)	Infertility duration, intercourse frequency and regularity, coital technique, knowledge about fertile period

ART, assisted reproductive technologies; STD, sexually transmitted disease

regular in frequency and with frequent sexual intercourse throughout the cycle.

It is also relevant to ask how much the couple knows about the fertile period during the menstrual cycle. Recent data have shown that the best period for the sperm to penetrate the female reproductive tract is prior to ovulation. This period may last for up to 6 days, and immediately after ovulation the cervical mucus becomes hostile to sperm, mostly due to a progestational effect[5].

Information regarding the sexual act itself is paramount to understanding the mechanisms underlying infertility. Lubricants used during sexual intercourse are usually spermicidal or determine lower sperm motility, and therefore it is necessary to know whether they are used. The most common lubricants used are K-Y®Jelly, Lubrifax®, Keri" lotion or even saliva[6–8].

Previous fatherhood, albeit not a guarantee of current fertility, may reveal the reproductive potential of the male partner. Varicocele has been pointed out as the leading cause of secondary infertility[9]. Any previous investigation and treatment will help the evaluation to progress and spare the couple repeating examinations, thus saving time and money. A very productive and meaningful manner of evaluating patient history is through a work-up sheet that addresses anamnesis in a chronological fashion. This will give information regarding the male partner throughout different stages of his development.

Prenatal exposure to drugs, pharmaceuticals or environmental agents should be assessed. Fetal exposure to diethylstilbestrol (DES) may lead to epididymal cysts, an increased incidence of cryptorchidism and altered semen variables in adult life[10]. Patients with hypospadias may present endogenous endocrine abnormalities, including altered testosterone biosynthesis[11]. On the other hand, it is important to emphasize the role that endocrine disruptors play in male infertility. These substances and their by-products, used in the phytopharmaceutical industry, may affect serum endocrine levels, or alter hormone action, production, release and/or elimination. These deleterious effects have been demonstrated in animal models, and an increased concern about their effects in humans has arisen due to a greater incidence of reproductive-tract abnormalities and decreased sperm concentration in many areas worldwide[12].

In the near future, even information regarding how the patient was conceived will be necessary. Since ICSI may allow children to carry the same genetic defects as their fathers, such as Y-chromosome microdeletions, infertility has ironically become an inheritable clinical condition.

Cryptorchidism may affect 2–5% of born male children, and as such is an important cause of infertility[13]. Studies have demonstrated that 30% of children with unilateral cryptorchidism and 50% with bilateral cryptorchidism will present important semen alterations when adults. It is also noteworthy that, contrary to early indications, orchiopexy, even if performed while still very young, will not prevent future infertility[14].

Still during childhood, inguinal hernias, and their surgical correction, may play a role in infertility. Inguinal herniorrhaphy is the leading cause of iatrogenic obstruction of the vas deferens and testicular atrophy due to impaired blood supply to the testis[15,16]. An estimated 0.8–2% of inguinal herniorrhaphies performed in children lead to iatrogenic lesions of the deferent ducts, while in adults that risk decreases to about 0.3%[17,18]. Furthermore, there is no doubt that the actual number of iatrogenic lesions to the vas deferens is larger, but since the surgical procedure is usually unilateral, fertility is not always affected.

Ejaculatory disturbances may be caused by surgery performed during childhood on the bladder neck, in the pelvis or in the retroperitoneum. In the early 1960s, many children presenting with urethral defects were submitted to a surgical procedure known as YV plastic repair of the bladder neck. This surgery causes serious lesions to the internal sphincter, causing bladder-neck closure defects. In adult life these patients present with a decreased ejaculate volume (< 1 ml), and retrograde ejaculation. This diagnosis may be confirmed by finding sperm in the urine after ejaculation.

Puberty usually occurs between the ages of 11 and 12 years in boys. If puberty onset is precocious, this may indicate an adrenogenital syndrome. On the other hand, if puberty is delayed, it may be secondary to an endocrinopathy, such as in Klinefelter's syndrome or idiopathic hypogonadism.

Testicular torsion may occur in the newborn, infant or adolescent, and may lead to testicular atrophy. An estimated 30–40% of men with a history of testicular torsion have difficulty in achieving parenthood, due to the alterations in semen variables[19,20]. Although in the past changes of spermatogenesis were attributed to a possible rupture in the blood–testis barrier, testicular biopsies in contralateral testes have shown that these also present with histological alterations, supporting the hypothesis that testes prone to torsion, as well as their contralateral counterpart, already demonstrate defects in spermatogenesis[21].

Between adolescence and adult life, information regarding sexual behavior and risks related to STDs is very important. Even though its importance has declined, urethritis is still an important source of infection to the prostate, epididymides and testes. The most common urethritis-causing agents are: *Neisseria gonorrhoeae*, *Chlamydia trachomatis*, *Ureaplasma urealyticum* and *Trichomonas vaginalis*. In the United States, *C. trachomatis* is the principal agent in causing non-gonococcic urethritis and acute epididymitis, and 10–25% of men are asymptomatic, sometimes presenting with an increase in seminal leukocytes[22].

Viral orchitis may also impair testicular function, especially if the onset is postpubertal. Mumps may cause unilateral orchitis in 30% of male patients and bilateral orchitis in 10%, and these patients will possess a decrease in testicular volume and consistency[23].

An important reminder is that a prolonged fever on its own can be a source of damage to spermatogenesis. Therefore, these effects will not be observed immediately, since the duration of the spermatogenic cycle is 74 days in men, a period during which type B spermatogonia will differentiate into mature sperm, in addition to 15 days of sperm transport through the excretory system until they are ready for ejaculation. Thus, if damage to the testis from fever or medication is suspected, seminal analysis should be performed after 90 days.

Substance abuse has been linked to male infertility in many studies, and it is well documented that alcohol[24,25], tobacco[26], marijuana[27], cocaine[28,29] and anabolic steroids[30,31] may also cause testicular dysfunction. Alcohol has been shown to decrease serum testosterone levels, and this is due to its effects on three different levels: the hypothalamus, the pituitary gland and the testicular Leydig cells. While it directly alters Leydig cell function, and thus leads to the observed lower testosterone levels, alcohol may also have a negative impact on hypothalamic hormone production and the pituitary production, release and function of luteinizing and follicle stimulating hormones[24,25].

Tobacco, on the other hand, may cause a number of alterations, such as testicular atrophy, altered sperm morphology, low sperm motility, decreased semen volume, impaired spermatogenesis, poor acrosome reaction and sperm-penetrating ability, increased amounts of oxidative DNA damage, a higher risk for chromosome 13 aneuploidies and elevated serum prolactin and estradiol levels[26]. Marijuana and cocaine have both been shown to interfere with spermatogenesis, decreasing sperm concentration and motility and increasing the number of sperm with altered morphology[27,28], while high doses of cocaine may cause erectile dysfunction[29]. Finally, exogenous testosterone and its metabolite, estrogen, lead to the suppression of gonadotropin releasing hormone (GnRH) production in the hypothalamus. This leads to a decreased release of luteinizing hormone (LH) from the pituitary gland, and thus to lower testicular testosterone production in the Leydig cells[31]. After ceasing use of these substances, spermatogenesis is expected to be back to normal within 3–6 months. Although uncommon, the pituitary suppression caused by steroidal drugs may be irreversible[32].

There are medications that may interfere with spermatogenesis, affecting quality and quantity of the ejaculate. Antidepressive therapy may increase blood prolactin levels, which in turn will decrease the production of gonadotropins[33]. Calcium channel blocker antihypertensives (nifedipine, diltiazem) may block the acrosome reaction and prevent sperm–egg binding[34,35], while alpha-blocker antihypertensives (prazosin, terazosin, phenoxybenzamine) may lead to retrograde ejaculation or even aspermia[36]. Other drugs are known to impair spermatogenesis, depending on the dosage and length of treatment. Some examples are sulfasalazine[37,38] and cimetidine[39].

Testicular cancer, Hodgkin's disease and leukemia represent three of the most frequent oncological diseases in young adult males. Their incidence is highest in the age group 15–35 years. A growing number of young men are treated successfully for cancer by chemotherapy and radiotherapy. Testicular cancer, for example, a major concern in male infertility, is currently treated by orchiectomy associated with chemotherapy, radiotherapy and retroperitoneal lymphadenectomy, with survival rates reaching upwards of 90%[40]. The benefits of these therapies come at a price, and this may be temporary or permanent infertility[41].

Testicular damage caused by cytotoxic drugs was first described in humans in 1948, when azoospermia was reported in men following treatment with nitrogen mustard[42]. Many other drugs have been shown to be gonadotoxic, and the agents most commonly implicated are: alkylating agents (cyclophosphamide, chlorambucil, busulfan, procarbazine, mustine, melphalan), antimetabolites (cytarabine, 5-fluorouracil, methotrexate), vinca alkaloids (vinblastine, vincristine), cisplatin and analogs, and topoisomerase-interactive agents (bleomycin, doxorubicin, danorubicin, actinomycin)[43]. Although efforts have been made to modify protocols in order to minimize effects on fertility, the chances of fathering children after treatment remain difficult to predict[44].

Alkylating agents are known to be the drugs most deleterious to spermatogenesis, and they cause a cumulative effect. When a dose of > 400 mg/kg of alkylating agents is used, 30% of prepubertal boys and 70–95% of adult men will present with gonadal dysfunction[45,46]. Radiotherapy, on the other hand, may cause permanent azoospermia if doses of > 400 cGy are used, while a dose of > 300 cGy may cause various degrees of oligozoospermia[47]. These deleterious effects of chemo- and radiotherapy on spermatogenesis may last for up to 4 or 5 years, and therefore seminal analyses performed before this period of time should be considered inconclusive.

Statistically, 50% of patients with a history of testicular cancer are oligozoospermic, and 7–10% azoospermic before receiving any treatment[48]. Post-therapeutic spermatogenic output will depend on the type of chemo- or radiotherapy utilized. Cryopreservation of sperm has provided hope for fertility preservation in cancer patients. These men should be referred to a licensed sperm-banking unit as soon as possible, to collect one or various samples for freezing. Sperm banking is currently the only proven method of preserving fertility in cancer patients, although hormonal manipulation to enhance spermatogenic recovery and banking of testicular germ cells are both possibilities for the future[43].

Besides the negative effects of chemo- and radiotherapy on testicular function, retroperitoneal lymphadenectomy may cause ejaculatory dysfunction. Most of these patients will present with aspermia due to interruption of the sympathetic nodal nervous chain or its peripheral nerves, such as the sacral plexus or the hypogastric nerves[49]. Recently, nerve-sparing techniques have been used more, and these side-effects have become less common[50].

Patients presenting with postsurgical aspermia or, more rarely, retrograde ejaculation may revert to anterograde ejaculation after treatment with sympathomimetic drugs (e.g. ephedrine sulfate)[51]. If the pharmaceutical approach fails, semen can simply be retrieved from the urine and, after pH and osmolarity control, be used for intrauterine insemination (IUI) or ICSI. Nevertheless, the best way to preserve fertility in a male patient with testicular cancer during reproductive age is through gamete cryopreservation prior to the oncological treatment, especially with the advent of ICSI, which allows the use of very few sperm to achieve fertilization.

Finally, systemic diseases may also affect the male reproductive tract. Diabetes and multiple sclerosis may both cause ejaculatory and sexual dysfunction, for example. Respiratory diseases associated with infertility may be caused by immotile cilia syndrome, or Kartegener's syndrome, in which sperm concentration is normal but they are immotile due to defects in the flagellum.

PHYSICAL EXAMINATION

A general physical examination should consider weight, height and arm span. Careful observation of all the systems may reveal important signs contributing to male-factor infertility diagnosis. This is especially true since altered function in many organs may alter reproductive potential in the man. As an example, an infertile patient without any specific complaint presenting with inadequate virilization, such as sparse facial and pubic hair and gynecomastia, may have hypogonadism or Klinefelter's syndrome. On the other hand, inadequate virilization and anosmia are associated with Kallmann's syndrome.

Although chronic diseases are not usually found when evaluating a patient for infertility, early or mild alterations in adrenal function, chronic alcoholism or diabetes may be detected by careful physical examination. However, the genital physical examination, performed under ideal temperature ($> 23°C$) and light conditions, will provide the most important information regarding the pathogenesis of infertility in the male partner.

The examination initiates with the patient in the upright position. This will allow better evaluation of the penis, scrotal size, testicular position, symmetry of testicular structures and, no less important, the venous return condition in the pampiniform plexus. Regarding the penis, insertion of the urinary meatus is the most important aspect, since hypospadias renders the patient unable to place the ejaculate within the vaginal vault.

A small scrotum or the scrotum of an obese man is more difficult to palpate, and therefore these patients may require scrotal ultrasonography. When examining the testes, size, consistency and regularity should be recorded. Patients with normal seminal analysis usually have testicles of 4.5 cm in length by 2.5 cm in height, with a minimum volume of 15 ml, as assessed by the Prader orchidometer. Not surprisingly, testicular volume and consistency usually predict seminal analysis results, especially taking into account that 85% of testicular volume is represented by the seminiferous epithelium.

On the other hand, patients with small testes tend to present with varying degrees of oligozoospermia or even with azoospermia. If during the prepubertal phase the boy does not undergo normal gonadal development, in adult life he will most likely present with small (< 8 ml) and hardened testes. Such is true in Klinefelter's syndrome. However, if the gonads develop normally but suffer injuries, such as in viral or bacterial orchitis, they show decreased size and consistency.

Following examination of the testes, the epididymides should be evaluated using one hand to hold the testis while the other gently palpates the epididymal head, body and cauda between the thumb and the index finger. Epididymal volume, consistency, regularity, cysts and distance between the testis and the epididymis should be noted at this time. The further is the epididymis from the testis the more prone it is to abnormalities, while epididymal volume reflects testicular production and effusion.

It is quite common to observe cysts in the epididymal head, but they are usually smaller than 0.7 cm and have no clinical meaning. However, when these cysts are larger or more numerous they may obstruct the epididymis and block sperm passage.

Moving on through the male reproductive tract, the deferent ducts should be evaluated. These are firm, cylindrical structures measuring 3 mm in diameter, and are easily distinguished from the other structures in the spermatic cord. Under ideal room-temperature conditions and with a cooperative patient the deferent ducts are always identified. For that reason, deferent duct agenesis is, in most cases, diagnosed solely through the physical examination, and ancillary examinations and exploratory surgery are not necessary. Various degrees of epididymal malformation, as well as agenesis or hypoplasia of the seminal vesicles, usually accompanies uni- or bilateral absence of the vas deferens. If the physical examination shows a thickening or hardening of the vas deferens, this may be a sign of previous infection, usually caused by STDs. Vasectomized patients present with dilated and painful epididymides.

The last structure analyzed in the physical examination is the pampiniform plexus of the spermatic cord, observing possible asymmetries, bulges or growths. With the patient in the upright position, testicular volumes are measured and expected to be symmetrical. A grade II or III varicocele, usually on the left side, will reduce the testis volume and shift its axis from vertical to horizontal. Admitting that varicocele causes alterations in spermatogenesis, seminiferous tubule diameter will decrease, as well as testicular volume. It is common to find testicular asymmetry in unilateral varicocele patients, and the ipsilateral testis will be at least 2 ml smaller in volume than its contralateral counterpart.

For diagnosis of a grade I varicocele, the patient will have to perform a Valsalva maneuver. Careful examination before and during a Valsalva maneuver will allow the examiner to palpate any engorgement of the pampiniform plexus. Subclinical varicoceles are not diagnosed by a physical examination, and their clinical meaning is currently questioned. The spermatic cord should be examined up to the point at which it exits the scrotum, and any abnormality, such as a spermatic cord cyst or inguinal–scrotal hernia, should be observed.

The history and physical examination, with especial attention paid to the genitalia, are essential components not only in diagnosing male factor infertility but also in determining the management and prognosis for the infertile couple. Although seminal analysis is still the most important examination in male factor evaluation, it does not possess the necessary standardization, due to the lack of proper guidance given to the patient when ordering the examination and the lack of protocol and quality assurance among different laboratories. As a result, comparisons from different laboratories are very difficult. It is important to keep in mind that seminal analysis will not determine whether a man is fertile or not, especially because fertility is a couple phenomenon, of which pregnancy is the ultimate proof. Detailed descriptions of the current methodologies and interpretation of semen analysis are discussed in other chapters.

Although semen analysis initiates the investigation of the infertile man, it cannot provide all the answers to questions regarding his fertility potential. It is never enough to repeat that semen analysis alone will not allow determination of the patient's true fertility potential, but the average results from separate seminal analyses will allow the physician to estimate this potential. With these considerations in mind, in our institution we group patients into three categories (Table 8.2), according to their potential for natural conception.

This table should serve only as a starting point for discussing the patient's condition, and, as mentioned previously, the cut-off rates shown are still widely debatable. According to the World Health Organization, the reference value for semen volume is 2.0 ml[52]. If the patient produces no semen at all after an orgasm, he has aspermia. This may be due to clinical issues, such as bilateral sympathectomy, bilateral retroperitoneal lymphadenectomy, antihypertensive drugs which block the sympathetic tone, transurethral or open surgical resections of the bladder neck or prostate, extensive pelvic surgery and diabetic neuropathy.

Table 8.2   Semen classification based on an average between two samples

Variables	Potential for natural conception		
	High	Moderate	Low
Volume (ml)	> 2	1–2	< 1
Concentration ($\times 10^6$/ml)	> 20	10–20	< 10
Motility (% motile)	> 50	40–50	< 40
Morphology (% normal)	> 14*	4–14*	< 4*
	> 30**	20–30**	< 20**

*Classified according to Kruger strict criteria, 1986;
**classified according to World Health Organization, 1999

Hypospermia without spermatozoa in semen with a pH of less than 7.4 could be due to ejaculatory duct obstruction or congenital absence of seminal vesicles. Hypospermia with spermatozoa in the ejaculate with a pH of less than 7.4 could be due to obstruction of the seminal vesicle opening by a mucus-like plug; this obstruction may dissolve spontaneously[53].

MALE REPRODUCTIVE ENDOCRINOLOGY

From the clinical point of view, the most important hormones related to male fertility are follicle stimulating hormone (FSH), luteinizing hormone (LH) and testosterone. FSH acts primarily on Sertoli cells, stimulating the production of androgen-binding protein (ABP), which in turn binds to testosterone and intensifies its action on the seminiferous tubules[54]. Sertoli cells also produce inhibins A and B, which inhibit pituitary secretion of FSH, and even if the testis presents only spermatogonia, inhibin production is sufficient to decrease FSH levels to normal. FSH levels are therefore limited in predicting spermatogenic integrity[55]. LH acts on Leydig (or interstitial)

cells, where it stimulates the synthesis of testosterone. Only 2% of circulating testosterone is in the unbound form (free testosterone), and thus capable of producing its effects. Around 30% of circulating testosterone is bound to a specific globulin – sex hormone-binding globulin – and 68% is bound to albumin and other non-specific proteins[56]. Testosterone will, in the same manner as FSH, stimulate Sertoli cell function and therefore promote spermatogenesis. Testosterone is also converted into dihydrotestosterone in peripheral tissue, where it is responsible for the manifestation of secondary male sex characteristics[57].

Prolactin is secreted by the pituitary gland, and its production is inhibited by dopamine and stimulated by thyroid stimulating hormone (TSH). Although prolactin does not exert a direct action on spermatogenesis, chronic hyperprolactinemia is known to alter GnRH action, leading to altered secretion of FSH and LH and, consequently, decreased libido, sexual dysfunction, gynecomastia and alterations of spermatogenesis[58].

The male endocrine profile (FSH, LH and testosterone) is not necessary in patients with a normal seminal analysis. Patients with a sperm concentration as low as 10×10^6 cells/ml have been shown to be able to achieve paternity by natural conception[59]. On the other hand, patients with a sperm concentration of fewer than 5×10^6 cells/ml demonstrate significantly lower fertility rates[60]. A hormonal profile is therefore useful in severely oligozoospermic and azoospermic patients, as shown in Table 8.3.

If we consider only circulating FSH levels, a few practical conclusions related to oligozoospermia or azoospermia may be reached:

- Normal FSH: the alteration is either post-testicular (obstructive) or testicular (normo-gonadotropic hypogonadism). If post-testicular, hormonal treatment is unnecessary, and fertilization may be achieved through vasectomy reversal or ICSI (e.g. congenital bilateral absence of the vas deferens) using epididymal or testicular (TESE) aspiration[61]. If the

Table 8.3 Association between serum hormone levels and origin of oligozoospermia or azoospermia

Type of oligozoospermia or azoospermia	Serum hormone levels
Post-testicular (obstructive) Vasectomy Congenital bilateral absence of the vasa deferentia	FSH, LH and testosterone usually normal
Pre-testicular (usually from hypothalamic or hypophyseal disorders, also known as hypogonadotropic hypogonadism) Tumors Hyperprolactinemia Kallmann's syndrome	Low FSH, usually low LH and testosterone
Testicular (hypergonadotropic hypogonadism) Genetic syndromes (Klinefelter's, myotonic dystrophy) Embryological malformations (cryptorchidism) Cytotoxic drugs (chemotherapy) Sequelae from viral diseases (mumps)	Elevated FSH, variable LH and testosterone
Testicular (normogonadotropic hypogonadism) Androgen resistance Sertoli cel only syndrome and maturation arrest Y-chromosome microdeletions	Normal FSH, elevated LH and testosterone Normal FSH, LH, and testosterone Normal FSH, LH, and testosterone

FSH, follicle stimulating hormone; LH, luteinizing hormone

alteration is testicular, thus signifying androgen resistance, hormonal treatments could be beneficial to the patient. If this is not the case, sperm could be retrieved by masturbation (if oligozoospermic) or TESE (if azoospermic) for ICSI[62].

- Low FSH: the alteration may be either hypothalamic or hypophyseal, and treatment involves correcting these primary alterations. Sometimes, simultaneous hormonal treatment is necessary, such as in Kallmann's syndrome.

- High FSH: anamnesis and karyotyping may both help to define diagnosis in these patients, and treatment will depend on the etiology and presence of sperm in the ejaculate or in the testis[63]. If viable sperm are found, fertilization may be achieved through ICSI. If not, the couple may have to use donor semen or adoption as an option for constituting a family.

IMAGING THE REPRODUCTIVE TRACT

There are several imaging resources that may be used to investigate the male reproductive tract for abnormalities, but the most frequently used are ultrasonography[64] and nuclear magnetic resonance (NMR)[65]. Computerized tomography has been less and less indicated in clinical practice, due mainly to the fact that, besides using ionizing radiation, it does not render superior pelvic images when compared with transrectal ultrasound (TRUS) or magnetic resonance imaging (MRI). Nowadays deferentography is hardly used, mostly because there is a risk of iatrogenic deferent lesions at the puncture site. However, when there is doubt regarding vas deferens injury from previous hernia repair, deferentography is the imaging method of choice for confirming the clinical suspicion.

Scrotum

With the patient in a standing position in a warm room, an attentive physician is able to inspect and examine all the structures inside the scrotum. These include testicular and epididymal volume, consistency and regularity, the presence or absence of the vasa deferentia as well as their diameters and clinical varicocele. Since the role of subclinical varicocele is currently rather controversial[66], and physical examination of the scrotum provides most of the information we need, imaging resources are not used very often to evaluate scrotal content. As an exception, scrotal ultrasonography may be helpful when evaluating obese patients or patients with a short scrotum.

Ductal obstruction

Although complete obstruction of the deferent ducts is very rare, it should be investigated because it is treatable[67]. A good imaging resource in this situation is high-frequency transrectal ultrasonography (TRUS), because it produces excellent images of the ejaculatory ducts, seminal vesicles and prostate[68]. It is also considered a simple, readily available and inexpensive examination. Another imaging approach is MRI, which can be performed either with or without a rectal probe. Although it offers very good spatial reconstitution of the necessary structures, it is not readily accessible, and costs will be significantly increased. However, in contrast to TRUS, MRI does not depend on examiner skill[69].

Patients with a normal scrotum examination who present with a low volume of ejaculate (< 1 ml) and seminal fluid devoid of fructose and coagulation might have complete ejaculatory duct obstruction. If submitted to TRUS, they may exhibit dilated ejaculatory ducts and/or seminal vesicles (greater than 1.5 cm in anteroposterior diameter). But it is important to keep in mind that normal vesicle size does not necessarily rule out the possibility of ductal obstruction. Under TRUS guidance, seminal vesicle aspiration and

vesiculography can be performed[70]. A large number of spermatozoa in the seminal vesicle fluid reinforce the diagnosis. While complete ejaculatory duct obstruction is relatively easy to diagnose and is accepted by everyone, partial duct obstruction is suggested by some, and is not as easy to demonstrate. Usually, when a patient is oligozoospermic and/or asthenozoospermic with a lower ejaculate volume, without any other clinical or laboratory finding, he is investigated for partial ejaculatory duct obstruction. Aspiration puncture of the seminal vesicles could be important in these patients, especially if performed immediately following ejaculation, because the partial obstruction will lead to impaired efflux from the seminal vesicles, and a large number of sperm may be found in the aspirate.

Pituitary gland

In male infertility, the most common indication for carrying out computerized tomography or MRI of the brain is in imaging the pituitary gland for diagnosis of hypogonadotropic hypogonadism[65]. Even if very unusual in an infertility-clinic setting, hypogonadism associated with gonadotropic insufficiency deserves special attention, as it is one of the few alterations in male infertility with specific and effective clinical treatment.

VARICOCELE

Varicocele is defined as an abnormal increase in scrotal volume due to dilated veins in the pampiniform plexus. Although it is present in 15–25% of the male population, its prevalence can reach 40% in infertile men[71,72]. Most patients are asymptomatic, but some may present with testicular pain which increases following physical activities or long periods in the upright position. However, the pain is relieved upon adopting the supine position, which explains why patients do not usually refer to pain in the morning.

Diagnosis is performed through careful physical examination in a warm room (> 23°C), with the patient in the upright position. If there is an observable or palpable dilatation in the pampiniform plexus before or during a Valsalva maneuver, diagnosis is confirmed, and the varicocele classified as grade I, II or III, according to the intensity of the dilatation:

- Grade I varicoceles are visible with difficulty, but easily palpable during a Valsalva maneuver;

- Grade II varicoceles are visible, and there is significant venous gorging during the Valsalva maneuver;

- Grade III varicoceles are easily visible, with great reflux during the Valsalva maneuver.

There is enough evidence in the literature to demonstrate that varicocele can cause macroscopic, microscopic and functional alterations to the testes[73,74]. Varicocele usually develops earlier and more intensely on the left side, because venous return is more difficult due to anatomical peculiarities in the internal spermatic drainage system on this side[75,76]. Macroscopic alterations are evident in adolescents, because these patients present with a delay in development of the left testis. This delay will eventually lead to testicular asymmetry, a difference in volume of more than 2 ml between the testes in the adult[77,78].

Histologically, patients with varicocele demonstrate a loss of maturational stratification, characterized by: loss of desmosomes, adluminal compartment structural disorganization, maturation arrest in the different stages of spermatogenesis, early release of spermatids into the lumen and, as a consequence, thinning of the seminiferous epithelium and increase of the tubular lumen[79,80].

As far as testicular function is concerned, the consequences of venous ectasia may be observed in two compartments: interstitial and intratubular. The World Health Organization (WHO), through a multicentric study comparing young patients with and without varicocele, observed that varicocele patients possess lower blood testosterone levels, characterizing impaired steroidogenesis and Leydig cell dysfunction. Alterations in the seminiferous tubules cause changes in seminal variables and lead to a decrease in sperm concentration, motility and normal morphology[81]. There is also evidence showing that sperm from patients with varicocele possess a lower ability to bind tightly to the human oocyte zona pellucida[82].

The negative effects of varicocele on the testes have been shown over the past few decades, either through clinical[83,84] or experimental studies[85]. Although many theories have been proposed and much has been hypothesized, it is not known how venous reflux and ectasia lead to testicular malfunction. Many studies regarding varicocele and infertility evaluate variables between men with and without varicocele or assess pre- and post-varicocelectomy data, but a definite explanation for the negative impact of varicocele on gametogenesis or for its bilateral effects has yet to be found[86].

Etiology

Testicular blood flow and hyperthermia

The involvement of testicular blood flow in varicocele etiopathogeny is highly concordant with studies related to hyperthermia, but many controversies have yet to be explained[87,88]. Some groups have shown that this increase in blood flow is present on both sides, even in unilateral varicoceles[89]. Even though a change in testicular blood flow direction associated with varicocele has not been defined, it is very important to recognize that an increase in blood flow is most compatible with hyperthermia, and that contralateral organs may respond in a similar fashion to their ipsilateral counterparts when an injury is present, due to hormonal and neural mechanisms.

Testicular hyperthermia is considered the most important mechanism leading to the secondary alterations associated with varicocele[90]. The scrotum is maintained at a lower temperature than body temperature owing to five important anatomical traits: (1) dartos muscle, (2) cremaster muscle, (3) countercurrent heat-exchange mechanism, (4) the absence of adipose tissue and (5) the presence of many sweat glands. Two systems play a main role in thermal regulation. The scrotal system, with the dartos and cremaster muscles, assists the countercurrent heat-exchange mechanism. This in turn allows heat exchange from the arterial to the venous system, thus maintaining thermal homeostasis[90]. Varicocele impairs this heat-exchange mechanism, and therefore hinders the cooling of arterial blood before it enters the testis. This alteration in blood flow prevents the testis from maintaining a lower temperature.

An increase in testicular temperature may have a direct effect on spermatogenic germ cells, altering metabolism, Sertoli cell function, DNA synthesis, apoptosis rates and nutrient content and oxygen tension in the testicular environment, as well as decreasing enzymatic activity and leading to vascular alterations due to an increase in arteriovenous shunting[91,92]. The higher testicular temperature associated with androgenic suppression will also act concurrently, altering different stages of spermatogenesis, generally lowering the sperm concentration[93].

Spermatogenesis and apoptosis

Spermatogenesis is a continuous proliferative process that leads to the production of millions of sperm each day. Apoptosis, or programmed cell death, is present in both physiological and pathological situations, and will determine, during gametogenesis, the sperm concentration in fertile and infertile men. Apoptosis is associated with nuclear DNA fragmentation[94], and is present throughout spermatogenesis, occurring in spermatogonia, spermatocytes and spermatids[95].

Since the process of apoptosis has been extensively studied and documented[96–102], and although it is known that heat stress, androgen deprival and accumulation of toxic substances in the testes all contribute to increase, apoptosis

rates, more studies regarding the molecular mechanisms underlying varicocele-induced activation of apoptosis need to be done[103].

Apoptosis-induced DNA fragmentation can currently be evaluated through many different techniques, of which the TUNEL (terminal deoxynucleotide transferase-mediated dUTP nick-end labeling) and the Comet (or single cell gel electrophoresis) assays are noteworthy. In a recent study, DNA fragmentation rates were significantly increased in adolescents with grades II and III bilateral varicocele[104].

Sperm motility

Many men with varicocele present lower sperm motility, and this may or may not be accompanied by alterations in other sperm variables[105]. Most studies have focused on three basic causes of this lower sperm motility: an increased concentration of reactive oxygen species (ROS), the presence of antisperm antibodies and deficient mitochondrial activity[106].

ROS concentration in sperm is inversely related to motility[107]. Although ROS are normally present, and even necessary at low concentrations, excessive ROS are present during leukospermia or an increased presence of abnormal sperm, such as sperm with cytoplasmic droplets[108]. Men with varicocele present a higher concentration of ROS and a lower antioxidant capability[109]. This is demonstrated by the fact that these men demonstrate a defect in mitochondrial oxidative phosphorylation, with a low concentration of the mitochondrial coenzyme Q10, an important antioxidant[110], and a deficiency in superoxide dismutase (SOD) and catalase[111].

Sperm morphology

Although classical alterations in sperm morphology associated with varicocele are an increase in fusiform and amorphous cells[112], recent data assessed through strict criteria demonstrate that there is a decrease in normal sperm morphology[113]. Specific studies evaluating sperm donors exposed to cadmium, shown to cause stress to the testes, demonstrated an increase in the expression of heat shock protein (HSP), which, among other characteristics, possesses actin-like sequences. Since it is not yet known whether HSPs act as protectors of actin or inhibit its polymerization[114], and since patients with varicocele exposed to environmental agents possess higher cadmium concentrations, future studies may help us to understand how HSPs participate in sperm morphology determination.

Another important finding is an increase in cells with midpiece cytoplasmic droplets, which lead to lower sperm motility in these patients with varicocele[115].

It is also important to assess the acrosome reaction in patients with varicocele, along with functional tests that evaluate the acrosome and its ability to bind to the zona pellucida. A study of adolescents with varicocele found that sperm from these patients possessed decreased binding capacity to the zona pellucida (hemizona assay, HZA), when compared with adolescents without varicocele[82].

Acrosome reaction

Alterations of sperm function seem to be more relevant than morphology and concentration in varicocele patients, and this involves the acrosome reaction and zona pellucida binding[116].

Sperm from patients with varicocele demonstrate an altered calcium influx mechanism[117]. Cofactors such as metals may exacerbate this alteration, and there is a wide variety of individual response, ranging from no alteration to infertility. Since this variability may be explained by qualitative and quantitative differences in protein expression, studies have set out to find candidate genes, to evaluate susceptibility for this defect[118].

The acrosome reaction is calcium-dependent, and few motile sperm are able to complete this exocytosis[119]. Following cholesterol efflux there is an influx of calcium ions, which will stimulate

mannose receptor externalization and initiate exocytosis through myosin activity[117]. Calcium influx is controlled by voltage-dependent channels[120], and it has been demonstrated that men with varicocele exhibit a deletion of amino acids in the calcium channel pore, thus providing a genetic cause for infertility. These channels may be altered when environmental agents are present, since they may also transport zinc, cadmium, cobalt, nickel, lead and aluminum[121]. Since the testicular cadmium concentration is higher and the zinc concentration lower in men with varicocele[118], it has been suggested that cadmium may negatively affect calcium channels. It has not yet been defined whether varicocelectomy or zinc supplementation will reverse the effects of cadmium on these channels[106].

In spite of the enormous progress that has been achieved related to varicocele and its consequences on spermatogenesis, many doubts still remain. Prospectively designed studies, which are currently scarce, would not only help us to understand better the intrinsic mechanisms through which varicocele affects male fertility, but also shed light on the present uncertainties regarding treatment.

AZOOSPERMIA

Defined as the complete absence of sperm in the seminal fluid after centrifugation, azoospermia represents a very important topic in male infertility, and, as such, deserves special attention. It is present in 1% of all men and in approximately 15% of infertile men[122,123]. The first issue regarding azoospermia is to be certain that we really are dealing with azoospermia and not severe oligozoospermia. The distinction between these two entities is not only a semantic issue but rather fundamental, since the presence of just a few spermatozoa could represent the difference between being a genetic father or not.

This has become particularly true since the introduction of ICSI in 1992. For this reason, the WHO guideline recommends that if no spermatozoa are found in three aliquots of 10 μl of semen, the whole specimen should be centrifuged at $3000\,g$ for 15 min and the resulting pellet examined thoroughly[52]. Moreover, it is not unusual to detect sperm in the specimen of a patient initially considered azoospermic[124]. Therefore, azoospermia should not be definitely assumed unless two separate samples are scrutinized in this way.

Azoospermia may be due to a variety of conditions, and a history, physical examination, hormonal profile, genetic and imaging resources will be necessary not only to establish the cause but also to direct the couple towards the best treatment option suitable. Some causes are potentially correctable; other conditions are irreversible but still possibly treatable by assisted reproductive techniques using the husband's semen; and, finally, some causes are irreversible and not amenable to any form of treatment, demanding donor semen or adoption in order to constitute a family.

This section discusses the evaluation of some specific conditions associated with azoospermia.

Azoospermia with small testicles

Azoospermia associated with bilateral small testicles may be caused by either primary or secondary testicular failure. The differentiation between these two very distinct clinical situations is feasible using the initial results of the endocrine tests. Patients who sustain elevated FSH and LH and low testosterone levels have primary testicular insufficiency in both Leydig and germ-cell compartments. Elevated gonadotropins distinguish primary testicular failure from hypothalamic–pituitary diseases. Klinefelter's syndrome and its variants represent a typical example of primary testicular failure. These alterations, confirmed by karyotyping, account for 14% of these cases of azoospermia[125]. On the other hand, some patients might present azoospermia with elevated FSH but normal LH and testosterone. Although they do not exhibit total panhypogonadal dysfunction,

from a therapeutic perspective they are similar to patients with primary testicular failure, and, as such, are not clinically treatable. Finally, patients with low FSH, LH and testosterone have secondary hypogonadism, and represent one of the very few occasions where specific therapy may be effective. However, patients with congenital or acquired hypogonadotropic hypogonadism are rarely seen in an infertility clinic, but when they do present they should be tested for deficiencies of other pituitary hormones (thyroid-stimulating, adrenocorticotropic and growth hormones)[126].

Patients with an altered gonadotropin profile and anosmia or hyposmia are candidates for Kallmann's syndrome. A careful neurological examination, including visual field testing, serum prolactin measurements and radiological images of the pituitary fossa may reveal a pituitary adenoma. It is especially noteworthy that, although it is unusual for infertility due to hyperprolactinemia to occur in men without impotence and hypoandrogenization, hyperprolactemia does occur without any detectable hypothalamic or sellar alteration.

Congenital absence of vasa deferentia

Considering that the scrotal contents are very easily reached and knowing that the vas deferens is a fairly solid structure, 3 mm in diameter, the diagnosis of unilateral or bilateral vasal agenesis is possible through physical examination. Ancillary examinations or even surgical exploration is not necessary to confirm the diagnosis, but may be useful for seeking associated abnormalities. Approximately 25% of men with unilateral vasal agenesis and 10% of men with congenital bilateral absence of the vasa deferentia (CBAVD) have unilateral renal agenesis documented by abdominal ultrasonography[127]. Moreover, since the seminal vesicles and vasa deferentia are formed by the Wolffian ducts, a variable degree of seminal vesicle abnormalities is expected. Most patients with vasal agenesis submitted to transrectal ultrasonography (TRUS) will exhibit seminal-vesicle hypoplasia or agenesia. For the same embryological reasons, it is possible to explain why a patient with unilateral absence of the vas deferens may have segmental abnormality of the contralateral vas deferens and seminal vesicle and present with azoospermia. In terms of seminal analysis, patients with CBAVD commonly show a decrease in ejaculate volume, fructose content and semen pH[128,129].

Another remarkable clinical aspect about CBAVD is its association with mutations of the cystic fibrosis transmembrane conductance regulator (CFTR) gene. Almost all patients manifesting cystic fibrosis have CBAVD, and almost 70% of men with CBAVD have mutation of the CFTR gene. It is also important to mention that routine laboratory methods may fail to identify all CFTR abnormality in a man with CBAVD, and the presence of a mutation cannot be ruled out.

Assuming that we cannot be a 100% sure that a man with CBAVD does not harbor a genetic abnormality in the CFTR gene, if his semen is to be used, it is very important to test his wife for CFTR gene mutations. The chance that she may be a carrier is estimated to be 4%[130].

Azoospermia due to obstruction/spermatogenesis failure

When bilateral testicular atrophy and vasal agenesis are excluded, azoospermia may occur due to ductal obstruction at some level in the reproductive system, or abnormal spermatogenesis. To determine the etiology of the azoospermia, we must rely upon FSH measurements, ejaculate volume and testicular biopsy.

Normal ejaculate volume

Patients with normal ejaculate volume may present either ductal obstruction or abnormalities of spermatogenesis, and the FSH level could be used to direct the next step. If the FSH level is high (greater than twice the upper limit range), the patient has severe germ- and Sertoli-cell dysfunction, and there is no need to perform a testicular biopsy for diagnostic purposes. However, if

testicular sperm extraction with ICSI is being considered, a testicular biopsy may be indicated, initially, for prognostic purposes. On the other hand, patients should be warned that the presence of sperm in a previous biopsy specimen does not assure that sperm will be found on the day of ICSI. For that reason, the role of prognostic biopsy in patients with a very high FSH concentration has been considered rather controversial. However, when a patient has a normal serum FSH level, a testicular biopsy can lead to the diagnosis, as normal serum FSH levels do not guarantee normal spermatogenesis. Testicular biopsy may be unilateral or bilateral, and a consensus about this issue has not yet been reached. If performed unilaterally, a testicular biopsy should be done on the best testis.

Testicular biopsy can be performed either by a standard open incision technique or by percutaneous methods. An open surgical biopsy performed under general anesthesia can provide enough testicular tissue for histological and cryopreservation purposes. The presence of sperm in the fresh specimen may avoid the need for repeat surgery. If normal testicular histology is confirmed, obstruction at some level in the semen pathway must be present, and the location of the obstruction may be determined.

Vasectomy is, without any doubt, the most common cause of ductal obstruction. After that, bilateral epididymal obstruction is considered the most important cause of obstructive azoospermia and microscopic surgical exploration may show dilated epididymal tubules.

Low ejaculate volume

Patients with azoospermia and a very low ejaculate volume (< 1 ml) may have gonadotropin insufficiency, CBAVD or ejaculatory duct obstruction (EDO). Ejaculatory dysfunction does not cause azoospermia, but rather aspermia or hypospermia with oligozoospermia.

The determination of additional seminal parameters, such as pH and fructose concentration, may be useful in determining the presence of total EDO, as the seminal vesicles produce an alkaline secretion containing fructose. However, caution should be taken, because the results of semen pH and fructose testing may be misleading if they are not properly performed. The method of choice for determining EDO is transrectal ultrasonography (TRUS)[70,131]. Although vasography is considered an alternative method, TRUS is minimally invasive and prevents the possible risk of vasal injury associated with vasography. For a more detailed description, the reader is directed to the above section on 'Imaging the reproductive tract'.

GENETIC EVALUATION

Screening for genetic alterations in infertile men is usually recommended in cases of severe oligozoospermia, non-obstructive azoospermia and in azoospermia due to congenital bilateral absence of the vasa deferentia. The most common genetic tests used for evaluating the origin of these alterations are: karyotyping, screening for Y-chromosome microdeletions and mutations in the cystic fibrosis genes. Genetic screening may also be recommended for patients with varicocele or cryptorchidism, since more than one factor may be present.

Karyotype

It has been known for decades that constitutional chromosome abnormalities are more prevalent in infertile men than in fertile men[132], and these are inversely related to sperm concentration. An estimated 5% (2–8%) of infertile men present with chromosomal alterations[132–134], but in the azoospermia group this number may reach 15%, and this is mostly due to 47,XXY aneuploidy, or Klinefelter's syndrome, the most common chromosomal abnormality in men with severe infertility[135]. Almost all men with a 47,XXY karyotype are azoospermic, while 46,XY/47,XXY mosaic men may show a limited number of sperm in their ejaculates. During testicular sperm extraction

(TESE), sperm is found in 50% of 47,XXY men[136], and most of them are 23,X or 23,Y, although there is an increase in 24,XX or 24,XY cells. While the majority of chromosome alterations in azoospermic men are sex chromosome-related, a wide array of abnormalities has been described, such as reciprocal and Robertsonian translocations, inversions, duplications and deletions.

Some preliminary studies have shown that there is an increase in prenatally detected sex chromosome abnormalities during gestations from ICSI, when compared with gestations from natural conception[137]. It has also been well described that infertile men possess an increase in chromosome alterations both in somatic cells and in gametes[138,139]. Knowing that when men possess these alterations there is an increased risk of abortion, or of children being born with genetic and congenital alterations, karyotyping is recommended for patients presenting with azoospermia or with severe oligozoospermia before performing ICSI.

Y-chromosome microdeletions

Since the original work by Tiepolo and Zuffardi[140], many studies have demonstrated an association between male infertility and the presence of microdeletions in the long arm of the Y-chromosome (Yq)[141,142]. Karyotyping will not reveal these microdeletions, and therefore molecular techniques such as the polymerase chain reaction (PCR) must be used.

There are three loci (chromosomal regions) associated with spermatogenesis in this region, and they have been termed azoospermia factors: AZFa, AZFb and AZFc. Many candidate genes have been isolated in infertile men: DBY and USPY9 in AZFa[143,144], RBMY1 in AZFb[145] and DAZ in AZFc[146]. Other genes have been identified in Yq, but their contribution to the AZF phenotype has yet to be determined.

Y-chromosome microdeletions may lead to primary testicular insufficiency, which is characterized by azoospermia or severe oligozoospermia.

Around 60% of Y-chromosome microdeletions occur in region AZFc, while 15% occur in AZFb and 5% in AZFa. The other 20% involve more than one AZF region[141]. Between 10 and 15% of infertile men present Yq microdeletions[142]. In patients with idiopathic severe oligozoospermia this figure may rise to 18%, and in idiopathic azoospermia to 20%. The region in which the microdeletion occurs may also determine how spermatogenesis will be affected. AZFa microdeletions are associated with complete absence of germ cells, in a syndrome known as Sertoli cell only syndrome (SCOS). AZFb microdeletions, on the other hand, determine maturation arrest. Finally, AZFc microdeletions, unlike AZFa and AZFb, are not associated with any specific phase of spermatogenesis. Phenotypical alterations may range from azoospermia to, more typically, oligozoospermia[147]. The presence of AZFa and AZFb microdeletions greatly decreases the chances of finding sperm in the testes, and therefore screening for Y-chromosome microdeletions is very useful in determining the prognosis for patients with non-obstructive azoospermia[148]. Men with important seminal alterations associated with clinical conditions such as varicocele or cryptorchidism may also present Yq microdeletions[149–151].

Patients carrying AZFc microdeletions are not necessarily azoospermic, and thus are candidates for ICSI using sperm from the ejaculate or the testes. In these cases, Y chromosome-bearing sperm will transport the microdeletions. Male children born from these patients will therefore also possess these deletions[152–154]. Some recent articles have suggested an increased risk of altered gonadal formation and Turner's syndrome (45,X0) in children from Yq-microdeletion patients[155–158], and this leads to important ethical issues.

Patients with non-obstructive azoospermia or severe oligozoospermia should be screened for Y-chromosome microdeletions even if signs of testicular lesions are present, since both may occur simultaneously, and ICSI may allow transmission of these deletions. On the other hand, patients with a sperm count of more than 10×10^6 sperm/ml do not need to be screened, since Yq microdeletions are very rare in this case.

CFTR gene

Cystic fibrosis (CF) is one of the most common recessive autosomal diseases in Caucasians, with a prevalence of one affected person per 2500 births. One in 25 individuals is an asymptomatic heterozygote. CF is caused by a mutation in the gene encoding for the cystic fibrosis transmembrane conductance regulator protein (CFTR). The most common mutation in the CFTR gene is the deletion of a phenylalanine in position 508 (Δ508), but more than 1000 different mutations have been identified, according to the CFTR online database (www.genet.sickkids.on.ca/cftr). Congenital bilateral absence of the vasa deferentia (CBAVD) is in many cases considered an incomplete or mild form of CF. Around 70–80% of these men are heterozygotes for CFTR mutations[159,160]. Another mutation associated with CBAVD is the presence of five thymines in intron 8 (the 'wild-type' has seven or nine), designated the '5T allele'. This alteration leads to the non-transcription of exon 9, and thus to low levels of CFTR[161]. CBAVD is diagnosed in 1.5% of all cases of male infertility. Most (60%) heterozygote mutations are compound mutations (different mutations in each copy of the CFTR gene)[162]. Congenital unilateral absence of the vas deferens (CUAVD) is also related to CFTR mutations. Although the prevalence of mutations in these patients varies significantly (10–73%)[163,164], it has been established that the occurrence of CUAVD is due in part to the production of a defective CFTR protein. Therefore the clinical manifestation of patients with a CFTR mutation may be azoospermia or oligozoospermia, associated with CBAVD and CUAVD, respectively.

It is important to note that these patients demonstrate normal spermatogenesis. They are therefore candidates for ICSI by collecting sperm from the epididymides or the testes. If their female partner is a heterozygote for the CFTR mutation, their children are at risk of presenting classic cystic fibrosis. Therefore, if a patient presents with CBAVD or CUAVD, both partners in the couple should be investigated for CFTR mutations, and appropriate genetic counseling should be provided.

CONCLUSIONS

We may expect that 30% of infertile couples are so due to a significant isolated male factor, and associated male and female factors are present in an additional 20%. Although male factors contribute to half of the cases of infertility, the pathophysiological mechanisms of male infertility are so poorly understood that most infertile men are described as idiopathic oligo/astheno/teratozoospermia rather than having an etiological diagnosis. As a consequence, there is no scientific basis for clinical treatment, except for gonadotropin deficiency. The use of assisted reproductive technologies, particularly ICSI, has become the rule, instead of the exception, and physicians and patients have shifted focus from the cause of infertility to the ultimate goal, pregnancy. To reverse the present situation, we need to improve current male-factor diagnostic tools, emphasizing genetics and post-receptor mechanisms, which will open new venues for protein- or gene-based therapies directed towards the underlying cause and mechanisms of male infertility.

REFERENCES

1. Thonneau P, et al. Incidence and main causes of infertility in a resident population (1.850.000) of three French regions (1988–1989). Hum Reprod 1991; 6: 811
2. Palermo G, et al. Pregnancies after intracytoplasmic injection of a single spermatozoon into an oocyte. Lancet 1992; 340: 17
3. Stein ZA. A woman's age: child bearing and child rearing. Am J Epidemiol 1985; 121: 327
4. Sharlip ID, et al. Best practice policies for male infertility. Fertil Steril 2002; 77: 873
5. Wilcox AJ, Weinberg CR, Baird DD. Timing of sexual intercourse in relation to ovulation: effects on the probability of conception, survival of pregnancy, and sex of the baby. N Engl J Med 1995; 333: 1517
6. Goldenberg RL, White R. The effect of vaginal lubricants on sperm motility in vitro. Fertil Steril 1975; 26: 872
7. Tagatz GE, Okagaki T, Sciarra JJ. The effect of vaginal lubricants on sperm motility and viability in vitro. Am J Obstet Gynecol 1972; 113: 88
8. Tulandi T, Plouffe L Jr, McInnes RA. Effect of saliva on sperm motility and activity. Fertil Steril 1982; 38: 721
9. Gorelick JI, Goldstein M. Loss of fertility in men with varicocele. Fertil Steril 1993; 59: 613
10. Whitehead ED, Leiter E. Genital abnormalities and abnormal semen analyses in male patients exposed to diethylstilbestrol in utero. J Urol 1981; 125: 47
11. Klip H, et al. Hypospadias in sons of women exposed to diethylstilbestrol in utero: A cohort study. Lancet 2002; 359: 1102
12. Sharpe RM. Environment, lifestyle and male infertility. Baillieres Best Pract Res Clin Endocrinol Metab 2000; 14: 489
13. Thompson ST. Preventable causes of male infertility. World J Urol 1993; 11: 111
14. Lee PA. Fertility in cryptorchidism: does treatment make a difference? Endocrinol Metab Clin North Am 1993; 22: 479
15. Pollack R, Nyhus LM. Complications of groin hernia repair. Surg Clin North Am 1983; 63: 1363
16. Wantz GE. Complications of inguinal hernial repair. Surg Clin North Am 1984; 64: 287
17. Lynn, HB, Johnson, WW. Inguinal herniorrhaphy in children. Arch Surg 1961; 83: 573
18. Sparkman RS. Bilateral exploration in inguinal hernia in juvenile patients. Review and appraisal. Surgery 1962; 51: 393
19. Bartsch G, et al. Testicular torsion: Late results with special regard to fertility and endocrine function. J Urol 1980; 124: 375
20. Anderson JB, Williamson RC. Fertility after torsion of the spermatic cord. Br J Urol 1990; 65: 225
21. Hadziselimovic F, et al. Testicular histology in children with unilateral testicular torsion. J Urol 1986; 136: 208
22. Karam GH, et al. Assymptomatic Chlamydia trachomatis infections among sexually active men. J Infect Dis 1986; 154: 900

23. Werner CA. Mumps orchitis and testicular atrophy, occurrence. Ann Intern Med 1950; 32: 1066

24. Emanuele MA, Emanuele NV. Alcohol's effect on male reproduction. Alcohol Health Res World 1998; 22: 195

25. Kucheria K, Saxena R, Mohan D. Semen analysis in alcohol dependence syndrome. Andrologia 1985; 17: 558

26. Sofikitis N, et al. Effects of smoking on testicular function, semen quality and sperm fertilizing capacity. J Urol 1995; 154: 1030

27. Kolodny RC, et al. Depression of plasma testosterone levels after chronic intensive marihuana use. N Engl J Med 1974; 290: 872

28. Bracken MB, et al. Association of cocaine use with sperm concentration, motility, and morphology. Fertil Steril 1990; 53: 315

29. George VK, et al. Effects of long-term cocaine exposure on spermatogenesis and fertility in peripubertal male rats. J Urol 1996; 155: 327

30. Alen M, Reinila M, Vihko R. Response of serum hormones to androgen administration in power athletes. Med Sci Sports Exerc 1985; 17: 354

31. Dohle GR, Smit M, Weber RF. Androgens and male fertility. World J Urol 2003; 21: 341

32. Jarow JP, Lipshultz LI. Anabolic steroid-induced hypogonadotropic hypogonadism. Am J Sports Med 1990; 18: 429

33. Porter RJ, Mulder RT, Joyce PR. Baseline prolactin and L-tryptophan availability predict response to antidepressant treatment in major depression. Psychopharmacology (Berl) 2003; 165: 216

34. Endres G. Clinical approaches to male infertility with a case report of possible nifedipine-induced sperm dysfunction. J Am Board Fam Pract 1997; 10: 131

35. Aaberg RA, et al. Effects of extracellular ionized calcium, diltiazem and cAMP on motility of human spermatozoa. J Urol 1989; 141: 1221

36. Hommonai ZT, Shilon M, Paz GF. Phenoxybenzamine – an effective male contraceptive pill. Contraception 1984; 29: 479

37. Delaere KP, Strijbos WE, Meuleman EJ. Sulphasalazine-induced reversible male infertility. Acta Urol Belg 1989; 57: 29

38. Fukushima T, et al. Effects of sulfasalazine on sperm acrosome reaction and gene expression in the male reproductive organs of rats. Toxicol Sci 2005; 85: 675

39. Van Thiel DH, et al. An evaluation of the antiandrogen effects associated with H2 antagonist therapy. Scand J Gastroenterol Suppl 1987; 136: 24

40. Meistrich ML. Effects of chemotherapy and radiotherapy on spermatogenesis. Eur Urol 1993; 23: 136

41. Giwercman A, Petersen PM. Cancer and male infertility. Bailliere's Best Pract Res Clin Endocrinol Metab 2000; 14: 453

42. Spitz S. The histological effects of nitrogen mustard on human tumours and tissues. Cancer 1948; 1: 383

43. Howell SJ, Shalet SM. Testicular function following chemotherapy. Hum Reprod Update 2001; 7: 363

44. Chung K, et al. Sperm cryopreservation for male patients with cancer: an epidemiological analysis at the University of Pennsylvania. Eur J Obstet Gynecol Reprod Biol 2004; 113(Suppl 1): S7

45. Petersen PM, et al. Dose-dependent impairment of testicular function in patients treated with cisplatin-based chemotherapy for germ cell cancer. Ann Oncol 1994; 5: 355

46. Brougham MF, et al. Male fertility following childhood cancer: current concepts and future therapies. Asian J Androl 2003; 5: 325

47. Naysmith TE, et al. Do men undergoing sterilizing cancer treatments have a fertile future? Hum Reprod 1998; 13: 3250

48. Pont J, Albrecht W. Fertility after chemotherapy for testicular germ cell cancer. Fertil Steril 1997; 68: 1

49. Kedia KR, Markland C, Fraley EE. Sexual function following high retroperitoneal lymphadenectomy. J Urol 1975; 114: 237

50. Jewett MAS, et al. Retroperitoneal lymphadenectomy for testis tumor with nerve sparing for ejaculation. J Urol 1988; 139: 1220

51. Fossa SD, et al. Post-treatment fertility in patients with testicular cancer. I. Influence of retroperitoneal lymph node dissection on ejaculatory potency. Br J Urol 1985; 57: 204

52. World Health Organization. WHO Laboratory Manual for the Examination of Human Semen and Sperm–Cervical Mucus Interaction, 4th edn. New York: Cambridge University Press, 1999

53 Jeyendran RS. Interpretation of Semen Analysis Results. A Practical Guide, 1st edn. Cambridge: Cambridge University Press, 2000

54. Means AR, et al. Follicle stimulating hormone, the Sertoli cell and spermatogenesis. Recent Prog Horm Res 1976; 32: 477

55. Bergmann M, Behre HM, Nieschlag E. Serum FSH and testicular morphology in male infertility. Clin Endocrinol 1994; 40: 133

56. Dunn JF, Nisula BC, Rodbard D. Transport of steroid hormones: binding of 21 endogenous steroids to both testosterone-binding globulin and corticosteroid-binding globulin in human plasma. J Clin Endocrinol Metab 1981; 53: 58

57. Griffin JF., Wilson JD. Disorders of the testes and male reproductive tract. In Wilson JD, Foster DW, eds. Textbook of Endocrinology, 17th edn. Philadelphia: WB Saunders, 1985: 259

58. Carter JN, et al. Prolactin-secreting tumors and hypogonadism in 22 men. N Engl J Med 1978; 299: 847

59. Jouanet P, et al. Male factors and the likelihood of pregnancy in infertile couples. I. Study of sperm concentration. Int J Androl 1988; 11: 379

60. Burini AS, et al. A low sperm concentration does not preclude fertility in men with isolated hypogonadotrophic hypogonadism after gonadotropin therapy. Fertil Steril 1988; 50: 343

61. De Croo I, et al. Fertilization, pregnancy, and embryo implantation rates after ICSI in cases of obstructive and non-obstructive azoospermia. Hum Reprod 2000; 15; 1383

62. Devroey P, et al. Pregnancies after testicular sperm extraction and intracytoplasmic sperm injection in non-obstructive azoospermia. Hum Reprod 1995; 10: 1457

63. Jezek D, Knuth UA, Schulze W. Successful testicular sperm extraction (TESE) in spite of high serum follicle stimulating hormone and azoospermia: correlation between testicular morphology, TESE results, semen analysis and serum hormone values in 103 infertile men. Hum Reprod 1998; 13: 1230

64. Kuligowska E, Fenlon HM. Transrectal US in male infertility: spectrum of findings and role in patient care. Radiology 1998; 207: 173

65. Parsons RB, et al. MR imaging in male infertility. Radiographics 1997; 17: 627

66. Eskew LA, et al. Ultrasonographic diagnosis of varicoceles. Fertil Steril 1993; 60: 693

67. Jarow JP. Transrectal ultrasonography of infertile men. Fertil Steril 1993; 60: 1035

68. Littrup PJ, et al. Transrectal US of the seminal vesicles and ejaculatory ducts: clinical correlation. Radiology 1988; 168: 625

69. Schnall MD, et al. The seminal tract in patients with ejaculatory dysfunction: MR imaging with an endorectal surface coil. AJR Am J Roentgenol 1992; 159: 337

70. Belker AM, Steinbock GS. Transrectal prostate ultrasonography as a diagnostic and therapeutic aid for ejaculatory duct obstruction. J Urol 1990; 144: 356

71. Pryor JL, Howards SS. Varicocele. Urol Clin North Am 1987; 14: 499

72. Meacham RB, et al. The incidence of varicoceles in the general population when evaluated by physical examination, gray scale sonography and color Doppler sonography. J Urol 1994; 151: 1535

73. Pinto KJ, Kroovand RL, Jarow JP. Varicocele related testicular atrophy and its predictive effect upon fertility. J Urol 1994; 152: 788

74. Sigman M, Jarow JP. Ipsilateral testicular hypotrophy is associated with decreased sperm counts in infertile men with varicoceles. J Urol 1997; 158: 605

75. Shafik A, Bedeir GA. Venous tension patterns in cord veins. I. In normal and varicocele individuals. J Urol 1980; 123: 383

76. Buschi AJ, et al. Distended left renal vein: CT/ sonographic normal variant. AJR Am J Roentgenol 1980; 135: 339

77. Haans LC, et al. Testis volumes, semen quality and hormonal patterns in adolescents with and without a varicocele. Fertil Steril 1991; 56: 731

78. Sawczuk IS, et al. Varicoceles: effect on testicular volume in prepubertal and pubertal males. Urology 1993; 41: 466

79. Dubin L, Hotchkiss RS. Testis biopsy in subfertile men with varicocele. Fertil Steril 1969; 20: 51

80. Cameron DF, et al. Ultrastructural alterations in the adluminal testicular compartment in men with varicocele. Fertil Steril 1980; 33: 526

81. World Health Organization. The influence of varicocele on parameters of fertility in a large group of men presenting to infertility clinics. Fertil Steril 1992; 57: 1289

82. Cedenho AP, et al. Adolescents with varicocele have an impaired sperm–zona pellucida binding capacity. Fertil Steril 2002; 78: 1339

83. Chehval MJ, Purcell MH. Deterioration of semen parameters over time in men with untreated varicocele: evidence of progressive testicular damage. Fertil Steril 1992; 57: 174

84. Villanueva-Diaz CA, et al. Sperm dysfunction in subfertile patients with varicocele and marginal semen analysis. Andrologia 1999; 31: 263

85. Turner TT. The study of varicocele through the use of animal models. Hum Reprod Update 2001; 7: 78

86. Naughton CK, Nangia AK, Agarwal A. Pathophysiology of varicoceles in male infertility. Hum Reprod Update 2001; 7: 473

87. Saypol DC, et al. Influence of surgically induced varicocele on testicular blood flow, temperature, and histology in adult rats and dogs. J Clin Invest 1981; 68: 39

88. Ross JA, Watson NE Jr, Jarow JP. The effect of varicoceles on testicular blood flow in man. Urology 1994; 44: 535

89. Green KF, Turner TT, Howards SS. Varicocele: reversal of the testicular blood flow and temperature effects by varicocele repair. J Urol 1984; 131: 1208

90. Dahl EV, Herrick JF. A vascular mechanism for maintaining testicular temperature by counter-current exchange. Surg Gynecol Obstet 1959; 108: 697

91. Mieusset R, Bujan L. Testicular heating and its possible contributions to male infertility: a review. Int J Androl 1995; 18: 169

92. Simsek F, et al. Role of apoptosis in testicular tissue damage caused by varicocele. Arch Esp Urol 1998; 51: 947

93. Lue Y, et al. Testicular heat exposure enhances the suppression of spermatogenesis by testosterone in rats: the 'two-hit' approach to male contraceptive development. Endocrinology 2000; 141: 1414

94. Batistatou A, Greene LA. Internucleosomal DNA cleavage and neuronal cell survival/death. J Cell Biol 1993; 122: 523

95. Hikin AP, et al. Spontaneous germ cell apoptosis in humans: evidence for ethnic differences in susceptibility of germ cells to programmed cell death. J Clin Endocrinol Metab 1998; 83: 152

96. Nagata S, Golstein P. The Fas death factor. Science 1995; 267: 1449

97. Lee J, et al. The Fas system is a key regulator of germ cell apoptosis in the testis. Endocrinology 1997; 138: 2081

98. Nicholson DW, Thornberry NA. Caspases: Killer proteases. Trends Biochem Sci 1997; 22: 299

99. Moll UM, Zaika A. Nuclear and mitochondrial apoptotic pathways of p53. FEBS Lett 2001; 493: 65

100. Kroemer G, Reed JC. Mitochondrial control of cell death. Nat Med 2000; 6: 513

101. Antonsson, B, Martinou JC. The Bcl-2 protein family. Exp Cell Res 2000; 256: 50

102. Nagata S. Apoptotic DNA fragmentation. Exp Cell Res 2000; 256: 12

103. Baccetti B, Collodel G, Piomboni P. Apoptosis in human ejaculated sperm cells. J Submicrosc Cytol Pathol 1996; 28: 587

104. Bertolla RP, et al. Apoptosis and varicocele: sperm cell DNA fragmentation. J Urol 2003; (Suppl 1)169: 417

105. Schlesinger MH, Wilets IF, Nagler HM. Treatment outcome after varicocelectomy. A critical analysis. Urol Clin North Am 1994; 21: 517

106. Marmar JL. The pathophysiology of varicoceles in the light of current molecular and genetic information. Hum Reprod Update 2001; 7: 461

107. de Lamirande E, Gagnon C. Reactive oxygen species and human spermatozoa. I. Effects on the motility of intact spermatozoa and on sperm axonemes. J Androl 1992; 13: 368

108. Aitken RJ, et al. Differential contribution of leukocytes and spermatozoa to the generation of reactive oxygen species in the ejaculates of oligozoospermic patients and fertile donors. J Reprod Fertil 1992; 94: 451

109. Barbieri ER, et al. Varicocele-associated decrease in antioxidant defenses. J Androl 1999; 20: 713

110. Mancini A, et al. Coenzyme Q10 concentrations in normal and pathological human seminal fluid. J Androl 1994; 15: 591

111. Gagnon C, et al. Reactive oxygen species and human spermatozoa. Ann NY Acad Sci 1991; 637: 436

112. MacLeod J. Seminal cytology in the presence of varicocele. Fertil Steril 1965; 16: 735

113. Schatte EC, et al. Varicocelectomy improves sperm strict morphology and motility. J Urol 1998; 160: 1338

114. Kantengwa S, et al. Heat shock proteins: an autoprotective mechanism for inflammatory cells? Semin. Immunol 1991; 3: 49

115. Zini A, et al. Effect of varicocelectomy on the abnormal retention of residual cytoplasm by human spermatozoa. Hum Reprod 1999; 14: 1791

116. Virgil P, et al. Assessment of sperm function in fertile and infertile men. Andrologia 1994; 26: 55

117. Benoff S, et al. The effect of calcium ion channel blockers on sperm fertilization potential. Fertil Steril 1994; 62: 606

118. Benoff S, et al. A potential role for cadmium in the etiology of varicocele-associated infertility. Fertil Steril 1997; 67: 336

119. Benoff S, et al. Classification of male factor infertility relevant to in vitro fertilization insemination strategies using mannose ligands, acrosome status and anti-cytosketetal antibodies. Hum Reprod 1996; 11: 1905

120. Benoff S, et al. Variation in region IS6 of the L-type voltage-dependent calcium (Ca+2) channel (L-VDCC) alpha-1 subunit in testis and sperm: implications for role of cadmium (Cd+2) in

varicocele-associated infertility (VAI). Fertil Steril 2000; 74: 555

121. Platt B, Busselberg D. Combined actions of Pb+2, Zn+2 and Al+3 on voltage-activated calcium channel currents. Cell Mol Neurobiol 1994; 14: 831

122. Willott GM. Frequency of azoospermia. Forensic Sci Int 1982; 20: 9

123. Jarow JP, Espeland MA, Lipshultz LI. Evaluation of the azoospermic patient. J Urol 1989; 142: 62

124. Odival T Jr, et al. Search and identification of spermatozoa and spermatids in the ejaculate of nonobstructive azoospermic patients. Int Braz J Urol 2005; 31: 42

125. Rao MM, Rao DM. Cytogenetic studies in primary infertility. Fertil Steril 1977; 28: 209

126. Sokol RZ, Swerdloff RS. Endocrine evaluation. In Lipshultz LI, Howards SS, eds. Infertility in the Male, 3rd edn. St Louis: Mosby-Year Book, 1997: 210

127. Schlegel PN, Shin D, Goldstein M. Urogenital anomalies in men with congenital absence of the vas deferens. J Urol 1996; 155: 1644

128. Anguiano A, et al. Congenital bilateral absence of the vas deferens. A primarily genital form of cystic fibrosis. JAMA 1992; 267: 1794

129. Chillon M, et al. Mutations in the cystic fibrosis gene in patients with congenital absence of the vas deferens. N Engl J Med 1995; 332: 1475

130. The Male Infertility Best Practice Policy Committee of the American Urological Association, and the Practice Committee of the American Society for Reproductive Medicine. Report on evaluation of the azoospermic male. Fertil Steril 2004; 82 (Suppl): 131

131. Jarow JP. Seminal vesicle aspiration in the management of patients with ejaculatory duct obstruction. J Urol 1994; 152: 899

132. Chandley AC. The chromosomal basis of human infertility. Br Med Bull 1979; 35: 181

133. Hargreave T. Genetically determined male infertility and assisted reproduction techniques. J Endocrinol Invest 2000; 23: 697

134. Gckas J, et al. Chromosomal factors of infertility in candidate couples for ICSI: an equal risk of constitutional aberrations in women and men. Hum Reprod 2001; 16: 82

135. de Braekeleer M, Dao TN. Cytogenetic studies in male infertility: a review. Hum Reprod 1991; 6: 245

136. Palermo GD, et al. Births after intracytoplasmic injection of sperm obtained by testicular extraction from men with nonmosaic Klinefelter's syndrome. N Engl J Med 1998; 338: 588

137. Van Opstal D, et al. Determination of the parent of origin in nine cases of prenatally detected chromosome aberrations found after intracytoplasmic sperm injection. Hum Reprod 1997; 12: 682

138. Meschede D, et al. Chromosome abnormalities in 447 couples undergoing intracytoplasmic sperm injection – prevalence, types, sex distribution and reproductive relevance. Hum Reprod 1998; 13: 576

139. Colombero LT, et al. Incidence of sperm aneuploidy in relation to semen characteristics and assisted reproductive outcome. Fertil Steril 1999; 72: 90

140. Tiepolo L, Zuffardi O. Localization of factors controlling spermatogenesis in the nonfluorescent portion of the human Y-chromosome long arm. Hum Genet 1976; 34: 119

141. Foresta C, Moro E, Ferlin A. Y-chromosome microdeletions and alterations of spermatogenesis. Endocr Rev 2001; 22: 226

142. Pryor JL, et al. Microdeletions in the Y-chromosome of infertile men. N Engl J Med 1997; 336: 534

143. Foresta C, Ferlin A, Moro E. Deletion and expression analysis of AZFa-genes on the human Y-chromosome revealed a major role for DBY in male infertility. Hum Mol Genet 2000; 9: 1161

144. Sun C, et al. An azoospermic man with a de novo point mutation in the Y-chromosomal gene USP9Y. Nat Genet 1999; 23: 429

145. Elliott DJ, et al. Expression of RBM in the nuclei of human germ cells is dependent on a critical region of the Y-chromosome long arm. Proc Natl Acad Sci USA 1997; 94: 3848

146. Reijo R, et al. Diverse spermatogenic defects in humans caused by Y-chromosome deletions encompassing a novel RNA-binding protein gene. Nat Genet 1995; 10: 383

147. Vogt PH. Molecular genetics of human male infertility: from genes to new therapeutic perspectives. Curr Pharm Des 2004; 10: 471

148. Hopps CV, et al. Detection of sperm in men with Y-chromosome microdeletions of the AZFa, AZFb and AZFc regions. Hum Reprod 2003; 18: 1660

149. Moro E, et al. Y-chromosome microdeletions in infertile men with varicocele. Mol Cell Endocrinol 2000; 161: 67

150. Foresta C, et al. Y-chromosome microdeletions in cryptorchidism and idiopathic infertility. J Clin Endocrinol Metab 1999; 84: 3660

151. Krausz C, et al. A high frequency of Y-chromosome deletions in males with nonidiopathic infertility. J Clin Endocrinol Metab 1999; 84: 3606

152. Kent-First MG, et al. The incidence and possible relevance of Y-linked microdeletions in babies born after intracytoplasmic sperm injection and their infertile fathers. Mol Hum Reprod 1996; 2: 943

153. Page DC, Silber S, Brown LG. Men with infertility caused by AZFc deletion can produce sons by intracytoplasmic sperm injection, but are likely to transmit the deletion and infertility. Hum Reprod 1999; 14: 1722

154. Oates RD, et al. Clinical characterization of 42 oligospermic or azoospermic men with microdeletion of the AZFc region of the Y-chromosome, and of 18 children conceived via ICSI. Hum Reprod 2002; 17: 2813

155. Siffroi JP, et al. Sex chromosome mosaicism in males carrying Y-chromosome long arm deletions. Hum Reprod 2000; 15: 2559

156. Jaruzelska J, et al. Mosaicism for 45,X cell line may accentuate the severity of spermatogenic defects in men with AZFc deletion. J Med Genet 2001; 38: 798

157. Papadimas J, et al. Ambiguous genitalia, 45,X/46,XY mosaic karyotype, and Y-chromosome microdeletions in a 17-year-old man. Fertil Steril 2001; 76: 1261

158. Patsalis PC, et al. Effects of transmission of Y-chromosome AZFc deletions. Lancet 2002; 360: 1222

159. Quinzii C, Castellani C. The cystic fibrosis transmembrane regulator gene and male infertility. J Endocrinol Invest 2000; 23: 684

160. Casals T, et al. Heterogeneity for mutations in the CFTR gene and clinical correlations in patients with congenital absence of the vas deferens. Hum Reprod 2000; 15: 1476

161. Chu CS, et al. Genetic basis of variable exon-9 skipping in cystic fibrosis transmembrane regulator mRNA. Nat Genet 1993; 3: 151

162. Patrizio P, et al. Aetiology of congenital absence of vas deferens: genetic study of three generations. Hum Reprod 1993; 8: 215

163. Dork T, et al. Distinct spectrum of CFTR gene mutations in congenital absence of vas deferens. Hum Genet 1997; 100: 365

164. Casals T, et al. Extensive analysis of 40 infertile patients with congenital absence of the vas deferens: In 50% of cases only one CFTR allele could be detected. Hum Genet 1995; 95: 205.

9

The basic semen analysis

Roelof Menkveld

INTRODUCTION

The scientific approach to establish a male's fertility potential by means of the semen analysis started in 1677, with van Leeuwenhoek's letter to the Royal Society of London describing the discovery of the human spermatozoon by Johan Ham. According to Schirren[1], van Leeuwenhoek stated that in the case of a sterile marriage, the microscope could solve the problem as to the responsible partner. A more scientific approach to the semen analysis procedure was introduced by the end of the 19th century, when Lode[2] performed the first dilutions of semen samples before performing a sperm count with the aid of a hemocytometer, finding a mean sperm concentration of 60.88×10^6/ml for the four males investigated. In 1941, Hotchkiss[3] published a basic grading system for sperm motility evaluation that was modified by MacLeod and Heim[4] in 1945 to a system in which the motility and progressive activities were recorded separately, the motility in 10% units and the forward progression on a scale of 0–4.

Belding[5] made one of the first contributions towards sperm morphology evaluation as we know it today by suggesting a classification for abnormalities of the head, midpiece and tail, which could be indicated as a single abnormality or a combination of abnormalities. This was followed by a description of the acrosome and the presence of vacuoles in the sperm head by Williams *et al.* in 1934[6]. Over this time period, different methods were proposed for the evaluation of semen samples with the inclusion of various semen parameters and standards for normality[4,5,7–12].

Further standardization and minimum requirements for the methodology of a semen analysis performance and 'normal' semen variable standards were established in 1951 by the American Fertility Association[13]. This was followed by the contributions of MacLeod and Gold[14], Freund[15,16] in the 1960s and Eliasson in the 1970s[17,18], especially with regard to sperm morphology. In order to obtain better world standardization of semen analysis, the first World Health Organization (WHO) manual was published in 1980[19], followed by the 1987[20], 1992[21] and 1999 editions[22].

Requirements for a complete extended semen analysis as performed today are undergoing changes according to the demands of time and new developments in the fields of spermatology and andrology, as well as assisted reproductive technologies (ART). Today, a complete basic semen analysis must also include screening tests for the presence of antisperm antibodies, such as the mixed antiglobulin reaction (MAR) test[23], and a leukocyte peroxidase test[24] aimed at identifying the presence of polymorphonuclear leukocytes.

Other tests are still mentioned in the 1999 WHO manual[22], including the sperm–mucus penetration test[25], performed with good periovulatory human cervical mucus or with human mucus replacements such as bovine mucus[26] or hyaluronate[27], the sperm–cervical mucus contact test[28], the zona-free hamster-ovum penetration test[29] and the hemizona assay test[30], which are performed to a lesser and more selective extent, for example when indicated by unexplained poor ART results. Newly developed tests such as the DNA status of the spermatozoa[31], the acrosome reaction test[32], the reactive oxygen species (ROS) activity of the spermatozoa and especially leukocytes[33] and the antioxidation capacity of seminal plasma[34] have recently attracted more attention.

However, owing to new developments and advances in ART procedures, especially intracytoplasmic sperm injection (ICSI), McDonough[35] doubted the future role of the standard basic semen analysis, and wrote: 'Traditional sperm analysis as a clinical test may become nothing more than an ancestral heirloom. It may be performed spasmodically by those who know how to do it, like a 1940-air show or laparotomy, to remind us of the good old days. We have come to the end of something. Surely someone will want to carve a headstone for traditional sperm analysis or perhaps a mausoleum will be more fitting.'

It is difficult to agree with the above concepts. Even in the light of new developments such as *in vitro* fertilization (IVF) and especially ICSI, semen analysis has and will be the most important test in the initial investigation of a male's fertility potential. It is therefore extremely important that a semen analysis should be performed skillfully and properly. If the necessary background data are known, including a short personal and medical history, so that the results can be interpreted correctly, the basic (complete) semen analysis will always remain the cornerstone of the initial investigation of a male's fertility potential, as part of a couple's basic infertility investigation.

A complete semen analysis can be divided into the following four categories: (1) background

data, (2) physical analysis, (3) microscopic analysis and (4) additional procedures. Biochemical analyses and functional tests should be performed on repeated semen analysis when indicated, for instance after unexpected poor results with ART.

THE BASIC SEMEN ANALYSIS

Specimen handling

Semen samples present a possible biohazard since they may contain harmful viruses, e.g. human immunodeficiency virus (HIV), hepatitis B and herpes. Therefore, semen samples should always be handled with care, as if infected, and the wearing of protective gear is advised (gloves, masks and spectacles). Further information is given in the 1999 WHO manual[22], based on the work of Schrader[36].

Background data

A semen analysis cannot be interpreted unless some basic facts are known, namely the method by which the sample was produced, the time lapse between production and analysis, days of abstinence and the type of container used, as these factors can have an influence on the results, as discussed below. These factors are the so-called background data, and should also include data from a succinct medical history taken when the semen sample was received.

Methods for the production of semen

Today, it is expected that the semen sample should be collected in a specially equipped, and if necessary air-conditioned, room at or in close proximity to the laboratory, especially when special tests are involved[37,38]. This method has the advantage that the exact time of semen production and the time lapse between production and investigation are known, and observations such as the presence of coagulation and the occurrence of liquefaction can be made. The way in which the sample is produced is also controlled. Many patients may produce a sample by coitus interruptus or by using a spermicidal condom if the sample is produced at home. Coitus interruptus has the disadvantage that the first part of the sample may be lost. An indication that the sample may have been produced by coitus interruptus will be the presence of vaginal epithelium cells[38].

When the patient collects the sample at the laboratory, a relationship can be built with the patient, information is easy to obtain and the patient's enquiries can be answered. It often happens that a sample is brought to the laboratory and left on a counter without any information. The results of such a semen analysis cannot be evaluated or interpreted because the method of production, days of abstinence and time of ejaculation are not known.

For patients having problems producing a semen sample by masturbation, a wide range of special condoms are available, such as silastic condoms (e.g. Seminal Collection Device™, HDC Corp., Milipitas, CA, USA)[39], the Seminal Pouch™ made of polyethylene (Milex Products Inc., Chicago, USA), condoms made of polyurethane (Male-Factor Pak™; FertiPro NV, Beernem, Belgium) and complete kits (Hy-gene™ Kit, FertiPro) for transportation of the sample to the laboratory[22]. Normal latex condoms should not be used for semen collection as they may impair sperm motility due to their spermicidal properties.

Semen samples should thus be produced by masturbation into a clean plastic container that is sterile-packed at shipment, or otherwise should be separately sterilized at the laboratory. The patient is instructed to urinate and then to wash his hands with soap and water and the glans of the penis with water alone, before producing the sample.

The patient should be asked about the precise period of abstinence, as well as a short medical history. Questions regarding his medical history should include information on the occurrence of any previous infections or illnesses, especially in the past 3 months, if it is his first visit, or since his previous semen analysis when a repeat analysis is being performed. Also included in this medical history should be questions on any recent medication or anesthesia in the past 3 months, any previous history of operations of the urogenital tract, especially involving the bladder, an orchidopexy, orchiectomy, varicocelectomy or testicular biopsy, or whether he has had any severe injuries of the testicles or orchitis. A note should also be made about his smoking and drinking habits[40].

Containers

In the early years, glass containers were used, but this practice should be discouraged, owing to the possibility of virus contamination and the fact that the glass containers have to be washed and sterilized after use. There is also the possibility that the container may break while being washed, or even when the man is producing the semen sample[40]. The ideal container is a 60–100-ml wide-mouth plastic jar made of polypropylene, with a screw cap that fits tightly to prevent any loss of semen when it is transported. In our experience, some types of plastic (e.g. polystyrene) have the disadvantage that they may cause increased viscosity, or may be toxic to the spermatozoa and may influence motility. Before the introduction of new containers in a laboratory, these should always first be tested for any negative effects on the semen sample and ART outcome[39,40].

Abstinence

The profound effect of abstinence on semen parameters, especially semen volume and sperm concentration, is well known[41]. It is therefore important that a fixed period of abstinence should be prescribed so that optimum results can be expected, the semen analysis is performed according to more standardized conditions and the results of different semen analyses can be compared with each other. If this is not done, it is impossible to know whether differences between semen parameters of different semen samples from the same patient are due to normal variation, a difference in days of abstinence or both. The variation of 2–7 days suggested in the WHO manual[22] is too long[42], and should be standardized to 3–4 days[40,43]. The question is now raised whether the period of abstinence should be expressed as days or the exact number of hours[42]. For routine semen analysis the number of days will be acceptable, but for medical trials the exact number of hours is advised.

After production of the semen sample the container is placed in an incubator at 37°C until complete liquefaction has occurred. The sample is then ready for evaluation, and is usually transferred to a graduated conical test-tube for further processing.

Physical parameters

Parameters describing the appearance of the sample are classified by Freund[44] and Zaneveld and Polakoski[45] as physical parameters, and include the color, liquefaction and viscosity, while coagulation and odor can also be added to this category. Although strictly speaking a biochemical characteristic, pH is also included in this group. All these parameters are simple to evaluate and are mainly determined by visual examination.

Coagulation

This is an important aspect of semen analysis that is ignored by many investigators, mainly because many semen samples are still produced at home instead of at the laboratory. Human semen is ejaculated in a liquefied state, but is quickly transformed into a semisolid state or coagulum, probably under the influence of the enzyme protein kinase[46] secreted by the seminal vesicles. In a normal situation, nearly the whole sample is transformed into the coagulated state, and only a very small part remains liquefied. This is generally regarded as the first portion of the ejaculate, containing the major part of the motile sperm fraction. In cases where coagulation does not occur it may be the result of congenital absence of the vas deferens and the seminal vesicles, as the coagulating enzymes originate from the seminal vesicles,

and is then also associated with the absence of fructose in the seminal plasma.

Liquefaction

In a normal sample, liquefaction occurs within 10–20 minutes. This is caused by a proteolytic enzyme fibrinolysin secreted by the prostate[47], as well as two other proteolytic enzymes, fibrinogenase and aminopeptidase[48]. Liquefaction therefore serves as an indicator of normal prostatic function.

After complete liquefaction the sample will appear homogeneous in composition and color. Small roundish particles may still be present in some samples; however, this can be regarded as normal, and they will usually dissolve within an hour. If liquefaction takes more than 20 minutes or does not occur at all, it is a sign that the prostate is not functioning normally, usually as a result of previous prostatitis. In some cases this non-liquefaction of semen may be a cause of infertility, as the spermatozoa are not released from the coagulum[40].

Viscosity

As long ago as 1934, Cary and Hotchkiss[7] described the consistency of semen as slightly more viscous than water. The most convenient way to determine viscosity is by means of a modified pipette method[37]. The semen is drawn into a Pasteur pipette and slowly released in a drop-wise fashion. The viscosity is regarded as normal when single drops are formed that are released within a distance of 20 mm from the point of the pipette. If threads are longer than 20 mm the viscosity can be regarded as increased[40].

It is also important to distinguish between a delayed period of liquefaction (non-homogeneous appearance) and an increase in the viscosity (homogeneous but 'sticky'). Increased viscosity may be the result of abnormal prostatic function due to an infection in the genital tract, prostate or seminal vesicles[49], or an artifact as a result of the use of an unsuitable type of plastic container, frequent ejaculation or the psychological state of the patient. A constant increase in viscosity may be regarded as a cause of infertility[45] for *in vivo* conception, and can also have an adverse effect on the determination of spermatozoa concentration and motility.

Biochemical means should be used to reduce high semen viscosity, for example α-amylase[50] and chymotrypsin[51], while another method is the addition of an equal volume of a medium such as saline, phosphate-buffered saline or culture medium, followed by repeat pipetting with a wide-bore pipette[52]. In these cases, care should be taken that the sperm concentration is correctly calculated, taking into consideration the extra dilution effect of the added fluid[53].

Volume

The most common method still used today to determine the volume is by transferring the sample to a 15-ml graduated conical tube and reading the volume to the nearest 0.1 ml. Determination of the volume can also be performed by means of weighing samples, taking the total weight of the sample and container minus the container weight determined beforehand. The weight is expressed as the nearest 0.1 ml, taking 1 g equal to 1 ml[53].

The normal volume of an ejaculate after 3–5 days of sexual abstinence is 2–6 ml. Hotchkiss[11] stressed the importance of a normal volume, as this is needed for good buffering function of the seminal pool against the acid secretions of the vagina. If the volume of a semen sample is smaller than 1.0 ml, it is important to establish whether a complete sample was collected. This is important, as the first portion containing the major amount of sperm with the best motility is often lost. A low volume may, however, also be the result of an obstruction due to a previous infection of the genital tract, or of congenital absence of the seminal vesicles and vas deferens; this condition will be associated with the absence of fructose[45]. A small volume may also be due to retrograde ejaculation, especially if the patient has had any previous surgery of the prostate or the bladder neck.

Retrograde ejaculation can be diagnosed by investigation of the urine after ejaculation.

Color

By paying attention to the color of the semen sample, an indication of possible pathology of the semen can already be obtained. Cary and Hotchkiss[7] described the color of normal semen as opaque and grayish, which will change to yellowish with an increase in the days of abstinence. Hotchkiss[11] noticed that fresh blood will give semen a reddish color and old blood a brownish color, which may be caused by recent inflammation. In cases of inflammation a more yellowish color may exist, while samples with a low sperm concentration will usually have a transparent and watery consistency. Schirren[1] found that certain types of medicine such as antibiotics might discolor the semen.

Odor

Although semen has a strong, distinctive odor, derived from the prostatic secretions, this parameter is seldom used. The odour is sometimes compared to that of the flowers of the chestnut or St John's bread tree. It is thought that the odor is caused by oxidation of the spermine secreted by the prostate. Only with absence of the odor or when an uncharacteristic odor is present should a note be made, as this is usually associated with an infection[45], or is the result of a long period of abstinence[37].

pH

Preference should be given to pH measurement using a special pH indicator paper (range 6.4–8.0; Merck #9557), for hygiene reasons and also the possibility that sexually transmitted diseases may be transferred when using the glass-electrode method. After liquefaction, a drop of semen is placed on the indicator strip and immediately compared against a color scale. The pH of a normal ejaculate may vary between 7.2 and 7.8[22].

In cases of acute prostatitis, vesiculitis or bilateral epididymitis, the pH will always be more than

8.0[45]. In cases of chronic infection of the above organs, the pH will always be below 7.2, and can be as low as 6.6. With an obstruction of the ejaculatory duct or in cases where only prostatic fluids are secreted, the pH will also be less than 7.0, and if the sample is azoospermic this low pH may also indicate the presence of bilateral congenital absence of the vas deferens[22].

Microscopic analysis

Wet preparation examination

After completion of the physical examination, the centrifuge tubes are placed on a cradle or roller system[39] for the duration of all subsequent procedures. This can be done at room temperature or at 37°C. After 10 minutes of gentle mixing, a drop of semen is taken with a positive-displacement pipette and placed on a precleaned glass slide kept at 37°C until use. The size of the drop of semen will depend on the size of the coverslip used, so that the depth of fluid between the microscope slide and the coverslip is about 20 μm, to allow maximum free movement of the spermatozoa and still optimum visibility with a 40× objective. The standard drop size most often used is 10 μl for a 20×20-mm coverslip. Complete guide tables for different sizes of coverslips and corresponding drop sizes to be used can be found in several publications[22,39,53]. The preparation is left for a few minutes to stabilize before examination.

General appearance All examinations of wet preparations are done with phase-contrast optics, first at a 100× or 150× or low-power field (LPF) magnification (with 10× or 15× objectives) to obtain an overall view, and then at 400× or high-power field (HPF) magnification (with a 40× objective). The examination starts with scanning through ten LPFs to get an impression of the general appearance of the sample. The impression obtained here will dictate all subsequent procedures, such as the performance of a MAR test[23] if enough motile spermatozoa are present, or a vital staining test[54] when the motility is low. An estimation of the number of spermatozoa per HPF is made, which will be used to determine the dilution of the sample for calculation of the sperm concentration and drop size to be used for preparing smears for sperm morphology evaluation.

Agglutination and presence of other cells The sample is also examined for the presence of sperm agglutination. Two types of agglutination can be observed. In the first instance, agglutination can be due to non-specific factors where, in most cases, non-motile spermatozoa adhere to cells present in the seminal plasma; when this occurs it is termed aggregation[39]. The second is specific agglutination, caused by antisperm antibodies, which consists mostly of motile spermatozoa clumps with only minimal involvement of other cells or debris[39]. Agglutination is described as negative (−), occasional (±), slight (+), moderate (++) or severe (+++)[40], or as an appropriate percentage to the nearest 5%[39,53]. A note is also made of the presence of other cells, such as round cells, and the presence of spermine phosphate crystals, recorded in the same way as for agglutination. The presence of any organisms is also recorded.

Analysis of quantitative parameters

The parameters classified under this heading are those that are regarded by many investigators to constitute a complete or standard semen analysis, and include estimation of the percentage and grade of sperm motility, the vital staining procedure to determine the percentage of live spermatozoa, if indicated due to poor motility, the spermatozoa concentration and the morphology of the spermatozoa. The MAR test[23] and a leukocyte peroxidase test[24] should now also be included as routine procedures[55].

Motility and forward progression Motility is now mostly determined in one of two manners. The first is by manual observation of the sample with phase-contrast optics. More recently, automated computer-assisted semen analysis (CASA) techniques have been introduced with varying degrees of success[22,39]. This is discussed briefly under a separate heading dealing with CASA.

For the manual method, the wet preparation slide, as prepared for the initial examination, can be used and the evaluation is performed as described in the WHO[22] and European Society for Human Reproduction and Embryology (ESHRE)[53] manuals. The exact aliquot of semen to provide a depth of 20 μm is of importance due to the rotary and spiral movement pattern of progressive motile spermatozoa. If the time interval between the initial wet preparation and observation for motility is too long, a new preparation should be made, and examination of the wet preparation should begin as soon as the flow of the semen drop has ceased. If this has not occurred within a minute, a new preparation should be made and examined[53].

Spermatozoa are classified according to the rapidity of their forward progressive motility into four grades, from grade a to grade d, as follows:

- Grade a = rapid progressive motility;
- Grade b = slow or sluggish progressive motility;
- Grade c = non-progressive motility;
- Grade d = immotile.

Definitions of rapid and slow forward motility will differ, depending on whether the motility evaluation is performed at room temperature or at 37°C by means of a hot stage fitted on the microscope. For rapid motility at 37°C, the spermatozoa should travel ≥ 25 μm per second, and at room temperature ≥ 20 μm per second, i.e. the distance of five and four sperm heads, respectively, as spermatozoa move more rapidly at 37°C[22]. If the forward progression is < 5 μm per second, for both room temperature and 37°C determinations, spermatozoa are regarded as having a non-progressive grade c motility. Between these limits, spermatozoa will be regarded as having a grade b or slow forward motility.

At least 200 spermatozoa should be counted in five separate high-power magnification fields with the aid of phase-contrast microscopy. The percentages of the different categories must add up to 100%. The count should be repeated on a separate wet preparation. The results of the two counts are then averaged, provided that they are within acceptable limits that can be calculated according to a method provided in the ESHRE manual[53].

Poor motility or asthenozoospermia can be caused by several factors. One reason may be artifacts caused by the wrong method of collection, such as use of a condom which may be sperm-toxic, contamination by vaginal secretions, the use of lubricants[56], an incomplete sample, a long delay in transportation of the sample to the laboratory or exposure to extreme temperatures. Artifacts can also be caused by technical factors such as cold shock due to use in the laboratory of cold containers, slides and pipettes, the use of unsuitable, contaminated or wet containers, storage of the sample at an adverse temperature[57,58] or wrong thickness of the wet preparation (< 10 μm), hindering the free rotational movement of the spermatozoa[59]. Poor motility can also be due to structural abnormalities of the midpiece[60], or the short-tail[61] and immotile cilia or Kartagener's syndrome[62]. Poor motility may also be caused by unfavorable environmental conditions during the formation and maturation of spermatozoa before they are released from the Sertoli cells[63,64], or during transport through the epididymis[65] and ductal system, or via abnormal functions of the prostate or seminal vesicles caused by acute infections or inflammation of the accessory glands. Other factors that can cause poor motility are the presence of hematospermia, a varicocele, chromosomal aberrations, bacterial infections and an abnormal pH[58,66], as well as the presence of certain metals or metal ions[67].

Sperm concentration In 1929, the well-known article of Macomber and Sanders[68] was published in which their sperm counting technique, which forms the basis for most of the techniques still used today, was described. A 1:20 dilution was made with the aid of a white blood-cell pipette, and the count performed on a hemocytometer. The diluting fluid consisted of a 5% sodium bicarbonate solution to which 1% formalin was added.

Over the years, the pipettes used to prepare the dilutions have changed, with the aim of measuring and delivering the semen aliquot to be diluted as accurately as possible. Concern about delivering the true measured volume of the semen aliquot is due to the higher viscosity of semen compared with water. Instead of the white blood-cell pipette, Eliasson[18] used micropipettes to make a 1:50, 1:100 or 1:200 dilution. Van Zyl[69] introduced the use of a glass tuberculin syringe instead of the white blood-cell pipette. With this method it is possible to make a 1:10, 1:20 or a 1:100 dilution. Menkveld et al.[70] demonstrated that the results of the tuberculin syringe method compared well with the results of the white blood-cell pipette (WCP) method. In 1979, Makler introduced a special sperm-counting chamber, which was improved in 1980[71]. With the Makler chamber it is possible to carry out sperm counts directly on undiluted semen samples, after immobilization of the spermatozoa in a hot water bath at ±60°C. The exact amount of semen delivered to the chamber for this apparatus is not as critical as for the preparation of dilutions for counting using the standard hemocytometer.

Depending on the observed sperm number per high-power field, a 1:10, 1:20 or a 1:50 dilution will be made, while some laboratories also make use of a 1:100 dilution[40]. It is now advised that positive-displacement pipettes should be used to deliver the semen aliquot, and a normal air-displacement pipette to deliver the dilution fluid[22,53]. For a 1:10 dilution, 900 μl of the dilution fluid is placed in a small tube and 100 μl of the semen sample is transferred to the dilution fluid by means of the positive-displacement pipette. The sperm suspension is thoroughly mixed by vortex, and both sides of a hemocytometer with improved Neubauer ruling is carefully filled without spilling

the suspension over the sides of the chamber. The hemocytometer is left in a moist Petri dish for about 10 minutes for the spermatozoa to settle on the bottom of the chamber[40]. The number of spermatozoa in the upper left corner block (consisting of 16 smaller blocks) of the central grid, used for counting red blood cells, is counted, to determine the proportion of blocks from the 25 in the grid that should be considered for counting.

A reference table is given in the WHO[22] and ESHRE[53] manuals indicating the number of blocks from the 25 to be included so that in all instances the number of spermatozoa counted will be more than 200. The counting procedure is repeated on the other side. By the use of a table also provided in the two manuals[22,53], the actual concentrations are calculated, depending on the initial dilution and the number of blocks counted per side of the hemocytometer. It is very important to note that the two tables with conversion factors in the WHO[22] and ESHRE[53] manuals differ, due to the fact that the WHO manual (incorrectly) first obtains the mean of the two counts. The two counts obtained are compared to establish whether the results are within acceptable limits by means of a formula also provided in the two manuals. If the counts are not within acceptable limits, the whole counting procedure should be repeated. Estimation of the sperm concentration with the aid of computerized equipment (CASA) is gaining ground, and is now used as the routine method in many laboratories[22,39].

Differences still exist as to what can be regarded as a normal sperm concentration, and many different so-called normal cut-off values have been proposed, including 60×10^6 by Macomber and Sanders[68], 20×10^6 by Eliasson[18] and by MacLeod and Gold[72] and 10×10^6/ml by Van Zyl[69] and Van Zyl et al.[73,74].

Sperm morphology evaluation   The 1999 WHO manual[22] recommends that sperm morphology evaluation should be performed according to strict Tygerberg criteria. The principles for the evaluation of sperm morphology by strict Tygerberg criteria were laid down by Menkveld[41] and Menkveld et al.[75], while the clinical application for the in vitro situation was demonstrated by Kruger et al.[76]. In a follow-up study Kruger et al.[77] also described the prognostic categories with strict criteria for in vitro fertilization outcome, i.e. the poor-prognosis or P-group with ≤ 4% morphologically normal spermatozoa, the good-prognosis or G-group with 5–14% morphologically normal spermatozoa and the normal group with ≥ 15% morphologically normal spermatozoa[76,77].

Sperm morphology evaluation according to strict criteria uses a holistic approach, starting with the preparation of clean microscope slides, the correct preparation of thin semen smears, the correct methodology for evaluation of the slides, i.e. the correct optics and magnification to be used, the correct number of spermatozoa to be evaluated and, most important of all, the criteria for a morphological normal spermatozoon as based on biological evidence[41,78,79]. Morphological evaluation of the semen smear can also include evaluation of the semen cytology. Therefore, two slides are prepared, one thicker smear for semen cytology evaluation and a thin smear for sperm morphology evaluation. It may also be beneficial to prepare one or two extra smears that can be kept in case the original smear is unsuitable for evaluation, or for back-up purposes[18,73].

Morphological evaluation of spermatozoa The morphological evaluation of spermatozoa as discussed here is based on the methodology described by Menkveld[41], Kruger et al.[76], Menkveld et al.[75] and Menkveld and Kruger[78]. If indicated, due to oiliness or dirt, slides must be thoroughly cleaned before use, first washed in a detergent, rinsed in clean water and then rinsed in alcohol and air-dried[78]. For the morphology evaluation smear, a small drop of semen is used so that a very thin smear is prepared. As a result, all the spermatozoa will be within one focus level and each sperm can be visualized separately and no more than 5–10 spermatozoa will be present per visual field at oil magnification (1000 or 1250×). The size of the

drop will depend on the sperm concentration; for high concentrations a small drop is used (~5 μl), for normal concentrations a drop of ~10 μl will be used and for low concentrations a drop of not more than 15 μl, as with these thicker smears the semen may wash off with the staining procedure[78]. The thickness of the smear can also be controlled by altering the angle and speed of the microscope slide used to make the smear[11,17].

The slides are left until they appear to be just air-dried, i.e. only a few minutes, and are then immediately fixed in methanol or ether–alcohol (50:50) and can be stored for later reference or until staining. The modified Papanicolaou technique should be the preferred method for staining the smears[22,39,75]. Alternative staining methods exist, such as the rapid blood-staining methods[80], and the Spermac stain method[81,82]. The Spermac stain is also a rapid staining method and gives excellent staining of the acrosome region and sperm tails[81]. The rapid blood-staining methods, such as Diff-Quik®[80], cause the spermatozoa to swell slightly, and thereby may cause slight alterations to the form of the spermatozoa giving rise to bigger size measurements, which should be kept in mind when using these stains. Problems with background staining can also occur when too much seminal plasma is present on the slide[83].

The criteria used for a morphologically normal spermatozoon are based on the appearance of spermatozoa seen in good cervical mucus drawn from the endocervical canal shortly after intercourse for the performance of a postcoital test. These spermatozoa have a very homogeneous appearance, with only small biological variations[75,78,84]. According to the strict Tygerberg criteria[41,75], a normal spermatozoon is defined as one having an oval form with a smooth contour and a clearly visible and well-defined acrosome, with homogeneous light blue staining. The tail should be apically inserted without any abnormalities of the neck/midpiece region; there should be no tail abnormalities; and there should be no cytoplasmic residues at the neck region or on the tail. Measurements for an abnormal cytoplasmic droplet and normal sperm size as seen with Papanicolaou staining are based on those described by Eliasson in 1971[17]. The size of a normal acrosome was described as covering between 40 and 70% of the anterior part of the sperm head, with abnormal cytoplasmic droplets being present when larger than 50% of a normal-sized sperm head, which will measure 3.0–5.0 µm in length and 2.0–3.0 µm in width. The midpiece should not be longer than 1.5 times the length of a normal head and about 1 µm thick. The tail should be about 45–50 µm long and without any sharp bends[17]. For a spermatozoon to be classified as morphologically normal, with strict Tygerberg criteria[41,75], the whole spermatozoon must be normal, as suggested by Eliasson[17]. However, in contrast to the views of earlier workers[14,15,17], borderline or slightly abnormal spermatozoa are considered to be abnormal according to strict Tygerberg criteria[41,75]. This was proposed to keep allowable sperm morphology variations as small as possible, in agreement with biological variations seen in the cervical mucus[75].

However, the measurements as proposed by Eliasson[17] and in other publications[22,75] are in need of re-evaluation, as the range allowed especially for the normal head length of 3.0–5.0 µm is probably too wide. Our own experience indicates that the head length for normal spermatozoa may vary between 4.0 and 4.5 µm, with a mean of 4.07 ± 0.19 µm and a mean width of 2.98 ± 0.14 µm, as measured with a built-in microscope eyepiece micrometer (Menkveld, unpublished data). We have shown in several publications that males presenting with large-headed spermatozoa of > 5.0 µm in length, and with a proportional increase in width, and/or large acrosomes can be associated with poor *in vitro* fertilization results[76,85] and decreased sperm functional abilities[85].

The presence and size of, and terminology for, cytoplasmic droplets or cytoplasmic residues are also controversial. Originally, it was stated by Eliasson[17], the WHO manuals[19,20] and Menkveld *et al.*[75] that a normal cytoplasmic droplet present on spermatozoa should be < 50% of a normal sperm head. This has been changed to < 30% in the 1999 WHO manual[22]. Recently, Cooper *et al.*[86] and Cooper[87] addressed this issue of the presence and size of the cytoplasmic bodies, as well as the correct terminology to be used. From the publication by Cooper[87], it is clear that the retention of cytoplasmic material on spermatozoa as seen in air-dried and stained smears can be associated with impaired sperm function. It is also clear from this article and from our own experience[34] that no amount of cytoplasmic material should be present on a normal spermatozoon at all, and if observed it should be regarded as an abnormality, regardless of the size or amount of cytoplasmic material present. In the article by Cooper[87], it is suggested that the correct term to use if cytoplasmic material is present should be 'excess cytoplasmic residues', or just cytoplasmic residues.

At least 200 spermatozoa should be evaluated in duplicate per slide with the highest magnification possible, i.e. 1000×, but preferably 1250×. In case of any doubt about the dimensions of a spermatozoon, the size can be measured with a micrometer. The spermatozoa should preferably not be evaluated in one area but in several areas, to increase the accuracy of the evaluation[78].

The latest WHO manuals[21,22] recommend that spermatozoa should be classified only as normal or abnormal. A note should be made if a specific abnormality occurs in a frequency of > 20%. However, as indicated above, an abnormal spermatozoon can have only one specific abnormality or any combination of two or up to four abnormalities. To reflect this, the teratozoospermia index (TZI) was introduced as an indication of the mean number of abnormalities per abnormal spermatozoon[21,22]. The TZI value will therefore always be between 1 and 4. However, in the 1999 WHO manual[22], cytoplasmic residues were omitted as an abnormality, and the TZI value was indicated as being between 1 and 3. This was in contrast to the ESHRE manual, which maintained that this is not correct and the value should be between 1 and 4[53].

Evaluation of semen cytology For the evaluation of the semen cytology, i.e. investigation of the presence of different cells and organisms, a thicker smear is prepared. A small drop of egg albumin may be added to ensure better adherence of the cells to the slide. However, the more intense staining of the albumin background can sometimes make it difficult to identify the round cells present. The smears are fixed immediately in 1:1 solution of ether–alcohol for 30 minutes and stained together with the slide for morphology evaluation[78]. The slides are screened at a low magnification (15×), and if any cells or organisms are observed a 40× objective is used to make a better diagnosis. Cells looked for are especially polymorphonuclear white blood cells, monocytes and epithelium cells. With good staining, germinal epithelium cells, sometimes called precursors, can also be identified. The presence of identified cells, especially polymorphonuclear white blood cells (WBC) is recorded separately in a semiquantitative way by means of plus and minus signs as follows: no cells/HPF −; occasional cells/HPF ±; 1–5 cells/HPF +; 5–10 cells/HPF ++; > 10 cells/HPF +++[78]. A good correlation has been found between WBC identified in this manner and granulocyte white blood cells counted by means of the leukocyte peroxidase method, with ≥ +WBC/HPF correlating to ≥ 0.25×10^6 leukocytes/ml semen, a value found to be of pathological importance[78,88]. More details of the cytological evaluation of semen smears and the origin[89] of different cell types and the identification of these cells have been published by others[55,89–91].

The mixed antiglobulin reaction (MAR) test A MAR test as described by Jager *et al.*[23] must be included in all semen analysis as a routine procedure, as a screening test for the possible presence of antispermatozoa antibodies if a sufficient number of motile spermatozoa are present. The original MAR test as described by Jager *et al.*[23] makes use of a suspension of sensitized R_1R_2 erythrocytes. The erythrocytes are sensitized by washing them three times with a phosphate-buffered saline

(PBS) solution, pH 7.5. The suspension is mixed 5:1 with a strong incomplete anti-D serum (Behring ORRA 20/21) and incubated at 37°C for 30 minutes. After incubation the suspension is again washed three times in PBS and suspended to a hematocrit of 5–10%. This suspension can be kept at 4°C for a few days[23]. However, today, most laboratories make use of commercial products (MarScreen®, Bioscreen, New York, USA; SpermMar, FertiPro)[22], in which the erythrocytes are substituted by latex particles[92].

For the latex MAR test, a drop of semen is placed on a clean glass slide followed by a drop of antiserum to human immunoglobulin (IgG) and a drop of the sensitized latex particle suspension. Care should be taken that the drops do not touch each other, as this can influence the outcome of the test. The drops are thoroughly mixed with a coverslip and then covered by the same coverslip. The test is read after 10 minutes at room temperature. No interpretation is made if latex agglutinates are not observed. The test is reported as negative if no latex particles are observed bound to motile spermatozoa, doubtful when < 10% of motile sperm have latex particles bound to them, positive if 10–90% of motile spermatozoa show latex particles bound and strongly positive if > 90% of motile spermatozoa show latex particles bound. In all cases of a positive MAR test (> 10% binding), blood and seminal plasma can be obtained for subsequent testing of antisperm antibody titers with the microagglutination[93] and immobilization[94] tests at a later stage.

However, these tests are now also performed very rarely in most modern andrology laboratories, and have been substituted by the Immunobead test for IgA, IgG and IgM (Irvine Scientific, Santa Anna, USA; Laboserv GmbH, Am Boden, Staufenberg, Germany)[53]. Commercial kits are also available for the direct determination of IgA and IgM antisperm antibodies in semen, although IgM antibodies are seldom found on spermatozoa and the clinical relevance is not clear. IgA, on the other hand, is the antisperm antibody of most clinical importance, as spermatozoa coated with IgA antibodies are not capable of penetrating the cervical mucus *in vivo*, and may be an important reason for long-standing unexplained infertility, which is easily treatable by intrauterine insemination (IUI) of the husband's washed spermatozoa. Some laboratories perform the IgG and IgA MAR test simultaneously on the semen sample, while others only do the IgA MAR test if the IgG MAR test is positive, as IgA anti-sperm antibodies are seldom found on their own[95].

Detection and role of leukocytes   Ejaculates usually contain cells other than spermatozoa, called round cells, compiled of, for example, white blood cells and germinal epithelium cells, the latter con-tributing up to 90% of all round cells in fertile males, with a mean concentration of 0.12×10^6/ml semen, as found by Ariagno *et al.*[96]. The inclusion of a test for the identification of granular white blood cells must now be regarded as part of the standard basic routine semen analy-sis, as the presence of leukocytes is associated with the production of ROS[55], causing DNA damage and reduced pregnancy rates with ART[33]. Many procedures are available for the detection of leuko-cytes in semen, but, based on the available litera-ture, the leukocyte peroxidase test is indicated as a basic test for this purpose[24].

Peroxidase test for detecting leukocytes. The solu-tion for performing the leukocyte peroxidase test (Endtz test)[97] is prepared by dissolving 125 mg benzidine and 150 mg cyanosine (phloxine) in 50 ml 95% alcohol which is then further diluted with 50 ml distilled water. This solution can be stored in a light-protected bottle. A 3% hydrogen peroxide solution is also prepared. Before the test is performed, 250 μl of the stock solution is mixed with 20 μl of the peroxide solution. For the test itself, one drop of semen is mixed with one drop of the above working solution on a clean glass slide, covered with a coverslip and examined microscopically after 2 minutes, and the number of brown cells per high-power field estimated. Neutrophil granulocytes (leukocytes) stain brown.

Granules of basophil and eosinophil granulocytes stain reddish brown to violet, while lymphocytes and precursors stain light pink, as they are peroxidase-negative[22,24]. The concentration of peroxidase-positive cells can be counted with the aid of a hemocytometer, and expressed as 10^6/ml semen. The WHO manual[22] suggests that the pre-sence of $> 1 \times 10^6$ granulocytes/ml semen should be regarded as the presence of leukocytospermia, possibly based on the work of Comhaire *et al.*[98].

Other methods for the detection of leukocytes. The suitability of the leukocyte peroxidase test as a screening test for leukocytes has been questioned, and more sophisticated methods have been pro-posed[55]. However, it has been demonstrated that polymorphonuclear granulocytes are the most prevalent WBC in semen[22,55], and these cells are mainly responsible for the production of ROS[99,100]. As the leukocyte peroxidase test detects only granular WBC, the procedure can be consid-ered a suitable and reliable routine test for this purpose[97].

The identification of lymphocytes and mono-cytes is possible with the aid of monoclonal anti-bodies against the common leukocyte antigen CD45, whereby granulocytes, lymphocytes and macrophages can be detected, while other mono-clonal antibodies allow the selective staining of other WBC subpopulations[101–104]. According to Wolff[99], immunocytochemistry can be considered the gold standard for the detection of WBC, but these methods are time-consuming and labor-intensive, and thus more suitable as a research tool than a routine method.

The use of flow cytometry with the aid of monoclonal antibodies can also be considered. Ricci *et al.*[105] described this method as a simple, reproducible procedure, capable of accurately detecting leukocytes in semen and categorizing the different WBC subpopulations without any preliminary purification procedures of the semen samples. Another (indirect) method is the detection of polymorphonuclear leukocyte (PMN) elastase. This enzyme is released by activated granulocytes, and can be measured in fresh or frozen seminal plasma. The method is objective, but costly and time-consuming. A strong correlation has been found between elastase levels and WBC numbers in semen[106]. Esfandiari et al.[107] used the nitroblue tetrazolium reduction test for the identification of leukocytes and the assessment of ROS production by leukocytes and spermatozoa.

The most basic way of detecting WBC in semen samples is by direct observation of semen smears using bright-field light microscopy with the aid of the Papanicolaou, or the Bryan–Leishman staining[108] technique, as discussed in the preceding morphology section. However, the cytological identification of leukocytes and germinal epithelium cells has always been regarded as an insufficient method in much of the literature[109]. The argument is the inability of most observers to diagnose accurately the various leukocyte subpopulations, or even the inability to distinguish between the different WBC forms and immature germinal epithelium cells. However, positive identification of both groups is possible with a good staining method such as Papanicolaou, although thorough theoretical knowledge, practical training and extensive experience are required[78,89–91,110–112].

Cut-off values for leukocytospermia. Controversy exists about what can be regarded as leukocytospermia. The WHO manual defines leukocytospermia as the presence of excessive numbers of white blood cells (WBC) or leukocytes in the human ejaculate, which are predominantly granulocytes and more specifically of the neutrophil subtype, and states that in a normal ejaculate the number of WBC should be $< 1 \times 10^6$/ml[21,22]. Politch et al.[113] already concluded that more research is needed to establish thresholds for pathological levels of WBC in semen for both a mono-antibody-based immunohistological method and the peroxidase method. New cut-off values as low as 0.25×10^6 and even 0.2×10^6 WBC/ml have been proposed[88,108].

Controversy about leukocytospermia. The fact that the presence of leukocytes in semen may have a negative impact on semen parameters and sperm function was addressed as early as 1980 by Comhaire et al.[98] and in 1982 by Berger[114], and in 1990 by Wolff et al.[115]. However, in 1992 and 1993, Tomlinson et al. published three articles with an opposite view[103,104,116]. The first article indicated that seminal leukocytes may play a positive role in male fertility by the removal of morphologically abnormal spermatozoa, the second suggested that the presence of immature germ cells but not leukocytes in semen is associated with reduced success of *in vitro* fertilization and the third, a prospective study, suggested that leukocytes and leukocyte subpopulations in semen are not a cause for male infertility[103,104,116]. In 1995, Aitken and Baker concluded that there does not appear to be a convincing case for believing that seminal leukocytes are 'good Samaritans'. They mentioned that on the other hand leukocytes may often be present without an obvious effect but that it must always be kept in mind that WBC may pose a risk depending on the circumstances that led to their infiltration of the semen sample and that the potentioal of WBC to act as negative terrorists must not be ignored[117].

Since then, several more articles with opposing views have been published, as well as reports suggesting that inflammation of the male reproductive tract causing leukocytospermia may be a temporary and self-limiting episode, and that this phenomenon is probably common even in fertile males[118,119].

Matters are further complicated by reports of a very poor relationship between the presence of bacteriospermia and leukocytospermia and male genital tract inflammation[120]. Comhaire et al. reported that leukocytospermia may be associated with inflammatory reactions of the male genital tract due to the presence of bacteria, and found that ejaculates with $> 10^6$ peroxidase positive cells/ml semen contained significantly more pathogenic bacteria isolates, compared with a group of men with $< 10^6$ peroxidase-positive cells/ml semen[98]. Punab et al. also found a positive correlation between the WBC count and the number of different micro-organisms, and also between the WBC count and the total count of micro-organisms in the semen samples they investigated for both leukocytospermia and bacteriospermia[108].

In contrast, Rodin et al. found that leukocytospermia was a poor marker for the presence of bacteriospermia[121], while Eggert-Kruse found no significant association between leukocytospermia and bacteriospermia[122], and neither did Cottell et al.[123].

The origin of bacteriospermia is still complex. Bacteriospermia usually occurs due to one or more of the following three reasons: (1) normal colonization, (2) contamination of the semen sample or (3) a urogenital infection[123]. The male genital tract is usually bacteria-free, but the urethra may be colonized by a variety of micro-organisms. It is not clear to what extent these bacteria, which are usually considered as commensal organisms, can contribute to an inflammatory process[124]. Matters are furthermore complicated due to the possibility of contamination of semen samples by non-pathogenic commensals of the skin or glans penis[123]. It is therefore not clear to what extent bacteriospermia is indicative of male genital infection per se, and different results for the relationship between leukocytospermia and bacteriospermia have been published, as mentioned above.

To add to the controversy, the incidence of leukocytospermia as found in different infertile male populations varies widely from 6.8 to 44.3%[125].

Influence of leukocytospermia on semen parameters and sperm function. As mentioned in the above paragraph on 'Controversies about leukocytospermia', contradictory reports have been published in the literature on the effect of leukocytospermia or even the presence of leukocytes on semen parameters and the functional ability of spermatozoa.

For instance, Kaleli et al. found a significant positive correlation between leukocyte counts, as determined using the leukocyte peroxidase test, and increased hypo-osmotic swelling test scores, higher sperm concentrations and enhanced acrosome reactions[126]. These favorable effects were especially noted at seminal leukocyte concentrations of between 1 and 3×10^6/ml semen. Kiessling found that semen samples with evaluated concentrations of leukocytes contained a significantly higher frequency of spermatozoa with ideal morphology[127].

Eggert-Kruse et al. did not find any significant association between the presence of leukocytospermia and the production of antisperm antibodies in semen of the IgA and IgG types as detected using the red blood-cell MAR test[122]. Neither did Rodin et al. find a negative or positive effect on semen parameters and sperm function in the presence of leukocytospermia[121].

Many reports on the negative effects of leukocytospermia on sperm function have been published, for instance by Chan et al., who showed that, in the presence of leukocytospermia, hyperactivation of spermatozoa, but not sperm motility, was negatively affected[128]. Negative correlations between leukocyte concentrations and progressive sperm motility, normal sperm morphology and the hypo-osmotic swelling test have also been reported[129], as well as a negative effect on normal sperm morphology, with an increase in the incidence of the stress-related phenomenon of elongated spermatozoa[112].

From the most recent literature, it is now clear that the main negative effect of leukocytospermia is the production of ROS, causing DNA fragmentation and damage of spermatozoa as detected with the TUNEL (terminal deoxynucleotide transferase-mediated dUTP nick-end labeling) and sperm chromatin structure assays[31,33,130,131]. Henkel et al. found that DNA fragmentation due to leukocytospermia did not correlate with in vitro fertilization rates, but found a significantly reduced pregnancy rate in IVF and ICSI patients inseminated with spermatozoa for semen samples containing high numbers of TUNEL-positive spermatozoa. This would imply that spermatozoa with damaged DNA are able to fertilize an oocyte, but at the time that the parental genome is switched on, further development of the embryo stops, leading to a lower pregnancy rate[31,33]. This is in agreement with earlier work published by Aitken *et al.* showing that the incidence of spontaneous pregnancies was negatively correlated with the generation of ROS in a prospective study performed in a group of oligozoospermic patients, where about half the population exhibited increased ROS activity[132], and is also confirmed by the work of Fedder[110]. Therefore, the main negative effect of the presence of leukocytospermia seems to be high ROS production, especially by the WBC but also by spermatozoa themselves, which then causes poor sperm functional ability either by ROS action on the sperm membrane where they interact with polyunsaturated fatty acids or by DNA damage or fragmentation.

Source of leukocytospermia. According to Barratt *et al.* leukocytospermia has a heterogeneous etiology, including infections, inflammations and autoimmunity, making the immediate cause for this condition quite complex and unclear[133]. In most cases, leukocytes present in semen are presumed to originate from some sort of infection in the male genital tract, but most men with leukocytospermia have negative cultures of samples obtained from the seminal tract[134,135]. Purvis and Christiansen found that, often, the source of white blood cells in semen is the testicle/epididymis, and that this may be of significance, since spermatozoa are exposed to the potentially damaging influence of leukocytes for much longer periods in the epididymis than in other parts of the tract, leaving more time for DNA damage to occur[136]. It is thought that in some males the origin of leukocytospermia may be sources outside the genital tract, and a wide range of these factors that may cause leukocytospermia have been reported[109,118,120,136–141].

Trum *et al.* reported that leukocytospermia was associated with a history of gonorrhea[120]. Close *et al.* found that current cigarette smokers, marijuana users and heavy alcohol users showed a statistically significant greater number of leukocytes in the seminal fluid than did non-users, in a group of 164 men investigated for infertility

problems[142]. The increase in round cells and leukocytes in semen samples from smokers was confirmed by a study of Trummer *et al.*[143]. It has also been reported that clomiphene citrate treatment of a group of males with low serum testosterone levels may have led to leukocytospermia[144]. Although it was not correlated with the presence of leukocytospermia, Bieniek and Riedel reported that the same bacteria could be found in the semen samples of men who were diagnosed with bacterial foci in their teeth, oral cavities and jaws, and that after 6 months, following dental treatment in about two-thirds of these men, their semen samples proved to be sterile and the semen parameters such as sperm concentration, motility and morphology had clearly improved, while the semen parameters of the control group remained poor[137].

Treatment of leukocytospermia. In many reports, antibiotics have routinely been used to treat leukocytospermia, but this is also a controversial matter as several studies have obtained differing results[118,134].

A meta-analysis of the effectiveness of treatment with broad-spectrum antibiotics of men suffering from leukocytospermia and/or bacteriospermia was performed by Skau and Folstad[139]. In total, 23 clinical studies were identified, but only 12 studies were included for analysis. Their results indicated that the most used antibiotics were doxycycline, erythromycin and trimethoprim in combination with sulfamethoxazole, and treatment resulted in significant improvements in semen quality. When improvements in the results for different semen parameters were expressed as weighted effect size, the smallest effect was found for sperm concentration, with a mean weighted effect size of 0.16, followed by semen volume and sperm motility, with a mean weighted effect of 0.20, followed by an improvement in normal sperm morphology, with a weighted effect size of 0.22, and the best response to antibiotic treatment was a significant reduction in the concentration of leukocytes in semen samples, with a mean weighted effect size of 0.23.

A literature survey with emphasis on antibiotic treatment for leukocytospermia only was performed, and 12 articles dealing with the topic were identified[110,118,119,145–153]. Ten of the articles reported a positive response, that is, a reduction in seminal leukocyte concentrations[110,118,145–147,149–153]. Some of the articles also reported an improvement in semen parameters, and four[110,118,145,153] reported the occurrence of pregnancies as a result of the antibiotic treatment. In a case study of a male with azoospermia, antibiotic treatment for leukocytospermia resulted not only in a decrease of the leukocyte concentration, but also in the appearance of spermatozoa; however, two ICSI treatment cycles were unsuccessful[150]. Interesting was the observation by Branigan and Muller that higher ejaculation frequencies enhanced the disappearance of leukocytes from semen samples[145], and this was confirmed by Yamamoto et al.[152]. Only two articles reported that significant reductions in the leukocyte concentrations were not obtained[119,148].

There may be several reasons for not obtaining a positive response with antibiotic treatment for leukocytospermia. One reason may be that different end-points are set for successful treatment results, as illustrated by the two cases found in the literature survey referred to above, reporting a negative result. Although there was a (significant) reduction in seminal leukocyte concentrations after antibiotic treatment, this did not meet the end-point of total eradication of leukocytospermia set by the authors[119,148].

Other reasons may be as postulated by Purvis and Christiansen, who proposed two reasons for difficulties in showing positive antibiotic treatment-effects in infertile males presenting with leukocytospermia[118]. The first is that the therapy may not have been appropriate for the organism(s) responsible for the infection, or that the dose or duration may have been inadequate. According to the authors, only certain antibiotics, the most important being ciprofloxacin, have the capacity to penetrate the accessory sex glands in high enough concentrations. The encouragement of frequent ejaculation during antibiotic treatment is important, as the higher turnover of secretions would be anticipated to encourage passage of the antibiotics into the glandular lumen of affected organs and thereby increase the efficiency of the treatment. The second is that pathological changes in the reproductive tract, due to the presence of infection and responsible for poor semen quality, may become permanent (e.g. epididymal stenosis causing a delay in transit time of spermatozoa or seminiferous tubule failure caused by orchitis). Antibiotic treatment can therefore be expected to have a positive effect on sperm quality only if the chronic infection is still active and the pathological organism is still present, and where the degree of damage is still limited.

Eggert-Kruse et al. are of the very forcible opinion that patients with symptoms of genital tract infections (leukocytospermia) should be treated as soon as possible, often as partner therapy, to avoid the severe sequelae of ascending infections[102]. However, they and others warn strongly that antibiotic treatment should be used with caution and used only when clearly indicated, especially in healthy individuals[102,154,155], the reasons being that the non-critical use of antibiotics may result in resistant strains of bacteria, and that certain antibiotics may also have a possible toxic effect on spermatogenesis.

The working mechanism of antibiotic treatment in the improvement of semen parameters is not yet quite clear. One mechanism suggested by Skau and Folstad is that antibiotic treatment may cause a reduction in the level of cytotoxic cells present in the testes, causing a reduction in immune activity in the testes, resulting in a higher number of morphologically normal spermatozoa, and less DNA damage[139]. The effect of treatment can also lead to pregnancies without clear alterations in semen quality but after the disappearance of leukocytes from the ejaculate, possibly because the source of ROS production and thus DNA damage has been eliminated.

Sperm vital staining test   Where previously it was normal procedure to perform a vital staining test on every semen sample with a sperm concentration of $> 1.0 \times 10^6$/ml, it is now mostly performed in cases with progressive sperm motility of $< 30\%$. The method as described by Eliasson[54], based on the method described by Blom[156], is generally used. A drop of semen is placed on a spot plate and mixed with one drop of 1% aqueous eosin Y solution. After 15 seconds two drops of 10% aqueous nigrosin solution are added and thoroughly mixed. A drop of this mixture is transferred to a clean glass slide and a thin smear made and air-dried. The smears are examined with a 100× oil magnification. Red cells or any sperm cells not totally white are regarded as dead, and the results are expressed as the percentage of live (white) sperm. It is important to note that, although the staining solutions are referred to as aqueous eosin Y and nigrosin solutions, this refers to the type of eosin Y and nigrosin. Both eosin Y and nigrosin should be dissolved in phosphate-buffered solutions to prevent hypo-osmotic swelling of the sperm tails and the induction of sperm death due to the hypo-osmotic stress caused when the solutions are prepared with water, which thus can give false-negative (low vitality) results[157].

The performance of a vital stain technique is an important tool to distinguish between live but motionless and dead spermatozoa. Motionless but still alive spermatozoa can be found, for example, in cases of Kartagener's syndrome, or may be caused by cold shock. In cases where all spermatozoa are found to be dead by vital staining, the condition is called necrozoospermia.

Additional procedures

Azoospermia

When examination of the wet preparation indicates that the semen sample contains no spermatozoa, i.e. azoospermia, the following steps are performed. The sample is centrifuged in a conical disposable plastic centrifuge tube for 10 minutes at $3000\,g$. The supernatant is carefully drawn off and discarded, and the pellet suspended in a small amount of medium and re-examined microscopically using phase-contrast optics. The results are interpreted as follows:

- No spermatozoa observed = azoospermia;

- Spermatozoa present = cryptozoospermia, or sometimes called severe oligozoospermia ($< 1 \times 10^6$ spermatozoa/ml)[39].

Moderate oligozoospermia

In cases where the spermatozoa concentration is $< 5.0 \times 10^6$/ml, the remaining semen after completion of all procedures can be centrifuged at $\pm 200\,g$ for 10 minutes. The pellet is suspended in a small volume of medium and a small drop used to prepare a standard smear. The smear is air-dried and stained for use in cases where there are too few spermatozoa present on the original morphology smear.

Semen biochemistry

Semen biochemistry is not usually performed as part of the standard basic semen analysis procedure. However, in cases of azoospermia, or in the presence of round cells in the wet preparation, certain tests can be performed to aid in the diagnosis of azoospermia, or identification of granular white blood cells when round cells are present. These biochemical tests are usually carried out on seminal plasma obtained by centrifugation of the semen sample in a conical disposable test-tube at $3000\,g$ for 30 minutes.

A test for α-glucosidase can be performed to identify a possible obstruction at the site of the epididymis, as this enzyme is produced exclusively by the epididymis[158]. When the α-glucosidase value is reduced, it can be interpreted that the azoospermia may be due to an obstruction at the level of the epididymis. In cases of azoospermia, the fructose content of the seminal plasma can also be determined, either biochemically or directly on the semen sample as a bench test (as discussed below). Fructose is *inter alia* an indicator of the secretory function of the seminal vesicles, and low fructose levels may indicate congenital dysgenesis (absence) of the seminal vesicles and vas deferens. A kit (Fructose Test; FertiPro) for the spectrophotometric determination of fructose in semen/seminal plasma is commercially available[22].

In cases where round cells are observed in the wet preparation, a PMN-elastase assay can be performed[159]. This enzyme is secreted by activated granulocytes, and can be measured in fresh or frozen seminal plasma. The method is objective and convenient, but costly and time-consuming, as 20 samples must be tested at the same time, but a strong correlation has been found between elastase levels and WBC numbers in semen. An increased value of > 290 ng/ml semen is a strong indication of the presence of leukocytes, or a silent inflammation of the genital tract[106,160].

Colorimetric bench method for fructose determination

A bench method for the quick determination of fructose has been described by Amelar, based on the Selivanoff method[161]. In this test, 5 mg of resorcinol is added to 33 ml of concentrated hydrochloric acid and diluted to 100 ml with distilled water. An aliquot of 0.5 ml semen is added to 5 ml of the reagent in a heat-resistant glass tube and heated to boiling point. In the presence of fructose, an orange-red coloring will appear within 60 seconds after boiling. Special care should be taken when performing this procedure by wearing protective clothing, especially glasses for protection of the eyes, due to the vicious boiling[161].

Semen cultures

In all cases where a semen analysis is done for the first time, swabs should be prepared for culturing of aerobic bacteria and for *Ureaplasma* and *Mycoplasma,* especially in cases for ART procedures. The patient should be instructed to pass urine and then to wash his hands with soap and water and the glans penis with water alone. The semen is produced into individually packed and sterilized containers. Unfortunately there is poor correlation between bacteriospermia and leukocytospermia, and the validity of culturing semen samples has been questioned[55]. It is also evident that it is difficult to culture semen samples, and some laboratories prescribe specialized procedures in order to obtain optimal results[22].

Computer-assisted semen analysis

The past decade has seen the development of many computer-based systems to analyze semen samples more accurately, objectively and efficiently. Although systems for the measurement of sperm concentration[22,39,162,163] and normal morphology[164] exist, the motility parameter has received the most attention[22,163]. These systems have primarily enabled the critical analysis of sperm head kinematics, while flagellar kinematics remains a future challenge. To date, numerous parameters of sperm head motion have been identified, of which 11 have been officially accepted and standardized. Computer-assisted semen analysis (CASA) has also been invaluable in the characterization of hyperactivated motility[22].

Three of the most generally used CASA parameters are: (1) curvilinear velocity (VCL), i.e. the measure of the rate of travel of the centroid of the sperm head over a given time period (this is calculated from the sum of the straight lines joining the sequential positions of the sperm head along the sperm's track); (2) straight-line velocity (VSL) (this represents the straight-line distance between the first and last centroid positions for a given time period); (3) linearity of forward progression (LIN) (this is reported as the ratio VSL/VCL expressed as a percentage, and represents the value of 100 cells swimming in a perfectly straight line)[22,39,163].

In an attempt to standardize CASA results stringent guidelines for the correct operational procedures for CASA systems have been proposed by the ESHRE Andrology Special Interest

Group[165,166]. The guidelines include several recommendations, namely, the need for internal and external quality control, adequate training, including that offered by the different manufacturers, and correct operational procedures. The group have advised that in any manuscript or report the technical operational procedures should be clearly spelled out. These should include the image acquisition rate, which is recommended as 50 Hz, tract sampling time, recommended to be a minimum of 0.5 seconds, indication of the type of smoothing algorithm employed, the number of cells sampled, recommended to be > 200 in at least six fields, the type of chamber used, recommended depth 10–20 μm, and also some data on the instrument used, such as the model and software version numbers and microscope optics and magnification[22,39,156,166].

Quality control in the andrology laboratory

In the modern andrology laboratory, the importance of a distinct quality assurance (QA) policy has become very evident in the past decade, and every laboratory should have such a program in place, including measures for quality control (QC). QA is the larger picture of QC and examines overall laboratory quality, including good laboratory administration of personnel and laboratory procedures, communications skills between all role players and introduction of remedial actions taken when indicated, and documentation of procedures and programs. Detailed descriptions of QA and QC programs and methods can be found in the WHO 1999 manual[22], the ESHRE manual[53] and various articles[165,166] and textbooks[39].

The 1999 WHO manual[22] and the ESHRE manual[53] also place great emphasis on especially QC, which must include an internal (IQC) and an external (EQC) leg. The IQC program should include aspects of control of equipment and replicate assessments of the main semen parameters between and within technologists. It can also include sampling of monthly averages and other more sophisticated actions such as assessing systematic differences between technicians.

There are several EQC programs in different countries and continents run by governments, for example UK NEQAS (UK National External Quality Assessment Service), or national and international society programs such as those of the European Academy of Andrology (EAA) and ESHRE. These programs are limited due to practical logistical difficulties in sending out large numbers of the same samples as well as cost factors.

A problem encountered with the different programs is that the standards between them differ, and also they do not all follow the same procedures with regard to standardization. It is known that some national programs use Diff-Quik™-stained smears and others Papanicolaou-stained smears, which may give different results. Other problems have been encountered with sperm morphology as demonstrated by Cooper et al.[167], indicating that users of the ESHRE EQC program are much more strict in their sperm morphology scoring compared with users of the EAA and UK NEQAS programs. Disagreements between motility grades a and b have also been found between the three schemes. Better standardization can be achieved by continued training of laboratory personnel, as done by the ESHRE Special Interest Group in Andrology with their basic semen analysis training program[168], but continued interaction between laboratories and the training facility is also important to assure continued standardization[169].

INTERPRETATION OF SEMEN ANALYSIS RESULTS

As mentioned previously, a semen analysis result cannot be interpreted correctly unless all factors that may have an influence on the results are known. It is also important when repeat semen analyses are performed and compared with previous results that there are a number of factors that may add to the normal biological variation of the results[170]. Some of them are discussed below.

Sources of variation affecting semen parameters

Many sources of variation are known, but only some of those that can cause large variations in semen parameters, such as sexual abstinence, seasonal influences or illness, are discussed briefly.

Today, it is an accepted fact that abstinence can have a pronounced but varied effect on the semen parameters. This can vary from a small influence on sperm morphology to a statistical significant effect on sperm motility, sperm concentration and semen volume. This is due to the fact that production of spermatozoa and the secretions of the accessory glands that form the seminal plasma are daily ongoing processes[37,40,41,45].

It is generally accepted that the human is not a seasonal breeder and that spermatogenesis is a continuous and active process throughout the year. However, a few studies have been reported in which a possible seasonal influence has been investigated[171–175]. From the literature, it appears that this influence is the result of increased summer temperatures and is mainly an influence on sperm concentration and/or sperm morphology. On the other hand, it has also been speculated that day length rather than temperature may be a reason for seasonal fluctuations[175]. Henkel *et al.* found significant seasonal changes in chromatin condensation and sperm count[175]. Best chromatin-intact values with a mean maximum value of 86.2% aniline blue-negative spermatozoa were found in January, and the highest mean sperm concentration of 68.75×10^6/ml semen was found in April in a group of patients investigated in Germany. For a control group of patients from the Southern hemisphere, a seasonal change shift by 4–5 months was observed for maximum chromatin condensation, but no trend for sperm concentration could be observed.

Mention is often made in articles or chapters on male infertility that a common cold, a bout of influenza or other febrile illnesses will have an adverse effect on spermatogenesis. Therefore, it is important that this is queried in the questionnaire to be completed with every semen analysis[1,37]. MacLeod published several articles demonstrating the effect of a viral infection with an increased body temperature as well as the effect of chickenpox on semen quality[176,177]. He found that sperm concentration, motility, forward progression and morphology were all impaired.

The same effect was observed by Menkveld and Kruger[40,41]. The effect can be quite drastic, and is an important factor when evaluating semen analysis results. Two cases presented by Menkveld and Kruger[40,41] illustrated that the motility, speed of forward progression and percentage of morphologically normal spermatozoa were the first parameters to show negative effects of the illness. The sperm concentration was not immediately negatively affected, probably due to storage of spermatozoa in the genital tract. This may suggest, therefore, that sperm morphology and movement can be altered while in the genital tract, especially the epididymis[65,178]. The negative effect of the illness is longest reflected in the sperm morphology, which may indicate that spermatogenesis and spermiogenesis are very sensitive as far as the whole process of morphogenesis is concerned.

The adverse environmental effects investigated above seem to have their most pronounced effects on sperm morphology[40,41,179]. Menkveld *et al.*[40,41,179], like MacLeod[14,176,177], came to the conclusion that sperm morphology is a very sensitive parameter that will reflect any adverse influence on the body/testes in a short time. Menkveld and Kruger speculated that any illness or infection might cause a temporary decrease in the percentage of morphologically normal forms, after which it will return to its original value[40,41]. However, if the testes are repeatedly attacked by adverse influences or conditions, this may start to cause histological changes in the lamina propria and basal membrane or Sertoli cell function, which will then adversely influence spermatogenesis. This negative effect will first be reflected in a gradual lowering of the percentage of morphologically normal spermatozoa[179,180], with an increase in the percentage of elongated sperm as well as an increase in the number of immature forms. This will then be followed by a decrease in the sperm concentration[40,41,180].

Number of semen analyses to be performed

Zaneveld and Polakoski[45] advocated that if a patient produces a normal sample with the first semen analysis, then there is no need to perform a further semen analysis. However, if the sample is a borderline case or classified as abnormal according to the specific laboratory's standards, it will be necessary to do more semen analyses before a final diagnosis can be made. In these cases they recommend that three semen analyses, with 3–5 weeks' intervals, should be carried out. Some authors feel that there will always be some variation from sample to sample, and that it is therefore necessary to perform at least two semen analyses before a diagnosis can be made[181–183]. Others have stated that several or 3–4 semen analyses over a period of 3 months, representing a complete cycle of spermatogenesis, are required to make an estimation of a patient's fertility potential[18,37,73].

An aspect that must now seriously be considered is the cost factor. Due to the increasing costs, the tendency is to keep the number of semen analyses per patient to a minimum. A good policy, therefore, in a case where the first semen sample is classified as normal according to the specific laboratory's standards, will be to suffice with one semen analysis and to repeat the semen analysis only if indicated due to a long time interval or due to a recent medical event. In a case where the semen analysis is abnormal, the analysis can be repeated two or three times within a period of 3 months so that a good semen profile of the patient can be obtained.

Interpretation of results

The evaluation of a semen specimen must be based on an overall picture that relates seminal volume, spermatozoa concentration, motility and sperm morphology and the results of additional tests such as the MAR test[23], leukocyte peroxidase test and biochemical results[24]. It must be kept in mind that even when results are far below the normal values of a laboratory, conceptions can still occur, although the time to reach this goal may be longer in such cases compared with cases where normal semen values are observed[39,184].

A distinction should also be made according to the reason the semen analysis was requested. Results of a semen analysis that may establish a poor prognosis for *in vivo* fertilization may still be adequate for *in vitro* fertilization. Calculating an index of the total concentration of morphologically normal motile spermatozoa may be of use for *in vitro* fertilization but is of little relevance for *in vivo* fertilization, as volume plays an important part in these calculations. It is known that oligozoospermia is frequently associated with a large semen volume, which must be regarded as an abnormal parameter, and this abnormal factor can therefore not be used to calculate such an index and compensate for the low sperm concentration. Large semen volumes are associated with semen loss from the vagina after intercourse, resulting in a large percentage of the available spermatozoa also being lost.

Much has been written about interrelationships between semen parameters and the compensating interaction of semen parameters[37,185]. Although there may be a general tendency[186] that high sperm concentrations are associated with higher percentages of motility and normal morphology, Menkveld *et al.*[41,75,180] have shown that there are exceptions, especially as far as sperm morphology is concerned. With regard to the compensating interaction of semen parameters, the above-mentioned argument also holds true. In cases where the volume is within the normal range, a certain degree of compensating interaction may occur, but this will be limited. It was observed[43,73] while calculating normal values and minimal values for conception, based on the occurrence of conceptions in an infertile population (which incidentally should be used and not so-called 'normal populations'), that a single and consistently very abnormal semen parameter could be associated with no, or only a sporadic, occurrence of conception in apparently normal women[43,187].

Standards for normal semen parameters and fertility

Normal standards of semen parameters for the basic semen features, i.e. volume, motility, sperm concentration and morphology, have from time to time been published[43] and also reviewed in the WHO manuals[19–22]. In the 1999 WHO manual[22], the term 'normal values' was changed to 'reference values'. The values published in the WHO manuals[19–22] were mostly obtained through studies done on so-called normal or fertile populations, and were not the lowest values necessary to achieve spontaneous pregnancies. This means that spontaneous pregnancies in normal relationships can also be obtained with lower semen parameter values than those indicated in the manuals. Many authors, especially those not working in the field of andrology, do not take this fact into consideration, and confuse normality with fertility. This results in a situation whereby if the semen parameters (variables) are not within the normal range, as given in the WHO manuals[19–22], males are regarded as infertile, i.e. not capable of conception. This can lead to social problems and stress among couples, for example in cases where spontaneous pregnancies actually occur after such a pronouncement has been made.

The differences between standards for normality and fertility have been demonstrated by Van Zyl[188], Van Zyl et al.[73,74] and Menkveld and Kruger[41,43]. Results of semen analyses of males who had recently impregnated their wives were classified according to the then internationally accepted normal standards[17] by Van Zyl et al.[73] and according to the 1987 WHO manual[20] normal values by Menkveld and Kruger[41,43], and compared with classifications based on the values used for fertility at Tygerberg Hospital[189]. Van Zyl et al.[73] found that only 18.8% of the men were classified as normal or fertile according to the then normal international criteria, as against 68.4% of men according to the Tygerberg values. Menkveld and Kruger[41,43] found corresponding values of 20.5% and 64.5%, respectively. The Tygerberg normal values were based on comparison of the values of each separate semen parameter with those in spontaneous pregnancies obtained in a group of apparently normal women attending the infertility clinic at Tygerberg Hospital[73,74,187]. The lowest value for each semen parameter, above which no significant increase in pregnancy rate per interval group occurred, was taken as the normal value for fertility for each semen parameter. It was found that, based on these semen parameter values, males could be divided into one of three groups, fertile or normal, subfertile and infertile. Fertile is regarded as an optimal chance for spontaneous conception *in vivo*, subfertile as a reduced chance and infertile as a small chance. These values were found to be also applicable to *in vitro* fertilization[189].

Recently, a number of studies have been published in which the semen parameter values of males from so-called fertile populations were compared with the semen parameter values of males from subfertile populations, in order to determine minimum cut-off values for the different semen parameters, to establish a male's fertility potential[190–194].

Guzick et al.[192], similar to Van Zyl et al.[73,74], Menkveld[41] and Menkveld and Kruger[189], found that men's fertility potential could be classified into one of three groups based on their semen parameters as possibly fertile or normal, subfertile and infertile. A summary of the proposed values for the different classes as found in the various

Table 9.1   Cut-off values of semen parameters for the classification of a male's possible fertility potential, as found in the recent literature, based on a comparison of fertile versus subfertile populations. The Tygerberg Hospital values are based on pregnancies observed

Author/semen parameters	Infertile	Subfertile	Fertile
Ombelet et al.[190]			
concentration (10^6/ml)			34.0
progressive motility (%)			45.0
morphology (% normal)			10.0 (SC)
Guzick et al.[192]			
concentration (10^6/ml)	< 13.5	13.5–48.0	> 48.0
motility (% motile)	< 32.0	32.0–63.0	> 63.0
morphology (% normal)	< 9.0	9.0–12.0	> 12.0 (SC)
Günalp et al.[193]			
concentration (10^6/ml)		9.0	
progressive motility (%)		14.0	42.0
morphology (% normal)		5.0	12.0 (SC)
Menkveld et al.[194]			
motility (% motile)		20.0	45.0
morphology (% normal)		21.0	31.0 (WHO)
morphology (% normal)		3.0	4.0 (SC)
AI (% normal)		3.0	3.0
TZI (0–4)		2.09	1.64
Tygerberg Hospital values*			
concentration (10^6/ml)	< 2.0	2.0–9.9	≥ 10.0
motility (% motile)	< 10.0	10.0–29.0	≥ 30.0
morphology (% normal)	< 5.0	5.0–14.0	≥ 15.0
volume (ml)		< 1.0 and > 6.0	1.0–6.0

*Based on publications of Van Zyl[69,188], Van Zyl et al.[73,74,187], Menkveld[41], Menkveld and Kruger[40,43,189] and Kruger et al.[76,77]; AI, acrosome index; TZI, teratozoospermia index; SC, strict Tygerberg Criteria[41,75]; WHO, 1992 World Health Organization criteria[21]

studies[190,192–194] is presented in Table 9.1. For the Tygerberg classification, the male is categorized based on his poorest semen parameter[189]. It is believed that in the subfertile group some compensating interaction between the different semen parameters may occur. However, if a specific semen parameter falls in the infertile category, the impairment is so severe that one or even more good semen parameters cannot compensate for the single poor parameter[189]; nevertheless, even in these cases, a spontaneous *in vivo* pregnancy is still possible.

REFERENCES

1. Schirren C. Practical Andrology. Berlin: Verlag Brüder Hartman, 1972: 10
2. Lode A. Untersuchungen über die Zahlen und Regene Rationsverhältnisse der Spermatozoiden bei Hund und Mensch. Arch Gesamte Physiol 1891; 50: 278
3. Hotchkiss RS. Factors in stability and variability of semen specimens – observations on 640 successive samples from 23 men. J Urol 1941; 45: 875
4. MacLeod J, Heim LM. Characteristics and variations in semen specimens of 100 normal young men. J Urol 1945; 54: 474

5. Belding DL. Fertility in the male: I. Technical problems in establishing standards of fertility. Am J Obstet Gynecol 1933; 26: 868

6. Williams WW, McGugan A, Carpenter HD. The staining and morphology of the human spermatozoon. J Urol 1934; 32: 201

7. Cary WH, Hotchkiss RS. Semen appraisal. A differential stain that advances the study of cell morphology. JAMA 1934; 102: 587

8. Pollak OJ, Joël CA. Sperm examination according to the present state of research. JAMA 1939; 113: 395

9. Davis CD, et al. Therapy of seminal inadequacy. I. Use of pituitary chorionic and equine gonadotropins. J Clin Endocrinol 1943; 3: 268

10. Harvey C, Jackson MH. Assessment of male fertility by semen analysis. An attempt to standardise methods. Lancet 1945; 2: 99,134

11. Hotchkiss RS. Fertility in Man. London: William Heineman Medical Books, 1945

12. Williams WW. Routine semen examinations and their interpretation. Trans Am Soc Stud Steril 1946; 139

13. Abarbanel AR, et al. Evaluation of the barren marriage. Minimal procedures. Fertil Steril 1951; 2: 1

14. MacLeod J, Gold RZ. The male factor in fertility and infertility. IV. Sperm morphology in fertile and infertile marriage. Fertil Steril 1952; 2: 394

15. Freund M. Standards for the rating of human sperm morphology. Int J Fertil 1966; 11: 97

16. Freund M. Semen analysis. In Behrman SJ, Kistner SW, eds., Progress in Infertility, 2nd edn. Boston: Little, Brown & Co, 1968: 593

17. Eliasson R. Standards for investigation of human semen. Andrologie 1971; 3: 49

18. Eliasson R. Analysis of semen. In Behrman SJ, Kistner SW, eds. Progress in Infertility, 2nd edn. Boston: Little, Brown & Co, 1968: 691

19. World Health Organization. WHO Laboratory Manual for the Examination of Human Semen and Sperm–Cervical Mucus Interaction, 1st edn. Singapore: Press Concern, 1980

20. World Health Organization. WHO Laboratory Manual for the Examination of Human Semen and Sperm–Cervical Mucus Interaction, 2nd edn. Cambridge: Cambridge University Press, 1987

21. World Health Organization. WHO Laboratory Manual for the Examination of Human Semen and Sperm–Cervical Mucus Interaction, 3rd edn. Cambridge: Cambridge University Press, 1992

22. World Health Organization. Laboratory Manual for the Examination of Human Semen and Sperm–Cervical Mucus Interaction. 4th edn. Cambridge: Cambridge University Press, 1999

23. Jager S, Kremer J, Van Slochteren-Draaisma T. A simple method of screening for antisperm antibodies in the human male – detection of spermatozoal surface IgG with the direct Mixed Antiglobulin Reaction carried out on untreated fresh human semen. Int J Fertil 1978; 23: 12

24. Nahoum CR, Cardozo D. Staining for volumetric count of leukocytes in semen and prostate-vesicular fluid. Fertil Steril 1980; 34: 68

25. Kremer J. A simple sperm penetration test. Int J Fertil 1965; 10: 209

26. Zavos PM, Cohen MR. Bovine mucus penetration test: an assay for fresh and cryopreserved human spermatozoa. Fertil Steril 1980; 34: 175

27. Mortimer D, et al. A simplified approach to sperm–cervical mucus interaction testing using a hyaluronate migration test. Hum Reprod 1990; 5: 835

28. Kremer J, Jager S. The sperm–cervical mucus contact test: a preliminary report. Fertil Steril 1976; 27: 335

29. Yanagimachi R, Yanagimachi H, Rogers BJ. The use of zona-free hamster ova as a test-system for the assessment of the fertilizing capacity of human spermatozoa. Biol Reprod 1976; 15: 471

30. Franken DR, et al. Hemizona assay and teratozoospermia: increasing sperm insemination concentrations to enhance zona pellucida binding. Fertil Steril 1990; 54: 497

31. Henkel R, et al. DNA fragmentation of spermatozoa and ART. Reprod Biomed Online 2003; 7: 477

32. Kruger TF, Menkveld R. Acrosome reaction, acrosin levels, and sperm morphology in assisted reproduction. Assist Reprod Rev 1996; 6: 27

33. Henkel R, et al. Effect of reactive oxygen species produced by spermatozoa and leukocytes on sperm functions in non-leukocytospermic patients. Fertil Steril 2005; 83: 635

34. Rhemrev JPT, et al. The acrosome index and the fast TRAP as protection of IVF outcome. Hum Reprod 2001; 16: 1885

35. McDonough P. Editorial comment: has traditional sperm analysis lost its clinical relevance? Fertil Steril 1997; 67: 585

36. Schrader SM. Safety guidelines for the andrology laboratory. Fertil Steril 1989: 51; 387

37. Mortimer D. The male factor in infertility. Part I: Semen analysis. Curr Probl Obstet Gynecol Fertil 1985; 8: 4

38. Alexander NJ. Male evaluation and semen analysis. Clin Obstet Gynecol 1982; 25: 463

39. Mortimer D. Practical Laboratory Andrology. Oxford: Oxford University Press 1994

40. Menkveld R, Kruger TF. Basic semen analysis. In Acosta AA, Kruger TF, eds. Human Spermatozoa in Assisted Reproduction, 2nd edn. Carnforth: Parthenon Publishing, 1996: 53

41. Menkveld R. An investigation of environmental influences on spermatogenesis and semen parameters. PhD dissertation (in Afrikaans), Faculty of Medicine, University of Stellenbosch, South Africa, 1987

42. Elzanaty S, Malm J, Giwercman A. Duration of sexual abstinence: epididymal and accessory sex gland secretions and their relationship to sperm motility. Hum Reprod 2005; 20: 221

43. Menkveld R, Kruger TF. Basic semen analysis. In Acosta AA, et al. eds. Human Spermatozoa in Assisted Reproduction. Baltimore: Williams and Wilkins, 1990: 68

44. Freund M. Performance and interpretation of the semen analysis. In Rolands M, ed. Management of the Infertile Couple. Springfield: Charles C Thomas, 1968: 48

45. Zaneveld LJD, Polakoski KL. Collection and the physical examination of the ejaculate. In Hafez ESE, ed. Techniques of Human Andrology. Amsterdam: Elsevier, North-Holland Biomedical Press, 1977: 147

46. Mandal A, Bhattacharyya AK. Studies on the coagulational characteristics of human ejaculates. Andrologia 1985; 17: 80–6

47. Amelar RD. Coagulation, liquefaction and viscosity of human semen. J Urol 1962; 87: 187

48. Mann T. Biochemical appraisal of human semen. In Joël CA, ed. Fertility Disturbances in Men and Women. Basel: Karger, 1971: 146

49. Portnoy L. The diagnosis and prognosis of male infertility: a study of 44 cases with special reference to sperm morphology. J Urol 1946; 48: 735

50. Vermeiden JPW, et al. Pregnancy rate is significantly higher in in vitro fertilization procedure with spermatozoa isolated from nonliquefying semen in which liquefaction is induced by α-amylase. Fertil Steril 1989; 51: 149

51. Tucker M, et al. Use of chymotrypsin for semen preparation in ART. Mol Androl 1990; 2: 179

52. Hancock P, McLaughlin E. British Andrology Society guidelines for the assessment of post vasectomy semen samples. J Clin Pathol 2002; 55: 812

53. Kvist U, Björndahl L. Manual on Basic Semen Analysis. ESHRE Monographs. Oxford: Oxford University Press, 2002

54. Eliasson R. Supravital staining of human spermatozoa. Fertil Steril 1977; 28: 1257

55. Menkveld R. Leukocytospermia. In Daya S, Harrison RF, Kempers RD, eds. Advances in Fertility and Reproductive Medicine. International Congress Series. Amsterdam: Elsevier, 2004; 1266: 218

56. Goldenberg RL, White R. The effect of vaginal lubricants on sperm motility in vitro. Fertil Steril 1975; 26: 872

57. Carruthers GB. Assessment of the semen. In Philipp EE, Carruthers, GB, eds. Infertility. London: William Heinemann Medical Books, 1981: 195

58. Appell RA, Evans PR. The effect of temperature on sperm motility and viability. Fertil Steril 1977; 28: 1329

59. Makler A. The thickness of microscopically examined seminal samples and its relationship to sperm motility estimation. Int J Androl 1978; 1: 213

60. Folgerí T, et al. Mitochondrial disease and reduced sperm motility. Hum Reprod 1993; 8: 1863

61. Barthelemy C, et al. Tail stump spermatozoa: morphogenesis of defect. An ultrastructural study of sperm and testicular biopsy. Andrologia 1989; 22: 417

62. Eliasson R, et al. The immotile-cilia syndrome. A congenital ciliary abnormality as an etiologic factor in chronic airway infection and male sterility. N Engl J Med 1977; 297: 1

63. Atherton RW. Evaluation of sperm motility. In Hafez ESE, ed. Techniques of Human Andrology. Amsterdam: Elsevier, North-Holland Biomedical Press, 1977: 173

64. MacLeod J, Pazianos A, Ray BS. Restoration of human spermatogenisis by menopausal gonadotrophins. Lancet 1964; 1: 196

65. Purvis K, Brekke I, Tollefsrud A. Epididymal secretory function in men with asthenoteratozoospermia. Hum Reprod 1991; 6: 850

66. Bar-Sagie D, Mayevsky A, Bartoov B. A fluorometric technique for simultaneous measurement of pH and motility in ram semen. Arch Androl 1981; 7: 27

67. Kesserü E, León F. Effect of different solid metals and metallic pairs on human sperm motility. Int J Fertil 1974; 19: 81

68. Macomber D, Sanders MB. The spermatozoa count. Its value in the diagnosis, prognosis and treatment of sterility. N Engl J Med 1929; 200: 981

69. Van Zyl JA. A review of the male factor in 231 infertile couples. S Afr J Obstet Gynecol 1972; 10: 17

70. Menkveld R, Van Zyl JA, Kotze TJvW. A statistical comparison of three methods for the counting of human spermatozoa. Andrologia 1984; 16: 554

71. Makler A. The improved ten-micrometer chamber for rapid sperm count and motility evaluation. Fertil Steril 1980; 33: 337

72. MacLeod J, Gold RZ. The male factor in fertility and infertility. II. Spermatozoa counts in 1000 men of known fertility and in 1000 cases of infertile marriage. J Urol 1951; 66: 436

73. Van Zyl JA, et al. The importance of spermiograms that meet the requirements of international standards and the most important factors that influence semen parameters. In Proceedings of the 17th Congress of the International Urological Society. Paris: Diffusion Dion Editeurs, 1976; 2: 263

74. Van Zyl JA, et al. Oligozoospermia: a seven-year survey of the incidence, chromosomal aberrations, treatment and pregnancy rate. Int J Fertil 1975; 20: 129

75. Menkveld R, et al. The evaluation of morphological characteristics of human spermatozoa according to stricter criteria. Hum Reprod 1990; 5: 586

76. Kruger TF, et al. Sperm morphologic features as a prognostic factor in in vitro fertilization. Fertil Steril 1986; 46: 1118

77. Kruger TF, et al. Predictive value of abnormal sperm morphology in in vitro fertilization. Fertil Steril 1988; 49: 112

78. Menkveld R, Kruger TF. Evaluation of sperm morphology by light microscopy. In Acosta AA, Kruger TF, eds. Human Spermatozoa in Assisted Reproduction, 2nd edn. Carnforth: Parthenon Publishing, 1996: 109

79. Mortimer D, Menkveld R. Sperm morphology assessment – historical perspectives and current opinions. J Androl 2001; 22: 192

80. Kruger TF, et al. A quick, reliable staining technique for human sperm morphology. Arch Androl 1987; 18: 275

81. Oettlé EE. Using a new acrosome stain to evaluate sperm morphology. Vet Med 1986; 81: 263

82. Menkveld R. Appendices. In Menkveld R, et al., eds. Atlas of Human Sperm Morphology. Baltimore: Williams & Wilkins, 1991: 115

83. Menkveld R, et al. Effect of different staining and washing procedures on the results of human sperm morphology evaluation by manual and computerised methods. Andrologia 1997; 29: 1

84. Menkveld R, et al. Basic principles and practical aspects. In Menkveld R, et al., eds. Atlas of Human Sperm Morphology. Baltimore: Williams & Wilkins, 1991: 6

85. Menkveld R, et al. Acrosomal morphology as a novel criterion for male fertility diagnosis: relation with acrosin activity, morphology (strict criteria) and fertilization in vitro. Fertil Steril 1996; 65: 637

86. Cooper TG, et al. Cytoplasmic droplets are normal structures of human sperm but are not well preserved by routine procedures for assessing sperm morphology. Hum Reprod 2004; 19: 2283

87. Cooper TG. New debate. Cytoplasmic droplets: the good, the bad or just confusing? Hum Reprod 2005; 20: 9

88. Menkveld R, Kruger TF. Sperm morphology and male urogenital infections. Andrologia 1998; 30 (Suppl 1): 49

89. Johanisson E, et al. Evaluation of 'round cells' in semen analysis: a comparative study. Hum Reprod Update 2000; 6: 404

90. Riedel H-H, Semm K. Leucospermia and male fertility. Arch Androl 1980; 5: 51

91. Riedel H-H. Techniques for the detection of leukocytospermia in human semen. Arch Androl 1980; 5: 287

92. Mahmoud A, Comhaire F. Debate continued. Antisperm antibodies. Use of the mixed agglutination reaction (MAR) test using latex beads. Hum Reprod 2000; 15: 231

93. Friberg J. A simple and sensitive micro-method for demonstration of sperm-agglutinating activity in serum from infertile men and women. Acta Obstet Gynecol Scand 1974; 36 (Suppl): 21

94. Isojima S, Shun T, Ashitaka Y. Immunologic analysis of sperm-immobilizing factor found in sera of women with unexplained sterility. Am J Obstet Gynecol 1968; 101: 677

95. Menkveld R, et al. Detection of sperm antibodies on unwashed spermatozoa with the immunobead test: a comparison of results with the routine method and seminal plasma TAT and SCMC test. Am J Reprod Immunol 1991; 25: 88

96. Ariagno J, et al. Shedding of immature germ cells. Arch Androl 2002; 48: 127

97. Endtz AW. A rapid staining method for differentiating granulocytes from 'germinal cells' in Papanicolaou-stained semen. Acta Cytol 1974; 18: 2

98. Comhaire F, Verschraegen G, Vermeulen L. Diagnosis of accessory gland infection and its possible role in male infertility. Int J Androl 1980; 3: 32

99. Wolff H. Methods for the detection of male genital tract inflammation. Andrologia 1998; 30 (Suppl 1): 35

100. Shekarriz M. Positive myeloperoxidase staining (Endtz test) as an indicator of excessive reactive oxygen species formation in semen. J Assist Reprod Genet 1995; 12: 70

101. Wolff H, Anderson DJ. Immunohistologic characterization and quantitation of leukocyte subpopulations in human semen. Fertil Steril 1988; 49: 497

102. Eggert-Kruse W, et al. Differentiation of round cells by means of monoclonal antibodies and relationship with male fertility. Fertil Steril 1992; 58: 1046

103. Tomlinson MJ, et al. The removal of morphologically abnormal sperm forms by phagocytes: a positive role for seminal leukocytes? Hum Reprod 1992; 10: 517

104. Tomlinson MJ, et al. Round cells and sperm fertilizing capacity: the presence of immature germ cells but not seminal leukocytes are associated with reduced success of in vitro fertilization. Fertil Steril 1992; 58: 1257

105. Ricci G, et al. Leukocyte detection in human semen using flow cytometry. Hum Reprod 2000; 15: 1329

106. Ludwig M, et al. Evaluation of seminal plasma parameters in patients with chronic prostatitis or leukocytospermia. Andrologia 1998; 30 (Suppl 1): 41

107. Esfandiari N, et al. Utility of nitroblue tetrazolium test for assessment of reactive oxygen species production by seminal leukocytes and spermatozoa. J Androl 2003; 24: 862

108. Punab M, et al. The limit of leukocytospermia from the microbiological viewpoint. Andrologia 2003; 35: 271

109. Wolff H. The biological significance of white blood cells in semen. Fertil Steril 1995; 63: 1143

110. Fedder J. Nonsperm cells in human semen: with special reference to seminal leukocytes and their possible influence on fertility. Arch Androl 1996; 36: 41

111. Leib Z, et al. Reduced semen quality caused by chronic abacterial prostatitis: an enigma or reality? Fertil Steril 1994; 61: 1109

112. Menkveld R, et al. Morphological sperm alternations in different types of prostatitis. Andrologia 2003; 35: 288

113. Politch JA, et al. Comparison of methods to enumerate white blood cells in semen. Fertil Steril 1993; 60: 372

114. Berger RE, et al. The relationship of pyospermia and seminal fluid bacteriology to sperm function as reflected in the sperm penetration assay. Fertil Steril 1982; 37: 557

115. Wolff H, et al. Leukocytospermia is associated with poor semen quality. Fertil Steril 1990; 53: 528

116. Tomlinson MJ, Barratt CLR, Cooke ID. Prospective study of leukocytes and leukocytes subpopulations in semen suggest they are not a cause of male infertility. Fertil Steril 1993; 60: 1069

117. Aitken RJ, Baker HWG. Seminal leukocytes: passengers, terrorists or good Samaritans? Hum Reprod 1995; 10: 1736

118. Purvis K, Christiansen E. Infection in the male reproductive tract. Impact, diagnosis and treatment in relation to male fertility. Int J Androl 1993; 16: 1

119. Yanushpolsky EH, et al. Antibiotic therapy and leukocytospermia: a prospective, randomised, controlled study. Fertil Steril 1995; 63: 142

120. Trum JW, et al. Value of detecting leukocytospermia in the diagnosis of genital tract infection in subfertile men. Fertil Steril 1998; 70: 315

121. Rodin DM, Larone D, Goldstein M. Relationship between semen cultures, leukospermia, and semen analysis in men undergoing fertility evaluation. Fertil Steril 2003; 79 (Suppl 3): 1555

122. Eggert-Kruse W, et al. Induction of immunoresponse by subclinical male genital tract infection? Fertil Steril 1996; 65: 1202

123. Cottell E, et al. Are seminal fluid microorganisms of significance or merely contaminants? Fertil Steril 2000; 74: 465

124. Willén M, et al. The bacterial flora of the genitourinary tract in healthy fertile men. Scand J Urol Nephrol 1996; 30: 387

125. Omu AE, et al. Seminal immune response in infertile men with leukocytospermia: effect on antioxidant activity. Eur J Obstet Gynecol Reprod Biol 2000; 86: 195

126. Kaleli S, et al. Does leukocytospermia associate with poor semen parameters and sperm function in male fertility? The role of different seminal leukocytes concentrations. Eur J Obstet Gynecol Reprod Biol 2000; 89: 185

127. Kiessling AA, et al. Seminal leukocytes: friends or foes? Fertil Steril 1995; 64: 196

128. Chan PJ, et al. White blood cells in semen affect hyperactivation but not sperm membrane integrity

in the head and tail regions. Fertil Steril 1994; 61: 986

129. Arata de Bellabarba G, et al. Nonsperm cells in human semen and their relationship with semen parameters. Arch Androl 2000; 45: 131

130. Aitken RJ, et al. Differential contribution of leukocytes and spermatozoa to generation of oxygen species in the ejaculates of oligozoospermic patients and fertile donors. J Reprod Fertil 1992; 94: 451

131. Alvarez JG, et al. Increased DNA damage in sperm from leukocytospermic semen samples as determined by the sperm chromatin structure assay. Fertil Steril 2002; 78: 319

132. Aitken RJ, Irvine DS, Wu FC. Prospective analysis of sperm oocyte fusion and reactive oxygen species generation as criteria for the diagnosis of infertility. Am J Obstet Gynecol 1991; 164: 542

133. Barratt CLR, Bolton AE, Cooke ID. Functional significance of white blood cells in the male and female reproductive tract. Hum Reprod 1990; 5: 639

134. Anderson DJ. Should male infertility patients be tested for leukocytospermia? Fertil Steril 1995; 63: 246

135. Hillier SL, et al. Relationship of bacteriologic characteristics to semen indices in men attending an infertility clinic. Obstet Gynecol 1990; 75: 800

136. Purvis K, Christiansen E. The impact of infection on sperm quality. J Br Fertil Soc 1995; 1: 31

137. Bieniek KW, Riedel H-H. Bacterial foci in teeth, oral cavity, and jaw – secondary effects (remote action) of bacterial colonies with respect to bacteriospermia and subfertility in males. Andrologia 1993; 25: 159

138. Busolo F, Zanchetta R, Cusinato R. Microbial flora in semen of asymptomatic infertile men. Andrologia 1984; 16: 269

139. Skau PA, Folstad I. Do bacterial infections cause reduced ejaculate quality? A meta-analysis of antibiotic treatment of male infertility. Behavioral Ecol 2003; 14: 40

140. Eggert-Kruse W, et al. Antisperm antibodies and microorganisms in genital secretions – a clinical significant relationship? Andrologia 1998; 30 (Suppl 1): 61

141. Mićić S, Petrovic S, Dotlić R. Seminal antisperm antibodies and genitourinary infections. Urology 1990; 35: 54

142. Close CE, Roberts PA, Berger RE. Cigarettes, alcohol and marijuana are related to pyospermia in infertile men. J Urol 1990; 144: 900

143. Trummer H, et al. The impact of cigarette smoking on human semen parameters and hormones. Hum Reprod 2002; 17: 1554

144. Matthews GJ, Goldstein M, Schlegel HJM. Nonbacterial pyospermia: a consequence of clomiphene citrate therapy. Int J Fertil Menopaus Stud 1995; 40: 187

145. Branigan EF, Muller CH. Efficacy of treatment and recurrence rate of leukocytospermia in infertile men with prostatitis. Fertil Steril 1994; 62: 580

146. Branigan EF, Spadoni LR, Muller CH. Identification and treatment of leukocytospermia in couples with unexplained infertility. J Reprod Med 1995; 40: 625

147. Erel TE, et al. Antibiotic therapy in men with leukocytospermia. Int J Fertil 1997; 42: 206

148. Krisp A, et al. Treatment with levofloxacin does not resolve asymptomatic leukocytospermia – a randomised controlled study. Andrologia 2003; 35: 244

149. Maruyama DK, et al. Effects of white blood cells on the in vitro penetration of zona-free hamster eggs by human spermatozoa. J Androl 1985; 6: 127

150. Montag M, Van der Ven H, Haidl G. Recovery of ejaculated spermatozoa for intracytoplasmic sperm injection after anti-inflammatory treatment of an azoospermic patient with genital tract infection: a case report. Andrologia 1999; 31: 179

151. Malallah YA, Zissis NP. Effect of minocycline on the sperm count and activity in infertile men with high pus cell counts in their seminal fluid. J Chemother 1992; 4: 286

152. Yamamoto M, et al. Antibiotic and ejaculation treatments improve resolution rate of leukocytospermia in infertile men with prostatitis. Nagoya J Med Sci 1995; 58: 41

153. Ekwere PD, Etuk EH. Semen quality among subfertile males following treatment with ofloxacin. Curr Ther Res 1991; 50: 425

154. Bar-Chama N, Goluboff E, Fisch H. Infection and pyospermia in male infertility. Is it really a problem? Urol Clin North Am 1994; 21: 469

155. Schlegel PN, Chang TSK, Marshall FF. Antibiotics: potential hazard to male fertility. Fertil Steril 1991; 55: 235

156. Blom E. A one-minute live–dead sperm stain by means of eosin–nigrosin. Fertil Steril 1950; 1: 176

157. Björndahl L, et al. Andrology Lab Corner. Why the WHO recommendations for eosin–nigrosin staining techniques for human sperm vitality assessment must change. J Androl 2004; 25: 671

158. Comhaire F, et al. Why do we continue to determine α-glucosidase in human semen? Andrologia 2002; 34: 8

159. Maegawa M, et al. Concentration of granulocyte elastase in seminal plasma is not associated with sperm motility. Arch Androl 2001; 47: 31

160. Blenk H, Hofstetter A. Complement C3, coeruloplasmin and PMN-elastase in the ejaculate in chronic prostato-adnexitis and their diagnostic value. Infections 1991; 19 (Suppl 3): 138

161. Amelar RD. Infertility in Men. Philadelphia: FA Davies, 1966: 13

162. Knuth UA, Yeung C-H, Nieschlag E. Computerized semen analysis: objective measurement of semen characteristics is biased by subjective parameter setting. Fertil Steril 1987; 48: 118

163. Mortimer D, Goel N, Shu MA. Evaluation of the CellSoft automated semen analysis system in a routine laboratory setting. Fertil Steril 1988; 50: 960

164. Kruger TF, et al. A new computerized method of reading sperm morphology (strict criteria) is as efficient as technician reading. Fertil Steril 1993; 59: 202

165. ESHRE Andrology Special Interest Group. Guidelines on the application of CASA technology in the analysis of spermatozoa. Hum Reprod 1998; 13: 142

166. ESHRE Andrology Special Interest Group. Consensus workshop on advanced diagnostic andrology techniques. Hum Reprod 1996; 11: 1463

167. Cooper TG, et al. Semen analysis and external quality control schemes for semen analysis need global standardization. Int J Androl 2002; 25: 306

168. Björndahl L, et al. ESHRE basic semen analysis courses 1995–1999: immediate beneficial effects of standardized training. Hum Reprod 2002; 17: 1299

169. Franken DR, et al. Monitoring technologist reading skills in a sperm morphology quality control program. Fertil Steril 2003; 79 (Suppl 3): 1637

170. Álvarez C, et al. Biological variation of seminal parameters in health subjects. Hum Reprod 2003; 18: 2082

171. Mortimer D, et al. Annual patterns of human sperm production and semen quality. Arch Androl 1983; 10: 1

172. Tjoa WS, et al. Circannual rhythm in human sperm count revealed by serially independent sampling. Fertil Steril 1982; 38: 454

173. Saint Pol P, et al. Circannual rhythms of sperm parameters of fertile men. Fertil Steril 1989; 51: 1030

174. Rojansky N, Brzezinski A, Schenker JG. Seasonality in human reproduction: an update. Hum Reprod 1992; 7: 735

175. Henkel R, et al. Seasonal changes in human sperm chromatin condensation. J Assist Reprod Genet 2001; 18: 371

176. MacLeod J. The clinical implications of deviations in human spermatogenesis as evidenced in seminal cytology and experimental production of these deviations. In Proceedings of the Fifth Congress on Fertility and Sterility, Stockholm, June 16–22. Excerpta Medica International Congress Series. 1966; 133: 563

177. MacLeod J. Effect of chickenpox and of pneumonia on semen quality. Fertil Steril 1951; 2: 523

178. Fredricsson B. On the development of different morphologic abnormalities of human spermatozoa. Andrologia 1978; 10: 43

179. Menkveld R, et al. Possible changes in male fertility over a 15-year period. Arch Androl 1986. 17: 143

180. Menkveld R, Kotze TJvW, Kruger TF. Relationship of human sperm morphology with other semen parameters as seen in different reference populations. Hum Reprod 1992; 6 (Suppl 1): 96

181. Mehan DJ, Chehval MJ. A clinical evaluation of a new silastic seminal fluid collection device. Fertil Steril 1977; 28: 689

182. Amelar RD, Dubin L, Schoenfeld C. Semen analysis: an office technique. Urology 1973; 2: 605

183. Taylor PJ, Martin RH. Semen analysis in the investigation of infertility. Can Fam Phys 1981; 27: 113

184. Jouannet P, et al. Male factors and the likelihood of pregnancy in infertile couples. 1. Study of sperm characteristics. Int J Androl 1988; 11: 379

185. MacLeod J, Gold RZ. The male factor in fertility and infertility. VIII. A study of variation in semen quality. Fertil Steril 1952; 7: 387

186. MacLeod J. A possible factor in etiology of human male infertility. Fertil Steril 1962; 13: 29

187. Van Zyl JA, Kotze TJvW, Menkveld R. Predictive value of spermatozoa morphology in natural fertilization. In Acosta AA, et al., eds. Human Spermatozoa in Assisted Reproduction. Baltimore: Williams & Wilkins, 1990: 319

188. Van Zyl JA. The infertile couple. Part II. Examination and evaluation of semen. S Afr Med J 1980; 57: 485

189. Menkveld R, Kruger TF. Basic semen analysis: the Tygerberg experience. In Acosta AA, et al., eds. Human Spermatozoa in Assisted Reproduction. Baltimore: Williams & Wilkins, 1990: 164

190. Ombelet W, et al. Semen parameters in a fertile versus infertile population: a need for change in the interpretation of semen testing. Hum Reprod 1997; 12: 987

191. Zinaman MJ, et al. Semen quality and human fertility: a prospective study with healthy couples. J Androl 2000; 21: 145

192. Guzick DS, et al. Sperm morphology, motility and concentration in fertile and infertile men. N Engl J Med 2001; 345: 1388

193. Günalp S, et al. A study of semen parameters with emphasis on sperm morphology in a fertile population: an attempt to develop clinical thresholds. Hum Reprod 2001; 16: 110

194. Menkveld R, et al. Semen parameters including WHO and strict criteria morphology, in a fertile and subfertile population: an effort towards standardisation of in vivo thresholds. Hum Reprod 2001; 16: 1165

10

Advances in automated sperm morphology evaluation

Kevin Coetzee, Thinus F Kruger

INTRODUCTION

Normal sperm morphology has been shown to be predictive of male fertility, independent of other semen parameters. Two literature surveys were conducted to assess this value, both confirming the superior value of percentage normal sperm morphology, as compared with any other manually evaluated semen parameter[1,2], when evaluated using standardized methodology under controlled conditions.

In humans, normal fertile ejaculates contain spermatozoa exhibiting considerable morphological variations not only in the size and shape of the head and the acrosome, but also in the degree of nuclear vacuolation, size of persisting cytoplasmic droplets, midpiece disturbances and tail abnormalities[1]. Since 1950 many investigators have tried to create a standardized set of criteria for the assessment of human sperm morphology[3–9]. The major shortcoming underlying the universal acceptance of any of these criteria and/or guidelines has been the large interobserver, intraobserver and interlaboratory coefficients of variation observed. The value of manually evaluated sperm morphology outcomes has been questioned by many, owing to the lack of precision and reliability observed. Most of the variation inherent to manual evaluations can be attributed to the subjective nature of evaluation and methodological inconsistencies. Despite the lack of confidence in the manually evaluated sperm morphology outcomes, the majority of clinics persist in the use of the standard, manually evaluated semen analysis[1,10].

Automated systems have the power to increase the objectivity, precision and reproducibility of sperm morphology evaluations, and add further value by providing accurate sperm kinematics measures. As attractive as this option may seem, not many automated systems have been introduced into routine andrology laboratories. The majority of systems currently in operation are used in more experimental situations, because of the objective biological resolution of the systems. The probable reasons for the resistance to routine application of the systems are: (1) the cost of the systems, (2) technical limitations of some of the systems (software and hardware) and (3) the limited number of technical and clinical studies published per system to prove their value[11]. Only through continued demonstration of the value of objective automated semen analysis outcomes in relation to fertility in large prospective randomized studies will the incentive increase to introduce automated systems into routine andrology laboratories[12].

AUTOMATED SYSTEMS

Although this chapter's focus is on automated systems, manual techniques and semiautomatic systems have been developed that can also be classified as objective systems. These techniques and systems are important in that they are often simple and economical to set up and use. Calamera *et al.*[13] modified and described a manual method using only a video camera, monitor and microscope. An acetate overlay mask of normal sperm morphology was created by three independent observers using World Health Organization (WHO) 1992[14] guidelines and strict criteria. Similarly, Goulart *et al.*[15] in a comparative study (manual vs. semiautomatic vs. automatic) developed a manual system in which the operator controlled all the settings (strict criteria) and the evaluation procedure, using a computer mouse. Semiautomatic methods for classifying human sperm based on objective measurements of head shapes and sizes have also been developed[15,16], in which the operator can interactively control the evaluation procedure. In the study by Goulart *et al.*[15], the semiautomatic system was found to be the most reliable and secure method for performing sperm analysis, as such a system allowed the operator to confirm or correct possible computer misidentification. Although these systems have demonstrated a certain degree of accuracy and reliability in the evaluation of sperm morphology, the limitation is the time required per evaluation.

True automated systems consist of a microscope, a video camera, a computer, a frame grabber and morphology software. The systems work as follows. The video camera delivers the image (digitization) to the frame grabber, which stores it for analysis, and the image is evaluated by the morphology software and included for statistical analysis. Recognition of spermatozoa and exclusion of other cells depend on the software specifications (gates) for sperm shape, size and color (stain) intensity. Once spermatozoa are recognized

and separated from debris and other cells, metric measurements are performed on the sperm head, midpiece, acrosome and other cytological features. The software is normally programmed to recognize spermatozoa according to dimensions and criteria required by the authors[17]. These may depend on the staining procedure used (e.g. Papanicolaou vs. Diff-Quik®) and the range of values of the classification systems used (e.g. strict criteria, WHO guidelines, biological selection criteria, etc.).

Many variations (hardware and/or software) of the above configuration can be developed to eliminate a weakness and/or exploit a strong point (Table 10.1). Sofitikis *et al.*[18] used a confocal laser scanning microscope instead of a normal light microscope to evaluate sperm morphology quantitatively. They were therefore able to use unstained semen samples to define the normal ranges of sperm morphometric parameters, to exclude the effect of the staining procedure.

The initial systems relied only on morphometric measurements to classify spermatozoa into groups. Evaluation precision was improved by the Hamilton Thorne Research integrated visual optical system (IVOS), which introduced the signature method of including evaluation of the sperm head shape, shown to be of most clinical significance[19,32]. The ability of the systems to evaluate shape is important, because the correct cell head aspect ratio does not always guarantee normality. Other systems have also incorporated shape analysis methods in their evaluation procedure, for example the Hobson Sperm Tracker[20].

The sperm head automated morphometric analysis system (SHAMAS) used by Garrett *et al.*[33] included another classification parameter, %Z: the percentage of sperm with characteristics which conform to those of sperm that bind to the zona pellucida of the human oocyte. These 'zona pellucida preferred' values indicate axial symmetry, narrow neck and large acrosomal area as important for sperm–zona binding, and therefore normal fertilizing potential.

Table 10.1 Automated sperm morphology analyzers. Modified from reference 31

Software	Authors	Company	Instrument	Criteria and measurements
FERTECH SMA	Coetzee et al.[17] Kruger et al.[19,21,22] Laquet et al.[23] Menkveld et al.[24]	FERTECH, Norfolk, VA	IVOS, Hamilton Thorne Research, Beverly, MA	Strict criteria: head size and shape (signature method) and acrosome size
CellForm-Human	Davis et al.[12], Davis and Gravance[25]	Microsoft Corp., Bellview, WA	Combination system	WHO 1987: length, width, area, perimeter and width/length ratio
HDATA	MacLeod and Irvine[26]	Pyramid Technical Consultants, Waltham, MA	HTM-S 2030, Hamilton Thorne Research, Beverly, MA	WHO 1987: length, width and area
Morphologizer II	Wang et al.[27,28]	Cryo Resources Ltd	Combination system	WHO 1987: area, perimeter, length/width ratio, roundness, length and width
MOP-Videoplan	Mundy et al.[29]	Kontron	Combination system (SEM)	NG: area, perimeter, head maximum diameter, head width, midpiece width, midpiece length and tail length
Microsoft Professional Basic 7.0	Garret and Baker[30]	Microsoft Corp., Redmond, WA	Combination system	WHO 1992: set of 32 morphometric parameters (size, shape and staining heterogeneity)
NG	Sofikitis et al.[18]	NG	Confocal scanning laser microscope, Lasertec, Yokohama, Japan	±2SD of fertile men: length, width, length of midpiece, length of principle piece of sperm tail
Hobson Sperm Tracker	El-Ghobashy and West[20]	Hobson Tracker United, Sheffield, UK	Combination system	WHO 1999: head length 4–5 μm, width 2.5–3.5 μm, length/width ratio 1.5–1.75 and acrosome size 40–70% of total, including tail and acrosomal vacuoles
Zeiss image-processing system KS400 (Zeiss-Vision)	Goulart et al.[15]	Zeiss, Germany	Combination system	Strict criteria, head size and shape

NG, not given; SEM, scanning electron microscope; WHO, World Health Organization

SLIDE PREPARATION AND STAINING

In a world-wide survey conducted by Ombelet *et al.*[34], it was confirmed that a wide variety of different methodologies were being followed for the evaluation of sperm morphology. The adopted and adapted methods included procedures for the preparation of semen samples and staining of sperm cells, as well as classification systems used to identify normal and abnormal cells. Ombelet *et al.*[34] concluded that an urgent need to standardize sperm morphology evaluation methodology existed. Just as in the case of the visual evaluation of sperm morphology, users of computer-assisted sperm morphology analyzers must recognize that the principles of standardization and quality control are paramount to accurate evaluations[35].

Sample preparation and staining may significantly influence the precision and reliability of sperm morphology evaluations. The variation that may result from these procedures can to a large extent be overcome by an experienced technician using visual evaluation, but this may not be possible when an automated system is used[24]. By the very nature of the evaluation process in automated systems, there is no means of compensating for preparation defects and artifacts. For example, small differences in background shading relative to cell staining intensity can result in digitization errors, leading to incorrect classification or the inability to identify the cell as a sperm.

Davis and Gravance[25] found that the percentage of normal sperm detected by the CellForm-Human method was not different for washed specimens compared with unwashed controls. The technical variability arising from semen preparation and slide staining methods could, however, be reduced when specimens were washed and resuspended to a standard concentration ($150–200 \times 10^6$) before smearing. Lacquet *et al.*[23] also preferred using washed semen samples resuspended at a concentration of 100×10^6 cells/ml. Thin, evenly spread smears were made from this solution to ensure that approximately five cells were available per screen for analysis. It is now preferred practice to prewash the semen sample and to adjust the concentration of the resultant sperm sample. A single- or double-wash procedure can be followed. If a single wash is performed the sample must be adequately diluted ($\geq 1:5$, semen/medium) prior to centrifugation. Washing the semen sample may be essential for two reasons: (1) to remove as much of the acellular constituents (plasma) of the semen as possible and (2) to concentrate the sperm sample[11]. The presence of a high concentration of seminal plasma results in intense background staining and flaking during the staining procedure. A droplet, its size depending on the concentration of the resultant sperm sample, must be thinly smeared across a clean slide and allowed to air-dry (room temperature). This capability of being able to adjust the concentration of sample is especially important for oligozoospermic samples. The sample processing procedure must result in between 10 and 20 sperm per high-field magnification (5–10 sperm per computer screen) to optimize the reading time. The density of sperm required for automatic evaluations is therefore double that required for manual evaluations.

The most commonly used stains or staining methods used for the evaluation of sperm morphology are hematoxylin stain, the Papanicolaou method, the Shorr method, the Spermac method or the Diff-Quik method. Morphometric measurements were found to be more accurate and precise when sperm were stained with GZIN than when stained with Papanicolaou or hematoxylin[25]. Lacquet *et al.*[23] found no statistical difference in outcome between five different Diff-Quik (Hemacolor Kit, Merck) staining procedures. Menkveld *et al.*[24], in a study comparing the effect of washing and staining methods (Papanicolaou, Shorr, Diff-Quik and Spermac) on automated evaluation, obtained results comparable to manual evaluation by washing the semen samples once and staining with Diff-Quik stain. Wang *et al.*[27], using a simplified Shorr staining procedure, found that less shrinkage of the spermatozoa occurred compared with the Papanicolaou staining procedure, resulting in higher length, width and length/width ratio means. Different staining procedures therefore result in different chromatic and physical appearances of sperm cells. This is certainly true for the Papanicolaou and Diff-Quik staining methods[36].

Dimension-specific software (Papanicolaou and Diff-Quik) has therefore been loaded into the Hamilton Thorne Research (IVOS) system. A study was hence conducted to determine the agreement between computer-analyzed normal sperm morphology values (n = 97) stained according to the Papanicolaou and Diff-Quik methods[17]. A significant bias of 1.6% was obtained in favor of higher normal sperm morphology percentages when the Diff-Quik method was used. One of these two methods had to be selected to standardize methodology for future automated evaluation studies. The Diff-Quik staining procedure was selected as the preferred staining method, because of its simplicity, short staining time and good contrast. This difference seen when using different stains also illustrates the importance of ensuring that the software program is developed according to the method of cell staining used.

These results illustrate the importance of the standardization of procedures, and of selecting procedures that will result in optimal cell recognition and evaluation. The requirements are: thin, evenly spread smears (five sperm cells per screen) to ensure that all sperm are on the same focus plane, and a staining procedure that ensures minimal background staining, good contrast and good color differentiation. The reproducible production of high-quality slides will ensure that the time required to carry out normal sperm morphology evaluations is kept to the minimum.

EVALUATION PRECISION

The manual evaluation of sperm morphology still continues, resulting in inaccurate and valueless measures, even though a better alternative exists. The coefficients of variation for repeat estimates by manual evaluation of normal sperm have been observed to be as high as 100% within and between laboratories. The average coefficients of variation for most laboratories are probably in the range 30–60%[37]. This high possible level of variation may no longer be acceptable, with increasing pressure for laboratories to implement strict quality control programs and be accredited according to the guidelines and conditions of accreditation bodies. If automated systems represent the only alternative, the question would have to be whether the available versions have reached the level of precision acceptable for routine implementation.

Although inaccurate and imprecise, the visual evaluation of sperm morphology provides the only practical standard with which to compare the outcomes of automated evaluations of normal sperm morphology. For these systems to be accepted they must first demonstrate coefficients of variation smaller in magnitude than those obtained for visual evaluations. The strict criteria are unique in that the underlying philosophy of the classification system limits variation in the evaluation of sperm morphology. This is clearly illustrated by the study performed by Menkveld et al.[32], in which relatively low coefficients of variation were obtained for repeat manual evaluations by experienced technicians, ranging between 5.21 and 27.76%. The goal should therefore be to develop systems that will produce coefficients of variation of < 10%.

Davis et al.[12], measuring the same sperm repeatedly by computer, obtained a < 1% overall coefficient of variation for repeated measures. In their study, Kruger et al.[19] analyzed 255 cells three times in succession and obtained pairwise agreements of 0.85, 0.80 and 0.85 (K statistic > 0.75, i.e. excellent agreement). Davis et al.[12] also partitioned the variance among other factors and obtained the following coefficients of variation: between men 1.84–4.17%, between slides 0.6–1.38%, between repetitions 0.16–1.10% and between sperm 6.59–11.39%. Sperm morphology outcomes, as determined by an automated system using stained smears from washed samples, was shown in a study by Garrett and Baker[30] to have a coefficient of variation equaling < 4% for the same semen sample and < 7% with different batches of stain. The authors concluded that such results are superior to those of an experienced technician using manual evaluations. The average intraslide (three repeat measures) coefficient of variation for the automated evaluations of 100 cells and 200 cells was found to be 9.73% and 8.30%, respectively, when using the IVOS. The average inter-slide coefficient of variation obtained using the IVOS was, however, 15.39%[38]. The approximately 6–7% higher variation obtained for inter-slide evaluations, as compared with intraslide evaluations, may once again point to the importance of sample and slide preparation.

The average coefficient of variation for repeat evaluations is known to be a function of both the number of sperm evaluated and the percentage of normal forms[25,39], due to statistical presuppositions. Semen samples with low percentages of normal sperm (< 10%) will inherently exhibit higher variability in repeat analyses. Davis and Gravance[25] concluded that at least 200 cells should be evaluated to obtain a stable estimate of the percentage of normal sperm. Analyzing the group of patients in whom the average normal sperm morphology outcome across the three evaluations was ≤ 10%, a coefficient of variation of 13.9% and 10.63%, for 100 and 200 cells, respectively[38], was obtained. Greater confidence in normal sperm morphology outcomes will therefore be achieved if 200 or more cells are evaluated in patients with low normal sperm outcomes. The evaluation of 200 or more cells per sample (per slide) will become more feasible as the speed of processors used in automated systems increases.

In a study comparing sperm morphology analyzed by a computer equipped with a morphologizer with that using the traditional manual method, Wang et al.[27] found a significant correlation between the two methods ($r = 0.52$; $p < 0.0001$) for percentage of normal forms. Although the mean percentages of normal forms classified by the methods were not significantly different (72.4% vs. 72.3%), the limits of agreement were relatively large (−20.5% to +20.7%). Davis et al.[12], comparing manual with automated classification, obtained a 60% unambiguous agreement. They also found that the automated classification method always resulted in a lower percentage of normal sperm than the manual method: 50.9% compared with 61.9%. Kruger et al.[22], evaluating 43 slide preparations blindly, found that 84% of the FERTECH's evaluations compared well with the manual method. In a subsequent study, Kruger et al.[19] correlated the percentage normal morphology (strict criteria) outcomes between manual and automated evaluations and found the limits of agreement to be between 12.1 and −15.5%. In the percentage normal sperm morphology range 0–20%, the limits of agreement were, however, narrower (8.4 to −6.6%). The Spearman correlation coefficient for this study was 0.85, which was similar to the correlation ($r = 0.83$) obtained between two observers performing manual evaluations. Using the 14% fertility cut-off point for strict criteria, Kruger et al.[21] found that the automated system was able to classify 81.3% (65/80) of cases, similar to the manual method.

Four identical automated instruments (Cell-Trak-S), two each at two sites, were used to analyze (archive) videotape material[40]. The coefficients of variation obtained for repeated measures were between 1 and 8% for each variable measured on all instruments. Kruger et al.[41] examined intermachine variation for two IVOS set-ups (Tygerberg vs. Norfolk), evaluating the same slides. The comparison showed no difference in the mean percentage of normal forms (15.6% vs. 15.8%) produced by the two systems. Although a correlation coefficient of 0.92 was obtained, the coefficient of variation was, however, 20.65%. In a multicenter study in which 30 sperm morphology slides were evaluated at five independent centers using the IVOS, the magnitudes of variation (coefficients of variation) obtained ranged between 11.36 and 23.09%[42]. Although most of the major variables (sample preparation, cell staining and classification system) influencing the evaluation of sperm morphology were eliminated, a variation of > 15% was still obtained between outcomes produced at the different centers.

The results observed show that there is good agreement between an experienced manual observer's evaluations and automated evaluations. The results also show that the use of an automated system does not mean that all variation will be eliminated. The technologist performing the computer-assisted evaluation therefore still has an important role to play in limiting variation. Factors other than sample and slide processing that the technologist can control, and which may significantly influence outcomes, are focus and illumination.

FERTILITY PREDICTION VALUE

The primary objective for developing any diagnostic tool for *in vitro* or *in vivo* human fertility diagnosis is the ability to determine accurately the fertility potential, to provide the infertile couple with realistic advice with regard to conception potential. Replacement of manual evaluations of sperm morphology with automated evaluations, therefore, also requires unequivocal proof that the outcomes have predictive value.

Wang *et al.*[28] were among the first to assess the usefulness of automated sperm morphology evaluation to predict the outcome of human sperm fertilizing capacity. Multivariate discriminant analysis was used to analyze the ability to predict the outcome of the zona-free hamster-oocyte assay. The eight variables selected were able to predict fertility capacity with 74% accuracy, compared with 84% when the manual method was used. Kruger *et al.*[22] determined the prognostic value of the IVOS by evaluating 21 slides from Tygerberg Hospital and 21 slides from Norfolk's *in vitro* fertilization (IVF) program. The fertilization rates for the two fertility groups, < 14% and > 14% normal forms, were 33.3% (15/45) and 76.6% (46/60), respectively, for manual evaluations and 46.8%

(30/64) and 75.6% (31/41), respectively, for automated evaluations (Tygerberg slides). Evaluations performed on the Norfolk slides produced a similar result: 27.4% (14/51) and 90.0% (127/141) and 33.9% (18/53) and 88.4% (123/139) for the manual and computer analyses, respectively.

Sofitikis *et al.*[18], using fresh sperm and a confocal scanning laser microscope, found that when the percentage normal forms were ≥ 22%, fertilization occurred in 25 of 26 cases, while below this percentage only two of 15 cases fertilized oocytes. MacLeod and Irvine[26] examined the value of both manual and computer-assisted semen analysis (WHO 1987[43]) using the Hamilton Thorne HTM-S 2030 in predicting the *in vivo* fertility ('normal' women) of cryopreserved donor semen. When the post-thaw semen profiles were compared, pregnant versus not pregnant, there were differences in respect of both morphometry and movement characteristics determined by the HTM-S. When multiple logistic regression was used to predict the achievement of pregnancy, the conventional criteria of semen quality were of no value ($\chi^2 = 6.67$; $p = 0.353$). However, the automated assessment of morphometric and movement characteristics successfully predicted outcome in 86.9% of cases ($\chi^2 = 44.3$; $p = 0.0021$). The most important variables in the regression were morphometric attributes (mean minor axis, mean major axis and mean area), amplitude of lateral head displacement and average path velocity.

Kruger *et al.*[21], using an automated system, showed that in patients with ≤ 10×10^6 motile spermatozoa, normal sperm morphology and the number of oocytes were important predictors of fertilization. The normal sperm morphology outcomes produced by automated evaluations were also found to be significantly ($p = 0.0001$) correlated with fertilization by logistic regression. Except for one case, all other zero fertilization cases were found to be within the group with < 10^6/ml sperm and < 10% normal sperm morphology. The overall fertilization rates for the fertility subgroups were: 45.6% (37/81) for the group with ≤4% normal forms, 72.5% (87/120) for the 5–9% group, 82.1% (46/56) for the 10–14% group and 85.2% (69/81) for the > 14% group. In another study conducted by the Kruger group[44], the automated normal sperm morphology outcomes were found to be significant predictors of both fertilization ($p = 0.0419$) *in vitro* and pregnancy ($p = 0.0210$), using logistic regression models. The fertilization rates across the 5% normal sperm morphology fertility cut-off point were 39.4% (≤5%) and 62.9% (> 5%), while the pregnancy rates were 15.2% (≤5%) compared with 37.36% (> 5%). The significance of the 5% normal sperm morphology fertility cut-off point established by the manual evaluation of sperm morphology, using the strict criteria, has therefore been confirmed by computer-assisted evaluations.

In a study using the Hobson Sperm Tracker, a positive correlation was found between the fertilization rate (FR%) and the proportions of sperm with a normal (oval) head shape, sperm exhibiting acrosomal vacuoles, sperm with a normal acrosomal size (40–70% of total head area) and sperm undergoing the acrosome reaction (AR) after adding follicular fluid[20]. Multiple regression analysis revealed that by incorporating the above four parameters, the sensitivity of prediction of *in vitro* fertilization rate values was 79% and the specificity was 93%, with a positive predictive value of 96%. During 1997–99, 1191 infertile couples with no known barrier to conception were assessed by conventional semen analysis and automated measurements, including motility, concentration and morphology evaluations[33]. A SHAMAS (sperm head automated morphometric analysis system) analysis was performed on Shorr-stained smears of washed semen. The analysis measures %C, which is similar to conventional manual percentage normal morphology, and %Z, the percentage of sperm with characteristics conforming to those of sperm that bind to the zona pellucida of the human oocyte. Binding to the zona pellucida is essential for fertilization, and the process is highly selective for sperm with axial symmetry, a narrow neck and a large acrosomal area. Three factors were found to be independently and significantly related to natural pregnancy in a multivariate Cox regression analysis, of which %Z was the most important, followed by VSL (straight-line velocity) and female age[33].

More large prospective randomized studies using automated evaluations are required to establish the 'true' clinical value of these systems. These must be performed using standardized and controlled slide preparation and sperm cell staining methods. The appropriateness of the manually established normal sperm morphology thresholds may have to be re-examined, or new thresholds may have to be determined by regression analysis.

CONCLUSIONS

Automated systems have been shown to have the potential to eliminate the biases and subjectivity plaguing the manual evaluation of sperm morphology. Although they are objective, the accuracy of the results from these systems can also be compromised by methodological errors. Variables such as sperm preparation methods, sperm cell staining methods, focus, parameter settings and the soft- and hardware components used can have a significant effect on the precision of evaluations. To ensure comparative and reliable results, procedures and instruments must be standardized and quality control maintained.

The studies performed, at least with the use of the IVOS, have shown that its precision and the predictive value of its outcomes are at least equal to the outcomes produced by an experienced observer performing manual evaluations. The group of patients identified with <5% normal sperm morphology, as with the manual evaluation of sperm morphology, have been shown to have a significantly depressed fertilization and pregnancy probability. Further clinical studies are needed to determine the true value of the automated systems, whereby multiple parameters, morphometric and kinematic, are measured in relation to fertility outcomes to create predictive models.

REFERENCES

1. Ombelet W, et al. Sperm morphology assessment: historical review in relation to fertility. Hum Reprod Update 1995; 1: 543

2. Coetzee K, Kruger TF, Lombard CJ. Predictive value of normal sperm morphology: a structured literature review. Hum Reprod Update 1998; 4: 73

3. Eliasson R. Standards for investigation of human semen? Andrologia 1971; 3: 49

4. Williams WW, ed. Sterility, the Diagnostic Survey of the Infertile Couple. Springfield, MA: WW Williams, 1964

5. Freund M. Standards for the rating of human sperm morphology. A co-operative study. Int J Fertil 1996; 11: 97

6. David G, et al. Anomalies morphologiques du spermatozoïde humain. 1) Propositions pour un système de classification. J Gynécol Obstet Biol Reprod 1975; 4 (Suppl 1): 17

7. Fredericsson B. Morphologic evaluation of spermatozoa in different laboratories. Andrologia 1979; 11: 57

8. Hofmann N, Freundl G, Florack M. Die Formstörungen der Spermatozoen im Sperma und Zervikalschleim als Spiegel testikulärer Erkrankungen, Gynäkologe 1985; 18: 189

9. Kruger TF, et al. Sperm morphologic features as a prognostic factor in in vitro fertilization. Fertil Steril 1986; 46: 1118

10. Davis RO, Katz D. Computer-aided analysis: technology at a crossroads. Fertil Steril 1993; 59: 953

11. Coetzee K, Kruger TF. Accuracy and prognostic value of computer-assisted (IVOS) sperm morphology evaluations. Middle East Fertil Soc J 1999; 4: 222

12. Davis RO, et al. Accuracy and precision of the Cell-Form-Human* automated sperm morphometry instrument. Fertil Steril 1992; 58: 763

13. Calamera JC, et al. Development of an objective and manual technique to study the human sperm morphology. Andrologia 1994; 26: 331

14. World Health Organization. WHO Laboratory Manual for the Examination of Human Semen and Semen–Cervical Mucus Interaction, 3rd edn. Cambridge: Cambridge University Press, 1992

15. Goulart AR, de Alencar Hausen M, Monteiro-Leal LH. Comparison of three computer methods of sperm head analysis. Fertil Steril 2003; 80: 625

16. Moruzzi JF, et al. Quantification and classification of human sperm morphology by computer-assisted image analysis. Fertil Steril 1988; 50: 142

17. Coetzee K, et al. Comparison of two staining and evaluation methods used for computerized human sperm morphology evaluations. Andrologia 1997; 29: 133

18. Sofikitis NV, et al. Confocal scanning laser microscopy of morphometric human sperm parameters: correlation with acrosin profiles and fertilizing capacity. Fertil Steril 1994; 62: 376

19. Kruger TF, et al. Sperm morphology: assessing the agreement between the manual method (strict criteria) and the sperm morphology analyzer IVOS. Fertil Steril 1995; 63: 134

20. El-Ghobashy AA, West CR. The human sperm head: a key for successful fertilization. J Androl 2003; 24: 232

21. Kruger TF, et al. A prospective study on the predictive value of normal sperm morphology as evaluated by computer (IVOS*). Fertil Steril 1996; 66: 285

22. Kruger TF, et al. A new computerized method of reading sperm morphology (strict criteria) is as efficient as technician reading. Fertil Steril 1993; 59: 202

23. Lacquet FA, et al. Slide preparation and staining procedures for reliable results using computerized morphology (IVOS*). Arch Androl 1996; 36: 133

24. Menkveld R, et al. Effects of different staining and washing procedures on the results of human sperm morphology evaluation by manual and computerised methods. Andrologia 1997; 29: 1

25. Davis RO, Gravance CG. Standardization of specimen preparation, staining, and sampling methods improves automated sperm-head morphometry analysis. Fertil Steril 1993; 59: 412

26. MacLeod IC, Irvine DS. The predictive value of computer-assisted semen analysis in the context of a donor insemination programme. Hum Reprod 1995; 10: 580

27. Wang C, et al. Computer-assisted assessment of human sperm morphology: comparison with visual assessment. Fertil Steril 1991; 55: 983

28. Wang C, et al. Computer-assisted assessment of human sperm morphology: usefulness in predicting fertilizing capacity of human spermatozoa. Fertil Steril 1991; 55: 989

29. Mundy AJ, Ryder TA, Edmonds DK. Morphometric characteristics of motile spermatozoa in subfertile men with an excess of non-sperm cells in the ejaculate. Hum Reprod 1994; 9: 1701

30. Garret C, Baker HWG. A new fully automated system for the morphometric analysis of human sperm heads. Fertil Steril 1995; 63: 1306

31. Coetzee K, Kruger TF. Automated sperm morphology analysis: Quo Vadis. Assist Reprod Rev 1997; 7: 109

32. Menkveld R, et al. The evaluation of morphological characteristics of human spermatozoa according to stricter criteria. Hum Reprod 1990; 5: 586

33. Garrett C, et al. Automated semen analysis: 'zona pellucida preferred' sperm morphometry and straight-line velocity are related to pregnancy rate in subfertile couples. Hum Reprod 2003; 18: 1643

34. Ombelet W, et al. Results of a questionnaire on sperm morphology assessment. Hum Reprod 1997; 12: 1015

35. ESHRE Andrology Special Interest Group. Guidelines on the application of CASA technology in the analysis of spermatozoa. Hum Reprod 1998; 13: 142

36. Menkveld R, et al., eds. Atlas of Human Sperm Morphology. Baltimore: Williams & Wilkins, 1991

37. Davis RO, et al. Accuracy and precision of the Cell-Form-Human automated sperm morphometry instrument. Fertil Steril 1992; 58: 763

38. Coetzee K, Kruger TF, Lombard CJ. Repeatability and variance analysis on multiple readings performed by a computer semen analyser (IVOS). Andrologia 1999; 3: 165

39. Cooper TG, et al. Internal quality control of semen analysis. Fertil Steril 1992; 58: 172

40. Davis RO, Rothmann SA, Overstreet JW. Accuracy and precision of computer-aided sperm analysis in multicenter studies. Fertil Steril 1992; 57: 648

41. Kruger TF, et al. Computer assisted sperm analyzing system: an analysis of intermachine morphology evaluations and intraslide evaluations using IVOS (Dimension system version 3). Presented at the American Society for Reproductive Medicine Congress, Boston, November, 1996, S223

42. Coetzee K, et al. Assessment of inter- and intralaboratory sperm morphology readings using a Hamilton Thorne Research IVOS semen analyzer. Fertil Steril 1999; 71: 80

43. World Health Organization. WHO Laboratory Manual for the Examination of Human Semen and Semen–Cervical Mucus Interaction, 2nd edn. Cambridge: Cambridge University Press, 1987

44. Coetzee K, et al. Clinical value in using an automated semen morphology analyser (IVOS). Fertil Steril 1999; 71: 222

11

Sperm morphology training and quality control programs are essential for clinically relevant results

Daniel R Franken, Thinus F Kruger

INTRODUCTION

Primary knowledge and understanding of the morphological appearance, and bright-field microscopic configuration, of a normal human sperm cell form the basis of the evaluation method for sperm morphology in which more strict criteria are applied. Disagreement in the results can be caused by a variety of factors, such as discrepancy in the specific techniques used during the analysis.

Since more clinicians are becoming aware of the importance of training and subsequent quality control measurements, standardization in semen analysis methodologies has become mandatory. In close agreement with the present author's beliefs, Kvist and Bjorndahl have made an important contribution towards the standardization of techniques needed to obtain a globally accepted and World Health Organization (WHO)-recognized semen analysis result[1]. The techniques focus mainly on assessments of sperm concentration, sperm motility, sperm morphology and sperm vitality.

Several authors have stressed the value of the assessment of human sperm morphology during both *in vitro*[2–5] and *in vivo*[6] studies. Furthermore, assessment of human sperm morphology and sperm concentration can also serve as a variable in reproductive health studies involving endocrinology and environmental toxicology, when specific endocrine disruptors are present[7–11]. These statements were confirmed by Coetzee *et al.*[12], who summarized all the important articles in a meta-analysis.

Training of andrology technologists can be accomplished using different educational approaches, of which the one-to-one workshop is the most successful teaching method. Direct communication and input on a one-to-one basis with an experienced worker ensures that the trainee understands the basic concepts of sperm morphology. This method, however, has a disadvantage in that only a small number of trainees can be trained per session. Our experience has indicated that a maximum of ten students per teacher can be trained per session[13,14].

A second and also valuable teaching method is the so-called group consensus technique[15]. In this method, the trainer (usually an individual with ample experience in sperm morphology evaluation) uses computer or video images that are projected onto a screen during training sessions. The advantage of this method lies in the fact that large numbers of students can be trained during a single session. The disadvantage of this method lies in the mass communication style, and the individual is often lost during group discussions.

A third training method is the use of an interactive CD-ROM program. Such an interactive computer program contains a variety of high-quality images of numbered spermatozoa. Advantages of this method include training at the individual's own leisure and time, as he/she can repeat specific sections of the program where certain concepts are poorly understood.

During previous studies we have presented numerous sperm morphology workshops in Africa, the Middle East and Europe. The format of these workshops consisted generally of hands-on, one-on-one teaching, accompanied by various sessions of consensus training, as well as the use of a CD-ROM program (Strict 1-2-3®). During the group consensus training sessions, participants were requested to evaluate photomicrographic images of sperm cells projected onto a large non-reflecting screen. It is important to remember that the educational value of the training will be enhanced if trainees are exposed to all the above-described methods.

SPERM MORPHOLOGY QUALITY CONTROL

Sperm morphology evaluations have important clinical value only in cases where the evaluation of normal/abnormal cells is done with accuracy. In most cases, manual reading by light microscopy under high-power magnification (1000×) has been the method of evaluation. Several factors have been identified that can influence the outcome of sperm morphology readings. These factors include quality of the slide, and staining procedures. Typically, a poor slide consists of a thick semen layer with multiple sperm cells on top of one another, thus causing extensive overlapping of cell heads, tails and debris.

Each andrology laboratory should therefore have an internal as well as an external quality control program. For example, the results obtained from each technician on the quality control sample are tabulated and plotted on a graph against the sample number. The mean and standard deviation of the results for each sample are computed and also plotted against the sample number. As part of the internal quality control system, each andrology technician should be able to prepare high-quality sperm slides in order to provide repeatable and reliable morphology readings for the referring clinicians.

At Tygerberg, a protocol has been developed for the preparation of sperm slides that not only are of a high quality but also fulfill the requirements of the manual reading techniques for sperm morphology[16]. These slides adhere to the description for the preparation of semen smears supplied by the WHO[17–20].

Slide preparation

For each sample, at least two smears should be prepared from a fresh sample for duplicate assessments in case of poor staining. The slide should first be cleaned, washed in 70% alcohol and dried, before a drop of semen is applied to the slide (Figure 11.1)[20].

To ensure optimal slide quality, the following standard protocol should be used during slide preparations: (1) frosted, precleaned glass slides with grounded edges are used at all times; (2) sperm counts are used as a guide to determine the sperm droplet size eventually used to prepare the smear (if the sperm count is $> 60 \times 10^6$ cells/ml, a $< 10\text{-}\mu l$ droplet is used, while if the sperm count is $< 60 \times 10^6$ cells/ml, a $10\text{–}30\text{-}\mu l$ drop is used; the final number of sperm cells in both cases should

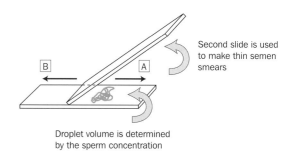

Second slide is used to make thin semen smears

Droplet volume is determined by the sperm concentration

Figure 11.1   Feathering method to prepare undiluted sperm morphology smears

produce 8–12 spermatozoa per high-power magnification); (3) the semen drop is typically placed in the middle of the slide at a point more or less 20% from the frosted end, using a micropipette fitted with disposable tips (Gilson P100; Lasec Laboratories, Cape Town, South Africa). The semen is gently touched at a 45° angle with the width side of a second slide; this allows the semen to spread evenly across the width of the first slide, after which the second slide is slightly pulled backwards and then pushed forwards while pushing downwards over the entire length of the first slide.

MONITORING THE TECHNICIAN'S SPERM MORPHOLOGY READING SKILLS

The Tygerberg approach

A typical Tygerberg sperm morphology training session consists of a multiple approach method that relies on hands-on, one-on-one individual training (experienced worker vs. inexperienced worker). We believe that this training method is imperative during the initial stages of teaching. Furthermore, we also use the consensus training and CD-ROM interactive programs. In our experience, after the training sessions, participants were enrolled on the continuous quality control (CQC) program. Participants received, on a quarterly basis, two Papanicolaou prestained sperm slides from normo-, terato- or severe teratozoospermic samples. The participant recorded the percentage of normal cells present on these slides, and the results were forwarded to the reference laboratory at Tygerberg Hospital. The 'correct' results according to the reference laboratory, i.e. the percentage of normal forms present on each of the slides, were subsequently supplied to the participating laboratory[13,14].

Due to the fact that the morphological slides used for evaluation of the standard of the trainees were random samples from different sperm donors, standardization was needed with respect to an index that is not dependent on the morphological level. On the assumption that the reference laboratory's morphology reading is the gold standard, an index was calculated using the following standardized statistical score:

> Standard deviation (SD) score = trainee score − reference laboratory score divided by SD test slides that were shipped to trainees[14]

As expected, the standard deviation decreases with lower levels of morphology, i.e. < 4% normal forms. The SD score reflects the number of SD units by which the measurement of the trainee differs from the gold standard for the specific slide. Each trainee can be evaluated according to the SD score for his/her level of agreement with the gold standard. Two SD score levels were chosen in order to evaluate poor readings, and for this purpose we selected the values ±0.5SD and ±0.2SD. The individual SD scores obtained from the training and follow-up contacts can be plotted against time on a graph that also indicates the limits.

An ongoing study at Tygerberg Hospital aims to record the value of quarterly monitoring and refresher courses on morphology reading skills of technicians over a period of 40 months. Nineteen individuals from 13 different andrology laboratories from Switzerland, Malaysia and Singapore were enrolled in a sperm morphology quality control program after initial training sessions. The mean values for the test slides (two slide sets) reported by each individual are presented in Figure 11.2. We regarded recordings outside the ±0.2SD score as a warning (Figure 11.2), and results outside the ±0.5SD score as an indicator for the individual to become concerned about his/her sperm morphology reading skills.

Five of the 19 participants (Figure 11.2 numbers 1, 7, 8, 9 and 19) attended annual refresher courses during the period. Participants 13 and 19 did not attend any refresher training, but maintained the reading skills acquired after one-to-one training. Adequate technician training is of paramount significance to achieve consistent results

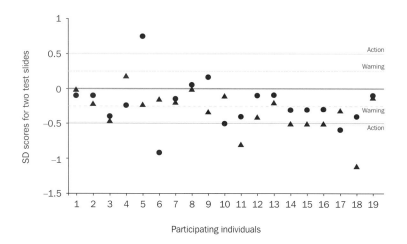

Figure 11.2   Mean standard deviation (SD) scores reported by 19 individuals from 13 andrology laboratories for test slides 1 and 2

within a given laboratory. Even when strict criteria are utilized[13,14], interlaboratory variation is probably the result of various factors, including (1) different semen and smear preparation techniques, (2) differences in interpretation and (3) technician experience[15].

Using specific criteria, we were able to classify the trainees according to their reported results.

Classification of reading skills

Poor reading skills

If 50% of readings recorded over the 40-month period were inside the limits of error, i.e. the ±0.5SD score, poor reading standards were assumed. Using the overall correctness of each individual, the results depicted in Figure 11.2 indicated that five (26%) participants (5, 6, 11, 17, 18) had poor reading skills during the evaluation period.

Marginal reading skills

If 51–59% of readings recorded over the 40-month period were within the ±0.5SD score, marginal reading skills were assumed.

Good reading skills

If 60–69% of the readings recorded over the 40-month period fell inside the limits of error, i.e. the ±0.5SD score, good reading standards were assumed. Five (26%) individuals (9, 12, 14, 15, 16) had good reading skills.

Excellent reading skills

If ≥70% of the readings recorded over the 40-month period were within the ±0.5SD score, excellent reading skills were assumed. Results in Figure 11.2 show that nine (47%) of the partaking individuals (1, 2, 3, 4, 7, 8, 10, 13, 19) maintained excellent reading skills.

Our results clearly illustrate that an external quality control program can be successfully implemented on condition that continuous monitoring is part of the program. In general, we were satisfied with the overall reading skills of the study group, since 73% maintained sperm morphology reading skills that were classified as good or excellent. We firmly believe that the technical maintenance of morphology readings is, apart from the initial training sessions, also dependent on annual refresher courses. The five participants, namely 1, 7, 8, 9 and 19 who randomly attended refresher courses were able to maintain their acquired reading skills. These individuals consistently produced reading skills that were within ±0.2SD score limits of error (Figure 11.3). This study also highlights the feasibility of initiating a global sperm morphology quality control program.

Finally, an important finding during the study was the significant role that the annual refresher courses played in the maintenance of morphology reading skills. Here, for the first time, we illustrated that those technicians who attended refresher courses were able to maintain their morphology reading skills over an extended period. In general, all participants (except refresher course attendees) showed a decline in reading at about 6–9 months after initial training. We believe that this is a tendency that will occur in any andrology unit, and laboratory directors should be aware of this phenomenon. Previous studies[21–23] concluded that the only way to ensure comparable interlaboratory results is through participation in a multicenter proficiency testing program[24]. Similar to the present study, Keel et al.[21] suggested that such a proficiency testing system should comprise an external interlaboratory quality program. During this program, simulated identical patient specimens are tested by participating individuals/laboratories.

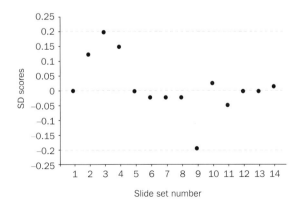

Figure 11.3 Standard deviation (SD) scores of an individual with excellent sperm morphology reading skills

REFERENCES

1. Kvist U, Bjorndahl L. Editorial. In Kvist U, Bjorndahl L, eds. Manual on Basic Semen Analysis. Oxford: Oxford University Press, 2002: v
2. Kruger TF, et al. Sperm morphologic features as a prognostic factor in in vitro fertilization. Fertil Steril 1986; 46: 1118
3. Kruger TF, et al. Predictive value of abnormal sperm morphology in in vitro fertilization. Fertil Steril 1988; 49: 111
4. Enginsu ME, et al. Evaluation of human sperm morphology using strict criteria after Diff-Quik staining: correlation of morphology with fertilization in vitro. Hum Reprod 1991; 6: 854
5. Ombelet W, et al. Teratozoospermia and in-vitro fertilization: a randomized prospective study. Hum Reprod 1994; 9: 1479
6. Eggert-Kruse W, et al. Clinical relevance of sperm morphology assessment using strict criteria and relationship with sperm–mucus interaction in vivo and in vitro. Fertil Steril 1995; 63: 612
7. Carlsen E, et al. Evidence for decreasing quality of semen during the past 50 years. Br J Med 1992; 303: 609
8. Auger J, et al. Decline in semen quality in fertile men in Paris during the past 20 years. N Engl J Med 1995; 332: 281
9. Irvine SE, et al. Evidence of deteriorating semen quality in the United Kingdom: birth cohort study in 577 men in Scotland over 11 years. Br J Med 1996; 312: 467
10. Auger J, Jouannet P. Evidence for regional differences of semen quality among French fertile men. Hum Reprod 1997; 12: 740
11. Swan SH, Elkin EP, Fenster L. The question of declining sperm density revisited: an analysis of 101 studies published 1934–1996. Environ Health Perspect 1997; 108: 961
12. Coetzee K, Kruger TF, Lombard CJ. Predictive value of normal sperm morphology: a structured literature review. Hum Reprod Update 1998; 4: 73
13. Franken DR, Barendson R, Kruger TF. A continuous quality control (CQC) program for strict sperm morphology. Fertil Steril 2000; 74: 721
14. Franken DR, et al. The development of a continuous quality control (CQS) programme for strict sperm morphology among sub-Saharan African laboratories. Hum Reprod 2000; 15: 667
15. Eustache F, Auger J. Inter-individual variability in the morphological assessment of human sperm: effect of

the level of experience and the use of standard methods. Hum Reprod 2003; 18: 1018

16. Menkveld R, et al. Effect of different staining and
    washing procedures on the results of human sperm
    morphology evaluation by manual and computerized
    method. Andrologia 1997; 29: 1

17. Menkveld R, et al. The evaluation of morphological
    characteristics of human spermatozoa according to
    stricter criteria. Hum Reprod 1990; 5: 586

18. Menkveld R, et al., eds. Atlas of Human Sperm Mor-
    phology. Baltimore: Williams & Wilkins, 1991

19. Menkveld R, Kruger TF. Evaluation of sperm mor-
    phology by light microscopy. In Acosta AA, Kruger
    TF, eds. Human Spermatozoa in Assisted Reproduc-
    tion. London: Parthenon Publishing, 1996: 189

20. World Health Organization. WHO Laboratory Man-
    ual for the Examination of Human Semen and
    Semen–Cervical Mucus Interaction, 4th edn. Cam-
    bridge: Cambridge University Press, 1999: 1

21. Keel BA, et al. Results of the American Association of
    Bio-analysts national proficiency testing programme
    in andrology. Hum Reprod 2000; 15: 680

22. Cooper TG, Atkinson AD, Nieschlag E. Experience
    with external quality control in spermatology. Hum
    Reprod 1999; 14: 765

23. Dunphy BC, et al. Quality control during the con-
    ventional analysis of semen, an essential exercise. J
    Androl 1989; 10: 378

24. Neuwinger J, Behre, HM, Nieschlag E. External
    quality control: the andrology laboratory: an experi-
    mental multicenter trial. Fertil Steril 1990; 54: 308

12

Role of acrosome index in prediction of fertilization outcome

Roelof Menkveld

INTRODUCTION

The clinical usefulness of the strict Tygerberg criteria for sperm morphology evaluation[1] for *in vitro* fertilization outcome and later for *in vivo* pregnancies has been demonstrated by Kruger *et al.*[2,3] and Van Zyl *et al.*[4], respectively, and thereafter has been confirmed in many publications[5]. However, even in the presence of the so-called P-pattern or in the poor-prognosis group ($\leq 4\%$ morphological normal forms), some men achieve fertilization of oocytes *in vitro*, and *in vivo* pregnancies occur occasionally[3,5]. Therefore, efforts to develop more sensitive predictors, especially for expected *in vitro* fertilization rates, are continuously being put forward. Some of these predictors are based on sperm biochemical tests such as the sperm chromatin dispersion test[6], the sperm chromatin structure assay[7] and the ubiquitin-based sperm assay[8], while others incorporate a combination of semen variables, for example the post-wash total progressively motile cell count[9], or have refined certain existing semen variables such as sperm morphology by the use of more specific sperm morphology parameters, namely the sperm deformity index[10] or the spontaneous acrosome reaction as seen with Spermac staining[11].

In this regard, Menkveld *et al.*[12] introduced the acrosome index (AI) as an additional tool in the prediction of *in vitro* fertilization outcome. It was

shown that the AI is another sensitive parameter, like normal sperm morphology evaluated according to strict criteria, in the prediction of *in vitro* fertilization rates of $\geq 50\%$, and that the AI is especially useful in the P-pattern group of patients. Since the AI can provide additional information, compared with normal sperm morphology, it can therefore be regarded as an independent parameter[13] for the prediction of assisted reproductive procedure outcomes. This additional role of the AI as a prognostic factor has been discussed in only a few publications[14–18], and is reviewed briefly in this chapter, with emphasis on the functional role played by the acrosome in the fertility pathway, particularly in relation to sperm binding to the zona pellucida, and its usefulness in assisted reproduction procedures, especially intracytoplasmic sperm injection (ICSI).

ROLE OF THE ACROSOME IN THE FERTILITY PATHWAY

The acrosome is formed by the Golgi apparatus during spermatogenesis, and can be described as a secretory granule situated at the apex of the sperm head, consisting of an inner acrosomal membrane that is closely associated with the nucleus of the sperm and which is continuous with the outer acrosomal membrane. The acrosomal matrix proper is located between the two membranes. The whole acrosome as well as the rest of the spermatozoon is covered by the plasma membrane. The acrosome contains a number of enzymes such as (pro)acrosin, which plays a vital role in the fertility pathway with regard to sperm binding to and penetration of the zona pellucida[19].

With contact of the spermatozoon to the zona pellucida, the acrosome undergoes the acrosome reaction, which can be described as an exocytotic event involving localized fusion between the outer acrosomal and plasma membranes, resulting in the formation of vesicles with the release of mainly the enzymes hyaluronidase and (pro)acrosin through the holes formed by the vesicles, and is one of the most important steps in sperm binding to and penetration of the zona pellucida[20,21]. It is now becoming increasingly evident that, for these functions to take place, especially with regard to sperm binding to the zona pellucida, normal sperm morphology and especially normal acrosomal morphology is essential[22,23]. Strong selection also takes place at the zona pellucida for spermatozoa with normal-sized acrosomes, as was nicely illustrated by Garrett and Baker[24].

Acrosomal size also plays an important role in the ability of the spermatozoon to undergo the acrosome reaction. Spermatozoa with large acrosomes were associated with a significantly higher percentage of live spontaneous acrosome-reacted spermatozoa, while spermatozoa with small acrosomes were associated with a high percentage of sperm death[25]. Semen samples containing a low percentage of spermatozoa with intact acrosomes were also associated with total fertilization failure[11], due to the inability of these spermatozoa to bind to the zona pellucida, as the acrosome reaction must take place at the time of binding to the zona pellucida. However, the inability of zona pellucida-bound spermatozoa to undergo the zona pellucida-induced acrosome reaction may also play an important role in non-fertilization[26,27]. According to Benoff et al.[28], the human sperm acrosome reaction occurs in vitro only in the most morphologically normal spermatozoa, and about

50% of all in vitro fertilization (IVF) failures are thought to be related to anomalies of acrosome structure and function.

MICROSCOPIC EVALUATION OF ACROSOMAL MORPHOLOGY

At first, the human sperm acrosome was deemed too small to be visualized by direct microscopy, and scanning electron and transmission electron microscopy were used or advocated[29]. However, the ability to evaluate acrosome morphology by light microscopy is now acknowledged[1,12].

Visual evaluation of sperm acrosomal morphology, performed with good bright-field optics at 1000× or preferably 1250× magnification on high-quality Papanicolaou-stained smears, is based on acrosomal size, its form and the staining characteristics of the acrosome, and can be performed simultaneously with the routine sperm morphology evaluation[1,12]. For classification as a morphologically normal acrosome, the same principles are applicable as for the classification of morphologically normal spermatozoa according to strict criteria, except that the postacrosomal area of the sperm head can be abnormal, but no neck/midpiece and tail abnormalities or cytoplasmic residues may be present[1]. If the spermatozoon is classified as normal, the acrosome must always be classified as normal. This means that the acrosome index will always be equal to, but in most cases greater than, the percentage of morphologically normal spermatozoa. When the acrosome evaluation is done simultaneously with the routine morphology evaluation, two laboratory counters are needed. On the first counter the sperm morphology is scored as normal or abnormal, and the second is used to keep a record of the acrosomes considered to be normal, or the whole range of acrosomal defects can be scored[1,12,30].

Acrosomal defects as seen with the light microscope can be classified as specific defects or as nonspecific alterations. Specific acrosomal defects, which are mostly concerned with acrosome size, are genetically caused[31,32], such as globozoospermia[19], and the miniacrosome defect[33]. However, genetic sperm defects are not limited to the acrosome only, but may affect any part of the spermatozoon, the short or stump tail defect being one observable by light microscopy[34]. These conditions are rare, but when they occur, are easy to detect using the light microscope.

However, acrosomes can also be classified as too large, an abnormality that may in some cases be associated with a higher rate of spontaneous acrosomal reactions[25] and decreased *in vitro* fertilization rates[2,12]. Staining defects may include irregular acrosomes, multiple vacuoles, cysts and 'empty' acrosomes[29]. These staining defects may indicate damage of the acrosome membranes, with subsequent leaking of (pro)acrosin from the acrosomes[35]. Jeulin *et al.*[29] found low fertilization rates of semen samples containing predominantly spermatozoa with acrosome staining defects, and postulated that the low *in vitro* fertilization rates associated with these increased acrosomal abnormalities might not be due to the presence of abnormal acrosomes *per se*, but due to a relationship between acrosomal abnormalities and nuclear immaturity of the spermatozoa. Sperm DNA abnormalities may be due to the production of reactive oxygen species (ROS) by the spermatozoa themselves, but mostly due to leukocytes present in semen samples[36].

ROLE OF THE ACROSOME INDEX IN ASSISTED REPRODUCTION

In 1986, Kruger *et al.*[2] reported that sperm morphology evaluated according to strict criteria[1] was a strong prognosticator of *in vitro* fertilization outcome in cases with a normal sperm concentration ($\geq 20 \times 10^6$/ml) and progressive motility ($\geq 30\%$ motility). A cut-off value at 15% morphologically normal spermatozoa was found to be associated with a fertilization rate of 37% in the $\leq 14\%$ group, but no pregnancies, and 82% in the $\geq 14\%$ group. In 1988, Kruger *et al.*[3] also reported

that a drastic drop in the fertilization rate (7.6%) occurred when < 4% morphologically normal spermatozoa was observed in a semen sample, while in the 4–14% group the fertilization rate was 63.9%.

In an initial investigation of the role of acrosomes and fertilization[30], it was observed that two distinct morphological acrosome patterns could be observed in the < 4% normal morphology group, whereby fertilization did and did not occur. In the few men with good fertilization, it was striking to observe a pattern of slightly and moderately elongated spermatozoa, but with morphologically normal (size and form) acrosomes. In one of the cases, four of four ova were fertilized *in vitro*, although there were only 2% morphologically normal spermatozoa present, but a total of 17% of spermatozoa had normal acrosomes. In a typical case in the group with no fertilization, of six ova inseminated *in vitro*, it was observed that small and/or abnormal acrosomes were mainly present. This case presented with only 1% morphologically normal spermatozoa and with a total of only 4% normal acrosomes.

In an ongoing study including 23 males, Menkveld *et al.*[35] found that when the acrosome morphology was classified into different groups, i.e. normal, small, staining defects and amorphous, and expressed as an acrosome index (percentage normal acrosomes), no fertilization occurred when the acrosome index was $\leq 15\%$. Important was the fact that, once again, cases were found where normal sperm morphology was < 5% but the acrosome index was > 15%. In those cases with an AI > 15% the fertilization rate was always $\geq 50\%$. The relationship between AI (percentage normal acrosomes) and fertilization rate was underlined by the observation that statistically significant differences were found for the acrosome index between groups with fertility rates of < 50% and $\geq 50\%$, i.e. $1.5 \pm 1.9\%$ and $28.5 \pm 11.6\%$ normal acrosomes, respectively[35].

When a receiver operating characteristic (ROC) curve analysis was performed on the IVF results of the 23 males[37], a cut-off value of $\geq 10\%$

(sensitivity 100% and specificity 100%) was obtained for the prediction of a fertilization rate of $\geq 50\%$. This result was confirmed in a follow-up study of 33 males[12]. A higher correlation between AI and fertilization rate ($r = 0.8631$; $p < 0.0001$) was found, compared with the correlation between morphology and fertilization rate ($r = 0.7953$; $p < 0.0001$). This means that the AI can be regarded as a more sensitive measurement of fertilization potential than sperm morphology, especially in the $< 5\%$ morphologically normal spermatozoa group. This may be attributed to the fact that spermatozoa with normal acrosomes but classified as abnormal according to the strict Tygerberg criteria, such as slightly abnormal, or slightly and moderately elongated spermatozoa, are more likely to bind to the zona pellucida[22,23] and to undergo the acrosome reaction[38], compared with spermatozoa from samples with a low AI ($< 10\%$ normal acrosomes).

In 1998, Menkveld et al.[39] reported on the predictive role of the AI and normal sperm morphology compared with that of the teratozoospermia index (TZI) as described in the 1992 WHO manual[40] in a study of 110 patients. It was found that the AI at a cut-off value of $\geq 9\%$ had a better predictive value to predict the possibility of a $> 50\%$ in vitro fertilization rate, compared with normal sperm morphology at $> 5\%$, and sperm morphology had a better predictability compared with the TZI at ≤ 1.46, by ROC curve analysis, with areas under the curve of 0.920, 0.739 and 0.634, respectively. In a study to define normal cut-off values based on data from fertile and subfertile populations, Menkveld et al.[41] determined the AI cut-off value to be at 8% normal acrosomes.

These results are in agreement with previous reports on the role of acrosomal morphology[11,23,28,29]. Liu and Baker[23] found that in cases with $< 30\%$ morphologically normal spermatozoa (according to WHO criteria), the acrosome status (percentage normal) was an important prognosticator of expected fertilization in vitro. Chan et al.[11] reported that semen samples with a low percentage ($< 40\%$) of spermatozoa with intact acrosomes were associated in 31% of cases with total fertilization failure (TFF). Benoff et al.[28] showed that by increasing the insemination concentration of spermatozoa to at least 25 000/ml acrosomally normal spermatozoa in patients with poor acrosomal morphology, fertilization rates and pregnancy rates reached similar levels compared with couples in whom the male presented with normal acrosomal morphology. These publications confirmed the fact that a minimum number or a minimum percentage of spermatozoa with normal acrosomes are needed for normal fertilization to occur in vitro, and underline the important physiological role played by acrosomes in the fertilization pathway[21].

Few reports by other investigators on the role of the AI per se have been published so far. Söderlund and Lundin[14] investigated fertilization of split sibling oocytes for IVF and ICSI in patients but with $< 5\%$ morphologically normal spermatozoa with $\geq 1 \times 10^6$/ml motile spermatozoa after a swim-up procedure. With the aid of ROC curve analysis for IVF rates of $\geq 50\%$, a cut-off value for the AI was determined at 7%. The 81 patients were divided into two groups: group A with AI $< 7\%$ included 42 patients, and group B with AI $\geq 7\%$ included 39 patients. The in vitro fertilization rate in group A was 43.5%, which was significantly lower compared with that of group B at 71.9% ($p = 0.001$). The study showed that in semen samples with $< 5\%$ morphologically normal spermatozoa and an AI $\geq 7\%$, the mean fertilization rate was about 70%, compared with the mean fertilization rate of 40% in the $< 7\%$ AI group. Rhemrev et al.[15] found no pregnancies in a group of 87 couples where the males presented with an AI $< 5\%$ and a fast total radical-trapping antioxidant procedure (TRAP) of < 1.14 mmol/l.

THE ACROSOME INDEX AND SELECTION OF PATIENTS FOR INTRACYTOPLASMIC SPERM INJECTION

With the introduction of ICSI[42], new doors have been opened for couples with severe male fertility problems, as with ICSI it is possible to overcome functional deficiencies, abnormal sperm morphology or shortage of adequate numbers of motile spermatozoa by placing a spermatozoon directly into the oocyte.

ICSI can be regarded as a very invasive procedure, and may also be more expensive in many centers compared with standard IVF. Furthermore, concern exists over the possible negative effects of ICSI, due to the injection of possibly genetically abnormal spermatozoa[43], on their offspring with regard to genetic and congenital abnormalities[44], increased spontaneous abortions, preterm deliveries and reduced birth weights[45]. ICSI should therefore be restricted to those couples with an unacceptably high risk of a low fertilization rate or total fertilization failure. However, a recent publication by Greco *et al.*[46] has shown that ICSI can also have a positive side, in so far as males with DNA-damaged (fragmented) spermatozoa in their semen samples, leading to decreased implantation and pregnancy rates but normal fertilization rates[47], can be successfully treated by ICSI with testicular spermatozoa. It was found that DNA fragmentation was significantly decreased in testicular spermatozoa, leading to a pregnancy rate of 44.4% and an implantation rate of 20.7%. An alternative to performing a testicular biopsy to obtain spermatozoa with low DNA damage may be to perform a selection procedure by the use of cervical mucus, as Bianchi *et al.*[48] have shown that spermatozoa able to cross a cervical mucus barrier possessed higher levels of DNA protamination and practically no signs of endogenous nick translations.

In cases of extreme oligozoospermia[49], cryptozoospermia, globozoospermia[50] or obstructive azoospermia, the choice of an ICSI procedure is self-evident, but problems in deciding between ICSI and IVF may arise when there is a chance of recovering sufficient numbers of motile spermatozoa after sperm preparation[15]. In the previous section dealing with *in vitro* fertilization, an oocyte fertilization cut-off value of ≥50% was used to determine the AI cut-off value[12,14]. However, an *in vitro* fertilization rate cut-off value point of 50% may be regarded as too high to decide between ICSI and IVF. A more appropriate fertilization cut-off point for ICSI may be regarded as a fertilization rate of <37% (two standard deviations (SDs) below the normal expected fertilization rate).

The only data so far available on this aspect were published by Menkveld *et al.* in 1999[51]. They conducted a prospectively designed study to investigate use of the AI as an additional parameter to sperm morphology evaluated by strict criteria in the selection of patients for ICSI. In this study, 134 semen samples were examined blindly on the day of IVF oocyte recovery. Sperm morphology and sperm acrosomal morphology were visually evaluated using light microscopy and expressed as the acrosome index (percentage normal acrosomes). ROC curve analysis indicated that for *in vitro* fertilization rates of ≤37% (2SD below their normal mean fertilization rate), the normal sperm morphology cut-off value was ≤3% (sensitivity 51%, specificity 89%, area under the curve 0.718) and for the acrosome index ≤7% (sensitivity 86%, specificity 86%, area under the curve 0.929). By lowering the fertilization rate cut-off points to <30% and <25%, with ROC curve analysis, the AI cut-off point was lowered to ≤6%, while for a fertilization rate of ≤20% the AI cut-off point increased to ≤7% again. In all instances the morphology cut-off point remained at ≤3%. With the AI cut-off points at ≤6% and ≥7%, fertilization rates were 22.4% (35/156 ova) and 74% (365/489 ova), respectively. According to the above results, the AI cut-off point can be set at ≤6% and be clinically helpful in the selection of patients who would need ICSI, especially in the group of patients showing P-pattern morphology (≤4%).

In the study by Söderlund and Lundin[14] there was no significant difference between the two AI groups (group A with AI < 7% and group B with AI ≥ 7%) when ICSI was performed, with fertilization rates of 65.8% and 63.5%, respectively. The study showed that in semen samples with < 5% morphologically normal spermatozoa and an AI ≥ 7% the mean fertilization rate was about 70%, compared with the mean fertilization rate of 40% in the < 7% AI group. The conclusion of Söderlund and Lundin was that evaluation of the sperm morphology and AI in combination with the total number of normal spermatozoa available after sperm preparation has a better predictive value for the choice of IVF or ICSI treatment than that of the basic semen parameters alone[14]. Rhemrev et al. suggested that patients with an AI < 5% may benefit from ICSI to prevent total fertilization failure and/or that males with < 2% morphologically normal spermatozoa should go for ICSI, and concluded that the evaluation of sperm morphology and AI in combination with the total number of motile sperm available after sperm preparation/separation may have a better predictive value for choice of IVF or ICSI treatment than the basic semen parameters alone[15].

CONCLUSIONS

The AI can play an important role in the decision-making process of assisted reproductive treatment procedures. Over time, the AI cut-off value for expected IVF rates of ≥ 50% has been lowered from ≥ 16% normal acrosomes to ≥ 9%, and determined to be at ≥ 8% to distinguish between a fertile and a subfertile population. However, the most important aspect is to decide whether to advise couples to undergo the ICSI procedure or not, and for this purpose a cut-off AI value of ≤ 6% normal acrosomes was determined by Menkveld et al.[51] as well as by Söderlund and Lundin[14], and < 5% by Rhemrev et al.[15]. Both Söderlund and Lundin, and Rhemrev et al. suggested that the combination of AI cut-off value

and total progressively motile spermatozoa number obtained after sperm preparation ($< 1.10 \times 10^6$/ml and $< 1.0 \times 10^6$/ml, respectively) are strong tools in the decision whether to perform ICSI[14,15].

REFERENCES

1. Menkveld R, et al. The evaluation of morphological characteristics of human spermatozoa according to stricter criteria. Hum Reprod 1990; 5: 586
2. Kruger TF, et al. Sperm morphological features as a prognostic factor in in vitro fertilization. Fertil Steril 1986; 46: 1118
3. Kruger TF, et al. Predictive value of abnormal sperm morphology in in vitro fertilization. Fertil Steril 1988; 49: 122
4. Van Zyl JA, Kotze TJvW, Menkveld R. Predictive value of spermatozoa morphology in natural fertilization. In Acosta AA, et al., eds. Human Spermatozoa in Assisted Reproduction. Baltimore: Williams & Wilkins, 1990: 319
5. Coetzee K, Kruger TF, Lombard CJ. Predictive value of normal sperm morphology: a structured literature review. Hum Reprod Update 1998; 4: 73
6. Fernández JL, et al. The sperm chromatin dispersion test: a simple method for the determination of sperm DNA fragmentation. J Androl 2003; 24: 59
7. Evenson DP, Larson KL, Jost LK. Sperm chromatin structure assay: its clinical use for detecting sperm DNA fragmentation in male infertility and comparisons with other techniques. J Androl 2002; 23: 25
8. Sutovsky P, Terada Y, Schatten G. Ubiquitin-based sperm assay for the diagnosis of male factor infertility. Hum Reprod 2001; 16: 250
9. Rhemrev JPT, et al. The postwash total progressive motile sperm cell count is a reliable predictor of total fertilization failure during in vitro fertilization treatment. Fertil Steril 2001; 76: 884
10. Aziz N, et al. The sperm deformity index: a reliable predictor of the outcome of oocyte fertilization in vitro. Fertil Steril 1996; 66: 1000
11. Chan PJ, et al. Spermac stain analysis of human sperm acrosomes. Fertil Steril 1999; 72: 124
12. Menkveld R, et al. Acrosomal morphology as a novel criterion for male fertility diagnosis: relation with acrosin activity, morphology (strict criteria), and fertilization in vitro. Fertil Steril 1996; 65: 637

13. Jeyendran RS, Zaneveld LJD. Controversies in the development and validation of new sperm assays. Fertil Steril 1993; 59: 726

14. Söderlund B, Lundin K. Acrosome index is not an absolute predictor of the outcome following conventional in vitro fertilization and intracytoplasmic sperm injection. J Assist Reprod Genet 2001; 18: 483

15. Rhemrev JPT, et al. The acrosome index, radical buffer capacity and number of isolated progressively motile spermatozoa predict IVF results. Hum Reprod 2001; 16: 1885

16. Kruger TF, Menkveld R. Acrosome reaction, acrosin levels, and sperm morphology in assisted reproduction. Assist Reprod Rev 1996; 6: 27

17. Mortimer D, Menkveld R. Sperm morphology assessment – historical perspectives and current opinions. J Androl 2001; 22: 192

18. Menkveld R. The use of the acrosome index in assisted reproduction. In Kruger TF, Franken DR, eds. Atlas of Human Sperm Morphology Evaluation. London: Taylor & Francis, 2004: 35

19. Schill W-B. Some disturbances of acrosomal development and function in human spermatozoa. Hum Reprod 1991; 6: 969

20. Mortimer D. Practical Laboratory Andrology. Oxford: Oxford University Press, 1994.

21. Wassarman PM. Fertilization in mammals. Sci Am 1988; 256: 52

22. Menkveld R, et al. Sperm selection capacity of the human zona pellucida. Mol Reprod Develop 1991; 30: 346

23. Liu DY, Baker HWG. Morphology of spermatozoa bound to the zona pellucida of human oocytes that failed to fertilize in vitro. J Reprod Fertil 1992; 94: 71

24. Garrett G, Baker WHG. A new fully automated system for the morphometric analysis of human sperm heads. Fertil Steril 1995; 63:1306

25. Menkveld R, et al. Relationship between human sperm acrosomal morphology and acrosomal function. J Assist Reprod Genet 2003; 20: 432

26. Bastiaan HS, et al. Relationship between zona pellucida-induced acrosome reaction, sperm morphology, sperm–zona pellucida binding, and in vitro fertilization. Fertil Steril 2003; 79: 49

27. Liu DY, Baker HWG. Disordered zona pellucida-induced acrosome reaction and failure of in vitro fertilization in patients with unexplained infertility. Fertil Steril 2003; 79: 74

28. Benoff S, et al. Numerical dose-compensated in vitro fertilization inseminations yield high fertilization and pregnancy rates. Fertil Steril 1999; 71: 1019

29. Jeulin C, et al. Sperm factors related to failure of human in-vitro fertilization. J Reprod Fertil 1986; 76: 735

30. Menkveld R, Kruger TF. Evaluation of sperm morphology by light microscopy. In Acosta AA, Kruger TF, eds. Human Spermatozoa in Assisted Reproduction. Carnforth: Parthenon Publishing, 1996: 89

31. Hofmann N, Haider SG. Neue Ergebnisse morphologisher diagnostik der Spermatogenesestörungen. Gynaköloge 1985; 18: 70

32. Baccetti B, et al. Genetic sperm defects and consanguinity. Hum Reprod 2001; 16: 1365

33. Baccetti B, et al. A 'miniacrosome' sperm defect causing infertility in two brothers. J Androl 1991; 12: 104

34. Favero R, et al. Embryo development, pregancy and twin delivery after microinjection of 'stump' spermatozoa. Andrologia 1999; 31: 335

35. Menkveld R, et al. Relationships between sperm acrosomal status, acrosin activity, morphology (strict Tygerberg criteria) and fertilization in vitro. Hum Reprod 1994; 9 (Suppl 4): 99

36. Henkel R, et al. Effect of reactive oxygen species produced by spermatozoa and leukocytes on sperm function in non-leukocytospermic patients. Fertil Steril 2005; 83: 635

37. Menkveld R, et al. Acrosomal morphology as an additional new criterion for male fertility diagnosis: relationship with sperm functional aspects. Hum Reprod 1995; 10 (Suppl 2): 100

38. Heywinkel E, Freudl G, Hofmann N. Acrosome reaction of spermatozoa with different morphology. Andrologia 1993; 25: 137

39. Menkveld R, Stander FSH, Kruger TF. Comparison between acrosome index and teratozoospermia index as additional criteria to sperm morphology in the prediction of expected in-vitro fertilisation outcome. Hum Reprod 1998; 13 (Abstr book 1): 52

40. World Health Organization. WHO Laboratory Manual for the Examination of Human Semen and Sperm–Cervical Mucus Interaction, 3rd edn. Cambridge: Cambridge University Press, 1992

41. Menkveld R, et al. Semen parameters including WHO and strict criteria morphology, in a fertile and subfertile population: an effort towards standardisation of in vivo thresholds. Hum Reprod 2001; 16: 1165

42. Palermo G, et al. Pregnancies after intracytoplasmic injection of a single spermatozoon into an oocyte. Lancet 1992; 340: 17

43. In't Veld PA, et al. Intracytoplasmic sperm injection (ICSI) and chromosomally abnormal spermatozoa. Hum Reprod 1997; 12: 752

44. Bonduelle M, et al. Incidence of chromosomal aberrations in children born after assisted reproduction through intracytoplasmic sperm injection. Hum Reprod 1998; 13: 781

45. Aytoz A, et al. Outcome of pregnancies after intracytoplasmic sperm injection and the effect of sperm origin and quality on this outcome. Fertil Steril 1998; 70: 500

46. Greco E, et al. Efficient treatment of infertility due to sperm DNA damage by ICSI with testicular spermatozoa. Hum Reprod 2005; 20: 266

47. Henkel R, et al. Influence of deoxyribonucleic acid damage on fertilization and pregnancy. Fertil Steril 2004; 81: 965

48. Bianchi PG, et al. Human cervical mucus can act in vitro as a selective barrier against spermatozoa carrying fragmented DNA and chromatin structural abnormalities. J Assist Reprod Genet 2004; 21: 97

49. Strassburger D, et al. Very low counts affects the results of intracytoplasmic sperm injection. J Assist Reprod Genet 2000; 17: 431

50. Coetzee K, et al. Short communication: an intracytoplasmic sperm injection pregnancy with a globozoospermia male. J Assist Reprod Genet 2001; 18: 311

51. Menkveld R, et al. The use of the acrosome index as an additional morphology parameter in the clinical selection of patients for ICSI. Hum Reprod 1999; 14 (Abstr book 1): 156

13

Acrosome reaction: physiology and its value in clinical practice

Daniel R Franken, Hadley S Bastiaan, Sergio Oehninger

INTRODUCTION

For successful fertilization of oocytes by spermatozoa, a set of functionally normal parameters with regard to oocyte and spermatozoon maturity is of paramount importance. In the spermatozoon, besides motility and zona binding, the occurrence of the acrosome reaction is of primary importance in the development of functional capability. However, before spermatozoa are able to undergo the acrosome reaction, essential modifications in cell physiology of the sperm, called capacitation, must occur. Numerous studies have tried to elucidate the precise biochemical and biophysical changes involved in the process determining a spermatozoon's fertilizing capacity. The normal progress of these changes may display important biomarkers of fertilizing ability, including the ability of the sperm to penetrate the cumulus oophorus, the corona radiata, the zona pellucida (ZP) and the vitelline membrane.

The ability to evaluate the human acrosome reaction is, however, restricted by a practical limitation. The loss of the human acrosome cannot be observed on living sperm by phase-contrast or differential interference-contrast microscopy, because of its relatively small size compared with that of other mammalian species. Initially, best results were obtained by electron microscopy; this method, however, is not suited for routine

analysis because of its expense and complexity. The need thus arose for a relatively simple test by which the human acrosome reaction could be quantified at the light microscope level. In addition, the labile nature of the human sperm acrosome makes analysis of the reaction problematic. The chosen procedure must therefore be able to distinguish between normal and degenerative reactions.

In addition to the above limitations, the existence of multifactorial induction and regulating systems and the individual perspectives and methods of measurement chosen by laboratories contribute to the uncertainty that still exists regarding the subject.

THE BIOCHEMISTRY OF CAPACITATION AND THE ACROSOME REACTION

The acrosome of a human spermatozoon is a membrane-bound organelle that develops during spermatogenesis as a product of the Golgi complex. It surrounds the anterior portion of the sperm nucleus and can be divided into the following components:

- Plasma membrane;
- Outer acrosomal membrane;

- Acrosomal matrix;

- Inner acrosomal membrane;

- Equatorial segment.

Factors inhibiting capacitation are incorporated into the membranes of sperm during maturation in the epididymis[1,2]. These factors include sialoglycoproteins, sulfoglycerolipids and steroid sulfates, which induce a significant increase in the net negative charge of the outer acrosomal membrane[3]. This state of decapacitation (stability) is maintained after ejaculation by the presence of inhibitory macromolecules in the seminal plasma[4] and in the lower areas of the female reproductive tract[1]. A specific glycoprotein has been identified as the primary decapacitator[1]; it is bound to the outer acrosomal membrane and can prevent interaction with extracellular signals as well as inhibit ion channel activity and/or enzymes[5]. This stability is further enhanced by the incorporation of cholesterol into the acrosomal membrane complex, preferentially into the plasma membrane.

Sperm acquire their fertilizing ability *in vivo* during their migration through the female genital tract. Capacitation can also be induced *in vitro* in chemically defined media[6]. The complete process, however, is not yet fully understood, but is thought to involve major biochemical and biophysical changes in the membrane complex, energy metabolism and ion permeability. The most significant changes are:

- Modification, redistribution and/or loss of the epididymal seminal plasma and cervical decapacitation factors – by exogenous or endogenous proteases specifically activated (plasmin, kallikrein and acrosin)[1,2];

- Net negative charge decrease by endogenous hydrolases (sterol sulfatase)[3];

- Membrane fluidity increase by the efflux of cholesterol, altering the cholesterol/phospholipid ratio and the influx of unsaturated fatty acids; these changes are thought to be serum albumin-mediated[3,7];

- Altered permeability allowing the increased uptake of calcium ions, glucose and oxygen, resulting in an elevated energy state, inducing hyperactivated motility and ability to undergo the acrosome reaction[8,9].

Notwithstanding the extent of these changes, capacitation is also thought to be a reversible event. The exact threshold of irreversibility, however, remains undefined, i.e. what constitutes the boundary between capacitation and the acrosome reaction. Many of these structural changes proposed to characterize capacitation may, however, be irreversible, which may lead to an untimely acrosome reaction. The acrosome reaction can therefore be seen as the end-point of capacitation.

Signals for initiation of the acrosome reaction are most likely received by one or more receptors on the plasma membrane surface, which transmit the message across the membrane. Zaneveld *et al.*[5] proposed a mechanism by which membrane receptor activation of guanosine triphosphate (GTP)-binding proteins stimulates second-messenger systems which regulate ion transport. An endogenous calcium ion threshold concentration has long been thought of as the primary inducer of the acrosome reaction[8,10]. Yanagimachi and Usui[11] showed that upon the addition of calcium, but not magnesium, guinea-pig sperm incubated for several hours in calcium-free medium underwent the acrosome reaction within 10 minutes. Since then, calcium has been implicated in many reactions leading to complete loss of the acrosome and eventually fertilization[10]:

- Activation of many enzymes (acrosin, hyaluronidase, phospholipase A2);

- Activation of enzyme messenger systems (adenylate cyclase);

- Neutralization of the net negative charge;

- Induction of hyperactivated motility[3].

Stock and Fraser[12] examined the extracellular Ca^{2+} requirements for the support of capacitation and the spontaneous acrosome reaction in human spermatozoa, and concluded that the optimal conditions for capacitation and the acrosome reaction in human spermatozoa require extracellular Ca^{2+} at 1.80 mmol/l with calcium channels providing a means of calcium entry. In contrast, White et al.[13] found that the acrosome reaction rates at 4 hours and 20 hours were little different in media with or without calcium, although the absence of calcium had a significant effect on the quality of motility.

The human sperm acrosome reaction is an exocytotic event characterized by significant ultrastructural changes leading to the complete loss of the outer acrosomal cap, following:

- Decondensation of the acrosomal matrix;

- Fenestration and vesiculation of the plasma membrane and outer acrosomal membrane;

- Dispersion of the vesicles;

- Release of the acrosomal content.

Nagae et al.[14] proposed a unique morphological sequence for this acrosome reaction. Vesicles established in the intermediate stage were formed by the invagination and pinching off of the outer acrosomal membrane and the plasma membrane. Stock et al. described a similar characterization[15]. In contrast, Yudin et al.[16] found that human sperm undergo an acrosome reaction similar to that of other mammals, in which the outer acrosomal and plasma membranes initially fuse by fenestration followed by vesiculation. The dispersion of these vesicles leaves the spermatozoon surrounded by a single, continuous membrane, i.e. the inner acrosomal membrane. In addition to these changes, the membrane proteins of the plasma membrane overlying the equatorial/postacrosomal region of the sperm head undergo a conformational change, resulting in activation[3]. This activation may facilitate fusion of the sperm with the oocyte vitelline membrane.

The loss of the membranes also releases or exposes activated lysins, assisting sperm penetration of the ZP^2. Acrosin, a trypsin-like serine protease found in the acrosome, has been implicated

in a number of events leading to fertilization. These include assisting sperm penetration of the ZP, triggering of the acrosome reaction[2] and activation of regulatory enzymes involved in Ca^{2+} transport[5]. Studies using p-aminobenzamidine (PABA)[17], an inhibitor of mouse sperm acrosin, have shown that acrosin is a necessary factor for dispersal of the acrosomal matrix, probably through the activation of proacrosin. In the presence of PABA, the membranes undergo normal vesiculation, but ZP penetration is inhibited.

MEASUREMENT OF THE ACROSOME REACTION IN HUMAN SPERMATOZOA

Capacitation and the acrosome reaction can be induced chemically, providing a controlled means for the evaluation of acrosomal exocytosis. Table 13.1 presents agents and methods commonly used to monitor and trigger the acrosome reaction. The acrosome reaction can be examined during basal conditions (incubating sperm under capacitating conditions) and/or following exogenous induction with pharmacological or physiological agonists. Inducers that have been analyzed in the clinical setting include the calcium ionophore

Table 13.1 Agents and methods commonly used to monitor the spontaneous and induced acrosome reaction

Inducers of the acrosome reaction
Calcium ionophore
Pentoxifylline
Follicular fluid
Progesterone
Solubilized zona pellucida

Methods to assess the acrosome reaction
Optical microscopy: triple-staining
Transmission electron microscopy
Chlortetracycline fluorescent assay
Fluorescent lectins
Labeling with antibodies
Flow cytometry

A23187[18–21], pentoxifylline[22,23], steroids[24–27], follicular fluid (FF)[28], solubilized ZP[29–31] and low temperature[20]. The methodologies used to examine acrosomal exocytosis have included triple staining (optic microscopy)[32], transmission electron microscopy[33], chlortetracycline fluorescent assay[34], fluorescent lectins[35,36], labeling with antibodies[37] and flow cytometry[38].

There are, however, inherent negative side-effects that must be taken into account, such as the possible negative effect on motility, and the fact that the means of induction overrides the normal processes involved in the acrosome reaction. For example, using a calcium ionophore, a toxic chemical substance, as the inducer, the time required for capacitation is minimized. The addition of complex biological fluids such as maternal cord serum, FF, granulosa cells, cumulus oophorus and ZP, even though uncontrolled in nature, is physiologically more correct. This is of particular relevance when future improvements in the treatment in male infertility are to be introduced into an assisted reproduction program, and also for furthering our knowledge of the *in vivo* regulatory system.

As mentioned above, several techniques have been employed to detect the acrosome reaction, each with its own level of characterization. Aitken and Brindle[39], however, showed that probes targeting different components involved in the acrosome reaction measure acrosomal loss at different rates. The labile nature of the acrosomal vesicle also requires a means of determining sperm viability and distinguishing between 'normal' and degenerative reactions. In the triple-stain technique according to Talbot and Chacon[35], trypan blue is used. Cross *et al.*[36] included the supravital stain Hoechst 33258, while Aitken *et al.*[21], in their protocol for assessing the ability of viable human spermatozoa to acrosome-react in response to A23187, employed a fluorescein-conjugated lectin in concert with the hypo-osmotic swelling test. The use of these different techniques may have a significant influence on the interpretation and comparison of results. This is illustrated by the often equivocal results obtained in acrosome reaction studies.

PHYSIOLOGICAL INDUCERS AND REGULATORS OF THE ACROSOME REACTION

Stock *et al.*[15] found that 32% of sperm coincubated with oocyte–cumulus complexes for 14–18 hours had initiated or completed the acrosome reaction. The effect of a number of female reproductive tract products on sperm fertilizing capacity was evaluated by coincubating fertile sperm samples with endometrial, oviductal, granulosa and cumulus cells, FF and maternal serum, by Bastias *et al.*[40]. Compared with control samples, endometrial and oviductal cell cultures did not alter sperm fertilizing capacity or their movement characteristics. Sperm coincubated with FF, granulosa cells or cumulus cells, however, exhibited a significantly higher ability to penetrate zona-free hamster ova. It is therefore reasonable to propose that secretions of cumulus cells could be involved in regulation of the sperm acrosome reaction.

Siegel *et al.*[41] concluded from their study that components within the FF might influence sperm physiology and enhance sperm fertilizing capacity by activating sperm proteinase systems involved in sperm reaction and interaction. An active Sephadex® G-75 fraction identified in FF was found to stimulate a rapid, transient increase in the intracellular free Ca^{2+} in human spermatozoa[42]. The ability of this fraction to induce the acrosome reaction led the authors to conclude that this influx of Ca^{2+} is responsible for the initiation of acrosomal exocytosis. Using indirect immunofluorescence, FF was found to induce the acrosome reaction rapidly after the sperm had been incubated for at least 10 hours[43]. Induction of the human acrosome reaction by whole FF and/or the active Sephadex G-75 component was found to satisfy the ultrastructural criteria known for physiological reactions, as shown by transmission electron microscopy[16].

Yudin *et al.*[16] also showed that human sperm capacitated for 6 hours at 40°C and then incubated with FF for 180 seconds resulted in 40% of the sperm reacting. Sperm incubated for 22 hours before FF treatment had their acrosome reaction rate enhanced six-fold, illustrating the potential effect of FF. An adequate preincubation period followed by FF treatment therefore seems to result in the synchronization of capacitation and facilitation of the acrosome reaction. In contrast, Stock *et al.*[44], examining the incidence of spontaneous acrosome reactions in human spermatozoa exposed to FF, found that FF can stimulate the acrosome reaction, but only after continuous exposure (> 6 hours) to 50% FF/medium. A short exposure (1 hour), even after 24 hours of preincubation, did not induce the reaction.

Recent studies have shown that the human sperm acrosome reaction-inducing activity in FF can be attributed to progesterone (P). Osman *et al.*[24] purified an active fraction from the fluid aspirated from preovulatory human follicles and identified it as 4-pregnen-3,20-dione (progesterone) and 4-pregnen-17α-ol-3,20-dione (17-hydroxyprogesterone). This was confirmed by Blackmore *et al.*[25], Foresta *et al.*[45] and Baldi *et al.*[46], who found that only P and 17-hydroxyprogesterone were able to induce a rapid, long-lasting, dose-dependent increase of intracellular free calcium, with maximum effect being obtained with 1.0 μg/ml. Sueldo *et al.*[27], however, found that 1.0 μg/ml of P enhanced the acrosome reaction only after 24 hours of incubation.

Luconi *et al.*[47] found several rapid non-genomic effects of P and estrogen (E) in human spermatozoa. They seem to be mediated by the steroids binding to specific receptors on the plasma membrane that are different from the classical ones. Progesterone, specifically, has been demonstrated to stimulate calcium influx, tyrosine phosphorylation of various sperm proteins, including extracellular signaling-regulated kinases, chloride efflux and cyclic adenosine monophosphate (cAMP) increase, finally resulting in the activation of spermatozoa through the induction of capacitation, hyperactivated motility and the acrosome reaction. On the other hand, E, which is present in micromolar levels in follicular fluid, seems to modulate sperm responsiveness to P. This occurs when E acts rapidly on calcium influx and on protein tyrosine phosphorylation.

In general, the isolation and characterization of the putative membrane receptors for P (mPR) and E (mER) in spermatozoa are still elusive. Luconi[47] obtained evidence supporting the existence and functional activity of mPR and mER in human spermatozoa. To characterize these membrane receptors, they used two antibodies directed against the ligand-binding domains of the classical receptors, namely c262 and H222 antibodies for PR and ER, respectively, hypothesizing that these regions should be conserved between non-genomic and genomic receptors. In Western blot analysis of sperm lysates, the antibodies detected a band of about 57 kDa for PR and 29 kDa for ER, excluding the presence of the classical receptors. On live human spermatozoa, both antibodies were able to block the calcium and AR response to P and E, respectively, whereas antibodies directed against different domains of the classical PR and ER were ineffective. Furthermore, c262 antibody also blocks *in vitro* the human sperm penetration of hamster oocytes. Taken together, all these data strongly support the existence of mPR and mER different from the classical ones, mediating rapid effects of these steroid hormones in human spermatozoa.

Siegel *et al.*[41] also found that FF obtained from different women under different stimulation regimens did not affect the fertilizing potential differently. Morales *et al.*[48], however, found that there was a positive, highly significant ($r = 0.72$; $p > 0.005$) correlation between the acrosome reaction-inducing activity and the P level of each FF sample.

Nevertheless, recent reports on the chemical nature of the acrosome reaction-inducing molecule present in FF have been contradictory. In contrast to the authors who attributed the acrosome reaction-inducing activity present in human

FF to P, Miska et al.[49] reported evidence to suggest that this substance is a protein. These authors identified a protein with a molecular mass of about 50 kDa and demonstrated the substance's sensitivity to unspecific proteases, increased temperature and pH changes. In a further study[50], the same authors identified the acrosome reaction-inducing substance (ARIS) as the progesterone-binding protein corticoid-binding globulin (CBG). Using anti-human CBG antibodies and dextran-coated charcoal they showed that only P bound to CBG could induce the acrosome reaction. CBG is a member of the SERPIN (serine proteinase inhibitor) superfamily that binds P tightly. Proteolysis by serine proteinases results in the release of this steroid hormone. This mechanism is thought to be essential in the activation of neutrophils by delivering high local concentrations of corticoids in inflammatory processes.

The serine proteinase involved in the spermatozoon is acrosin, localized at the plasma membrane, with inactive proacrosin located within the acrosome. During capacitation, proacrosin and acrosin are exposed at the plasma membrane. The CBG–progesterone complex, which may become bound on the plasma membrane, will therefore be proteolytically cleaved by exposed acrosin, leading to high local concentrations of P and subsequent induction of the acrosome reaction, confirming the important role of acrosin in physiological induction of the acrosome reaction. The exact mechanism underlying P-stimulated calcium entry in human sperm has, however, not been fully established. Another question to be answered concerns the source of CBG. Whether it is of liver origin, where it is known to be produced, and then is accumulated in FF, or whether the cumulus or granulosa cells can synthesize this protein, still have to be established.

The importance of the ZP for induction of the acrosome reaction, however, is well recognized[29–31,51–53]. Spermatozoa must penetrate this last barrier in the reacted state before they can penetrate and fertilize the oocyte. In vitro studies by Saling and Storey[54], using mouse sperm, were

the first to demonstrate a role for the ZP in the acrosome reaction. They incubated cumulus-free eggs with sperm suspensions in which > 50% of the population had undergone the acrosome reaction. After gradient centrifugation, only acrosome-intact sperm were detected on the ZP. They concluded that the acrosome reaction of a fertilizing mouse sperm occurs on the ZP. Saling et al.[55] and Bleil and Wassarman[56] maintained that, at least in the mouse, the acrosome reaction is induced by a ZP constituent, the glycoprotein ZP3. They proposed the following concept:

- Sperm attachment to the ZP;

- Specific and irreversible binding to the ZP;

- Physiological induction of the acrosome reaction;

- ZP penetration.

Cross et al.[36] used two approaches to test the ability of the human ZP to induce acrosomal exocytosis in human sperm. Non-viable human oocytes and acid-disaggregated zonae were used, and both the zona binding and exposure to disaggregated zona induced the acrosome reaction. Using the monoclonal antibody T-6, Coddington et al.[57] found that 93% of sperm bound to bisected human ZP exhibited immunofluorescent patterns indicative of the acrosome reaction. Hoshi et al.[58] observed that the acrosome reaction rate after sperm attachment to the zona for 6 hours was $35.7 \pm 17.7\%$, which was higher than in controls ($2.8 \pm 1.9\%$). The results so far indicate that the ability of spermatozoa to migrate to the ZP is a closely regulated process, ensuring that only sperm at the correct stage attach to and penetrate the ZP.

It has been shown that P exerts a priming effect on the ZP-stimulated acrosome reaction in the mouse[59] and in the human[60]. In the former studies, treatment with P followed by ZP led to maximal breakdown of phosphatidylinositol-4,5-bisphosphate (PIP2), signaling a priming role for P in the initiation of exocytosis. Cross et al.[29] were the first to report that treatment of human spermatozoa in suspension with acid-disaggregated human ZP (2–4 zonae pellucidae (ZP)/μl) increased the incidence of acrosome-reacted spermatozoa.

Lee et al.[30] demonstrated that pertussis toxin treatment of human spermatozoa inhibited the (solubilized) ZP-induced acrosome reaction. In contrast, acrosomal exocytosis induced by the calcium ionophore A-23187 was not inhibited by pertussis toxin pretreatment. Studies by Franken et al.[31] showed a dose-dependent effect of solubilized human ZP on the acrosome reaction in the range 0.25–1 ZP/μl, and also confirmed the involvement of G_i-protein during the ZP-induced acrosome reaction of human spermatozoa. More recently, Franken et al.[51] reported the validation of a new microassay using minimal volumes of solubilized, human ZP to test the physiological induction of the acrosome reaction in human spermatozoa (ZP-induced acrosome reaction test or ZIAR). In such studies, a dose-dependent effect of solubilized ZP on acrosomal exocytosis was observed, reaching maximal induction using 1.25–2.5 ZP/μl for both the microassay and the standard (macro)assay. Furthermore, the inducibility of the acrosome reaction by a calcium ionophore was similar in both assays.

Differences among species may account for the disparity in the results published, but the major differences among researchers are probably caused by the different experimental conditions and the varied assessment criteria. The *in vitro* conditions under which the work is performed can have a dramatic effect on the normal biochemical (metabolic and acrosomal) reactions of sperm, and also on the maturity of the oocyte–cumulus complexes and the molecules trapped in the complexes.

THE ACROSOME REACTION SITE

The precise site of the acrosome reaction still remains clouded by controversy. Three possible sites have been proposed[3]:

- The oviductal fluid of the ampulla;

- The cumulus matrix;

- The surface of the zona pellucida.

The majority of the initial sperm acrosome reaction site studies were performed on the cauda epididymal sperm of the golden hamster, because of its relatively large acrosomal cap. The progress of the acrosome reaction can therefore be followed by phase-contrast microscopy. Data from the oviductal studies are, however, equivocal. Cummins and Yanagimachi[61] studied the ampullary contents of female hamsters by phase-contrast microscopy, 4–10 hours after insemination with golden-hamster caudal epididymal sperm, and observed that 93 of 96 sperm swimming freely had modified and swollen acrosomal caps. In an earlier study, Yanagimachi and Phillips[62], also using phase-microscopy, found that only four of 14 free-swimming golden-hamster sperm had modified acrosomal caps.

Evaluating the cumulus matrix as the site of acrosomal reaction, Cummins and Yanagimachi[61] reported that all motile golden-hamster spermatozoa observed in the cumuli from oviducts had undergone or were undergoing the acrosome reaction. Yanagimachi and Phillips[62] reported that motile sperm, within the cumulus of golden-hamster cumulus-intact complexes from the ampulla, had modified acrosomes. However, in a videotaped study, Cherr et al.[63] found that only 3–6% of sperm had actually completed the acrosome reaction within the cumulus matrix, which was comparable to control levels of the acrosome reaction occurring in free-swimming sperm. Their study included both cumulus-intact and cumulus-free eggs, with a higher percentage of reacted sperm found in association with the zona pellucida of cumulus-intact eggs than with the ZP of cumulus-free eggs.

Tesarik[64] undertook a study to determine the site of the acrosome reaction of spermatozoa penetrating into freshly inseminated human oocytes. The inseminated oocytes were treated with an antiacrosin monoclonal antibody, and the bound antibody visualized at the ultrastructural level with the use of a second peroxidase-conjugated antibody. His findings indicated that the acrosome reaction of the fertilizing spermatozoon must be exactly synchronized with its penetration through the egg vestments by the action of specific acrosome reaction-promoting substances in the oocyte–cumulus complex. Quantitative analysis of the results showed that the number of spermatozoa within the ZP corresponded to the number of acrosin deposits associated with acrosomal ghosts on the ZP surface.

Using the triple-stain technique, the acrosomal status of sperm outside and within the cumulus during *in vitro* fertilization was examined[65]. The percentage of sperm undergoing the acrosome reaction increased significantly ($p < 0.05$) from 14.5 ± 1.5 to 24.5 ± 1.9 when incubated with a cumulus mass, and further increased to 49 ± 3.3 when incubated with mature expanded cumulus tissue containing an oocyte. White *et al.*[13] exposed prepared spermatozoa for 20–30 minutes to large pieces of human cumulus oophorus; while these spermatozoa were able to penetrate deep into the cumulus mass, none were found to have clearly undergone the acrosome reaction. From this study they also concluded that spermatozoa did not require a capacitation period for penetration.

In an *in vitro* system, depolymerization (softening) of the cumulus matrix may occur because of the high sperm concentration used. This may allow sperm to reach the zona pellucida with intact acrosomes. Cummins and Yanagimachi[61] therefore studied the ability of hamster sperm to penetrate intact cumulus matrices at low (3 : 1) sperm/egg ratios. Uncapacitated sperm were unable to penetrate the cumuli; at least 2 hours of preincubation were required. Of the 628 *in vitro* capacitated sperm seen in and on the cumuli, 270 could penetrate, of which only ten had intact unmodified acrosomes. They concluded that penetration of the cumulus was limited to a phase in capacitation before completion of the acrosome reaction, since sperm that had lost the acrosomal cap

penetrated poorly and showed reduced viability. Corselli and Talbot[66] also developed a system in which physiological sperm numbers (1–100) were used to challenge fresh hamster oocyte–cumulus complexes in capillary tubes. Their results showed that capacitated acrosome-intact hamster sperm can penetrate the extracellular matrix between the cumulus cells and can ultimately bind to the ZP. The results obtained by these two groups indicated that uncapacitated sperm tend to adhere to the cumulus cells on the periphery and are unable to penetrate, and that sperm that have lost the acrosomal cap also penetrate poorly.

The cumulus matrix may therefore be seen as a selection barrier, allowing only morphologically normal sperm that can undergo a normal acrosome reaction to penetrate the zona pellucida, and/or it may contain molecules that influence the ability of sperm to undergo the reaction. CBG and P, which are present in high concentrations in the cumulus matrix, have been proposed as the physiological stimulus for initiation of the acrosome reaction.

CLINICAL RELEVANCE OF THE ACROSOME REACTION

In two independent experiments, Barros *et al.*[67] and Singer *et al.*[68] using golden-hamster sperm and human sperm, respectively, found that sperm became infertile with prolonged incubation, as judged by their ability to bind to and penetrate the ZP. The reason for this decline in penetration with increasing incubation time was attributed to an increase in the percentage of acrosome-reacted sperm. In contrast, an increase in the penetration of zona-free hamster eggs was seen with increasing incubation time (increase in the acrosome-reacted population). Thus, acrosome-reacted sperm are prevented from penetrating the ZP. These results indicate that the fertilizing ability of spermatozoa is a time-dependent process.

Although only acrosome-reacted spermatozoa are capable of fusing with zona-free oocytes, there is no significant correlation between the proportion of acrosome-reacted cells and the levels of sperm–oocyte fusion observed. These two bioassays are thus measuring two different aspects of the sperm's ability to acrosome-react. White et al.[13] similarly concluded that there was no relationship between the acrosome reaction rate and the fertilization rate of normal human oocytes in vitro. In a study to assess whether patients who did not fertilize human oocytes in vitro could be identified by a lack of acrosomal response of their spermatozoa, Pampiglione et al.[69] found that patients who fertilized oocytes responded like fertile donors. It was also calculated that an acrosome reaction rate of < 31.3% predicted fertilization failure in 100% of cases. While spontaneous reactions bore no relation to fertility, the inducibility of the acrosome reaction (i.e. the difference between spontaneous and induced acrosome reaction), which describes the ability of viable sperm to undergo the acrosome reaction, was significantly reduced or absent in subfertile men, indicating acrosomal dysfunction as a likely cause of fertilization failure[19].

Henkel et al.[70] showed that inducibility should be at least 7.5% to be indicative of good fertilization. A > 13% level of acrosome-reacted sperm after induction of the acrosome reaction was also shown to have predictive value for fertilizing potential, because elevated levels of sperm able to lose their acrosome are necessary for successful fertilization. For diagnostic purposes, the kind of induction, be it physiological by means of the ZP glycoproteins or non-physiological by the application of a calcium ionophore or low temperature, is apparently not important. However, inducibility and appropriate timing of the acrosome reaction with the penetration of the ZP[61] are prerequisites for good fertilization[52,71].

Liu and colleagues[72,73] reported a sperm defect called disordered ZP-induced acrosome reaction (DZPIAR). This defect was the cause of failure of sperm penetration in a group of in vitro fertilization (IVF) patients with a long duration of infertility. These patients were previously diagnosed as having idiopathic infertility with repeated poor or no fertilization during IVF treatment.

Bastiaan et al.[52,71] and Esterhuizen et al.[53] reported similar findings in a study in which 164 andrology referrals were divided according to the percentage of normal spermatozoa in the ejaculate, namely < 4% normal forms ($n = 71$), 5–14% normal forms ($n = 73$) and > 14% normal forms ($n = 20$). ZIAR data for the < 4%, 5–14% and > 14% groups were 9.6 (± 0.6)%, 13.9 (± 0.5)% and 15.0 (± 1.1)%, respectively. The ZIAR result for fertile control men was 26.6 (± 1.4)%, which differed significantly from that of the three andrology referral groups. Likewise, significant differences were recorded during the hemizona assay, namely, 38.0% (< 4% normal forms), 54.5% (5–14% normal forms) and 62.6% (> 14% normal forms). Among the group with > 14% normal (Table 13.2) forms, five cases out of 21 (23%) had impaired ZIAR outcome (< 15%). Three (14%) of these men had normal morphology and sperm–zona binding, but showed a decrease in ZIAR results. The study concluded that ZIAR testing should become part of the second level of male fertility investigations, i.e. sperm functional testing, since 14% of andrology referrals revealed an impaired acrosome reaction response to solubilized ZP.

Table 13.2 Sperm–oocyte interaction results for five cases with impaired zona pellucida-induced acrosome reaction test (ZIAR)

Case	Sperm–zona binding (HZI)	Morphology (% normal forms)	ZIAR (%)
1	77	11	16
2	92	6	16
3	63	9	15
4	26	6	14
5	37	12	14

HZI, hemizona binding index

Liu and Baker[72] also studied the frequency of defective sperm–ZP interaction in oligozoospermic infertile men. Sperm–ZP binding and the ZP-induced acrosome reaction were performed in 72 infertile men with oligozoospermic semen (sperm count $< 20 \times 10^6$/ml). Oocytes that failed to fertilize in clinical IVF were used for the tests. Four oocytes were incubated for 2 hours with 2×10^6/ml motile sperm selected by swim-up from each semen sample. The number of sperm bound per ZP and the ZIAR were assessed. Under this condition, an average ≤ 40 sperm bound/ZP was defined as low sperm–ZP binding and a ZIAR $\leq 15\%$ was defined as low ZIAR. In the 72 oligozoospermic men, 28% had low sperm–ZP binding. Of those ($n = 52$) with normal sperm–ZP binding, 69% had low ZIAR. Overall, 78% had either low ZP binding or normal ZP binding but low ZIAR. Only 22% had both normal sperm–ZP binding and normal ZIAR. They concluded that oligozoospermic men have a very high frequency of defective sperm–ZP interaction, which may be a major cause of infertility or low fertilization rate in standard IVF.

Esterhuizen *et al.*[53] reported the ZP-induced acrosome reaction response (ZIAR) among 35 couples with normal and G-pattern (good prognosis) sperm morphology and repeated poor fertilization results during assisted reproduction treatment. Results were compared with *in vitro* fertilization rates of metaphase II oocytes. Interactive dot diagrams divided the patients into two groups, i.e. ZIAR $< 15\%$ and ZIAR $> 15\%$, with mean fertilization rates of 49% and 79%, respectively. The area under the curve was 99% and the 95% confidence interval did not include 0.5, demonstrating that the ZIAR test is able to predict fertilization failure among IVF patients.

CONCLUSIONS

The fertilizing spermatozoon undergoes a continuous reactionary process that is temporally and spatially regulated. Spermatozoa respond to signals during specific transformation stages and at defined sites that will ensure the binding to and penetration of the ZP. The asynchronous nature of the reaction may result in large-scale redundancy, because only the sperm in the right place at the right time will be able to penetrate the ZP and fertilize the oocyte. The *in vivo* situation appears to promote the probability of fertilization by ensuring that the maximum possible numbers of functionally competent spermatozoa reach the oocyte at the correct stage of capacitation.

We have shown that 14% of cases with unexplained infertility may have an impaired ZIAR, and should be treated with ICSI rather than IVF. The ZIAR[53] or DZPIAR[72] test has true diagnostic potential, as it can assist the clinician in identifying couples who will benefit from ICSI therapy. In the clinical management of infertility, allocation of patients between standard IVF and ICSI is mainly decided on the basis of specific sperm characteristics that play a role during fertilization. Patients with impaired sperm–zona interaction, i.e. zona pellucida binding and zona-induced acrosome reaction, have a higher success rate in the ICSI laboratory compared with IVF treatment[53,73]. Moreover, the implementation of these functional tests in the early stages of the work-up of men with subfertile basic sperm parameters or unexplained infertility should allow identification of those cases that ought to be directed to ICSI, avoiding loss of time secondary to the use of less successful options such as intrauterine insemination therapy.

REFERENCES

1. Oliphant G, Reynolds ALB, Thomas TS. Sperm surface components involved in the control of the acrosome reaction. Am J Anat 1985; 174: 269
2. Meizel S. Molecules that initiate or help stimulate the acrosome reaction by their interaction with mammalian sperm surface. Am J Anat 1985; 174: 285
3. Langlais J, Roberts KD. A molecular membrane model of sperm capacitation and the acrosome reaction of mammalian spermatozoa. Gamete Res 1985; 12: 183

4. Kanwar KC, Yanagimachi R, Lopata A. Effects of human seminal plasma on fertilization capacity of human spermatozoa. Fertil Steril 1979; 31: 321

5. Zaneveld LJD, et al. Human sperm capacitation and the acrosome reaction. Hum Reprod 1991; 6: 1265

6. Yanagimachi R. In vitro sperm capacitation and fertilization of golden hamster eggs in a chemically defined medium in in vitro fertilization and embryo transfer. In Hafez ESE, Semm K, eds. In Vitro Fertilization and Embryo Transfer. New York: Alan Liss, 1982: 65

7. Fleming AD, Yanagimachi R. Effect of various lipids on the acrosome reaction and fertilizing capacity of guinea pig spermatozoa, with special reference to the possible involvement of lysophospholipids in the acrosome reaction. Gamete Res 1981; 4: 253

8. Murphy SJ, Roldan ERS, Yanagimachi R. Effects of extracellular cations and energy substrates on the acrosome reaction of precapacitated guinea pig spermatozoa. Gamete Res 1986; 14: 1

9. Katz OF, Cherr GN, Lambert H. The evolution of hamster sperm motility during capacitation and interaction with the ovum vestments in vitro. Gamete Res 1986; 14: 333

10. Yanagimachi R. Calcium requirements for sperm–egg fusion in mammals. Biol Reprod 1978; 19: 949

11. Yanagimachi R, Usui N. Calcium dependence of the acrosome reaction and activation of guinea pig spermatozoa. Exp Cell Res 1974; 89: 161

12. Stock CE, Fraser LR. Divalent cations, capacitation and the acrosome reaction in human spermatozoa. J Reprod Fertil 1989; 87: 463

13. White DR, Phillips DM, Bedford JM. Factors affecting the acrosome reaction in human spermatozoa. J Reprod Fertil 1990; 90: 71

14. Nagae T, et al. Acrosome reaction in human spermatozoa. Fertil Steril 1986; 45: 701

15. Stock CE, et al. Human oocyte–cumulus complexes stimulate the acrosome reaction. J Reprod Fertil 1989; 86: 723

16. Yudin AI, Gottlieb W, Meizel S. Ultrastructural studies of the early events of the human sperm acrosome reaction as initiated by human follicular fluid. Gamete Res 1988; 20: 11

17. Fraser L. p-Aminobenzamidine, an acrosin inhibitor, inhibits mouse sperm penetration of the zona pellucida but not the acrosome reaction. J Reprod Fertil 1982; 66: 185

18. Jamil K, White IG. Induction of acrosomal reaction in sperm with ionophore A23187 and calcium. Arch Androl 1981; 7: 283

19. Cummins JM, et al. A test of the human sperm acrosome reaction following ionophore challenge: relationship to fertility and other seminal parameters. J Androl 1991; 12: 98

20. Sanchez R. A new method for evaluation of the acrosome reaction in viable human spermatozoa. Andrologia 1991; 23: 197

21. Aitken RJ, Buckingham DW, Fang HG. Analysis of the response of human spermatozoa to A23187 employing a novel technique for assessing the acrosome reaction. J Androl 1993; 14: 132

22. Tesarik J, Mendoza C, Carreras A. Effects of phosphodiesterase inhibitors caffeine and pentoxifylline on spontaneous and stimulus-induced acrosome reactions in human sperm. Fertil Steril 1992; 58: 1185

23. Tesarik J, Mendoza C. Sperm treatment with pentoxifylline improves the fertilizing ability in patients with acrosome reaction insufficiency. Fertil Steril 1993; 60: 141

24. Osman RA, et al. Steriod induced exocytosis: the human sperm acrosome reaction. Biochem Biophys Res Commun 1989; 160: 828

25. Blackmore PF, et al. Progesterone and 17-hydroxyprogesterone: novel stimulators of calcium influx in human sperm. J Biol Chem 1990; 265: 1376

26. Calvo L, et al. Acrosome reaction inducibility predicts fertilization success at in-vitro fertilization. Hum Reprod 1994; 9: 1880

27. Sueldo CE, et al. Effect of progesterone on human zona pellucida sperm binding and oocyte penetrating capacity. Fertil Steril 1993; 60: 137

28. Suarez SS, Wolf DP, Meizel S. Induction of the acrosome reaction in human spermatozoa by a fraction of human follicular fluid. Gamete Res 1986; 14: 107

29. Cross NL, et al. Induction of acrosome reactions by the human zona pellucida. Biol Reprod 1988; 38: 235

30. Lee MA, Check LH, Kopf GA. Guanine nucleotide-binding regulatory protein in human sperm mediates acrosomal exocytosis induced by the human zona pellucida. Mol Reprod 1992; 31: 78

31. Franken DR, Morales PJ, Habenicht UF. Inhibition of G protein in human sperm and its influence on acrosome reaction and zona pellucida binding. Fertil Steril 1996; 66: 1009

32. Talbot P, Chacon RS. A new technique for evaluating normal acrosome reactions of human sperm. J Cell Biol 1979; 83: 2089

33. Kohn FM, et al. Detection of human sperm acrosome reaction: comparison between methods using double staining, Pisum sativum agglutinin, concanavalin A

and transmission electron microscopy. Hum Reprod 1997; 12: 714

34. Lee MA, et al. Capacitation and acrosome reactions in human spermatozoa monitored by a chlortetracy-cline fluorescence assay. Fertil Steril 1987; 48: 649

35. Talbot P, Chacon RS. A triple-stain technique for evaluating normal acrosome reactions of human sperm. J Exp Zool 1981; 215: 201

36. Cross NL, et al. Two simple methods for detecting acrosome-reacted human sperm. Gamete Res 1986; 15: 213

37. Wolf DP, et al. Acrosomal status evaluation in human ejaculated sperm with monoclonal antibodies. Biol Reprod 1985; 32: 1157

38. Fenichel P, et al. Evaluation of the human sperm acrosome reaction using a monoclonal antibody, GB24, and fluorescence-activated cell sorter. J Reprod Fertil 1989; 87: 699

39. Aitken RJ, Brindle JP. Analysis of the ability of three probes targeting the outer acrosomal membrane or acrosomal contents to detect the acrosome reaction in human spermatozoa. Hum Reprod 1993; 8: 1663

40. Bastias MC, Kamijo H, Osteen KG. Assessment of human sperm functional changes after in vitro coincubation with cells retrieved from the human female reproductive tract. Hum Reprod 1993; 8: 1670

41. Siegel MS, Paulson RJ, Graczykowski JW. The influence of human follicular fluid on the acrosome reaction, fertilizing capacity and proteinase activity of human spermatozoa. Hum Reprod 1990; 5: 975

42. Thomas P, Meizel S. An influx of extracellular calcium is required for the initiation of the human sperm acrosome reaction induced by human follicular fluid. Gamete Res 1988; 20: 397

43. Fukuda M, et al. Correlation of the acrosomal status and sperm performance in the sperm penetration assay. Fertil Steril 1989; 52: 836

44. Stock CE, et al. Extended exposure to follicular fluid is required for significant stimulation of the acrosome reaction in human spermatozoa. J Reprod Fertil 1989; 86: 401

45. Foresta C, et al. Progesterone induces capacitation in human spermatozoa. Andrologia 1991; 24: 33

46. Baldi E, et al. Intracellular calcium accumulation and responsiveness to progesterone in capacitating human spermatozoa. J Androl 1991; 12: 323

47. Luconi M. Human spermatozoa as a model for studying membrane receptors mediating rapid nongenomic effects of progesterone and estrogens. Steroids 2004; 69: 553

48. Morales P, et al. The acrosome reaction-inducing activity of individual human follicular fluid samples is

highly variable and is related to the steroid content. Hum Reprod 1992; 7: 646

49. Miska W, Henkel R, Fehl P. Recent studies on the structure of the acrosome reaction-inducing substance (ARIS) in human follicular fluid. Mol Reprod Dev 1995; 42: 80

50. Miska W, Fehl P, Henkel R. Biochemical and immunological characterization of the acrosome reaction inducing substance (ARIS) of hFF. Biochem Biophys Res Commun 1994; 199: 125

51. Franken DR, Bastiaan HS, Oehninger SC. A microassay for sperm acrosome reaction assessment. J Assist Reprod Genet 2000; 17: 156

52. Bastiaan HS. Zona pellucida induced acrosome reaction (ZIAR), sperm morphology and sperm–zona binding assessments among subfertile men. J Assist Reprod Genet 2002; 19: 329

53. Esterhuizen AD, et al. Clinical importance of zona pellucida induced acrosome reaction (ZIAR test) in cases of failed human fertilization. Hum Reprod 2001; 16: 138

54. Saling PM, Storey BT. Mouse gamete interactions during fertilization in vitro: chlortetracycline as a fluorescent probe for the mouse acrosome reaction. J Cell Biol 1979; 83: 544

55. Saling PM, Irons G, Waibel R. Mouse sperm antigens that participate in fertilization. I. Inhibition of sperm fusion with the egg plasma membrane using monoclonal antibodies. Biol Reprod 1985; 33: 515

56. Bleil DJ, Wassarman PM. Sperm–egg interactions in the mouse: sequence of events and induction of the acrosome reaction by a zona pellucida glycoprotein. Dev Biol 1983; 95: 317

57. Coddington CC, et al. Sperm bound to zona pellucida in hemizona assay demonstrate acrosome reaction when stained with T-6 antibody. Fertil Steril 1990; 54: 504

58. Hoshi KH, et al. Induction of the acrosome reaction in human spermatozoa by human pellucida and effect of cervical mucus on zona-induced acrosome reaction. Fertil Steril 1993; 60: 149

59. Roldan ERS, Murase T, Shi Q-X. Exocytosis in spermatozoa in response to progesterone and zona pellucida. Science 1994; 266: 1578

60. Schuffner AA, et al. Zona pellucida-induced acrosome reaction in human sperm: dependency on activation of pertussis toxin-sensitive G(i) protein and extracellular calcium, and priming effect of progesterone and follicular fluid. Mol Hum Reprod 2002; 8: 722

61. Cummins JM, Yanagimachi R. Development of the ability to penetrate the cumulus oophorus by hamster

spermatozoa capacitated in vitro in relation to the timing of the acrosome reaction. Gamete Res 1986; 15: 187

62. Yanagimachi R, Phillips DM. The status of acrosomal caps of hamster spermatozoa immediately before fertilization in vivo. Gamete Res 1984; 9: 1

63. Cherr GN, Lambert H, Katz D. Completion of the hamster sperm acrosome reaction on the zona pellucida in vivo. J Cell Biol 1984; 99: 261

64. Tesarik J. Appropriate timing of the acrosome reaction is a major requirement for the fertilizing spermatozoon. Hum Reprod 1989; 4: 957

65. Carrell DT, et al. Role of the cumulus in the selection of morphologically normal sperm and induction of the acrosome reaction during human in vitro fertilization. Arch Androl 1993; 31: 133

66. Corselli J, Talbot P. An in vitro technique to study penetration of hamster oocyte–cumulus complexes by using physiological numbers of sperm. Gamete Res 1986; 13: 293

67. Barros C, et al. Relationship between the length of sperm preincubation and zona penetration in the golden hamster: a scanning electron microscopy study. Gamete Res 1984; 9: 31

68. Singer SL, et al. The kinetics of human sperm binding to the human zona pellucida and zona-free hamster oocyte in vitro. Gamete Res 1985; 12: 29

69. Pampiglione JS, Tan S, Cambell S. The use of the stimulated acrosome reaction test as a test of fertilizing ability in human spermatozoa. Fertil Steril 1993; 59: 1280

70. Henkel R, et al. Determination of the acrosome reaction in human spermatozoa is predictive of fertilization in vitro. Hum Reprod 1993; 8: 2128

71. Bastiaan HS, et al. The relationship between zona pellucida induced acrosome reaction (ZIAR), sperm morphology, sperm–zona pellucida binding and in vitro fertilization. Fertil Steril 2003; 79: 49

72. Liu DY, Baker HWG. Disordered acrosome reaction of spermatozoa bound to the zona pellucida: a newly discovered sperm defect causing infertility with reduced sperm–zona penetration and reduced fertilization in vitro. Hum Reprod 1994; 9: 1694

73. Liu DY, Garrett C, Baker HWG. Clinical application of sperm–oocyte interaction tests in in vitro fertilization–embryo transfer and intracytoplasmic sperm injection programs. Fertil Steril 2004; 82: 1251

14

Sperm–zona pellucida binding assays

Sergio Oehninger, Murat Arslan, Daniel R Franken

BIOLOGY OF FERTILIZATION

Obligatory requirements for the successful completion of normal fertilization include a mature, metaphase II oocyte and motile spermatozoa that have completed the process of capacitation. The newly formed zygote undergoes early cleavage divisions depending upon the oocyte's endogenous machinery, and at the 4–8-cell stage initiates transcription of the embryonic genome[1]. *In vivo*, these processes are synchronized with the preparation of the endometrial mucosa (window of implantation), thereby ensuring an adequate milieu receptive to the blastocyst.

Spermatozoa are highly differentiated cells whose main function is to activate the oocyte and deliver components, principally its DNA, leading to embryo development. In order to fertilize the oocyte successfully, the spermatozoon must be able to perform, at least, these functions: migration (allowing transport to the fertilization site through adequate motion patterns), recognition and binding to the zona pellucida (an event dependent upon specific receptor–ligand interactions), penetration of the zona pellucida (secondary to the release of enzymes following induction of the acrosome reaction by zona components), binding to the oolemma (also

dependent upon interaction of complementary gamete molecules), oocyte activation, nuclear decondensation and participation in pronuclear formation leading to syngamy (reviewed in reference 2).

Events leading to sperm–oocyte interaction

Only capacitated spermatozoa demonstrate the ability to respond to the adequate physiological stimuli that result in the display of adequate motion characteristics, acrosome reaction responsiveness and competence to interact with the oocyte and its vestments. Several cellular changes that are manifested during capacitation include, among others, removal or modification of surface proteins, efflux of cholesterol from the membranes, changes in oxidative metabolism, achievement of a hyperactivated pattern of motility and an increase in the phosphotyrosine content of several proteins. In addition to tyrosine phosphorylation of specific proteins, other modifications of cellular regulators occur, such as a decrease in calmodulin binding to proteins and an increase in calcium uptake, intracellular pH and cyclic adenosine monophosphate (cAMP) concentration[2,3].

Sperm–zona pellucida interaction: recognition, binding and induction of the acrosome reaction

The early events that occur during fertilization may be viewed as a special form of highly complex cell-to-cell recognition. Cell–cell recognition mechanisms in many somatic cell systems involve carbohydrate side-chains of membrane glycoproteins, and several observations indicate that similar molecules may have a role in spermatozoon–oocyte binding in mammals. Compelling evidence has now demonstrated that carbohydrate-binding proteins on the sperm surface mediate gamete recognition by binding with high affinity and specificity to complex glycoconjugates of the zona pellucida[2,4–6].

In the mouse, the best characterized species so far, tight binding is achieved through interaction of zona pellucida protein 3 (ZP3) and a putative complementary sperm-binding protein(s) present in the plasma membrane. ZP3 triggers the acrosome reaction that is then followed by a secondary binding process involving zona pellucida protein 2 (ZP2) and the inner acrosomal sperm membrane, leading to zona penetration[7,8]. Glycosylation appears to be mandatory for ZP3-ligand function. It has been demonstrated that O-glycosylation, and particularly terminal galactose residues of O-linked oligosaccharides, are essential for maintaining mouse gamete interaction. There is also some evidence that the amino sugar N-acetylglucosamine (NAG) is the key terminal monosaccharide involved in sperm–zona interaction in the mouse[9,10]. In contrast, the acrosome reaction-triggering activity of ZP3 seems to depend upon the integrity of the protein backbone (reviewed in references 5, 11 and 12). Peptides synthesized based upon the published DNA sequence of ZP3 proteins are able to induce acrosomal exocytosis in some species[13].

The molecular identity of the sperm surface receptor(s) for ZP3 has been the subject of intensive research. A number of candidate murine ZP3 receptor molecules have been proposed, including potential carbohydrate-binding proteins such as sp56, p95, β-1-4 galactosyltransferase and a D-mannosidase[9,14–18]. However, there has been confirmation neither of the structure or biological role of any of these molecules nor of their complementary ligand(s). The state of knowledge as related to the human is even more enigmatic.

In the mouse, ZP3-binding and ZP3-induced acrosomal exocytosis can be dissociated from each other, that is, they seem to represent two independent processes[19]. There are differences in the concentration-dependency of ZP3 to express sperm-binding activity and acrosome reaction-inducing activity. Specifically, the concentration response curve for ZP3 acrosome reaction-inducing activity is shifted to the right of the concentration response curve for ZP3-ligand activity. A model has been proposed predicting that ZP3 is composed of multiple 'functional ligands', and that the interaction of these ligands with the sperm surface is responsible for both the sperm-binding activity (through glycosylated epitopes) and the ability to induce a complete acrosome reaction[19]. Gamete recognition and adhesion probably depend upon a multivalent ligand interaction whereby the sperm protein receptor(s) bind to a number of different epitopes within the ZP3. These functional ligands do not necessarily have to be identical. The data concerning the involvement of either O- or N-linked glycosylation sites are also equivocal, particularly in the human. The lack of native human zona pellucida to perform direct carbohydrate analyses has made an unambiguous structural definition impossible so far.

We have proposed the hypothesis that, in the human, tight and specific sperm binding to the zona pellucida requires a 'selectin-like' interaction[6,20]. Hapten-inhibition tests, zona pellucida lectin-binding studies and removal/modification of functional carbohydrates by chemical and enzymatic methods have provided evidence for the involvement of defined carbohydrate moieties in initial binding. Our studies suggest the existence of distinct zona-binding proteins on human sperm that can bind to selectin ligands (reviewed in reference 21). Additionally, results suggest a possible convergence in the types of carbohydrate sequences recognized during initial human gamete binding and immune/inflammatory cell interactions (reviewed in reference 22). Full characterization of the glycoconjugates that manifest selectin-ligand activity on the human zona pellucida will allow a better understanding of human gamete interaction in physiological and pathological situations. Nevertheless, determination of the biochemical components and secondary structure of the human zona proteins has been hampered by the paucity of biological material.

For the past two decades, investigators have sought to identify an individual protein or carbohydrate side-chain as the 'sperm receptor'. Using 'knock-out' mice, in the absence of either ZP2 or ZP3 expression, a zona pellucida fails to assemble around growing oocytes and females are infertile. In the absence of ZP1 expression, a disorganized zona assembles around growing oocytes and females exhibit reduced fertility. These observations are consistent with the current model for zona pellucida structure in which ZP2 and ZP3 form long Z-filaments crosslinked by ZP1 (reviewed in reference 23).

However, recent genetic data in mice appear to be more consistent with the three-dimensional structure of the zona pellucida, rather than a single protein (or carbohydrate), determining sperm binding. Collectively, the genetic data indicate that no single mouse zona-pellucida protein is obligatory for taxon-specific sperm binding, and that two human proteins are not sufficient to support human sperm binding. An observed post-fertilization persistence of mouse sperm-binding to 'humanized' zona pellucida correlates with uncleaved ZP2. These observations are consistent with a model for sperm binding in which the supramolecular structure of the zona pellucida necessary for sperm binding is modulated by the cleavage status of ZP2[24–27].

Post-zona pellucida binding events: interaction between sperm and oocyte leading to fusion, oocyte activation, pronuclear formation and paternal contribution to early embryogenesis

Spermatozoa that have undergone the acrosome reaction after interaction with and penetration through the zona pellucida are able to bind to the plasma membrane of the oocyte (oolemma). This also seems to be a specific recognition event involving putative molecules located in the equatorial segment of the sperm (sperm fusion proteins) and yet-unidentified oocyte acceptors. Binding of the gametes leads to fusion of the membranes with incorporation of the entire spermatozoon into the ooplasm. Contact of the spermatozoon with the oocyte membrane triggers electrical membrane changes in the oocyte (membrane depolarization) and the release of cortical granules, which represent fast and delayed protective mechanisms against polyspermy (reviewed in reference 2).

There is still controversy as to the intimate mechanism(s) through which the spermatozoon activates the oocyte. Oocyte activation occurs in association with changes in the intracellular concentration of calcium ions, possibly modulated by a factor released by the spermatozoon once inside the oocyte. Unequivocal identification of this factor in the human and other species has not yet been achieved[28]. Sperm–oolemma binding and fusion are followed by activation of the oocyte's second-messenger systems (calcium, phosphatidylinositol-4,5-biphosphate (PIP2)), pH changes, protein synthesis, cyclin accumulation, DNA synthesis, nuclear envelope breakdown and the first cleavage division in some species. An increase in intracellular calcium is associated with microtubular rearrangement and pronuclear formation[2].

There is obviously extensive crosstalk between the spermatozoon and the oocyte. In addition to the effects secondary to membrane fusion and the release of oocyte activating factor(s) by the spermatozoon, the oocyte uses molecules that induce sperm head decondensation (male pronucleus growth factor) and the substitution of protamines by histones[2,29]. Fertilization is achieved after the oocyte completes meiosis, female and male pronuclei are formed and syngamy (pronuclei union) is accomplished.

ABNORMALITIES OF FERTILIZATION: CLINICAL LESSONS FROM *IN VITRO* FERTILIZATION AND INTRACYTOPLASMIC SPERM INJECTION SETTINGS

It has been reported that sperm–zona pellucida binding is a crucial step and that it reflects multiple sperm functions[30–32]. Many patients who are unable to fertilize oocytes under *in vitro* fertilization (IVF) conditions have a severe impairment of this functional step. A defective capacity to undergo the acrosome reaction is probably also a significant factor in some patients[33]. It has been shown recently that acrosomal exocytosis can be studied *in vitro* using small volumes of solubilized human zonae pellucidae and that G-proteins are involved as mediators[34]. This confirms previous studies that demonstrated the involvement of heterotrimeric G-proteins in induction of the acrosome reaction in other species[19]. It has also been demonstrated that functional/biochemical/morphological sperm immaturity (e.g. high content of creatine kinase) is present in many cases of male infertility, resulting in fertilization deficiencies[35].

In addition to a defective sperm–zona pellucida interaction, fertilization failure can also be due to sperm–oolemma fusion defects or to abnormal communication between the penetrating spermatozoon and the oocyte (e.g. lack or deficient sperm–oocyte activating factor, male pronucleus growth factor or other). Recent evidence from the intracytoplasmic sperm injection (ICSI) setting clearly demonstrates that post-gamete fusion abnormalities may occur. Advances in fluorescent imaging by laser scanning confocal microscopy and other novel techniques permit the sophisticated high-resolution examination of gametes and embryos, including the fate of the sperm centrosome, the oocyte's microtubule organizing center, mitochondrial distribution and the initiation of embryo cleavage[36]. We remain enthusiastic about ongoing studies that may help to elucidate the contribution of the gametes (functional, biochemical–molecular and genetic) to early embryogenesis, and identify specific molecules involved in fertilization disorders.

CLINICAL ASPECTS: MALE SUBFERTILITY AND SEMEN EVALUATION

Men consulting for infertility which is defined as male-factor typically present abnormalities of semen analysis consistent with varying degrees of oligoasthenoteratozoospermia, alone or in combination. In addition, other structural and biochemical sperm alterations can be demonstrated. From an anatomical point of view they can be divided into: membrane alterations (that can be assessed by tests of resistance to osmotic changes, translocation of phosphatidylserine and others), nuclear aberrations (abnormal chromatin condensation, retention of histones and presence of DNA fragmentation), cytoplasmic lesions (excessive generation of reactive oxygen species, loss of mitochondrial membrane potential or retention of cytoplasm, indicative of immaturity such as high creatine kinase content or presence of caspases) and flagellar disturbances (disturbances of the microtubules and the fibrous sheath). Some of these alterations are indicative of immaturity, the presence of an apoptosis phenotype, infection-necrosis or other unknown causes (reviewed in references 37–43).

Notwithstanding their occurrence and weak correlations with clinical outcomes, it is not clear how these abnormalities impact directly on sperm function, particularly gamete transportation, fertilization and contribution to embryogenesis. Furthermore, most such assays are still experimental, and more research is needed to validate their results in the clinical setting and to determine their true capacity to predict male fertility potential.

On the other hand, there are other specific and critical sperm functional capacities that can be more reliably examined *in vitro*. These functions include: motility, competence to achieve capacitation, zona pellucida binding, acrosome reaction, oolemma binding, decondensation and pronuclear formation. The assessment of some of these features is what is typically considered as sperm functional testing.

VALIDITY OF SPERM FUNCTION ASSAYS: RESULTS OF A META-ANALYSIS

The categories of functional assays that are usually considered include: (1) bioassays of gamete interaction (e.g. the heterologous zona-free hamster-oocyte test and homologous sperm–zona pellucida binding assays); (2) induced acrosome-reaction testing; and (3) computer-aided sperm motion analysis (CASA) for the evaluation of sperm motion characteristics[33,44–50].

We recently reported an objective, outcome-based examination of the validity of the currently available assays based upon the results obtained from 2906 subjects evaluated in 34 published and prospectively designed, controlled studies. The aim was carried out through a meta-analytical approach that examined the predictive value of four categories of sperm functional assays (computer-aided sperm motion analysis or CASA, induced acrosome-reaction testing, sperm penetration assay or SPA and sperm–zona pellucida binding assays) for IVF outcome[51].

Results of this meta-analysis demonstrated a high predictive power of the sperm–zona pellucida

binding and induced acrosome-reaction assays for fertilization outcome under *in vitro* conditions[51]. On the other hand, the findings indicated a poor clinical value of the SPA as a predictor of fertilization, and a real need for standardization and further investigation of the potential clinical utility of CASA systems. Although this study provided objective evidence in which clinical management and future research may be directed, the analysis also pointed out limitations of the current tests, and the need for standardization of present methodologies and the development of novel technologies. It is important to note that there are no studies addressing the validity and predictive power of these assays for natural conception.

DESIGN OF *IN VITRO* SPERM–ZONA PELLUCIDA BINDING ASSAYS

Our group has published extensively on the development and validation of an *in vitro* bioassay (the hemizona assay or HZA) for the assessment of tight human sperm binding to the homologous zona pellucida. The initial studies were based on the hypothesis that capacitated spermatozoa bind in a specific, tight and irreversible manner to the homologous, biologically intact zona pellucida, and undergo a physiologically induced acrosome reaction (exocytosis triggered by components of the zona pellucida). This hypothesis was tested by incubation of spermatozoa and the zona pellucida from microbisected human oocytes, followed by determination of the kinetics, sperm concentration-, sperm morphology- and time-dependency of binding, and sperm acrosomal status on tight binding.

The HZA was introduced as a novel diagnostic test for the binding of human spermatozoa to the human zona pellucida to predict fertilization potential[46]. In the HZA, the two matched zona hemispheres created by microbisection of the human oocyte provide three main advantages: (1) the two halves (hemizonae) are functionally equal surfaces, allowing controlled comparison of binding and reproducible measurements of sperm binding from a single egg; (2) the limited number of available human oocytes is amplified because an internally controlled test can be performed on a single oocyte; and (3) because the oocyte is split microsurgically, use of even fresh oocytes cannot lead to inadvertent fertilization and pre-embryo formation[46,52].

The two most common zona binding tests currently used are the HZA[46] and a zona pellucida-binding test[32,47]. Both bioassays have the advantage of providing a functional homologous test for sperm binding to the homologous zona pellucida, comparing populations of fertile and infertile spermatozoa in the same assay. The internal control offered by the HZA represents an advantage by decreasing the number of oocytes needed during the assay and diminishing the intra-assay variation[46,52–57].

Different sources of human oocytes can be used in the assay: oocytes recovered from surgically removed ovaries or postmortem ovarian tissue, and surplus oocytes from the IVF program. Since fresh oocytes are not always available for the test, various alternatives have been implemented for storage. Others have described the storage of human oocytes in dimethylsulfoxide (DMSO) at ultralow temperatures[58]. Additionally, Yanagimachi and colleagues showed that highly concentrated salt solutions provided effective storage of hamster and human oocytes such that the sperm-binding characteristics of the zona pellucida were preserved[59,60]. In developing the HZA, we have examined the binding ability of fresh and DMSO- and salt-stored (under controlled pH conditions) human oocytes, and have concluded that the sperm binding ability of the zona remains intact under all these conditions[53,61]. Subsequently, we have assessed the kinetics of sperm binding to the zona, showing maximum binding at 4–5 h of gamete coincubation, with similar binding curves for both fertile and infertile semen samples[46,53].

Detailed descriptions of oocyte collection, handling and micromanipulation, as well as

semen processing and sperm suspension preparations for the HZA, have been published elsewhere[46,53]. The assay has been standardized to a 4-h gamete coincubation, exposing each hemizona to a sperm droplet (50–100 μl of a dilution of 500 000 motile sperm/ml prepared after swim-up). Human tubal fluid supplemented with synthetic serum substitute or human serum albumin is usually the medium utilized for sperm preparation and gamete coincubation. After coincubation, the hemizonae are subjected to pipetting through a glass pipette in order to dislodge loosely attached sperm. The number of tightly bound spermatozoa on the outer surface of the zona is finally counted using phase-contrast microscopy (200×). Results are expressed as the number of sperm tightly bound to the hemizona for controls and patients, and also as the hemizona index (HZI), i.e. the number of sperm tightly bound, for the control sample (×100)[46].

The assay has been validated by a clear-cut definition of the factors affecting data interpretation, i.e. kinetics of binding, egg variability and maturation status, intra-assay variation and influence of sperm concentration morphology, motility and acrosome reaction status[53–55,57,62,63]. Because of the definition of the assay's limitations and its small intra-assay variation (less than 10%), the power of discrimination of the HZA has been maximized. Conversely, for other sperm–zona binding tests, several oocytes have to be used because of the high inter-egg variation, and in fact a high intra-assay coefficient of variation has been reported[32,47].

The specificity of the interaction between human spermatozoa and the human zona pellucida under HZA conditions is strengthened by the fact that the sperm tightly bound to the zona are acrosome-reacted[54,62]. Results of interspecies experiments performed with human, cynomolgus monkey and hamster gametes have demonstrated a high species specificity of human sperm–zona pellucida functions under HZA conditions, providing further support for the use of this bioassay in infertility and contraception testing[64].

PREDICTIVE VALUE OF THE HEMIZONA ASSAY FOR *IN VITRO* FERTILIZATION OUTCOME

In prospective, blinded studies, we have investigated the relationship between sperm binding to the hemizona and IVF outcome[31,56,65–67]. Results have shown that the HZA can successfully distinguish the population of male-factor patients at risk for failed or poor fertilization (Figure 14.1).

Powerful statistical results allow use of the HZA for prediction of the fertilization rate[67–70]. The HZA can distinguish a population of male-factor patients who will encounter low fertilization rates in IVF, and, when combined with the information provided by other sperm parameters (morphology and motion characteristics), gives reliable and useful information in the clinical arena. Of the basic sperm parameters, sperm morphology is the best predictor of the ability of spermatozoa to bind to the zona pellucida. Sperm from patients with severe teratozoospermia ('poor-prognosis' pattern or less than 4% normal sperm scores as judged by strict criteria) have an impaired capacity to bind to the zona pellucida under HZA conditions (membrane/receptor deficiencies?).

In our studies, when the HZA was removed from the regression analysis in order to identify the predictive value of other sperm parameters (sperm concentration, morphology and motion characteristics), percentage progressive motility was the second best predictor of *in vitro* fertilization outcome[31]. We speculated that the relationship between sperm morphology and IVF results depends upon an effect on zona pellucida binding. On the other hand, motility seemed to affect the rate of fertilization outside the prediction of the HZA. It would appear that, although important in achieving binding, motility may be more important for cumulus and zona pellucida penetration, factors not directly evaluated in the HZA. Logistic regression analysis provided a robust HZI range predictive of the oocyte's potential to be fertilized. This HZI cut-off value was approximately 35%. Overall, for failed vs. successful and poor vs. good fertilization rate, the correct predictive ability (discriminative power) of the HZA was 80% and 85%, respectively. Consequently, this information may be extremely valuable for counseling patients in the IVF setting (for example, considering a HZI below 35%, the chances of poor fertilization are 90–100%, whereas for a HZI over 35%, the chances of good fertilization are 80–85%) (Figure 14.1)[31,67,68,70].

The HZA has demonstrated excellent sensitivity and specificity with a low incidence of false-positive results. For a HZI of 35%, the positive predictive value of the HZA is 79% and its negative predictive value is 100% (considering good vs. poor fertilization rates). In the HZA, false-positive results can be expected, since other functional steps follow the tight binding of sperm to the zona pellucida and are essential for fertilization and pre-embryo development.

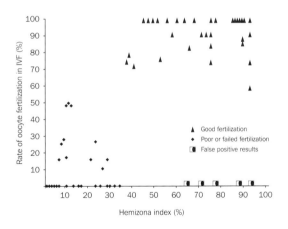

Figure 14.1 Cluster analysis of hemizona index (HZI) and rate of fertilization of mature oocytes in *in vitro* fertilization (IVF) considering a cut-off HZI of 35%. Cluster ▲: high HZI, successful fertilization in the range 50–100% of oocytes; cluster ◆: low HZI, failed or poor fertilization in the range 0–50% of oocytes; cluster ◼: false-positive results with high HZI but failed fertilization (< 15% of cases). For patients undergoing IVF treatment, and if HZI results are < 35%, the chances of poor fertilization are 90–100%, whereas for HZI results > 35%, the chances of good fertilization are 80–85%. Note the absence of false-negative results and evidence of 15% false-positive results. The cluster analysis was performed with combined data from references 56 and 66–68

PREDICTIVE VALUE OF THE HEMIZONA ASSAY FOR PREGNANCY OUTCOME IN INTRAUTERINE INSEMINATION THERAPY

The prediction of pregnancy in intrauterine insemination (IUI) cycles has been expected to be much more difficult than prediction of fertilization in IVF. This is due to the multifactorial nature of conception, as it depends upon the presence of many sperm functions and additional female parameters. For IUI therapy, the most significant female parameters are the quality or quantity of the oocyte(s) and the transportation of capacitated sperm to the fertilization site (e.g. effects of uterine and tubal environment, IUI preparation technique) (reviewed in reference 71). However, there are also other potential and more subtle female factors, such as exposure of spermatozoa to peritoneal and follicular fluid, that have been found to affect sperm binding to the zona pellucida and the ability to respond to physiological inducers of the acrosome reaction[72,73]. Sperm–zona pellucida binding is a crucial and common step in the journey leading to fertilization during both *in vivo* and *in vitro* models.

We therefore tested the power of the HZA to predict pregnancy outcome in patients undergoing IUI therapy using the husband's sperm. Only couples with a diagnosis of unexplained infertility and male factor infertility were asked to participate in the clinical trial. During a 3-year span, 82 couples who underwent 313 IUI treatment cycles and who were categorized into unexplained/male factor infertility agreed to participate. The male partner had a HZA within 3 months of the first IUI cycle, and couples underwent 1–6 IUI cycles within the next 12-month period. All female patients were subjected to controlled ovarian hyperstimulation using a similar gonadotropin protocol.

For all patients involved in the study, the HZI results ranged between 0 and 178%. Minimum and maximum HZI values that achieved a pregnancy were 17% and 109%, respectively. When we analyzed the data according to a 30–35% cut-off HZI range, which was proven optimum for prediction of successful fertilization in IVF[66,67], the HZA had a high negative predictive value (NPV) of almost 90% (i.e. patients with a HZI < 30% had a very low chance of conception) (Table 14.1). On the other hand, results demonstrated that the positive predictive value (PPV) of the test decreased in parallel with its NPV with increasing cut-off values ($r = -0.7$, $p < 0.05$ and $r = -0.8$, $p < 0.05$ for PPV and NPV, respectively). This was reflected as increased false-positive rates with higher HZI values (Figure 14.2). This result confirmed that a variety of pre- and post-sperm–zona pellucida binding factors play an active role in establishing a pregnancy: patients with high HZI values still may not be able to achieve conception.

In light of these findings, we re-examined the data in the range of HZI between 0 and 60%. This approach was also used in earlier IVF studies, where it was confirmed that successful fertilization occurred in nearly all patients with a HZI > 60% under optimal IVF conditions[74]. With a HZI cut-off value of 30–35%, we found a relatively higher PPV of 69%, but still a high incidence of false-positive results, with a very high negative predictive value of 93% (Table 14.1).

The data were also subjected to receiver operating characteristic (ROC) analysis to assess the contributions of all male and female parameters, for the overall population and also after categorization of patients according to the subgroup of etiology (male factor or unexplained). In this model, a HZI with cut-off value of 32% demonstrated significant power for the prediction of pregnancy in the male factor infertility subgroup, with 69% PPV and 93% NPV ($p = 0.005$). The average path velocity was the second male-factor parameter that had significance as predictor in this subgroup (30% PPV and 95% NPV with cut-off value of 46.5 µm/s, $p = 0.001$). The duration of infertility was a strong predictor of pregnancy in all patients and in both subgroups. Binary logistic regression analysis applied to all male and female

Table 14.1 Predictive value of hemizona assay (HZA) for pregnancy with intrauterine insemination (IUI) therapy considering a hemizona index (HZI) cut-off range of 30–35%. Predictive values were calculated for all patients and for patients who had HZI results in the range 0–60%

	All patients	Patients with HZI value between 0 and 60%
Positive predictive value (%)	40	69
False-positive rate (%)	69	42
False-negative rate (%)	11	11
Negative predictive value (%)	89	93

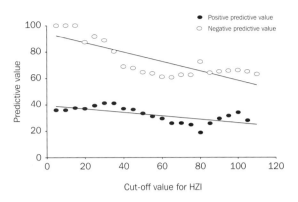

Figure 14.2 Relationship between different cut-off values of hemizona index (HZI) and corresponding positive and negative predictive values for conception in intrauterine insemination (IUI) therapy

parameters also confirmed the HZI as the most powerful and single parameter predictive of conception in couples with a diagnosis of male factor infertility (–2 log likelihood of 28.778 and χ^2 of 7.720, $p = 0.005$) (Table 14.2).

Although this evidence continues to encourage use of the HZA in the screening work-up of consulting couples before starting IUI therapy, larger prospective studies are still needed to confirm these favorable initial results.

PREDICTIVE VALUE OF THE HEMIZONA ASSAY FOR NATURAL CONCEPTION

It has been speculated that information from the semen analysis can be used to predict the likelihood that a couple will conceive within a period of time. This probability is influenced by a host of factors including semen quality, and studies in large groups or using simple models are required to overcome existing limitations[75]. The world literature has consistently used the World Health Organization (WHO) guidelines for normalcy cut-offs to address clinical situations. However, recent studies have raised doubts about such established guidelines.

Table 14.2 Results of logistic regression analysis of different sperm parameters and impact on pregnancy outcome in couples with diagnosis of male factor infertility undergoing intrauterine insemination (IUI) therapy

	$r^\dagger$	p Value
Morphology	0.19	0.07
Concentration	0.00	0.27
Motility	0.00	0.99
HZI	0.30	0.02*

†Partial contribution; *statistically significant; HZI, hemizona index

In a prospectively designed study, Ombelet and collaborators[76] compared a fertile and a subfertile population so as to define 'normal' values for different semen parameters. Semen analyses were performed according to WHO guidelines, except for sperm morphology (strict criteria). The authors used ROC curve analysis to determine the diagnostic potential and cut-off values for single and combined sperm parameters. Sperm morphology scored best, with a value of 78% (area under the ROC curve). Summary statistics showed a shift towards abnormality for most semen parameters in the subfertile population. Using the 10th centile of the fertile population as the cut-off value, the following results were obtained: 14.3×10^6/ml for sperm concentration, 28% for progressive motility and 5% for sperm morphology. Using ROC analysis, cut-off values were 34×10^6/ml, 45% and 10%, respectively. Cut-off values for normality were different from those described in the last edition of the WHO guidelines.

In addition, there are well-known variations in sperm parameters among different ejaculates from the same man, and differences among groups of patients[75]. To the best of our knowledge, there are scant data, if any at all, on the predictive value of any sperm structural–biochemical feature or sperm function test for the outcome of natural conception. Van der Merwe et al.[78] suggest that thresholds of < 5% normal sperm morphology, a concentration $< 15 \times 10^6$/ml and a motility < 30% should be used to identify the subfertile male. The lower threshold for morphology also fits IVF and IUI data calculated previously. Nevertheless, thresholds for natural conception (highly predictive of pregnancy within a given time-frame) need to be determined for the basic sperm parameters as well as for HZA and other functional tests.

DISCUSSION AND CONCLUSIONS

The high negative predictive value, but more important, the low false-negative rate (i.e. robust power to identify patients at high risk for fertilization failure in IVF and to fail conception in IUI), underscore the predictive ability of the HZA in the clinical setting.

Liu et al.[79] reported that sperm defects associated with poor sperm–zona pellucida binding or impaired zona pellucida-induced acrosome reaction and sperm–zona pellucida penetration are the major causes of failure of fertilization when all or most oocytes from a couple do not fertilize in

standard IVF. These authors further demonstrated that there is a high frequency of defective sperm–zona pellucida interaction in men with oligozoospermia ($< 20 \times 10^6$/ml) and severe teratozoospermia (strict normal sperm morphology ≤ 5%). According to these authors, sperm morphology correlated with sperm–zona pellucida binding, and sperm concentration correlated with zona pellucida-induced acrosome reaction in infertile men with a sperm concentration $> 20 \times 10^6$/ml. The authors suggested that a defective zona pellucida-induced acrosome reaction may cause infertility in up to 25% of men with idiopathic infertility. These patients would therefore require ICSI, despite the presence of an otherwise normal standard semen analysis[79–83].

The induced acrosome-reaction assays appear to be equally predictive of fertilization outcome in vitro as the sperm–zona pellucida binding tests, and are simpler in their methodologies[51]. Although the use of a calcium ionophore to induce the acrosome reaction is at present the most widely used methodology[84,85], the assay uses non-physiological conditions that may not accurately represent fertilization potential. The recent implementation of assays using small volumes of human solubilized zonae pellucidae[34,86], biologically active recombinant human ZP3[5,87,88] or active, synthetic ZP3 peptides[13] will probably allow the design of improved, physiologically oriented acrosome reaction assays.

Initially, it was believed that cloning of the human ZP3 gene would circumvent the obstacle manifested as a paucity of natural material, since a constant supply of recombinant protein would be available. However, several of the laboratories dedicated to this task have been generally unable consistently and reliably to purify a biologically active product so far (reviewed in reference 5). It seems clear that this is probably due to inadequate and heterogeneous glycosylation of the protein by the different cell lines used. Although we have been able to express and purify a human recombinant ZP3 that appears to demonstrate the full spectrum of biological activities, problems of

stable transfection, protein storage and maintenance of bioactivity have hampered progress[88].

Franken et al.[86] devised a new microassay that
is easy and rapid to perform, and facilitates the use
of minimal volumes of solubilized zonae pellucidae (even a single zona) for assessment of the
human acrosome reaction. The microassay has
been validated against standard macroassays, and
consequently offers a unique arena to test for the
physiological induction of acrosomal exocytosis by
the homologous zona pellucida. Moreover, initial
clinical studies using the microassay have demonstrated that the zona-induced acrosome reaction
(ZIAR) can predict fertilization failure in the IVF
setting. The microassay ZIAR can therefore refine
the therapeutic approach for male infertility prior
to the onset of therapy[89,90]. Bastiaan et al.[91,92]
prospectively evaluated the relationship between
sperm morphology, acrosome responsiveness to
solubilized zona pellucida using the microassay,
sperm–zona binding potential (HZA) and IVF
outcome. ROC curve analyses indicated ZIAR to
be a robust indicator for fertilization failure during IVF therapy, with a sensitivity of 81% and
specificity of 75%.

Sperm function tests may be of highest value in
order to direct the couple to assisted reproductive
technologies (ART). Assisted reproduction is usually indicated as a result of: (1) failure of urologi-
cal/medical treatments of the subfertile man (if
indicated); (2) the diagnosis of 'unexplained'
infertility in the couple; (3) the presence of 'basic'
sperm abnormalities of moderate–high degree; or
(4) abnormalities of sperm function as diagnosed
by predictive bioassays (such as the HZA or
ZIAR).

Typically, patients are selected for ICSI under
the following scenarios: (1) poor sperm parameters (i.e. $< 1.5 \times 10^6$ total spermatozoa with adequate progressive motility after separation, and/or
severe teratozoospermia with $< 4\%$ normal forms
in the presence of a borderline to low total motile
fraction); (2) poor sperm–zona pellucida binding
capacity with a hemizona assay index $< 30\%$,
and/or low ZIAR[67,70,91]; (3) failure of IUI therapy

in cases presenting with abnormal sperm parameters, including the presence of antisperm antibodies; (4) previous failed fertilization in IVF; and
(5) the presence of obstructive or non-obstructive
azoospermia, where ICSI is combined with sperm
extraction from the testes or the epididymis[51,93–95].
In the presence of severe oligoasthenoteratozoospermia, or if the outcome of sperm function
testing indicates a significant impairment of fertilizing capacity, couples should be immediately
directed to ICSI. This approach is probably more
cost-effective and will avoid loss of valuable time,
particularly in women aged > 35 years[94,96].

More research is needed to develop simpler
assays of sperm function that can be clinically useful for the prediction of both in vivo and in vitro
pregnancy outcomes. It is expected that advances
in molecular biology methodologies and novel
biotechnologies will help to achieve this goal.

REFERENCES

1. Braude P, Bolton V, Moore S. Human gene expression first occurs between the four- and eight-cell
   stages of preimplantation development. Nature 1988;
   332: 459

2. Yanagimachi R. Mammalian fertilization. In Knobil
   N, Neill JD, eds. The Physiology of Reproduction.
   New York: Raven Press, 1994: 189

3. Visconti PE, Kopf GS. Regulation of protein phosphorylation during sperm capacitation. Biol Reprod
   1998; 59: 1

4. Macek MB, Shur BD. Protein–carbohydrate complementarity in mammalian gamete recognition.
   Gamete Res 1988; 20: 93

5. Chapman NR, Barratt CLR. The role of carbohydrate in sperm–ZP3 adhesion. Mol Hum Reprod
   1996; 2: 767

6. Oehninger S. Molecular basis of human sperm–zona
   pellucida interaction. Cells Tissues Organs 2001;
   168: 58

7. Bleil JD, Wassarman PM. Mammalian sperm–egg
   interaction: identification of a glycoprotein in mouse
   egg zonae pellucidae possessing receptor activity for
   sperm. Cell 1980; 20: 873

8. Bleil JD, Wassarman PM. Sperm–egg interactions in
   the mouse: sequence of events and induction of the

acrosome reaction by a zona pellucida glycoprotein. Dev Biol 1983; 95: 317

9. Wassarman PM. Mammalian fertilization: molecular aspects of gamete adhesion, exocytosis and fusion. Cell 1999; 96: 175

10. Wassarman PM, Litscher ES. Towards the molecular basis of sperm and egg interaction during mammalian fertilization. Cells Tissues Organs 2001; 168: 36

11. Wassarman PM. Profile of a mammalian sperm receptor. Development 1990; 108: 1

12. Wassarman PM. Regulation of mammalian fertilization by zona pellucida glycoproteins. J Reprod Fertil 1990; 42: 79

13. Hinsch E, Oehninger S, Hinsch K. ZP3-6 peptide and acrosome reaction. Semen evaluation, testing and selection: a new look in the 2000s. Presented at the Andrology in the Nineties Precongress Training Course, Genk, Belgium, 1998, 25

14. Leyton L, Saling P. 95 kd sperm proteins bind ZP3 and serve as tyrosine kinase substrates in response to zona binding. Cell 1989; 57: 1123

15. Leyton L, Saling P. Evidence that aggregation of mouse sperm receptors by ZP3 triggers the acrosome reaction. J Cell Biol 1989; 108: 2163

16. Bleil JD, Wassarman PM. Identification of a ZP3-binding protein on acrosome-intact mouse sperm by photoaffinity crosslinking. Proc Natl Acad Sci USA 1990; 87: 5563

17. Cornwall GA, Tulsiani DR, Orgebin-Crist MC. Inhibition of the mouse sperm surface alpha-D-mannosidase inhibits sperm–egg binding in vitro. Biol Reprod 1991; 44: 913

18. Miller DJ, Macek MB, Shur BD. Complementarity between sperm surface beta-1,4-galactosyltransferase and egg-coat ZP3 mediates sperm–egg binding. Nature 1992; 357: 589

19. Kopf GS. Zona pellucida-mediated signal transduction in mammalian spermatozoa. J Reprod Fertil 1990; 42: 33

20. Patankar MS, et al. A revised structure for fucoidan may explain some of its biological activities. J Biol Chem 1993; 268: 21770

21. Oehninger S. Biochemical and functional characterization of the human zona pellucida. Reprod Biomed Online 2002; 7: 641

22. Clark GF, et al. The species recognition system: a new corollary for the human fetoembryonic defense system hypothesis. Cells Tissues Organs 2001; 168: 113

23. Wassarman PM, Jovine L, Litscher ES. Mouse zona pellucida genes and glycoproteins. Cytogenet Genome Res 2004; 105: 228

24. Rankin TL, et al. Human ZP3 restores fertility in Zp3 null mice without affecting order-specific sperm binding. Development 1998; 125: 2415

25. Rankin TL, et al. Fertility and taxon-specific sperm binding persist after replacement of mouse sperm receptors with human homologs. Dev Cell 2003; 5: 33

26. Castle PE, Dean J. Manipulating the genome to study reproduction. Mice with 'humanized' zonae pellucidae. Hum Reprod 1999; 14: 1927

27. Hoodbhoy T, Dean J. Insights into the molecular basis of sperm–egg recognition in mammals. Reproduction 2004; 127: 417

28. Fissore RA, Reis MM, Palermo GD. Isolation of the Ca2+ releasing component(s) of mammalian sperm extracts: the search continues. Mol Hum Reprod 1999; 5: 189

29. Thibault C, Gerard M, Menezo Y. Preovulatory and ovulatory mechanisms in oocyte maturation. J Reprod Fertil 1975; 45: 605

30. Oehninger S, et al. Failure of fertilization in in vitro fertilization: the 'occult' male factor. J In Vitro Fert Embryo Transf 1988; 5: 181

31. Oehninger S, et al. Prediction of fertilization in vitro with human gametes: is there a litmus test? Am J Obstet Gynecol 1992; 167: 1760

32. Liu DY, et al. A sperm–zona pellucida binding test and in vitro fertilization. Fertil Steril 1989; 52: 281

33. Fraser L, et al. Consensus workshop on advanced diagnostic andrology techniques. ESHRE Andrology Special Interest Group. Hum Reprod 1997; 12: 873

34. Franken DR, Morales PJ, Habenicht UF. Inhibition of G protein in human sperm and its influence on acrosome reaction and zona pellucida binding. Fertil Steril 1996; 66: 1009

35. Huszar G, Vigue L. Correlation between the rate of lipid peroxidation and cellular maturity as measured by creatine kinase activity in human spermatozoa. J Androl 1994; 15: 71

36. Schatten G. The centrosome and its mode of inheritance: the reduction of the centrosome during gametogenesis and its restoration during fertilization. Dev Biol 1994; 165: 299

37. Baccetti B, Collodel G, Piomboni P. Apoptosis in human ejaculated sperm cells (notulae seminologicae 9). J Submicrosc Cytol Pathol 1996; 28: 587

38. Baccetti B, et al. Recent advances in human sperm pathology. Contraception 2002; 65: 283

39. Barroso G, Morshedi M, Oehninger S. Analysis of DNA fragmentation, plasma membrane translocation of phosphatidylserine and oxidative stress in human spermatozoa. Hum Reprod 2000; 15: 1338

40. Marchetti C, et al. Study of mitochondrial membrane potential, reactive oxygen species, DNA fragmentation and cell viability by flow cytometry in human sperm. Hum Reprod 2002; 17: 1257

41. Oehninger S, et al. Presence and significance of somatic cell apoptosis markers in human ejaculated spermatozoa. Reprod Biomed Online 2003; 7: 469

42. Aitken RJ, Baker MA. Oxidative stress and male reproductive biology. Reprod Fertil Dev 2004; 16: 581

43. Huszar G, et al. Semen characteristics after overnight shipping: preservation of sperm concentrations, HspA2 ratios, CK activity, cytoplasmic retention, chromatin maturity, DNA integrity, and sperm shape. J Androl 2004; 25: 593

44. Yanagimachi R, Yanagimachi H, Rogers BJ. The use of zona-free animal ova as a test-system for the assessment of the fertilizing capacity of human spermatozoa. Biol Reprod 1976; 15: 471

45. Cross NL, et al. Two simple methods for detecting acrosome-reacted human sperm. Gamete Res 1986; 15: 213

46. Burkman LJ, et al. The hemizona assay (HZA): development of a diagnostic test for the binding of human spermatozoa to the human hemizona pellucida to predict fertilization potential. Fertil Steril 1988; 49: 688

47. Liu DY, et al. A human sperm–zona pellucida binding test using oocytes that failed to fertilize in vitro. Fertil Steril 1988; 50: 782

48. Mortimer D. Objective analysis of sperm motility and kinematics. In Keel BA, Webster BW, eds. Handbook of the Laboratory Diagnosis and Treatment of Infertility. Boca Raton: CRC Press, 1990: 97

49. Mortimer D, Curtis EF, Camenzind AR. Combined use of fluorescent peanut agglutinin lectin and Hoechst 33258 to monitor the acrosomal status and vitality of human spermatozoa. Hum Reprod 1990; 5: 99

50. World Health Organization. WHO Laboratory Manual for the Examination of Human Semen and Sperm–Cervical Mucus Interaction, 3rd edn. Cambridge: Cambridge University Press, 1992: 23

51. Oehninger S, et al. Sperm function assays and their predictive value for fertilization outcome in IVF therapy: a meta-analysis. Hum Reprod Update 2000; 6: 160

52. Hodgen GD, et al. The hemizona assay (HZA): finding sperm that have the 'right stuff'. J In Vitro Fert Embryo Transf 1988; 5: 311

53. Franken DR, et al. Hemizona assay using salt-stored human oocytes: evaluation of zona pellucida capacity for binding human spermatozoa. Gamete Res 1989; 22: 15

54. Franken DR, et al. Defining the valid hemizona assay: accounting for binding variability within zonae pellucidae and within semen samples from fertile males. Fertil Steril 1991; 56: 1156

55. Franken DR, et al. Comparison of sperm binding potential of uninseminated, inseminated-unfertilized, and fertilized-noncleaved human oocytes under hemizona assay conditions. Mol Reprod Dev 1991; 30: 56

56. Oehninger S, Acosta AA, Veeck L. Recurrent failure of in vitro fertilization: role of the hemizona assay (HZA) in the sequential diagnosis of specific sperm/oocyte defects. Am J Obstet Gynecol 1991; 164: 1210

57. Oehninger S, et al. Human preovulatory oocytes have a higher sperm-binding ability than immature oocytes under hemizona assay conditions: evidence supporting the concept of 'zona maturation'. Fertil Steril 1991; 55: 1165

58. Overstreet JW, Hembree WC. Penetration of the zona pellucida of nonliving human oocytes by human spermatozoa in vitro. Fertil Steril 1976; 27: 815

59. Yanagimachi R, et al. Retention of biologic characteristics of zona pellucida in highly concentrated salt solution: the use of salt-stored eggs for assessing the fertilizing capacity of spermatozoa. Fertil Steril 1979; 31: 562

60. Yoshimatsu N, Yanagimachi R. Zonae pellucidae of salt-stored hamster and human eggs: their penetrability by homologous and heterologous spermatozoa. Gamete Res 1988; 21: 115

61. Kruger TF, et al. Hemizona assay: use of fresh versus salt-stored human oocytes to evaluate sperm binding potential to the zona pellucida. J In Vitro Fert Embryo Transf 1991; 8: 154

62. Coddington CC, et al. Sperm bound to zona pellucida in hemizona assay demonstrate acrosome reaction when stained with T-6 antibody. Fertil Steril 1990; 54: 504

63. Coddington CC, et al. Functional aspects of human sperm binding to the zona pellucida using the hemizona assay. J Androl 1991; 12: 1

64. Oehninger S, et al. The specificity of human spermatozoa/zona pellucida interaction under hemizona assay conditions. Mol Reprod Dev 1993; 35: 57

65. Franken DR, et al. The hemizona assay (HZA): a predictor of human sperm fertilizing potential in in vitro fertilization (IVF) treatment. J In Vitro Fert Embryo Transf 1989; 6: 44

66. Oehninger S, et al. Hemizona assay: assessment of sperm dysfunction and prediction of in vitro fertilization outcome. Fertil Steril 1989; 51: 665

67. Oehninger S, et al. Clinical significance of human sperm–zona pellucida binding. Fertil Steril 1997; 67: 1121

68. Franken D, et al. The ability of the hemizona assay to predict human fertilization in vitro in different and consecutive IVF/GIFT cycles. Hum Reprod 1993; 8: 1240

69. Gamzu R, et al. The hemizona assay is of good prognostic value for the ability of sperm to fertilize oocytes in vitro. Fertil Steril 1994; 62: 1056

70. Oehninger S, Franken D, Kruger T. Approaching the next millennium: how should we manage andrology diagnosis in the intracytoplasmic sperm injection era? Fertil Steril 1997; 67: 434

71. Duran HE, et al. Intrauterine insemination: a systematic review on determinants of success. Hum Reprod Update 2002; 8: 373

72. Marin-Briggiler CI, et al. Effect of antisperm antibodies present in human follicular fluid upon the acrosome reaction and sperm–zona pellucida interaction. Am J Reprod Immunol 2003; 50: 209

73. Munuce MJ, et al. Modulation of human sperm function by peritoneal fluid. Fertil Steril 2003; 80: 939

74. Coddington CC, et al. Hemizona index (HZI) demonstrates excellent predictability when evaluating sperm fertilizing capacity in in vitro fertilization patients. J Androl 1994; 15: 250

75. Ford WC. Prediction of fecundability from semen analysis: problems in providing an accurate prognosis. Hum Fertil 1999; 2: 25

76. Ombelet W, et al. Semen parameters in a fertile versus subfertile population: a need for change in the interpretation of semen testing. Hum Reprod 1997; 12: 987

77. World Health Organization. WHO Laboratory Manual for the Examination of Human Semen and Sperm–Cervical Mucus Interaction, 4th edn. Cambridge: Cambridge University Press, 1999: 14

78. van der Merwe FH, et al. The use of semen parameters to identify the subfertile male in the general population. Gynecol Obstet Invest 2004; 59: 86

79. Liu de Y, Garrett C, Baker HW. Clinical application of sperm–oocyte interaction tests in in vitro fertilization–embryo transfer and intracytoplasmic sperm injection programs. Fertil Steril 2004; 82: 1251

80. Liu DY, Baker HWG. Disordered acrosome reaction of spermatozoa bound to the zona pellucida: a newly discovered sperm defect causing infertility with reduced sperm–zona penetration and reduced fertilization in vitro. Hum Reprod 1994; 9: 1694

81. Liu DY, Baker HW. Defective sperm–zona pellucida interaction: a major cause of failure of fertilization in clinical in-vitro fertilization. Hum Reprod 2000; 15: 702

82. Liu de Y, Baker HW. Frequency of defective sperm–zona pellucida interaction in severely teratozoospermic infertile men. Hum Reprod 2003; 18: 802

83. Liu de Y, Baker HW. High frequency of defective sperm–zona pellucida interaction in oligozoospermic infertile men. Hum Reprod 2004; 19: 228

84. Tesarik J. Appropriate timing of the acrosome reaction is a major requirement for the fertilizing spermatozoon Hum Reprod 1989; 4: 957

85. Cummins J, et al. A test of the human sperm acrosome reaction following ionophore challenge. J Androl 1991; 12: 98

86. Franken DR, Bastiaan HS, Oehninger S. Physiological induction of the acrosome reaction in human sperm: validation of a microassay using minimal volumes of solubilized, homologous zona pellucida. J Assist Reprod Genet 2000; 17: 374

87. van Duin M, Polman J, De Breet IT. Recombinant human zona pellucida protein ZP3 produced by Chinese hamster ovary cells induces the human sperm acrosome reaction and promotes sperm–egg fusion. Biol Reprod 1994; 51: 607

88. Dong KW, et al. Characterization of the biological activities of a recombinant human zona pellucida protein 3 (ZP3) expressed in human ovarian (PA-1) cells. Am J Obstet Gynecol 2001; 184: 835

89. Esterhuizen AD, et al. Clinical importance of a micro-assay for the evaluation of sperm acrosome reaction using homologous zona pellucida. Andrologia 2001; 33: 87

90. Esterhuizen AD, et al. Clinical importance of zona pellucida induced acrosome reaction (ZIAR test) in cases of failed human fertilization. Hum Reprod 2001; 16: 136

91. Bastiaan HS, et al. Zona pellucida induced acrosome reaction, sperm morphology, and sperm–zona pellucida binding assessments among subfertile men. J Assist Reprod Genet 2002; 19: 329

92. Bastiaan HS, et al. Relationship between zona pellucida-induced acrosome reaction, sperm morphology, sperm–zona pellucida binding, and in vitro fertilization. Fertil Steril 2003; 79: 49

93. Oehninger S. Clinical and laboratory management of male infertility: an opinion on its current status. J Androl 2000; 21: 814

94. Oehninger S. Place of intracytoplasmic sperm injection in clinical management of male infertility. Lancet 2001; 357: 2068

95. Oehninger S, Gosden RG. Should ICSI be the treatment of choice for all cases of in-vitro conception? No, not in light of the scientific data. Hum Reprod 2002; 17: 2237

96. Monzó A, et al. Outcome of ICSI in azoospermic patients: stressing the liaison between the urologist and reproductive medicine. Urology 2001; 58: 69

15

Detection of DNA damage in sperm

Ralf Henkel

INTRODUCTION

It has been reported that sperm DNA damage is predictive of fertilization and pregnancy after natural conception[1–3] and following the use of different techniques of assisted reproduction, namely intrauterine insemination (IUI)[4], *in vitro* fertilization (IVF)[5–8] and intracytoplasmic sperm injection (ICSI)[9–12]. This has important clinical implications for assisted reproduction techniques (ART), because the more invasive is the technique, the higher is the risk that a genetically damaged male genome will be transferred into the oocyte and fertilize the oocyte *in vitro*[10,13].

Normally, if the genetic damage in the male germ cell is severe, embryonic development stops at the time when the paternal genome is switched on, resulting in failed pregnancy[10]. However, genetic and biological protection mechanisms do not necessarily preclude further embryonic development, since Ahmadi and Ng[14] have demonstrated that fertilization with damaged spermatozoa can result in live-born (mouse) pups. This study also showed that the injection of a cytosolic sperm factor into the oocyte is a key point in the activation of oocytes. Since the DNA fragmentation rate is significantly higher in patients with poor semen quality, and DNA damage cannot be recognized while selecting spermatozoa to be injected for ICSI, the probability of

using defective spermatozoa in ICSI is much higher, which in turn increases the risk of transferring damaged DNA into oocytes. In addition, reports regarding increased chromosomal abnormalities, minor or major birth defects or childhood cancer suggest increased risks for babies born after ICSI[15–20], and have led to serious concerns about this technique.

For these grave reasons, various authors from different working groups have suggested that tests for DNA integrity and damage should be introduced into the routine andrological laboratory work-up[21–25]. Compared with other sperm parameters such as motility, Zini *et al.*[26] regard the evaluation of sperm DNA fragmentation as a particularly reliable assay because of its low biological variability. In the past, a number of test systems have been developed to investigate sperm DNA damage at different levels and different sites. Among these, some highly sophisticated assays examine chromosomal aberrations, including multicolor fluorescence *in situ* hybridization (FISH), or assays that probe for structural integrity of sperm DNA such as the sperm chromatin structure assay (SCSA), using flow cytometry. Other test systems for sperm nuclear maturity and condensation such as the aniline blue stain are rather simple, and are based on the evaluation of stained sperm smears by a technologist.

Since most of these assays are reportedly predictive of fertilization and pregnancy, this chapter contributes to an understanding of the currently available assays, so that the results of each can be better assessed. Moreover, in view of the varying financial capabilities of different andrology laboratories, this will then enable selection of which test systems can be employed to offer the most effective andrological diagnosis on the one hand, with optimum results following ART on the other. A summary of the test systems discussed in this chapter with a short description of the principle as well as main advantages and disadvantages is depicted in Table 15.1.

TEST SYSTEMS TO ASSESS DNA DAMAGE/FRAGMENTATION

Sperm DNA damage can occur at different levels, i.e. (1) direct damage of DNA in the form of strand breakages due to apoptosis, oxidative stress or radiation, (2) during chromatin condensation and packaging, resulting in immature nuclear condensation, or (3) at the chromosomal level in the form of chromosomal aberrations or aneuploidies. As each of these levels is important for the transmission of male genetic information and chromatin condensation, they reflect sites where damage that can have serious effects on fertilization and pregnancy may occur. Therefore, methods to measure such damage have been developed. Some of these assays have been tested for their predictive value for male infertility within the scope of an ART program.

Direct DNA damage can occur in the form of base modifications or single- and/or double-strand breakages. Base modifications are assessed through the measurement of 8-hydroxydeoxyguanosine, one of about 20 major biomarkers of oxidative DNA damage that has been shown to be representative, highly specific and potentially a mutagenic product. DNA strand breakages are often measured by means of the comet (single cell gel electrophoresis) assay, TUNEL (terminal deoxynucleotide transferase-mediated dUTP nick-end labeling) assay, in situ nick translation, the metachromatic shift of acridine orange fluorescence in the acridine orange staining test or the sperm chromatin structure assay.

Measurement of 8-hydroxydeoxyguanosine

8-Hydroxydeoxyguanosine (8-OHdG) occurs as substantial oxidative modification of DNA and is present in abundance in DNA[27] at levels of 2–4 per 100 000 deoxyguanosine molecules[28,29] in human spermatozoa. It can be measured in genomic DNA by means of high-performance liquid chromatography (HPLC), with subsequent electrochemical or gas chromatography–mass spectrometry detection. In order to perform this test, DNA has to be extracted from human sperm, followed by enzymatic digestion and detection by means of HPLC analysis. Since the method depends on sufficient extraction of 8-OHdG, quality of DNA digestion and detection limit of the HPLC, relatively high numbers of spermatozoa are necessary[30].

Several studies have revealed significantly higher amounts of 8-OHdG in the spermatozoa of smokers than in non-smokers, which are due to the high oxidative DNA damage. On the other hand, the intake of antioxidants such as vitamin C and its concentration in seminal plasma provide protection again this oxidative damage[29,31]. High amounts of 8-OHdG have also been linked to male infertility[32–34]. If this DNA damage is not repaired, 8-OHdG may be mutagenic and may cause embryonic loss, malformations or childhood cancers[3,28]. Despite that this test shows clear clinical significance, i.e. it is highly specific, quantitative and correlated with sperm function[30,35,36], the method is not commonly used because special equipment is required. Moreover, artifactual oxidation of deoxyguanosine can occur and lead to inaccurate results.

Table 15.1 Principles and main advantages and disadvantages of the most important test systems used to examine sperm DNA damage and chromosomal aberrations

Type of assay	Assay	Assay principle	Main advantages	Main disadvantages
DNA damage	Measurement of 8-hydroxydeoxy guanosine	Base modifications	• Clinically significant • High specificity • Quantitative • Correlates with sperm function	• Special equipment • Artifactual oxidation of deoxyguanosine • Large amount of sample
	Comet assay	DNA fragmentation, single- and double-strand breaks	• Simple to perform and cheap • Correlates with TUNEL assay • High sensitivity • Observation of individual cells • Small number of cells required • Correlates with fertility	• Fluorescence microscopy • Experienced observer • Not specific to oxidative damage
	TUNEL assay	DNA fragmentation, single- and double-strand breaks	• Clinically significant • High sensitivity and specificity • Correlates with sperm function and fertility	• Not specific to oxidative damage • More costly • Special equipment
	In situ nick translation	Single-strand DNA breaks	• Correlates with TUNEL assay • Specific for single-strand DNA breaks • Specific to endogenous DNA breaks	• Not specific to oxidative damage • Special equipment
	Acridine orange test	Differentiates between single- and double-stranded DNA and RNA	• Easy to perform • Low cost • Correlates with sperm function and fertility	• Distinction between differently labeled sperm not always easy • Special equipment
	Sperm chromatin structure assay (SCSA)	Susceptibility of nuclear DNA to denaturation	• Clinically significant • High sensitivity and specificity • Large number of sperm counted by flow cytometry • Unbiased quantitative assessment of DNA-bound acridine orange • Correlates with sperm function and fertility	• Special equipment • More expensive

Continued

Table 15.1   Continued

Type of assay	Assay	Assay principle	Main advantages	Main disadvantages
DNA condensation/ packaging	Aniline blue stain	Staining of lysine residues of remaining histones	• Clinically significant • High specificity and sensitivity • Low cost • Correlates with fertility in IVF • Easy to perform	• Correlation with other sperm parameters controversial • Inconsistencies due to subjective appraisal
	Toluidine blue stain	Binding to damaged dense chromatin	• Correlates with acridine orange stain, TUNEL assay and aniline blue stain • Easy to perform	• Clinical relevance not yet proven • Inconsistencies due to subjective appraisal
	chromomycin A_3 stain	Competing for same DNA binding site with protamines	• Clinically significant • High specificity and sensitivity • Correlates with fertility in IVF and ICSI	• Possible inconsistencies due to subjective appraisal
Chromosomal aberration and aneuploidy	Fluorescence *in situ* hybridization (FISH)	Detection of chromosomal abnormalities	• Clinically significant • High specificity and sensitivity • Correlates with fertility, pregnancy and disease of offspring	• Labor-intensive • Expensive • Special equipment

TUNEL, terminal deoxynucleotide transferase-mediated dUTP nick-end labeling; IVF, *in vitro* fertilization; ICSI, intracytoplasmic sperm injection

Comet assay

The single cell (micro)gel electrophoresis or 'comet' assay was developed to evaluate DNA integrity, including single- and double-strand breaks in somatic cells[37]. In 1988, Singh et al.[38] used alkaline conditions at pH > 13, a modification of the assay, which enables the detection of DNA single-strand breaks, alkali-labile sites, DNA–DNA/DNA–protein crosslinking and single-strand breaks associated with incomplete excision repair sites, and increased the sensitivity of the test. Since that time, the range of applications and the number of users have increased. In this assay, DNA strand breaks migrate in an agarose gel, and, depending on the amount of damaged DNA, create a bigger or smaller tail, which is visualized by means of DNA-specific fluorescent dyes, while intact, supercoiled, compact DNA remains in the nucleus[39]. The shape resembles a comet, and hence the name of the assay. For evaluation of the comet assay, the length of the tail, the percentage of DNA in the tail (intensity of tail staining) or the product of these two parameters, the tail moment, are taken into consideration.

With regard to male infertility and sperm function, several groups[40–43] have shown the clinical relevance of the comet assay. Although its predictive value has also been documented for fertilization and embryo development in both IVF and ICSI[7,44,45], the origin of such DNA damage remains obscure, and sources including apoptosis, improper DNA packaging and ligation during spermatogenesis or oxidative stress have been discussed. For the last, two different sources, reactive oxygen species (ROS) produced by leukocytes or by the spermatozoa themselves, seem possible (for review see reference 46). Interestingly, ROS that are normally found in the male reproductive tract can induce this DNA damage[47]. Moreover, DNA damage was reportedly increased after exposure to toxins (including cigarette-smoking), chemotherapy or radiation[48–51].

Unfortunately, to date, there is no standardized protocol to perform and evaluate this test, and it is therefore difficult to compare the results from different groups. While some authors calculate the percentage of comet-forming sperm, others report the average extent of the tails in a given sperm population[40,52,53]. On the other hand, the assay is easy to perform, is one of the most sensitive techniques available to measure DNA strand breaks[39] and correlates very well with results of the TUNEL assay[54].

TUNEL assay

Another test specific for broken sperm DNA is the TUNEL (terminal deoxynucleotide transferase-mediated dUTP nick-end labeling) assay[55]. The principle is based on the addition of labeled DNA precursors (dUTP: deoxyuridine triphosphate) at single- and double-strand DNA breaks by means of an enzymatically catalyzed reaction, using the template-independent terminal deoxynucleotide transferase (TdT). It incorporates biotinylated or fluorescinated dUTP to the 3'-OH ends of the DNA, which increase with the number of strand breaks. Compared with other methods to detect DNA damage, the TUNEL assay is more sophisticated, more expensive and more time-consuming. However, good-quality control parameters such as low intraobserver and interobserver variability have been demonstrated[56]. In addition, flow-cytometric measurement of the sperm sample analyzing a large amount of cells is possible.

Due to its high specificity and reproducibility, the TUNEL assay is one of the most frequently used test systems to investigate sperm DNA fragmentation. Its relevance in respect of sperm function[57–59] as well as fertilization and pregnancy has been proved repeatedly[4,5,8,60]. Sperm DNA fragmentation provides a clinical explanation even for early embryonic death[61] and recurrent pregnancy loss[62]. Moreover, Shoukir et al.[63] found a significantly lower blastocyst formation rate after ICSI compared with IVF, and postulated a negative paternal effect on preimplantation embryo development. The TUNEL assay evaluates DNA fragmentation, which is a rather late stage of apoptosis, and it cannot actually distinguish between apoptotic and necrotic cells[64,65]. This is even more important, as Sakkas *et al.*[66] found that TUNEL positivity and apoptotic markers such as the asymmetric distribution of phosphatidylserine in the sperm plasma membrane do not always exist in unison.

In situ nick translation

In contrast to the TUNEL assay, which detects both single- and double-strand DNA breaks, *in situ* nick translation detects only single-strand DNA breaks. This test quantifies the incorporation of labeled (biotinylated or fluorescinated) dUTP at the 3′-OH recessed termini of single-stranded DNA in a template-dependent enzymatic reaction by means of DNA polymerase I. Labeling with the *in situ* nick translation is indicative of endogenous nicks in the DNA[67,68]. Data obtained in human spermatozoa with both techniques, *in situ* nick translation and the TUNEL assay, are highly correlated[69]. In somatic cells, necrotic nuclei seem to be preferably stained by *in situ* nick translation, while the TUNEL assay appears to be rather indicative of apoptosis[70]. However, since spermatozoa do not show the typical morphological alterations characteristic of apoptosis in somatic cells, additional specific tests for other markers of apoptosis such as phosphatidylserine externalization, Fas expression or the presence of other active proapoptotic factors should be performed in order to distinguish clearly between apoptosis and necrosis.

Acridine orange test

The acridine orange test is a slide-based version of the original human sperm chromatin heterogeneity test[71] that was developed by Tejada *et al.*[72]. This test measures the susceptibility of sperm nuclear DNA to acid-induced denaturation by means of the metachromatic properties of acridine orange. This dye intercalates into the DNA as a monomer, which fluoresces green with double-stranded DNA, and binds to single-stranded DNA or RNA as an aggregate that emits red-orange light after excitation[73].

Due to its simplicity, several working groups have correlated the acridine orange test with different sperm functional parameters, including normal sperm morphology, as well as with male fertility in assisted reproduction programs. While Ibrahim and Pedersen[74] could not find a significant correlation between the acridine orange test and sperm motility and the penetration of zona-free hamster oocytes in the sperm penetration assay, others have demonstrated significant correlations with motility[75], sperm count[72], sperm–zona pellucida binding[76] and fertilization in an assisted reproduction program for IVF and ICSI[77–79]. Additionally, a significant correlation between chromatin integrity and normal sperm morphology as one of the most predictive sperm parameters for fertilization *in vitro* has been shown repeatedly[75,77].

Despite these mainly positive reports regarding the clinical value of the acridine orange test, concern has arisen about its reliability. This is mainly based on: (1) the poor conditions for the metachromatic shift from green to red-orange as the dye adsorbs on the glass surface, and (2) the difficulty in distinguishing between normal, green, and abnormal, red-orange, sperm heads accurately, especially if a sperm head contains both single- and double-stranded DNA. Furthermore, rapid fading of the fluorescence[80] and heterogeneous slide staining[81] are additional problems when performing this test. Thus, Evenson *et al.*[53,71] developed the more reliable sperm chromatin structure assay (SCSA).

Sperm chromatin structure assay

The SCSA is based on the same principle of metachromatic shift of the color of acridine orange as in the acridine orange test. However, in contrast to the acridine orange test, the detection method in the SCSA is flow cytometry. This approach makes it possible to measure large amounts of spermatozoa (typically 5000–10 000) per sample, which in turn renders the technique easy and highly reproducible[82]. Moreover, the inter- and intra-assay variability as well as the technical problems described for the acridine orange test are overcome by this automated reading. The interassay variability of the flow-cytometric detection of sperm chromatin damage has been shown to be less than 5%[83]. In addition to the advantages described thus far and summarized in Table 15.1, the flexibility of this assay needs to be mentioned. The test can be performed on fresh and frozen samples, which makes it easier to collect the specimen or even to ship them for evaluation[22].

A number of clinical studies have revealed the SCSA to be reliable and predictive for assessing the male fertility status. A percentage of chromatin-disturbed spermatozoa (red-orange stained sperm) higher than 30% is indicative of male infertility and poor fertilization in IUI, IVF and ICSI, including ongoing pregnancy[81,82,84–87]. Considering that sperm DNA integrity as measured by means of the SCSA is a more constant parameter over a longer period of time, compared with other sperm parameters[83], this assay has also been found suitable for effective use in epidemiological studies[88].

TEST SYSTEMS TO ASSESS SPERM DNA CONDENSATION/PACKAGING

Apart from test systems that directly assess the quality and integrity of the DNA itself, assays have been developed that probe DNA packaging and maturity. This is of particular importance because in spermatozoa, the histones, which are the predominant nuclear proteins in any somatic cell, are replaced during spermiogenesis by protamines in a multistep process. These protamines are disulfide bridge-stabilized, highly basic proteins that fit into the minor grooves of the DNA, neutralize the negative charges of the phosphate groups and thus enable the DNA to form linear arrays fitting into the major groove of the neighboring strand, instead of the voluminous supercoiled 'solenoids' present in somatic cells. This results in a highly condensed sperm nucleus in which the DNA takes up about 90% of the total volume. In contrast, the nuclear volume of the DNA in mitotic chromosomes is about 15%, and in somatic cells about 5%[89].

In the case of disturbed chromatin condensation, histones persist in the sperm nucleus and cause decondensation problems in the male genome after the spermatozoon enters the oocyte. Thus, patients showing abnormalities of this essential sperm maturation process during spermiogenesis are subfertile or infertile[90–92]. Various methods based on different principles for evaluation of the maturity grade of sperm chromatin condensation are available, and are discussed below.

Aniline blue stain

Immature, poorly chromatin-condensed sperm nuclei still contain the lysine-rich histones. In an acid–base reaction, acidic aniline blue binds to the basic lysine residues and thus discriminates between lysine-rich histones and arginine/cysteine-rich protamines. This test provides a positive blue staining of spermatozoa with disturbed chromatin condensation, while mature spermatozoa that contain protamines will not be stained. Terquem and Dadoune[93] originally described this simple and inexpensive slide-based test. However, owing to this feature, and the fact that the test is visually scored by a technologist, inconsistencies due to subjective assessment might arise, which in turn can compromise its repeatability. On the other hand, Franken et al.[94] have shown a coefficient of intra-assay variability for the aniline blue stain of less than 10%, indicating that it is a repeatable technique.

According to studies by Dadoune et al.[95] and Auger et al.[96], a normal ejaculate should contain at least 75% aniline blue-negative spermatozoa, which indicates normal chromatin condensation. These data were confirmed by Haidl and Schill[97] and Hammadeh[90], who showed that normal chromatin condensation is mandatory to induce fertilization. With regard to IVF and pregnancy, different groups[97–100] have demonstrated the clinical significance of this simple test, and the supplementation of routine semen analysis with this assay during andrological work-up has been suggested[100]. However, the question of whether the quality of sperm chromatin condensation contributes to poor fertilization and pregnancy rates after ICSI remains debated. While studies by Van Ranst et al.[101] and Hammadeh et al.[102] employing the aniline blue stain failed to predict the outcome of fertilization by ICSI, Sakkas et al.[103] showed, when applying the chromomycin A_3 (CMA$_3$) stain, a significantly higher percentage of spermatozoa with poorly packed chromatin in the ejaculate and only about half the fertilization rate in ICSI patients, compared with IVF patients. ICSI embryos even had a significantly lower developmental potential to reach the blastocyst stage. In a comparative study using the aniline blue and the CMA$_3$ stain, Razavi et al.[104] confirmed this result, as only the detection of sperm protamine deficiency by means of CMA$_3$ showed a significant effect on ICSI outcome. Thus, it appears that poor sperm chromatin condensation may contribute to the failure of fertilization after ICSI.

Toluidine blue stain

The toluidine blue stain is another slide-based simple and inexpensive test method to evaluate sperm DNA structure and packaging[105,106], which is based on the metachromatic and orthochromatic staining abilities for chromatin. Toluidine blue is basic thiazine nuclear dye that is intensively incorporated into damaged dense chromatin. Like acridine orange, after acid treatment of somatic apoptotic cells, this dye shows a metachromatic shift of color from light blue in normal sperm heads to purple-violet in nuclei with fragmented DNA[106]. To differentiate spermatozoa for DNA

integrity, Erenpreisa et al.[107] introduced this method. The same authors demonstrated a high correlation ($r = 0.63$–0.70; $p < 0.01$) between the toluidine blue stain, the acridine orange stain and the aniline blue stain, and concluded that the technique is sensitive enough to estimate in situ sperm DNA integrity. In addition, a significant correlation between the purple-violet staining pattern and the TUNEL assay could be revealed[108]. In an earlier study by Barrera et al.[109], it was found that sperm from fertile donors showed mostly the orthochromatic pale-blue staining pattern, whereas in oligozoospermic patients a high percentage of spermatozoa revealed the metachromatic purple-violet staining. Unfortunately, further direct clinical significance has not yet been proved. Therefore, one can rely only on the high correlation with acridine orange and on the experience with that test.

Chromomycin A_3 stain

Chromomycin A_3 (CMA$_3$) is a guanine–cytosine-specific fluorochrome that competes directly with protamines for the same binding site in the DNA. Like the aniline blue stain, the CMA$_3$ stain is a slide-based method that identifies poorly condensed DNA. Strongly stained sperm heads apparently lack protamines, whereas spermatozoa not stained by CMA$_3$ show normal chromatin condensation. Thus, the stain is indicative of an underprotamination of spermatozoa[67,68]. This was confirmed by the observation by Bizzaro et al.[110] that CMA$_3$ positivity of murine and human spermatozoa decreases after in situ protamination with salmon protamines. Moreover, these authors showed that the addition of increasing amounts of salmon protamines induced distinct morphological changes, so that initially deprotaminated sperm heads, which were decondensed, regained their original condensed appearance after the treatment.

With regard to other sperm parameters, the CMA$_3$ stain has been significantly and positively correlated with normal sperm morphology and negatively correlated with sperm count but not with sperm motility[94,111,112]. Manicardi et al.[68] revealed a significant association of CMA$_3$ positivity with the presence of endogenous nicks in sperm DNA, which in turn is an indication of disturbed spermiogenesis in specific patients, as these nicks normally occur during late spermiogenesis and disappear once sperm chromatin packaging is completed[113,114]. Since the test is also highly predictive of fertilization after IVF as well as after ICSI[104,112,115–117], and has been shown to be superior in predicting the outcome of ART as compared with aniline blue staining and the acridine orange test[117], it is suggested that determination of sperm chromatin condensation should be performed in a sequential andrological diagnosis program prior to any kind of assisted reproduction. Reportedly, the calculated cut-off value for the prediction of fertilization is 30%[117], i.e. at least 70% of the spermatozoa should be CMA$_3$-negative.

TEST SYSTEMS TO ASSESS CHROMOSOMAL ABERRATION AND ANEUPLOIDY

Apart from direct damage to sperm DNA resulting in strand breakages and the abnormal packaging of the male genome, chromosomal aberrations including aneuploidy or structural chromosome reorganizations have been identified as a cause of male infertility. Previous research has revealed that elevated genetic damage in spermatozoa is significantly increased in infertile men[118,119], and that aneuploidy is significantly higher in patients with recurrent pregnancy losses[120]. This is of particular importance, since it has been shown that chromosomal aneuploidy and diploidy in spermatozoa are negatively correlated with sperm count in the ejaculate and progressive motility[121,122], and concern about miscarriages and chromosomal abnormalities in the offspring has been raised, particularly

for ICSI[43,123,124]. The most frequently occurring aneuploidy syndromes are: triple X, Klinefelter's (XXY), Turner's (X instead of XX or XY), XYY, Patau's (trisomy of chromosome 13), Edward's (trisomy of chromosome 18) or Down's (trisomy of chromosome 21). A very rare disorder is the Jacobsen syndrome, in which a terminal deletion of chromosome 11q occurs. Others are the 'Cri du chat' syndrome, which is caused by deletion of part of the short arm of chromosome 5, or the Wolf-Hirschhorn syndrome, which is caused by partial deletion of the short arm of chromosome 4. The method of choice to investigate these chromosomal aberrations is fluorescence *in situ* hybridization (FISH).

Fluorescence *in situ* hybridization

The principle of FISH is the use of fluorochrome-labeled chromosome-specific probes that recognize a large section of the chromosome (0.2–2.0 Mb). These probes are hybridized with a sample of spermatozoa, and the labeled part of the chromosome appears as a fluorescent domain within the nucleus, where it can be identified by means of fluorescence microscopy[125]. Meanwhile, probes for all human and many rodent chromosomes are available, and can be used to identify such chromosomal aberrations by applying so-called multicolor FISH, whereby usually three or four differently fluorescing probes are hybridized in parallel. This is because the scoring has to be performed visually, and the eye is limited in distinguishing different fluorescing colors.

Although multicolor FISH has been shown to be highly specific with little or no error, and the specimen can be frozen even without cryoprotection until examination, the technique is currently highly labor-intensive and expensive. In this regard, Baumgartner et al.[126] recently developed a laser-scanning cytometry method for automated sperm analysis of the X chromosome, but the technique is still expensive and requires highly skilled personnel.

CONCLUSIONS

Generally, DNA damage can occur at different levels, i.e. direct breakage of the DNA, abnormal chromosome packaging and chromosomal aberrations. DNA damage has been proved to be of importance for human fertility as well as for the health of the offspring. Several techniques have been developed to examine such damage. Based on this knowledge, an andrological investigation should not only consist of routine spermiogram analysis, which includes sperm count, motility and morphology, but also incorporate more sophisticated testing, e.g. for DNA damage, as there is compelling evidence for its importance and clinical relevance. The practical question arising at this point is which test should be applied. This certainly depends on the personnel and financial capabilities of an ART program or andrology unit. Other questions arise concerning the standardization of such tests. The latter is an important issue because this is closely connected with the predictive value of the test in question.

Recently, more research has been performed, and understanding of the influence of the paternal genome on the reproductive process and methodology for examining such DNA damage have improved considerably. To date, various methods of testing sperm DNA integrity have been investigated with regard to their clinical value. Even though some of them are rather expensive and others are less reproducible, nowadays more information about male fertility status can and should be obtained, following which better strategies can be pursued to improve counseling and treatment of patients.

REFERENCES

1. Evenson DP, et al. Utility of the sperm chromatin structure assay as a diagnostic and prognostic tool in the human fertility clinic. Hum Reprod 1999; 14: 1039
2. Spano M, et al. Sperm chromatin damage impairs human fertility. Fertil Steril 2000; 73: 43
3. Loft S, et al. Oxidative DNA damage in human sperm influences time to pregnancy. Hum Reprod 2003; 18: 1265
4. Duran EH, et al. Sperm DNA quality predicts intrauterine insemination outcome: a prospective cohort study. Hum Reprod 2002; 17: 3122
5. Sun JG, Jurisicova A, Casper RF. Detection of deoxyribonucleic acid fragmentation in human sperm: correlation with fertilization in vitro. Biol Reprod 1997; 56: 602
6. Host E, Lindenberg S, Smidt-Jensen S. DNA strand breaks in human spermatozoa: correlation with fertilization in vitro in oligozoospermic men and in men with unexplained infertility. Acta Obstet Gynecol Scand 2000; 79: 189
7. Morris ID, et al. The spectrum of DNA damage in human sperm assessed by single cell gel electrophoresis (Comet assay) and its relationship to fertilization and embryo development. Hum Reprod 2002; 17: 990
8. Henkel R, et al. Influence of deoxyribonucleic acid damage on fertilization and pregnancy. Fertil Steril 2004; 81: 965
9. Lopes S, et al. Sperm deoxyribonucleic acid fragmentation is increased in poor-quality semen samples and correlates with failed fertilization in intracytoplasmic sperm injection. Fertil Steril 1998; 69: 528
10. Henkel R, et al. DNA fragmentation of spermatozoa and ART. Reprod Biomed Online 2003; 7: 477
11. Lewis SEM, et al. An algorithm to predict pregnancy in assisted reproduction. Hum Reprod 2004; 19: 1385
12. Tesarik J, Greco E, Mendoza C. Late, but not early, paternal effect on human embryo development is related to sperm DNA fragmentation. Hum Reprod 2004; 19: 611
13. Twigg JP, Irvine DS, Aitken RJ. Oxidative damage of DNA in human spermatozoa does not preclude pronucleus formation at intracytoplasmic sperm injection. Hum Reprod 1998; 13: 1864
14. Ahmadi A, Ng SC. Developmental capacity of damaged spermatozoa. Hum Reprod 1999; 14: 2279
15. In't Veld P, et al. Sex chromosomal abnormalities and intracytoplasmic sperm injection. Lancet 1995; 346: 773
16. Kurinczuk JJ, Bower C. Birth defects in infants conceived by intracytoplasmic sperm injection: an alternative interpretation. Br Med J 1997; 315: 1260
17. Ji BT, et al. Paternal cigarette smoking and the risk of childhood cancer among offspring of non-smoking mothers. J Natl Cancer Inst 1997; 89: 238

18. Aitken RJ, et al. Relative impact of oxidative stress on the functional competence and genomic integrity of human spermatozoa. Biol Reprod 1998; 59: 1037

19. Aitken RJ, Krausz C. Oxidative stress, DNA damage and the Y chromosome. Reproduction 2001; 122: 497

20. Aitken RJ, Sawyer D. The human spermatozoon – not waving but drowning. Adv Exp Med Biol 2003; 518: 85

21. De Jonge C. The clinical value of sperm nuclear DNA assessment. Hum Fertil 2002; 5: 51

22. Perreault SD, et al. Integrating new tests of sperm genetic integrity into semen analysis: breakout group discussion. Adv Exp Med Biol 2003; 518: 253

23. Sharma RK, Said T, Agarwal A. Sperm DNA damage and its clinical relevance in assessing reproductive outcome. Asian J Androl 2004; 6: 139

24. Tesarik J, Greco E, Mendoza C. Late, but not early, paternal effect on human embryo development is related to sperm DNA fragmentation. Hum Reprod 2004; 19: 611

25. Henkel R, et al. Sperm function and assisted reproduction technology. Reprod Med Biol 2005; 4: 7

26. Zini A, et al. Biologic variability of sperm DNA denaturation in infertile men. Urology 2001; 58: 258

27. Floyd RA. The role of 8-hydroguanine in carcinogenesis. Carcinogenesis 1990; 11: 1447

28. Fraga CG, et al. Ascorbic acid protects against endogenous oxidative DNA damage in human sperm. Proc Natl Acad Sci USA 1991; 88: 11003

29. Fraga CG, et al. Smoking and low antioxidant levels increase oxidative damage to sperm DNA. Mutat Res 1996; 351: 199

30. Shen HM, Ong CN. Detection of oxidative DNA damage in human sperm and its association with sperm function and male infertility. Free Rad Biol Med 2000; 28: 529

31. Shen HM, et al. Detection of oxidative DNA damage in human sperm and its association with cigarette smoking. Reprod Toxicol 1997; 11: 675

32. Kodama H, et al. Increased oxidative deoxyribonucleic acid damage in the spermatozoa of infertile male patients. Fertil Steril 1997; 68: 519

33. Ni ZY, et al. Does the increase of 8-hydroxyguanosine lead to poor sperm quality? Mutat Res 1997; 381: 77

34. Shen HM, Chia SE, Ong CN. Evaluation of oxidative DNA damage in human sperm and its association with male infertility. J Androl 1999; 20: 718

35. Chen CS, et al. Hydroxyl radical-induced decline in motility and increase in lipid peroxidation and DNA modification in human sperm. Biochem Mol Int 1997; 43: 291

36. Chen CS, et al. Maintenance of human sperm motility and prevention of oxidative damage through co-culture incubation. Andrologia 1997; 29: 227

37. Östling O, Johanson KJ. Microelectrophoretic study of radiation-induced DNA damages in individual mammalian cells. Biochem Biophys Res Commun 1984; 123: 291

38. Singh NP, et al. A simple technique for quantitation of low levels of DNA damage in individual cells. Exp Cell Res 1988; 175: 184

39. Collins AR, et al. The comet assay: what can it really tell us? Mutat Res 1997; 375: 183

40. Irvine DS, et al. DNA integrity in human spermatozoa: relationships with semen quality. J Androl 2000; 21: 33

41. Chan PJ, et al. A simple comet assay for archived sperm correlates DNA fragmentation to reduced hyperactivation and penetration of zona-free hamster oocytes. Fertil Steril 2001; 75: 186

42. Donnelly ET, et al. Assessment of DNA integrity and morphology of ejaculated spermatozoa from fertile and infertile men before and after cryopreservation. Hum Reprod 2001; 16: 1191

43. Schmid TE, et al. Genetic damage in oligozoospermic patients detected by fluorescence in-situ hybridization, inverse restriction site mutation assay, sperm chromatin structure assay and the Comet assay. Hum Reprod 2003; 18: 1474

44. Tomsu M, Sharma V, Miller D. Embryo quality and IVF treatment outcomes may correlate with different sperm comet assay parameters. Hum Reprod 2002; 17: 1856

45. Lewis SEM, et al. An algorithm to predict pregnancy in assisted reproduction. Hum Reprod 2004; 19: 1385

46. Henkel R. DNA fragmentation and its influence on fertilization and pregnancy outcome. In Kruger TF, Oehninger SC, eds. Male Infertility. London: Informa Healthcare, 2006: Ch 19

47. Aitken RJ. The Amoroso Lecture: The human spermatozoon – a cell in crisis? J Reprod Fertil 1999; 115: 1

48. Chatterjee R, et al. Testicular and sperm DNA damage after treatment with fludarabine for chronic

lymphocytic leukaemia. Hum Reprod 2000; 15: 762

49. Haines GA, et al. Increased levels of Comet-detected spermatozoal DNA damage following in vivo isotopic- or X-irradiation of spermatogonia. Mutat Res 2001; 495: 21

50. Migliore L, et al. Assessment of sperm DNA integrity in workers exposed to styrene. Hum Reprod 2002; 17: 2912

51. Belcheva A, et al. Effects of cigarette smoking on sperm plasma membrane integrity and DNA fragmentation. Int J Androl 2004; 27: 296

52. Hughes CM, et al. A comparison of baseline and induced DNA damage in human spermatozoa from fertile and infertile men, using a modified comet assay. Mol Hum Reprod 1996; 2: 613

53. Evenson DP, Larson KL, Jost LK. Sperm chromatin structure assay: its clinical use for detecting sperm DNA fragmentation in male infertility and comparisons with other techniques. J Androl 2002; 23: 25

54. Aravindan GR, et al. Susceptibility of human sperm to in situ DNA denaturation is strongly correlated with DNA strand breaks identified by single-cell electrophoresis. Exp Cell Res 1997; 236: 231

55. Gorczyca W, et al. Presence of DNA strand breaks and increased sensitivity of DNA in situ to denaturation in abnormal human sperm cells: analogy to apoptosis of somatic cells. Exp Cell Res 1993; 207: 202

56. Barroso G, Morshedi M, Oehninger S. Analysis of DNA fragmentation, plasma membrane translocation of phosphatidylserine and oxidative stress in human spermatozoa. Hum Reprod 2000; 15: 1338

57. Oosterhuis GJE, et al. Measuring apoptosis in human spermatozoa: a biological assay for semen quality? Fertil Steril 2000; 74: 245

58. Younglai EV, et al. Sperm swim-up techniques and DNA fragmentation. Hum Reprod 2001; 16: 1950

59. Shen HM, et al. Detection of apoptotic alterations in sperm in subfertile patients and their correlations with sperm quality. Hum Reprod 2002; 17: 1266

60. Benchaib M, et al. Sperm DNA fragmentation decreases the pregnancy rate in an assisted reproductive technique. Hum Reprod 2003; 18: 1023

61. Jurisicova A, Varmuza S, Casper RF. Programmed cell death and human embryo fragmentation. Mol Hum Reprod 1996; 2: 93

62. Carrell D, et al. Sperm DNA fragmentation is increased in couples with unexplained recurrent pregnancy loss. Arch Androl 2003; 49: 49

63. Shoukir Y, et al. Blastocyst development from supernumerary embryos after intracytoplasmic sperm injection: a paternal influence? Hum Reprod 1998; 13: 1632

64. Frankfurt OS, et al. Monoclonal antibody to single-stranded DNA is a specific and sensitive cellular marker of apoptosis. Exp Cell Res 1996; 226: 387

65. Didenko VV, Hornsby PJ. Presence of double-strand breaks with single-base 3' overhangs in cells undergoing apoptosis but not necrosis. J Cell Biol 1996; 135: 1369

66. Sakkas D, et al. Nature of DNA damage in ejaculated human spermatozoa and the possible involvement of apoptosis. Biol Reprod 2002; 66: 1061

67. Bianchi PG, et al. Effect of deoxyribonucleic acid protamination on fluorochrome staining and in situ nick-translation of murine and human mature spermatozoa. Biol Reprod 1993; 49: 1083

68. Manicardi GC, et al. Presence of endogenous nicks in DNA of ejaculated human spermatozoa and its relationship to chromomycin A3 accessibility. Biol Reprod 1995; 52: 864

69. Manicardi GC, et al. DNA strand breaks in ejaculated human spermatozoa: comparison of susceptibility to the nick translation and terminal transferase assays. Histochem J 1998; 30: 33

70. Gorczyca W, Gong J, Darzynkiewicz Z. Detection of DNA strand breaks in individual apoptotic cells by the in situ terminal deoxynucleotidyl transferase and nick translation assays. Cancer Res 1993; 53: 1945

71. Evenson DP, Darzynkiewicz Z, Melamed MR. Relation of mammalian sperm chromatin heterogeneity to fertility. Science 1980; 210: 1131

72. Tejada RI, et al. A test for the practical evaluation of male fertility by acridine orange (AO) fluorescence. Fertil Steril 1984; 42: 87

73. Rigler R. Microfluorometric characterization of intracellular nucleic acids and nucleoproteins by acridine orange. Acta Physiol Scand 1966; 67 (Suppl 1): 122

74. Ibrahim ME, Pedersen H. Acridine orange fluorescence as male fertility test. Arch Androl 1988; 20: 125

75. Shibahara H, et al. Clinical significance of the acridine orange test performed as a routine examination: comparison with the CASA estimates and strict criteria. Int J Androl 2003; 26: 236

76. Liu DY, Baker HWG. Sperm nuclear chromatin normality: relationship with sperm morphology, sperm–zona pellucida binding, and fertilization rates. Fertil Steril 1992; 58: 1178

77. Claassens OE, et al. The acridine orange test: determining the relationship between sperm morphology and fertilization in vitro. Hum Reprod 1992; 7: 242

78. Virant-Klun I, Tomazevic T, Meden-Vrtovec H. Sperm single-stranded DNA, detected by acridine orange staining, reduces fertilization and quality of ICSI-derived embryos. J Assist Reprod Genet 2002; 19: 319

79. Katayose H, et al. Use of diamide–acridine orange fluorescence staining to detect aberrant protamination of human ejaculated sperm nuclei. Fertil Steril 2003; 79 (Suppl 1): 670

80. Duran EH, et al. A logistic regression model including DNA status and morphology of spermatozoa for prediction of fertilization in vitro. Hum Reprod 1998; 13: 1235

81. Evenson DP, et al. Utility of the sperm chromatin structure assay as a diagnostic and prognostic tool in the human fertility clinic. Hum Reprod 1999; 14: 1039

82. Evenson DP, Larson KL, Jost LK. Sperm chromatin structure assay: its clinical use for detecting sperm DNA fragmentation in male infertility and comparisons with other techniques. J Androl 2002; 23: 25

83. Zini A, et al. Correlations between two markers of sperm DNA integrity, DNA denaturation and DNA fragmentation, in fertile and infertile men. Fertil Steril 2001; 75: 674

84. Larson KL, et al. Sperm chromatin structure assay parameters as predictors of failed pregnancy following assisted reproductive techniques. Hum Reprod 2000; 15: 1717

85. Spano M, et al. Sperm chromatin damage impairs human fertility. Fertil Steril 2000; 73: 43

86. Bungum M, et al. The predictive value of sperm chromatin structure assay (SCSA) parameters for the outcome of intrauterine insemination, IVF and ICSI. Hum Reprod 2004; 19: 1401

87. Virro MR, et al. Sperm chromatin structure assay (SCSA®) parameters are related to fertilization, blastocyst development, and ongoing pregnancy in in vitro fertilization and intracytoplasmic sperm injection cycles. Fertil Steril 2004; 81: 1289

88. Spano M, et al. The applicability of the flow cytometric sperm chromatin structure assay in epidemiological studies. Hum Reprod 1998; 13: 2495

89. Ward WS, Coffey D.S. DNA packaging and organization in mammalian spermatozoa: comparison with somatic cells. Biol Reprod 1991; 44: 569

90. Hammadeh ME. Association between sperm cell chromatin condensation, morphology based on

91. Braun RE. Packaging paternal genome with protamine. Nat Genet 2001; 28: 10

92. Steger K, et al. Round spermatids from infertile men exhibit decreased protamine-1 and -2 mRNA. Hum Reprod 2001; 16: 709

93. Terquem A, Dadoune JP. Aniline blue staining of human spermatozoa chromatin: evaluation of nuclear maturation. In André J, ed. The Sperm Cell. The Hague: Martinus Nijhoff, 1983: 249

94. Franken DR, et al. Normal sperm morphology and chromatin packaging: comparison between aniline blue and chromomycin A3 staining. Andrologia 1999; 31: 361

95. Dadoune JP, Mayaux MJ, Guilhard-Moscato ML. Correlation between defects in chromatin condensation of human, spermatozoa stained by aniline blue and semen characteristics. Andrologia 1988; 20: 211

96. Auger J, et al. Aniline blue staining as a marker of sperm chromatin defects associated with different semen characteristics between proven fertile and suspected infertile men. Int J Androl 1990; 13: 452

97. Haidl G, Schill WB. Assessment of sperm chromatin condensation: an important test for prediction of IVF outcome. Arch Androl 1994; 32: 263

98. Foresta C, et al. Sperm nuclear instability and staining with aniline blue: abnormal persistence of histones in spermatozoa in infertile men. Int J Androl 1992; 15: 330

99. Liu DY, Baker HWG. Sperm nuclear chromatin normality: relationship with sperm morphology, sperm–zona pellucida binding, and fertilization rates. Fertil Steril 1992; 58: 1178

100. Hammadeh ME, et al. Predictive value of sperm chromatin condensation (aniline blue staining) in the assessment of male fertility. Arch Androl 2001; 46: 99

101. Van Ranst H, et al. Chromatin condensation assessment in spermatozoa used for intracytoplasmic sperm injection. Hum Reprod 1994; 9 (Suppl 4): 24

102. Hammadeh ME, et al. The effect of chromatin condensation (aniline blue staining) and morphology (strict criteria) of human spermatozoa on fertilization, cleavage and pregnancy rates in an intracytoplasmic sperm injection programme. Hum Reprod 1996; 11: 2468

103. Sakkas D, et al. Spermnuclear DNA damage and altered chromatin structure: effect on fertilization

and embryo development. Hum Reprod 1998; 13 (Suppl 4): 11

104. Razavi S, et al. Effect of human sperm chromatin anomalies on fertilization outcome post-ICSI. Andrologia 2003; 35: 238

105. Erenpreisa J, Freivalds T, Selivanova G. Influence of chromatin condensation on the adsorption spectra of nuclei stained with toluidine blue. Acta Morph Hung 1992; 40: 3

106. Erenpreisa J, et al. Apoptotic cell nuclei favour aggregation and fluorescence quenching of DNA dyes. Histochem Cell Biol 1997; 108: 67

107. Erenpreisa J, et al. Comparative study of cytochemical tests for sperm chromatin integrity. J Androl 2001; 22: 45

108. Erenpreisa J, et al. Toluidine blue test for sperm DNA integrity and elaboration of image cytometry algorithm. Cytometry A 2003; 52A: 19

109. Barrera C, et al. Metachromatic staining of human sperm nuclei after reduction of disulphide bonds. Acta Histochem 1993; 94: 141

110. Bizzaro D, et al. In-situ competition between protamines and fluorochromes for sperm DNA. Mol Hum Reprod 1998; 4: 127

111. Bianchi PG, et al. Use of the guanine–cytosine (GC) specific fluorochrome, chromomycin A3, as an indicator of poor sperm morphology. J Assist Reprod Genet 1996; 13: 246

112. Lolis D, et al. Chromomycin A3-staining as an indicator of protamine deficiency and fertilization. Int J Androl 1996; 19: 23

113. McPherson SMG, Longo FJ. Localization of DNAse I-hypersensitive regions during rat spermatogenesis: stage dependent patterns and unique sensitivity of elongating spermatids. Mol Reprod Dev 1992; 31: 268

114. Sakkas D, et al. Relationship between the presence of endogenous nicks and sperm chromatin packing in maturing and fertilizing mouse spermatozoa. Biol Reprod 1995; 52: 1149

115. Esterhuizen AD, et al. Sperm chromatin packaging as an indicator of in-vitro fertilization rates. Hum Reprod 2000; 15: 657

116. Esterhuizen AD, et al. Chromatin packaging as an indicator of human sperm dysfunction. J Assist Reprod Genet 2000; 17: 508

117. Nasr-Esfahani MH, Razavi S, Mardani M. Relation between different human sperm nuclear maturity tests and in vitro fertilization. J Assist Reprod Genet 2001; 18: 221

118. Moosani N, et al. A 47,XXY fetus resulting from ICSI in a man with elevated frequency of 24,XY spermatozoa. Hum Reprod 1999; 14: 1137

119. Ohashi Y, et al. High frequency of XY disomy in spermatozoa of severe oligozoospermic men. Hum Reprod 2001; 16: 703

120. Carrell DT, et al. Elevated sperm chromosome aneuploidy and apoptosis in patients with unexplained recurrent pregnancy loss. Obstet Gynecol 2003; 101: 1229

121. Vendrell JM, et al. Meiotic abnormalities and spermatogenic parameters in severe oligoasthenozoospermia. Hum Reprod 1999; 14: 375

122. Vegretti W, et al. Correlation between semen parameters and sperm rates investigated by fluorescence in-situ hybridization in infertile men. Hum Reprod 2000; 15: 351

123. Lewis-Jones I, et al. Sperm chromosomal abnormalities are linked to sperm morphologic deformities. Fertil Steril 2003; 79: 212

124. Lathi RB, Milki AA. Rate of aneuploidy in miscarriages following in vitro fertilization and intracytoplasmic sperm injection. Fertil Steril 2004; 81: 1270

125. Shi QH, Martin RH. Aneuploidy in human sperm: a review of the frequency and distribution of aneuploidy, effects of donor age and lifestyle factors. Cytogenet Cell Genet 2000; 90: 219

126. Baumgartner A, et al. Automated evaluation of frequencies of aneuploid sperm by laser-scanning cytometry (LSC). Cytometry 2001; 44: 156

16

Chromosomal and genetic abnormalities in male infertility

Pasquale Patrizio, Jose Sepúlveda, Sepideh Mehri

BACKGROUND

About 15% of couples of reproductive age are affected by infertility, and in some 50% the male is the sole or main contributor[1]. The identification and initial classification of male infertility still rely on the results of semen analysis (i.e. azoospermia, oligozoospermia, asthenozoospermia, teratozoospermia or a combination), but this method alone is insufficient to determine a specific etiology of the disorder. A complete work-up, including detailed history and physical examination, hormonal and immunological assays, ultrasound or Doppler studies and genetic and chromosome testing is essential[2]. Recent advances in molecular genetics have greatly improved our understanding of many unexplained forms; however, 50% of cases still remain unclassified[3].

The advent of assisted reproductive techniques, namely intracytoplasmic sperm injection (ICSI), has provided the opportunity for severely infertile men to father their own offspring, but if genetic or chromosomal defects are responsible for infertility, then there is concern about transmitting genetic defects to the next generation[4].

There are different approaches to classifying male infertility on a genetic basis. In some textbooks the different forms are divided into pretesticular, testicular and post-testicular forms. A genetic or a chromosomal numerical or structural disorder can impair hormonal production or the stimulation of spermatogenesis (pretesticular event), or can impact upon control of the spermatogenic process itself (testicular event). In animal models and to some extent also in humans, genetic abnormalities affecting signaling cascades involved in the meiotic control of spermatogenesis are continuously being discovered and reported[5,6]. Other genetic/chromosomal disorders (for example cystic fibrosis and adult polycystic kidney disease) can affect sperm transport (post-testicular event).

In this chapter we utilize the following scheme of classification: (1) male infertility with a gene defect and (2) male infertility with chromosomal aberrations (either numerical or structural)[7].

MALE INFERTILITY WITH A GENE DEFECT

These disorders are caused by a mutation at a single-gene locus, and either can occur *de novo* or are inherited as autosomal (dominant or recessive) or X-linked. It is estimated that over 10 000 human diseases are monogenic. The global prevalence of all single-gene diseases at birth is approximately 10/1000[8]. Mendelian disorders observed in infertile men are detailed in Table 16.1. This list is by no means complete, but includes those

Table 16.1   Gene defects and male infertility

Condition	Gene involved (mapping)	Incidence	Phenotype	Inherited
Hemochromatosis	HFE (6p21.3) HFE (1q21)-juvenile	1:500	Organ failure (liver and testis) by iron overload	Autosomal recessive
Autosomal dominant polycystic kidney disease	PKD1 (16p13.3) PKD2 (4q21–23) PKD3 (?)	1:1000	Multiple cysts (kidney, liver, spleen, pancreas, testis, epididymis, seminal vesicle)	Autosomal dominant
Cystic fibrosis	CFTR (7q31.2)	1:2500	Respiratory infections, Wolffian duct anomaly, pancreatic insufficiency	Autosomal recessive
Congenital adrenal hyperplasia	P450C21 (6p21.3) 21-hydroxylase deficiency (most common)	1:5000	Variable, elevated ACTH, inhibited FSH/LH secretion, azoospermia	Autosomal recessive
Myotonic dystrophy	DMPK (19q13.2–3)	1:8000	Muscle wasting, cataracts; atrophic testes	Autosomal dominant
Usher's syndrome	USH1 (14q32) USH2 (1q41) USH3 (3q21–q25)	1:17 000	Low sperm motility, hearing loss, retinitis pigmentosa	Autosomal recessive
Prader–Willi syndrome	SNRPN (15q11q13)	1:20 000	Obesity, muscular hypotonia, mental retardation, hypogonadotropic hypogonadism	Autosomal dominant
Sex reversal syndrome	SRY (Yp11.3)	1:25 000	46,XX SRY(+) 46,XY SRY(−)	Y-linked
Kallman's syndrome	KAL1 (Xp22.3)[1] KAL2 (8p12)[2] KAL3 (?)[3]	1:30 000	Hypogonadotropic hypogonadism, anosmia	[1]X-linked recessive [2]Autosomal dominant [3]Autosomal recessive
Immotile cilia syndrome	DNAI1 (9p21–p13) DNAH5 (5p) 19q13.2, 16p2, 15q13	1:35 000	Sinusitis, bronchiectasis, immotile sperm	Autosomal recessive
Cerebellar ataxia	CLA1 (9q34–9) CLA3 (20q11–q13)	1:50 000	Eunuchoid phenotype, cerebellar impairment, atrophic testes	Autosomal recessive
Sickle cell anemia	HBB (11p15.5) (mutation)	1:58 000	RBC sickle shape, testicular microinfarctions	Autosomal recessive
Androgen insensitivity syndrome	AR (Xq11–q12)	1:60 000	Partial/complete testicular feminization	X-linked recessive
β-Thalassemia	HBB (11p15) (deletion)	1:114 000	Anemia; iron overload (pituitary and testis)	Autosomal recessive
Bardet–Biedl syndrome	BBS (11q13, 16q21, 3p12–q13, 15q22.3, 2q31, 20p12, 4q27, 14q32.11)	1:160 000	Retinal degeneration, obesity, cognitive impairment, GU malformations, polydactyly, hypogonadism	Autosomal recessive

Continued

Table 16.1   *Continued*

Condition	Gene involved (mapping)	Incidence	Phenotype	Inherited
Mixed gonadal dysgenesis??	WT1 (11p13) DAX1 (Xp21.3) testatin (20p11.2)	Rare	Unilateral testis (most common with SCO) and contralateral streak gonad, ambiguous external genitalia	Autosomal dominant X-linked recessive cytogenetic
Persistent Müllerian duct syndrome	AMH (19p13.3–p13.2) AMHR (12q13)	< 200 cases reported	Incomplete involution of Müllerian structures	Autosomal? X-linked
LH/FSH hormone and receptor mutations	LHβ (19q13.32) FSHβ (11p13)	Few male cases reported	Delayed puberty, arrested spermatogenesis	Autosomal recessive?
5α-Reductase deficiency	SRD5A1 (5p15) SRD5A2 (2p23)	Unknown	Male pseudohermaphroditism, severe hypospadias	Autosomal recessive

LH, luteinizing hormone; FSH, follicle stimulating hormone; ACTH, adrenocorticotropic hormone; RBC, red blood cell; GU, genitourinary; SCO, Sertoli cell-only syndrome

genetic conditions with the potential for clinical relevance.

Kallman's syndrome

Kallman's syndrome (KS) consists of congenital hypogonadotropic hypogonadism and anosmia. The gene responsible for the X-linked form of KS, KAL, encodes a protein, anosmin-1, that plays a key role in the migration of GnRH neurons and olfactory nerves to the hypothalamus. As a consequence of failed neuronal migration, the hypothalamus and anterior pituitary are unable to stimulate the testis. The hallmark of KS is delayed puberty and atrophic testes (< 2 cm). Clinical manifestations depend on the degree of hypogonadism, and in some cases the syndrome may present only with subfertility. Testicular biopsies display a wide range of findings from germ-cell aplasia to focal areas of complete spermatogenesis. In addition to X-linked pedigrees, autosomal dominant and recessive kindred with KS have also been reported[9].

Autosomal dominant KAL2 in 8p12 (FGFR-1, fibroblast growth factor receptor-1) and autosomal recessive KAL3 are associated with non-reproductive features, including cleft palate, mirror movements and dental agenesis[10].

Recent studies have confirmed that mutations in the coding sequence of the KAL1 gene occur in the minority of KS cases, while the majority of familial (and presumably sporadic) cases are caused by defects in at least two autosomal genes[11].

Congenital adrenal hyperplasia

Congenital adrenal hyperplasia (CAH) results from inherited defects in one of the five enzymatic steps required for the biosynthesis of cortisol from cholesterol. The most common form of CAH (95%) involves a deficiency of 21-hydroxylase located on 6p21.3[12].

Mutations in the cytochrome P450 21-hydroxylase gene (CPY21) tend to be transmitted in an autosomal recessive pattern. Deficiency of

21-hydroxylase occurs in three forms: (1) simple virilizing, (2) salt-wasting and (3) non-classical.

The simple virilizing and salt-wasting forms of 21-hydroxylase deficiencies are characterized by excess adrenal androgen biosynthesis *in utero*. This disorder in males is not recognized at birth; they have normal genitalia and are not diagnosed until later, often with a salt-wasting crisis. Cortisol and aldosterone production is low, but testosterone production is normal (peripheral conversion of androstenedione). Elevated adrenal androgen secretion (due to elevated adrenocorticotropic hormone, ACTH) in male CAH patients may suppress both follicle stimulating hormone (FSH) and luteinizing hormone (LH) secretion with resultant small testes, decreased spermatogenesis and testicular androgen production[13,14].

Prader–Willi syndrome

Prader–Willi syndrome (PWS) was the first human disorder attributed to genomic imprinting, whereby genes are expressed differentially based upon the parent of origin. PWS results from the loss of imprinted gene SNRPN on the paternal 15q11.2–13 locus with an autosomal dominant pattern. The loss of maternal genomic material at the same locus results in another imprinted disorder (Angelman's syndrome)[15]. Characteristics of this disorder include neonatal hypotonia, childhood-onset hyperphagia, obesity, mental retardation and short stature. A deficiency of GnRH is the postulated reason for the hypogonadism[16].

Bardet–Biedl syndrome

Bardet–Biedl syndrome (BBS) is a genetically heterogeneous disorder with linkage to eight loci[17,18] (Table 16.2). Although BBS was originally thought to be a recessive disorder[19], controversy exists about the presence of a recessive pattern 'with variable penetrance'[20].

Cardinal features include obesity, retinitis pigmentosa, polydactyly, hypogonadotropic hypogonadism, renal cystic dysplasia and developmental

Table 16.2 Chromosome localization of genes involved in Bardet–Biedl syndrome (BBS)

Gene involved	Mapping
BBS 1	11q13
BBS 2	16q21
BBS 3	3p12–q13
BBS 4	15q22.3
BBS 5	2q31
BBS 6	20p12
BBS 7	4q27
BBS 8	14q32.11

delay. Other associated clinical findings in BBS patients include diabetes, hypertension and congenital heart defects. The clinical diagnosis is based on the presence of at least four of these symptoms[21]. Some of the BBS genes are also involved in the function of the cilia and the formation of flagella, which can impair sperm motility and cause infertility[22].

Hemochromatosis

Hereditary hemochromatosis (HH) is an autosomal disorder characterized by excessive absorption of dietary iron, which may result in parenchymal iron overload and subsequent tissue damage[23]. Hypogonadotropic hypogonadism is the most frequent endocrinopathy associated with HH, secondary to iron deposition in the pituitary gonadotrophs, leading to loss of libido, impotence and body hair loss[24]. There are four types of HH, summarized in Table 16.3[25]. Type 1 is the most common; the other types of HH are considered to be rare and have been studied in only a small number of families[26].

Cerebellar ataxia and hypogonadism

Cerebellar ataxia and hypogonadism is a rare autosomal recessive condition most commonly

Table 16.3   Classification of hereditary hemochromatosis

Hereditary hemochromatosis	Locus	Inherited	Onset
Type 1 (classical)	6p21	Autosomal recessive	> 30 years
Type 2 (juvenile)	1q21	Autosomal recessive	< 30 years
Type 3	7q22	Autosomal recessive	4th–5th decade of life
Type 4	2q32	Autosomal dominant	> 60 years

observed in consanguineous unions, with onset at 20 years old. Clinical features include cerebellar impairment (speech and gait abnormalities), and eunuchoid phenotype with atrophic testis and low libido. Infertility is secondary to hypothalamic–pituitary dysfunction, possibly because of brain atrophy or hypoplasia. Genes involved are CLA1 (9q34–9) for the most common adult-onset type[27], and CLA3 (20q11–q13) for infant onset[28].

Other idiopathic hypogonadotropic hypogonadism

Some other forms of hypogonadotropic hypogonadism previously classified as idiopathic (IHH) have recently been associated with genetic mutations. They include the DAX1 gene, which encodes a nuclear transcription factor, leading to X-linked IHH associated with congenital adrenal hypoplasia (CAH)[11]. Another mutation in the prohormone convertase gene (PC1) has been linked to hypogonadotropic hypogonadism, in addition to extreme obesity, hypocortisolemia and deficient conversion of proinsulin to insulin[29]. Homozygous mutations in GPR54, a gene encoding G-protein-coupled receptor-54, have lately been reported as another cause of hypogonadotropic hypogonadism[30].

Immotile cilia syndrome

The immotile cilia syndrome (ICS) is a group of heterogeneous diseases with impaired or absent ciliary motility, and the most common is Kartagener's syndrome. Abnormalities in the motor apparatus or axoneme, due to either missing or very short dynein arms, cause a deficit in sperm motility. Clinical manifestations include chronic cough, sinus infection, nasal polyposis, bronchiectasis and infertility with asthenozoospermia[31]. While infertility is universal in patients with ICS, there is another condition known as fibrous sheath dysplasia, where teratozoospermia (short tails and thick flagella) is the cardinal feature and ejaculated sperm can be motile (more than 1000 polypeptides have been identified in the constitution of the cilium), and sperm concentrations can be normal or even high[32,33].

Although no specific genes have been linked to this disease, the inheritance pattern in family pedigrees suggests that it is likely to be autosomal recessive. ICS is caused by mutations on genes which encode dynein axoneme chains (DNAI). The ICS that maps 9p21–p13 (CILD1) is caused by a mutation in DNAI1. Another form (CILD2) is caused by mutation on 19q13.2–qter. Other loci for the disorder have been mapped to 5p (CILD3, DNAH5 gene), 16p12 and 15q13. Because the gene defect is usually recessive, offspring are likely to be normal; still, genetic counseling is recommended when assisted reproductive techniques are used[33].

Autosomal dominant polycystic kidney disease

Numerous large cysts of the kidneys, liver, pancreas and spleen, and a 10–40% chance of developing berry aneurysms in the brain, characterize this disorder. Because the syndrome is often asymptomatic until adulthood, affected men may initially present with infertility. Cysts in the epididymis and seminal vesicles or ejaculatory ducts can obstruct the ductal system and cause infertility. Three separate genetic loci have been associated with autosomal dominant polycystic kidney disease (ADPK). PKD1 accounts for 85% of the disease and has been mapped onto chromosome 16p13.3, where it encodes a receptor-like integral membrane protein involved in cell–cell and cell–matrix interaction. A mild form (PKD2) has been mapped to chromosome 4q21–23, and it encodes a non-specific calcium-permeable channel; another variant, PKD3, is currently unmapped[34].

An association between men with ICS and with ADPK disease has recently been observed. Electron microscopy studies have revealed abnormalities on both the flagellar dynein arms and the cilium of the kidney epithelium[33].

Cystic fibrosis transmembrane regulator mutations

Cystic fibrosis (CF) is the most common fatal autosomal-recessive disease in Caucasians, with an incidence of 1:2500 births and a carrier frequency of 1:25. Clinical features of CF include chronic pulmonary obstruction and infection, exocrine pancreatic insufficiency, neonatal meconium ileus and male infertility[35]. The CF gene, cystic fibrosis transmembrane regulator (CFTR; 7q31.2), encodes a protein that regulates the cyclic adenosine monophosphate chloride channel that controls the transport of electrolytes in many secretory epithelia. More than 1000 mutations have been identified in the CFTR gene[36], encompassing about 90% of cases of CF.

The CFTR gene also influences the formation of the seminal vesicles, the vas deferens and the distal two-thirds of the epididymis[37]. More than 95% of men with CF have abnormalities in Wolffian duct-derived structures, manifesting most commonly as congenital bilateral absence of the vas deferens (CBAVD).

Congenital bilateral absence of the vas deferens

This condition occurs in 1–2% of infertile men[38], and is considered a genital form of cystic fibrosis[39]. These patients exhibit the same spectrum of Wolffian duct defects as seen in those with full-blown cystic fibrosis, but generally lack the severe pulmonary, pancreatic and intestinal problems. Spermatogenesis is normal in approximately 90% of men with CBAVD[40]. Anatomically, the body and tail of the epididymis, the vas and the seminal vesicles may be absent, but the efferent ducts and the caput epididymis are almost always present[41].

It is thought that CBAVD is based on allelic patterns (homozygous and compound heterozygous) similar to typical CF but with less severe mutations[42]. The combination of the 5T (thymidines) allele in one copy of the CFTR gene (lack of exon 9), and a CF mutation (most commonly ΔF508) in the other copy, is peculiar for men with CBAVD. Therefore, it is important to include the 5T variants (intron 8) in the genetic screening for CF in patients and their partners before using assisted reproductive technologies (ART).

Congenital unilateral absence of the vas deferens

Another male infertility phenotype (possibly associated with CFTR mutations but still controversial) affects 0.5% of the general population, and only rarely presents with infertility[43]. Almost 40% of patients with congenital unilateral absence of the vas deferens (CUAVD) have been reported to have at least one mutation in CFTR. CUAVD is more frequent on the left side (70%), and may be associated with contralateral renal agenesis (75%). However, if CUAVD is associated with renal agenesis, the possibility of finding a CFTR mutation is lower (31%)[44].

Table 16.4	Syndromes associated with androgen receptor gene mutations	
Complete androgen insensitivity syndrome		*Partial androgen insensitivity syndrome*
Testicular feminization syndrome (Morris's syndrome)		Male pseudohermaphroditism
		Lub's syndrome
		Reifenstein's syndrome
		Gilbert–Dreyfus syndrome

Table 16.5	Exons of the androgen receptor gene (AR) involved in androgen sensitivity
Exon 1	Transactivation domain function (TAD) modulates transcriptional activity of AR downstream genes
Exons 2 and 3	Encode a peptide domain responsible for DNA-binding domain
Exons 4 and 8	Encode C-terminal peptide domain responsible for androgen binding

Androgen receptor gene mutations

The androgen receptor (AR) is a large steroid receptor whose gene is located on the X chromosome (Xq11–q12), and is essential for masculinization (fetal life) and virilization. AR mutations result in absent or structurally altered AR (functional impairment), causing partial or complete resistance to androgens (Table 16.4). The phenotype is variable, ranging from complete insensitivity (female phenotype) to normally virilized but infertile males. Clinical features include ambiguous genitalia, testicular atrophy, micropenis and hypospadias[45].

Over 300 distinct mutations have been reported in the AR. Mutations in exon 1 cause complete androgen insensitivity, while some mutations in the C-terminal ligand-binding domain (LBD) cause partial insensitivity[45]. Due to variable phenotypes, it has been proposed that as many as 40% of men with partial or totally impaired spermatogenesis may have subtle androgen insensitivity as an underlying cause[46].

A recent report found that only 2% of males with idiopathic infertility carried a significant variation within the AR gene[47]. The AR gene includes eight exons (three domains) (Table 16.5), and has a critical region on exon 1 of cytosine-adenosine-guanine (CAG) nucleotide repeats, formerly called the transactivation domain (TAD), usually between 15 and 30 repeats in number. Variation in length of this domain (> 40) results in severe spinal–bulbar muscular atrophy (Kennedy's disease)[48]. This debilitating, late-onset (after 30 years of age) disorder consists of progressive degeneration of the anterior motor neurons and muscular weakness, as well as infertility due to testicular atrophy[49].

Although still controversial, some men may have oligozoospermia and intermediate lengths of CAG repeats (i.e. > 30 but fewer than 40). In these instances, with the phenomenon of genetic anticipation, offspring may inherit a larger number of CAG repeats than those of their parent, and when they reproduce (second generation) may have a child with Kennedy's disease[50,51].

Myotonic dystrophy

Myotonic dystrophy (MD) is the most common cause of adult-onset muscular dystrophy, and usually presents with cataracts, muscle weakness and wasting, hypogonadism, electrocardiogram changes, diabetes (5% of cases) and cholelithiasis (25%). Symptoms usually become evident in the adult as early as in the second decade. The gene involved is located on the long arm of chromosome 19, region q13.2–3 (DMPK gene), and encodes the serine/threonine protein kinase family (myotonin-1). In MD there is an expansion (more than 35 repeat motifs) of the CTG sequence in the 3′-untranslated region of exon 5. Since reduced gene function correlates with the degree of repeat expansion, the severity of the condition varies with the number of repeats: normal individuals have between 5 and 35 CTG copies, mildly affected persons have between 50 and 80 copies and severely affected patients can have 2000 or more copies[52]. Like Kennedy's disease, this disorder is characterized by anticipation, in which amplification (anticipation) of the disease is observed in parent-to-child transmission, especially from mother to offspring[53]. Male infertility is observed in about 30% of subjects, whilst some degree of testicular atrophy occurs in at least 80% of males suffering from this disorder (seminiferous tubules are more involved (75%) than Leydig cells). FSH and LH levels are elevated, with normal testosterone levels. Despite these findings, 66% of married men with MD can conceive naturally. A recent report described an association between MD and defective sperm capacitation and the acrosome reaction[54].

Usher's syndrome

This is the most common cause of deafness–blindness in humans. This autosomal-recessive defect maps onto three chromosomes and results in three different phenotypes (US1 (14q32), US2 (1q41), US3 (3q21–q25)). Recently an association between Usher's syndrome and infertility has been reported[54]. The common denominator for these associations is an abnormality in the ciliary structure of the sperm and the photoreceptor cells, since they share docosahexaenoic acid (DHA). DHA blood levels are less than normal in patients

with retinitis pigmentosa (RP), and sperm of patients with RP have reduced motility and abnormal morphology. Patients with Usher's syndrome type II have the most pronounced reductions of DHA in the sperm[55,56].

β-Thalassemia and sickle cell anemia

Autosomal-dominant genomic deletions involving the β-globin gene (HBB), 11p15.4, account for approximately 10% of all β-thalassemia mutations. At least 60 different deletions have been described to date. Clinical features range from mild anemia (trait) to hemolytic anemia (transfusion-dependent) and iron overload (major thalassemia). Infertility results from the deposition of iron in the pituitary gland and testes. At the molecular level, it is hypothesized that iron overload may induce, via reactive oxygen species (ROS), sperm DNA oxidation and alter sperm membranes[57].

Sickle cell anemia is an autosomal-recessive genetic disease that results from the substitution of valine for glutamic acid at 11p15.5 of the HBB, responsible for a defective form of hemoglobin, hemoglobin S (HbS). Pituitary and testicular microinfarcts from sickle cell disease account for secondary hypogonadism and infertility[58].

SRY gene defects

SRY (sex determining region on Y chromosome) gene is located on the short arm of the Y chromosome (Yp11.3), and is important for determining 'maleness'. The SRY gene encodes a transcription factor, a member of the HMG-box family (DNA-binding proteins) formerly called testis-determining factor (TDF), which initiates male sex differentiation. Mutations in this gene (1 : 25 000) give rise to XY females (Xp22.11–p21.2) with gonadal dysgenesis (Swyer's syndrome); translocation of SRY to the X chromosome causes the XX male phenotype. All 46,XX men are sterile due to absence of the long arm of the Y chromosome containing the azoospermia factor (AZF) gene, which is necessary for normal spermatogenesis, but their external genitalia and testes are developed under the influence of the Y-chromosome genetic fragment present on the X chromosome[59].

5α-Reductase deficiency

A deficiency in the 5α-reductase type-2 isozyme produces a form of male pseudohermaphroditism (autosomal recessive) due to the lack of conversion of testosterone to dihydrotestosterone (DHT). There are two genes encoding 5α-reductase: type 1 has been mapped onto chromosome 5, while type 2 has been mapped onto chromosome 2p23 (SRD5A2 gene). Mutations in isozyme 2 are associated with low DHT (important for prostate and external genitalia development) in spite of high levels of testosterone. Clinical features include normal internal genital ductal structures and testes, but incompletely virilized external genitalia. Affected individuals exhibit perineoscrotal hypospadias and often a vaginal pouch. Generally, the testes are found in the labioscrotal folds or the inguinal canal, the seminal vesicles are rudimentary and the prostate may be absent[60].

Infertility results from the structural abnormalities of the external genitalia. Although spermatogenesis has been described in descended testes, natural fertility has not been reported[52].

Mixed gonadal dysgenesis

In males and females, mixed gonadal dysgenesis is a heterogeneous condition characterized by a unilateral testis on one side and a streak gonad on the opposite side. The phenotype ranges from normal males to patients with ambiguous external genitalia or females, depending on the amount of testosterone secreted by the testis. Genotypically, patients are usually 46,XY or 45,X/46,XY mosaicism (most common), both of which are associated with impaired gonadal development[61]. Since mutations in the SRY gene have not been detected (80% have normal SRY), gonadal

dysgenesis may be caused by cytogenetic mosaicism or by mutations in testis-organizing genes near to the SRY region. One of these genes may be the newly cloned human testatin gene (20p11.2), a putative cathepsin inhibitor that is expressed early in testis development, just after SRY expression[62]. Scrotal testes may be associated with inguinal hernias, and almost uniformly reveal seminiferous tubules with Sertoli cell-only and normal Leydig cells. The dysgenetic gonad is predisposed to malignant degeneration (one-third of patients) to gonadoblastoma or dysgerminoma, typically before puberty[63].

MALE INFERTILITY WITH CHROMOSOMAL ABERRATIONS

Chromosomal disorders are defined as the loss, gain or abnormal arrangement of genetic material at the chromosome level. These disorders can be further divided into numerical and structural abnormalities. Structural chromosome disorders can occur in single (deletions, duplications and inversions) or multiple (translocations) chromosomes. Usually they are a consequence of breakage that occurs during meiosis, and are becoming more frequently recognized as a contributing factor to male infertility (15% of azoospermic and 5% of oligozoospermic men)[64].

Klinefelter's syndrome

Klinefelter's syndrome (1 : 1000) is the most common genetic reason for azoospermia, accounting for about 14% of cases[65]. It is associated with a triad of clinical findings: small, firm testes (devoid of germ cells), azoospermia and possibly gynecomastia[52]. The phenotype can vary from a normal, virilized man to one with stigmata of androgen deficiency. Testicular histology shows hyalinization of the seminiferous tubules with Leydig cell hyperplasia[4].

This syndrome may also be associated with tall stature, female hair distribution, low intelligence quotient (IQ), lower-extremity varicosities, obesity, diabetes, increased incidence of leukemia and non-seminatous extragonadal germ-cell tumors, and breast cancer (20-fold higher than in normal males)[66]. About 90% of men have the classic 47,XXY genotype; the remaining (10%) are mosaic, with a combination of XXY/XY chromosomes (30 recognized mosaic patterns). Approximately 50% of XXY cases are paternally inherited, and a recent study suggested a relationship with advanced paternal age[67]. The extra X chromosome might originate in paternal meiosis I (nondisjunction of the XY bivalent in 50% of cases), or in maternal meiosis I or II (40% of cases), associated with maternal age[68]. Natural paternity with this syndrome is possible, but almost exclusively with the mosaic genotype[69]. Despite a uniformly abnormal somatic genotype, 75–100% of mature sperm from 47,XXY patients have a normal haploid sex chromosome complement (X or Y instead of XY or YY)[70]. The absence of significant gonosomal aneuploidy with somatic aneuploidy suggests that abnormal germ-cell lines are eliminated from further development at meiotic checkpoints within the testis[52].

XYY syndrome

The XYY syndrome has an incidence of 1:1000 live births. Fewer than 2% of men with the 47,XYY karyotype may be infertile[71]. The extra Y chromosome commonly (86%) originates through paternal meiotic II nondisjunction, while the remaining cases are due to postzygotic events[72]. The phenotype includes tall stature, aggressive and antisocial behavior and a higher risk of leukemia[3].

Studies that have focused on the chromosomal complements in mature sperm from XYY men show that very few sperm (< 1%) have sex-chromosomal disomy (YY, XX, XY)[73]. This finding supports the hypothesis that the extra Y chromosome is eliminated at meiotic checkpoints during spermatogenesis, and shows that men with 47,XYY syndrome can father offspring with normal karyotypes.

Noonan's syndrome

This syndrome is relatively common, with an estimated incidence of 1:1000–2500 live births. Noonan's syndrome (NS) patients are phenotypically equivalent to those with Turner's syndrome (XO), and share similar characteristics, i.e. webbed neck, short stature, lymphedema, low-set ears, wide-set eyes, cubitus valgus, cardiovascular disorders and pulmonary stenosis. This syndrome is inherited in an autosomal dominant pattern with karyotype 46,XY/XO mosaicism. A recently identified genetic locus at 12q24.2–q24.31 (PTPN11 candidate gene) could be involved in encoding a protein–tyrosine phosphatase that plays a role in the cellular response to extracellular signaling[74]. A second type of NS (type 2) appears to be transmitted in an autosomal recessive pattern. Typically, type 2 NS patients have hypertrophic obstructive cardiomyopathy, as opposed to 10–20% in the classical NS[75]. Fertility impairment is due to defects in spermatogenesis associated with cryptorchidism (77% at birth) and elevated FSH[76].

Chromosomal translocations

Chromosomal translocations are classified as Robertsonian (incidence 1:900) if they involve chromosome 13, 14, 15, 21 or 22, or reciprocal (incidence 1:625) if any other chromosome is involved. If there is no gain or loss of chromosome material, the translocation is considered to be 'balanced' (unaffected phenotype). The reproductive risk with a balanced translocation is that sperm can carry an unbalanced chromosome, leading to pregnancy loss.

Reciprocal translocations can lead to reduced fertility, spontaneous abortions or birth defects, depending on the chromosomes involved and the nature of the translocation[76].

Many translocations have been associated with male infertility. In particular, reciprocal and Robertsonian translocations (Robertsonian chromosomes are involved in as many as 15 different translocations) are at least 8.5-fold more common in infertile men than in randomly selected males. The most common Robertsonian translocation observed in infertile males is t(13q14q), where abnormal autosome rearrangement in meiosis causes spermatogenesis impairment. Carriers of another Robertsonian translocation involving chromosomes 14 and 21 (t(14;21)) are at risk for pregnancy loss and for offspring with Down's syndrome and birth defects[77].

Chromosomal inversions

An inversion occurs when a chromosome breaks in two places and the material between the breakpoints rotates 180°, hence reversing the order of the chromatin (incidence 1:1000). Such rearrangements may either interrupt important genes at the breakpoint, or interfere with normal chromosome pairing during meiosis, because of imbalances in chromosomal mass. Autosomal inversions, particularly those involving chromosome 9, are eight-fold more likely to occur in infertile than in fertile men. These types of chromosomal derangements tend to be balanced and result in phenotypically normal males, but with severe oligoasthenoteratospermia or azoospermia[1,76].

Y chromosome microdeletions

Structural changes (loss or microdeletions) of various regions of the short or long arm of the Y chromosome could result in the breakdown of spermatogenesis, and are the second most frequent genetic causes of infertility. Microdeletions derive from the homologous recombination of identical segments within palindromic sequences.

The spermatogenesis region on Yq11 associated with infertility is known as azoospermia factor (AZF). The AZF region is subdivided into AZFa (proximal), AZFb (central), AZFc (distal) and AZFd (actually AZFc proximal region), and the loss of any part of these regions can result in a variety of spermatogenic and infertility phenotypes[78]. Transcription units in these regions (Table

Table 16.6 Candidate genes involved in spermatogenesis

Region	Gene involved
AZFa	USP9Y, DBY, UTY
AZFb	RMBY, EIF1A, CDY
AZFc	DAZ
AZF, azoospermia factor	

16.6) encode proteins (mostly RNA-binding proteins) involved in the regulation of spermatogenesis via translational control. More than 30 Y-chromosome genes and gene families have been identified, although their function in spermatogenesis has not been completely detailed. Moreover, in the region of AZFc, the presence of partial deletions can also be observed in normal males[79].

Deletions are more frequent in the AZFc region (50–60%), involving the DAZ gene (deleted in azoospermia). In almost 50% of patients with DAZ deletions (AZFc) it is possible to find sperm in the ejaculate. For azoospermic patients, sperm can be retrieved by testicular biopsy (testicular sperm extraction or TESE)[80]. Incomplete spermatogenesis with no evidence of elongated spermatids or sperm in TESE has been reported in patients with a complete AZFb deletion (frequency 15%)[81]. Deletions in the AZFa region (frequency of 2–5%) are mostly associated with Sertoli cell-only (SCO) syndrome (75%), and overall, about 9% of men with SCO have a complete AZFa deletion[82].

Infertile men with non-obstructive azoospermia and those with sperm concentrations below 5 million/ml (severe oligozoospermia) should be offered testing for Y chromosome microdeletions. Overall, severe oligozoospermic patients have about a 4–6% risk of Y microdeletions[83], while patients with non-obstructive azoospermia have a 14% risk of Y microdeletions[84,85]. Y chromosome microdeletions may be passed on to a male offspring through ICSI[86]; thus, genetic counseling is recommended.

Some infertile men may actually be genetic mosaics and harbor DAZ deletions only in germ line (gamete) tissue and not in somatic cells[87], and thus many escape recognition with the common practice of DNA analysis from peripheral leukocytes.

Summary

The current genetic screening offered before ICSI reveals that 35% of men with non-obstructive azoospermia (20% abnormal karyotype and 15% genetic or Y deletions), and about 10% of men with severe oligozoospermia (5% abnormal karyotype and 5% genetic or Y deletions), have a genetic explanation for their absent or reduced spermatogenesis.

It is becoming clearer that abnormalities, both qualitative and quantitative, of spermatogenesis

may be the 'presenting symptoms' or phenotype of a variety of pathologies that can affect non-reproductive organs. Examples are men with congenital absence of the vas deferens whose etiology has been linked to cystic fibrosis; men with the immotile cilia syndrome and some of its variants (such as sperm fibrous sheath dysplasia), where the presenting symptoms can be chronic sinusitis or bronchiectasis; or male infertility associated with polycystic kidney disease or the rare spinobulbar muscular atrophy.

Many more forms of male infertility with a possible genetic etiology are still unrecognized. The time has come to associate phenotype with genotype in a more detailed and comprehensive manner. This requires the availability of modern molecular genetic testing and collaboration between andrologists/urologists, reproductive endocrinologists and genetic counselors. Notwithstanding the current limitations to identifying genetic 'syndromes' associated with male

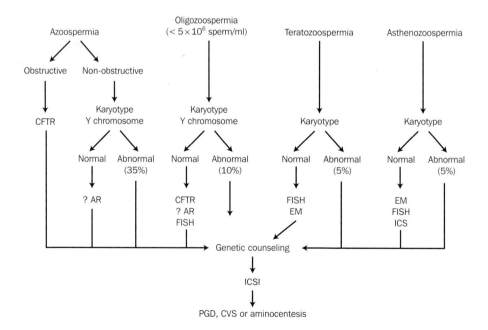

Figure 16.1   Algorithm for genetic evaluation of the infertile male undergoing intracytoplasmic sperm injection (ICSI). EM, electron microscopy; CFTR, cystic fibrosis transmembrane conductance regulator gene; AR, androgen receptor; PGD, preimplantation genetic diagnosis; CVS, chorionic villi sampling; FISH, fluorescence *in situ* hybridization; ICS, (gene screening for) immotile cilia syndrome or Kartagener's syndrome

infertility, a review of the literature on the health of offspring born after ICSI (for severe male infertility) has shown that the rate of chromosomal anomalies, compared with the general neonatal population, is increased. This slight increase is seen in the *de novo* sex aneuploidy rate (0.6% vs. 0.2%) and in structural autosomal abnormalities (0.4% vs. 0.07%), and is believed to be linked to the very reason for infertility in the fathers.

In summary, before undergoing ICSI, every male with idiopathic infertility should be fully evaluated and submitted to a minimum of genetic testing that includes karyotype, Y chromosome deletions and the androgen receptor. Additional genetic information could be gathered by using fluorescence *in situ* hybridization (FISH) on spermatozoa, since both azoospermic and oligozoospermic males have an increased risk of carrying a gene defect or aneuploid chromosomes. The algorithm shown in Figure 16.1 suggests a common genetic evaluation of the infertile male prior to and after ICSI.

REFERENCES

1. Shah K, et al. The genetic basis of infertility. Reproduction 2003; 126: 13
2. Brugh VM III, Lipshultz LI. Male factor infertility: evaluation and management. Urol Clin North Am 2004; 88: 367
3. Maduro MR, Lamb DJ. Understanding new genetics of male infertility. J Urol 2002; 168: 2197
4. Hargreave TB. Genetics and male infertility. Curr Opin Obstet Gynecol 2000; 12: 207
5. Nudell DM, Turek PJ. Genetic causes of male infertility: current concepts. Curr Urol Rep 2000; 1: 273
6. Rockett JC, et al. Gene expression patterns associated with infertility in humans and rodent models. Mutat Res 2004; 549: 225
7. Patrizio P, Broomfield D. The genetic basis of male infertility. In Glover TD, Barrat LR, eds. Male Fertility and Infertility. Cambridge: Cambridge University Press, 1999: 162
8. World Health Organization. Genes and Human Disease. Geneva: WHO, 2004
9. Pitteloud N, et al. Reversible Kallmann syndrome, delayed puberty, and isolated anosmia occurring in a single family with a mutation in the fibroblast growth factor receptor 1 gene. J Clin Endocrinol Metab 2005; 90: 1317
10. Dode C, et al. Loss-of-function mutations in FGFR1 cause autosomal dominant Kallmann syndrome. Nat Genet 2003; 33: 4463
11. Oliveira LM, et al. The importance of autosomal genes in Kallmann syndrome: genotype–phenotype correlations and neuroendocrine characteristics. J Clin Endocrinol Metab 2001; 86: 1532
12. Forest MG. Recent advances in the diagnosis and management of congenital adrenal hyperplasia due to 21-hydroxylase deficiency. Hum Reprod Update 2004; 10: 469
13. Cabrera MS, Vogiatzi MG, New MI. Long term outcome in adult males with classic congenital adrenal hyperplasia. J Clin Endocrinol Metab 2001; 86: 3070
14. Yang RM, Fefferman RA, Shapiro CE. Reversible infertility in man with 21-hydroxylase deficiency congenital adrenal hyperplasia. Fertil Steril 2005; 83: 223
15. Belinska B, et al. De novo deletions of SNRPN exon 1 in early human and mouse embryos result in a paternal to maternal imprint switch. Nat Genet 2000; 25: 74
16. Gunay-Aygun M, et al. The changing purpose of Prader–Willi syndrome clinical diagnostic criteria and proposed revised criteria. Pediatrics 2001; 108: e92
17. Mykytyn K, et al. Bardet–Biedl syndrome type 4 (BBS4)-null mice implicate Bbs4 in flagella formation but not global cilia assembly. Proc Natl Acad Sci USA 2004; 101: 8664
18. Kim JC, et al. MKKS/BBS6, a divergent chaperonin-like protein linked to the obesity disorder Bardet–Biedl syndrome, is a novel centrosomal component required for cytokinesis. J Cell Sci 2005; 118: 1007
19. Katsanis N, Lupski JR, Beales PL. Exploring the molecular basis of Bardet–Biedl syndrome. Hum Mol Genet 2001; 10: 2293
20. Burghes A, Vaessin H, Chapelle A. The land between mendelian and multifactorial inheritance. Science 2001; 293: 2213
21. Katsanis N. The oligogenic properties of Bardet–Biedl syndrome. Hum Mol Genet 2004; 13: 65
22. Beales P. Lifting the lid on Pandora's box: the Bardet–Biedl syndrome. Curr Opin Genet Dev 2005; 15: 315
23. McDermott H, Walsh CH. Hypogonadism in hereditary hemochromatosis. J Clin Endocrinol Metab 2005; 90: 2451

24. Walsh CH. Non-diabetic endocrinopathy in hemochromatosis. In Barton JC, Edwards CQ, eds. Hemochromatosis: Genetics, Pathophysiology, Diagnosis and Treatment. Cambridge: Cambridge University Press, 2000: 278

25. Franchini M, Veneri D. Recent advances in hereditary hemochromatosis. Ann Hematol 2005; 84: 347

26. Worwood M. Inherited iron loading: genetic testing in diagnosis and management. Blood Rev 2005; 19: 69

27. Delague V, et al. Nonprogressive autosomal recessive ataxia maps to chromosome 9q34–9qter in a large consanguineous Lebanese family. Ann Neurol 2001; 50: 250

28. Tranebjaerg L, et al. Genome-wide homozygosity mapping localizes a gene for autosomal recessive nonprogressive infantile ataxia to 20q11–q13. Hum Genet 2003; 113: 293

29. Silveira LF, MacColl GS, Bouloux PM. Hypogonadotropic hypogonadism. Semin Reprod Med 2002; 20: 327

30. Semple RK, et al. Two novel missense mutations in G protein-coupled receptor 54 in a patient with hypogonadotropic hypogonadism. J Clin Endocrinol Metab 2005; 90: 1849

31. Peeraer K, et al. Pregnancy after ICSI with ejaculated immotile spermatozoa from a patient with immotile cilia syndrome: a case report and review of the literature. Reprod Biomed Online 2004; 9: 659

32. Westlander G, et al. Different fertilization rates between immotile testicular spermatozoa and immotile ejaculated spermatozoa for ICSI in men with Kartagener's syndrome: case reports. Hum Reprod 2003; 18: 1286

33. Chemes HE. Phenotypes of sperm pathology: genetic and acquired forms in infertile men. J Androl 2000; 21: 799

34. Al-Bhalal L, Akhtar M. Molecular basis of autosomal dominant polycystic kidney disease. Adv Anat Pathol 2005; 12: 126

35. Daudin M, et al. Congenital bilateral absence of the vas deferens: clinical characteristics, biological parameters, cystic fibrosis transmembrane conductance regulator gene mutations, and implications for genetic counseling. Fertil Steril 2000; 74: 1164

36. Quinzii C, Castellani C. The cystic fibrosis transmembrane regulator gene and male infertility. J Endocrinol Invest 2000; 23: 684

37. Patrizio P, Salameh WA. Expression of the cystic fibrosis transmembrane conductance regulator (CFTR) mRNA in normal and pathological adult human epididymis. J Reprod Fertil Suppl 1998; 53: 261

38. Bernardino LF, Lima CE, Zats M. Analysis of mutations in the cystic fibrosis transmembrane regulator (CFTR) gene in patients with obstructive azoospermia. Genet Mol Biol 2003; 26: 1

39. Patrizio P, Zielenski J. Congenital absence of the vas deferens: a mild form of cystic fibrosis. Mol Med Today 1996; 2: 24

40. Silber SJ, Patrizio P, Asch RH. Quantitative evaluation of spermatogenesis by testicular histology in men with congenital absence of the vas deferens undergoing epididymal sperm aspiration. Hum Reprod 1990; 5: 89

41. Patrizio P, et al. Correlation between epididymal length and fertilization rate in men with congenital absence of the vas deferens. Fertil Steril 1994; 61: 265

42. Phillipson GTM, Petrucco OM, Matthews CD. Congenital bilateral absence of the vas deferens, cystic fibrosis mutation analysis and intracytoplasmic sperm injection. Hum Reprod 2000; 15: 431

43. Mulhall JP, Oates RD. Vasal aplasia and cystic fibrosis. Curr Opin Urol 1995; 32: 316

44. Casals T, et al. Heterogeneity for mutations in the CFTR gene and clinical correlations in patients with congenital absence of the vas deferens. Hum Reprod 2000; 15: 1476

45. Gottlieb B, et al. The androgen receptor gene mutations database (ARDB): 2004 update. Hum Mutat 2004; 23: 527

46. Aiman J, et al. Androgen insensitivity as a cause of infertility in otherwise normal men. N Engl J Med 1979; 300: 223

47. Hiort O, et al. Significance of mutations in the androgen receptor gene in males with idiopathic infertility. J Clin Endocrinol Metab 2000; 85: 2810

48. La Spada AR, et al. Androgen receptor gene mutations in X-linked spinal and bulbar muscular atrophy. Nature 1991; 352: 77

49. Pinsky L, Beitel LK, Trifiro MA. Spinobulbar muscular atrophy. In Scriver CR, et al., eds. Metabolic and Molecular Basis of Inherited Disease. New York: McGraw-Hill, 2000: 4147

50. Casella R, et al. Significance of the polyglutamine tract polymorphism in the androgen receptor. Urology 2001; 58: 651

51. Patrizio P, et al. Larger trinucleotide repeat size in the androgen receptor gene of infertile men with extremely severe oligozoospermia. J Androl 2001; 22: 444

52. Turek PJ, Pera RA. Current and future genetic screening for male infertility. Urol Clin North Am 2002; 29: 767

53. Vogt P. Molecular genetics of human male infertility: from genes to new therapeutic perspectives. Curr Pharm Des 2004; 10: 471

54. Hortas ML, Castilla JA, Gil MT. Decreased sperm function of patients with myotonic muscular dystrophy. Hum Reprod 2000; 15: 445

55. Connor WE, et al. Sperm abnormalities in retinitis pigmentosa. Invest Ophthalmol Vis Sci 1997; 38: 2619

56. Tosi MR, et al. Clinicopathologic reports, case reports, and small case series: Usher syndrome type 1 associated with primary ciliary aplasia. Arch Ophthalmol 2003; 121: 407

57. Perera D, et al. Sperm DNA damage in potentially fertile homozygous β-thalassaemia patients with iron overload. Hum Reprod 2002; 17: 1820

58. Barden EM, et al. Body composition in children with sickle cell disease. Am J Clin Nutr 2002; 76: 218

59. Layman LC. Human gene mutations causing infertility. J Med Genet 2002; 39: 153

60. Hedia S, et al. Male pseudo-hermaphroditism due partial 5 alpha-reductase deficiency, a case report. Tunis Med 2001; 79: 261

61. Alvarez-Nava F, Soto M, Borjas L. Molecular analysis of SRY gene in patients with mixed gonadal dysgenesis. Ann Genet 2001; 44:155

62. Eriksson A, et al. Isolation of the human testatin gene and analysis in patients with abnormal gonadal development. Mol Hum Reprod 2002; 8: 8

63. Chemes H, Muzulin PM, Venara MC. Early manifestations of testicular dysgenesis in children: pathological phenotypes, karyotype correlations and precursors stages of tumor development. APMIS 2003; 111: 12

64. Nudell DM, Pagani R, Lipshultz LI. Indications for genetic evaluation of men in a reproductive medicine program. Braz J Urol 2001; 27: 105

65. Rives N, et al. Assessment of sex chromosome aneuploidy in sperm nuclei from 47,XXY and 46,XY/47,XXY males: comparison with fertile and infertile males with normal karyotypes. Mol Hum Reprod 2000; 6: 107

66. Brugh VM III, Maduro MR, Lamb DJ. Genetic disorders and infertility. Urol Clin North Am 2003; 30: 143

67. Lowe X, et al. Frequency of XY sperm increases with age in fathers of boys with Klinefelter syndrome. Am J Hum Genet 2001; 69: 1046

68. Hargreave T. Genetic basis of male infertility. Br Med Bull 2000; 3: 650

69. Poulakis V, et al. Birth of two infants with normal karyotypes after intracytoplasmic injection of sperm obtained by testicular extraction from two men with nonmosaic Klinefelter. Fertil Steril 2001; 76: 1060

70. Bergère M, et al. Biopsed testis cells of four 47,XXY patients: fluorescence in-situ hybridization and ICSI results. Hum Reprod 2002; 17: 32

71. Prabhakara MG, et al. Genetic analysis of infertile males from Bangalore, India. Presented at the 54th Annual Meeting of the American Society of Human Genetics, Toronto, Canada, 2004, 920/T-182

72. Rives N, et al. Meiotic segregation of sex chromosomes in mosaic and non-mosaic XYY males: case reports and review of the literature. Int J Androl 2003; 26: 242

73. Wang IY, et al. Fluorescence in-situ hybridization analysis of chromosomal constitution in spermatozoa from a mosaic 47,XXY/46,XY male. Mol Hum Reprod 2000; 6: 665

74. Tartaglia M, et al. Mutations in PTPN11, encoding the protein tyrosine phosphatase SHP-2, cause Noonan syndrome. Nat Genet 2001; 29: 465

75. Van der Burgt I, Brunner H. Genetic heterogeneity in Noonan syndrome: evidence for an autosomal recessive form. Am J Med Genet 2000; 94: 46

76. Griffin DK, Finch KA. The genetic and cytogenetic basis of male infertility. Hum Fertil 2005; 8: 19

77. Antonelli A, et al. Chromosomal alterations and male infertility. J Endocrinol Invest 2000; 23: 677

78. Krausz C, Forti G, McElreavey K. The Y chromosome and male fertility and infertility. Int J Androl 2003; 26: 70

79. Hucklenbroich K, et al. Partial deletions in the AZFc region of the Y chromosome occur in men with impaired as well normal spermatogenesis. Hum Reprod 2005; 20: 191

80. Mulhall JP, et al. Azoospermic men with deletion of the DAZ gene cluster are capable of completing spermatogenesis: fertilization, normal embryonic development and pregnancy occur when retrieved testicular spermatozoa are used for intracytoplasmic sperm injection. Hum Reprod 1997; 12: 503

81. Hoops CV, et al. Detection of sperm in men with Y chromosome microdeletions of the AZFa, AZFb and AZFc regions. Hum Reprod 2003; 18: 1660

82. Kamp C, et al. High deletion frequency of the complete AZFa sequence in men with Sertoli-cell-only syndrome. Mol Hum Reprod 2001; 7: 987

83. Reijo R, et al. Severe oligozoospermia resulting from deletions of azoospermia factor gene on Y chromosome. Lancet 1996; 347: 1290

84. Reijo R, et al. Diverse spermatogenic defects in humans caused by Y chromosome deletions encompassing a novel RNA-binding protein gene. Nat Genet 1995; 10: 383

85. Foresta C, Moro E, Ferlin A. Y chromosome microdeletions and alterations of spermatogenesis. Endocr Rev 2001; 22: 226

86. Affara NA. The role of human and mouse Y chromosome genes in male infertility. J Endocrinol Invest 2000; 23: 630

87. Calogero AE, et al. Spontaneous transmission from father to his son of a Y chromosome microdeletion involving the deleted in azoospermia (DAZ) gene. J Endocrinol Invest 2002; 25: 631

17

Reactive oxygen species and their impact on fertility

R John Aitken, Liga E Bennetts

INTRODUCTION

Male infertility is a relatively common complaint that affects approximately one in 20 men in developed countries. Despite the prevalence of this condition, relatively little is known about the underlying pathophysiology. Indeed, since the advent of intracytoplasmic sperm injection (ICSI) as a therapeutic technique in 1992[1], the biomedical community has paid little attention to this problem. However, an appreciation of the etiology of male infertility will be essential if we are to optimize procedures for the management of this condition and contemplate strategies for its possible prevention.

Unlike female infertility, the male counterpart is not, predominantly, an endocrine condition; it is a pathology affecting germ cells. Most infertile men produce spermatozoa; however, these gametes are characterized by functional deficiencies stemming from defects occurring during spermatogenesis or sperm maturation. Interest in the origins of male infertility has recently been stimulated by data indicating that spermatozoa from such patients not only suffer from an impaired capacity for fertilization but also may exhibit high rates of DNA damage to both the mitochondrial and nuclear genomes[2–4]. One of the consequences of such damage is a possible increase in the mutational load carried by the

embryo as a consequence of aberrant DNA repair in the fertilized egg[5,6]. Thus, high rates of DNA damage in human spermatozoa have been associated with reduced rates of fertilization *in vivo* and *in vitro*, impaired preimplantation development of the embryo, increased rates of early pregnancy loss and high rates of morbidity in the offspring, including dominant genetic disease, infertility and cancer[7–15]. In light of these associations, attempts are now being made to define those factors responsible for the increased DNA damage and impaired functional competence seen in the spermatozoa of infertile males. As seen in the following section, of all the potential causes undergoing active consideration at the present time, oxidative stress appears to be amongst the most important.

One of the first mechanisms suggested for the induction of genetic damage in defective human spermatozoa involved endonuclease-mediated cleavage of the DNA as a result of incomplete apoptosis during spermatogenesis[16–18]. While plausible, recent analyses of putative apoptotic markers in spermatozoa, such as the plasma membrane translocation of phosphatidylserine, have suggested that aberrant apoptosis is not highly correlated with DNA fragmentation in the male germ line[19]. It has also been hypothesized that the DNA damage seen in defective human spermatozoa results from defective chromatin packaging during a critical stage of spermiogenesis. This proposal envisages that relief of the torsional stresses associated with chromatin packaging involves the repeated transient nicking of DNA by topoisomerase. Defects in the structure of the chromatin, or the activity of the topoisomerase system itself, may lead to the generation of gametes expressing high levels of DNA fragmentation[17,20].

In support of this hypothesis is the observation that errors of chromatin packaging are, indeed, commonly associated with DNA damage in the germ line[21]. A third hypothesis is that defective sperm function and DNA damage in the male germ line are both mediated by high levels of oxidative stress. Excessive production or exposure to reactive oxygen species (ROS) has been both statistically and causally associated with defective sperm function and DNA damage in a large number of independent studies[22–27]. Furthermore, nuclear DNA damage in spermatozoa appears to exhibit a tighter association with markers of oxidative stress than with apoptosis[19]. In order to examine this association between defective sperm quality and oxidative stress in more detail, the next section introduces the fundamental chemistry of ROS and reviews the mechanisms by which they exert their pathological effects.

REACTIVE OXYGEN SPECIES AND LIPID PEROXIDATION

The acronym ROS covers a wide range of metabolites derived from the reduction of molecular oxygen, including free radicals, such as the superoxide anion ($O_2^{-\bullet}$), and powerful oxidants such as hydrogen peroxide (H_2O_2). The term also covers molecules derived from the reaction of carbon centered radicals with oxygen, including peroxyl radicals ($ROO^\bullet$), alkoxyl radicals ($RO^\bullet$) and organic hydroperoxides ($ROOH$). It may also refer to other powerful oxidants such as peroxynitrite ($ONOO^-$) or hypochlorous acid ($HOCl$), as well as the highly biologically active free radical, nitric oxide ($^\bullet NO$).

The specific term 'free radicals' refers to any atom or molecule containing one or more unpaired electrons. As unpaired electrons are highly energetic, and seek out other electrons with which to pair, they confer upon free radicals considerable reactivity. Thus, free radicals and related 'reactive species' have the ability to react with, and modify the structure of, many different kinds of biomolecule, including proteins, lipids and nucleic acids. The wide range of targets that can be attacked by ROS is a critical aspect of their chemistry that contributes significantly to the pathological significance of these oxygen metabolites.

The most commonly encountered oxygen free radical in biological systems is $O_2^{-\bullet}$. When in aqueous solution, $O_2^{-\bullet}$ has a short half-life (1 ms) and is relatively inert. The radical is more stable and reactive in the hydrophobic environment provided by cellular membranes. The charge associated with $O_2^{-\bullet}$ means that this molecule is generally incapable of passing across biological membranes, although this molecule has been reported to exit cells using voltage-dependent anion channels. As a result of its lack of membrane permeability, $O_2^{-\bullet}$ may be more damaging if produced inside biological membranes than at other sites. It is also important to note that while $O_2^{-\bullet}$ can act as either a reducing agent or a weak oxidizing agent in aqueous solution, under the reducing conditions prevailing within cells, $O_2^{-\bullet}$ acts primarily as an oxidant.

Since most biological molecules only have paired electrons, free radicals are also likely to be involved in chain reactions that can propagate the damage induced by ROS. A classic example of such a chain reaction is the peroxidation of lipids in biological membranes. In this process, a ROS-mediated attack on unsaturated fatty acids generates peroxyl ($ROO^\bullet$) and alkoxyl ($RO^\bullet$) radicals that, in order to stabilize, abstract a hydrogen atom from an adjacent carbon, generating the corresponding acid ($ROOH$) or alcohol (ROH). The abstraction of a hydrogen atom from an adjacent lipid creates a carbon-centered radical that combines with molecular oxygen to recreate another lipid peroxide. In order to stabilize, the latter must again abstract a hydrogen atom from a nearby lipid, creating another carbon radical that combines with molecular oxygen to create yet another lipid peroxide. In this manner, a chain reaction is created that, if unchecked, would propagate the peroxidative damage throughout the plasma membrane, leading to a rapid loss of membrane-dependent functions[28].

The vulnerability of human spermatozoa to oxidative attack stems from the fact that these cells are particularly rich in unsaturated fatty acids[29]. Such an abundance of unsaturated lipids is necessary to create the membrane fluidity required by the membrane fusion events associated with fertilization, including acrosomal exocytosis and sperm–oocyte fusion. Unfortunately for spermatozoa, such unsaturated fatty acids are particularly prone to oxidative attack because the presence of a double bond weakens the C–H bonds on the adjacent carbon atoms, facilitating the hydrogen abstraction step and initiation of peroxidative damage, as indicated below:

Bis-allylic methylene group

Unsaturated fatty acid $R–CH=CH–CH_2–CH=CH–R'$

Hydrogen abstraction $OH^\bullet$ or $OOH^\bullet$

H_2O H_2O_2

Lipid radical $R–CH=CH–\overset{\bullet}{C}H–CH=CH–R'$

Such lipid peroxidation chain reactions can be promoted by the presence of transition metals such as iron and copper that can vary their valency state by gaining or losing electrons. Significantly, there is sufficient free iron and copper in human seminal plasma to promote lipid peroxidation once this process has been initiated[30]. When iron sulfate and ascorbate (added as a reductant to maintain the iron in a reduced state) are added to suspensions of human spermatozoa, large amounts of lipid peroxide are generated. A majority of these peroxides arise from the iron-catalyzed propagation, rather than *de novo* initiation, of lipid peroxidation cascades[31], according to the following equations:

$$ROOH + Fe^{2+} \rightarrow RO^\bullet + OH^- + Fe^{3+}$$
lipid hydroperoxide   alkoxyl radical

$$ROOH + Fe^{3+} \rightarrow ROO^\bullet + H^+ + Fe^{2+}$$
lipid hydroperoxide   peroxyl radical

Thus, the amounts of lipid peroxide generated on the addition of transition metals, such as iron, to human sperm suspensions will reflect the amount of lipid peroxide present in these cells at the moment the catalyst was added. The lipid peroxide content of these cells will, in turn, reflect differences in the amount of oxidative stress that the spermatozoa have suffered during their life history. Differences in susceptibility arise because of interindividual variation in (1) the presence and molecular composition of unsaturated fatty acids in the sperm plasma membrane, (2) the degree to which the spermatozoa have been exposed to ROS and transition metal catalysis during their life history and (3) the level of protection afforded by free radical scavengers, chain-breaking antioxidants and ROS-metabolizing enzymes in the vicinity of the spermatozoa during their sojourn in the male reproductive tract. Monitoring the generation of lipid peroxide breakdown products such as malondialdehyde and/or 4-hydroxy alkenals in the presence of ferrous ion promoters therefore generates a significant amount of information about the sperm population under investigation[32]. Such measurements of the 'lipoperoxidative potential' of human spermatozoa have clear diagnostic value[29,32].

Protection against lipid peroxidation includes membrane-associated antioxidants epitomized by α-tocopherol, a hydrophobic vitamin that is capable of intercepting alkoxyl and peroxyl radicals and terminating the peroxidation chain reaction[33]. This vitamin is extremely effective in breaking lipid peroxidation cascades, and has been shown to improve significantly the fertility of males selected on the basis of high levels of lipid peroxidation in their spermatozoa[34]. Moreover, this vitamin has been known since the 1940s to be essential for male reproduction. Of the small-molecular-mass scavengers involved in the protection of human spermatozoa, the most important are vitamin C, uric acid, tryptophan and taurine[35,36]. In terms of antioxidant enzymes, spermatozoa possess both the mitochondrial and cytosolic forms of superoxide dismutase (SOD) and the enzymes of the glutathione cycle, but very little catalase.

SOD catalyzes the dismutation of $O_2^{-\bullet}$, a reaction in which this molecule reacts with itself to generate H_2O_2. Such dismutation can occur spontaneously without SOD; however, the reaction proceeds much more slowly in the absence of this enzyme. There is sufficient SOD activity in the mitochondria and cytosol of human spermatozoa to account for most, if not all, of the H_2O_2 produced by these cells[37]. Although SOD is usually thought of in antioxidant terms, this is only true if this enzyme is tightly coupled with additional enzymes that can metabolize the H_2O_2 generated as a consequence of $O_2^{-\bullet}$ dismutation. In isolation, SOD converts a short-lived, rather inert, membrane-impermeant free radical ($O_2^{-\bullet}$) into a powerful, membrane-permeant oxidant, H_2O_2. Although the latter is not a free radical, it is, nevertheless, a potentially pernicious molecule. If not rapidly metabolized, it has the potential to initiate both lipid peroxidation in the sperm plasma membrane and trigger DNA damage to both the nuclear and mitochondrial genomes of these cells[3,38].

Some insight into the relative importance of $O_2^{-\bullet}$ and H_2O_2 in the initiation of peroxidative damage in human spermatozoa has come from studies employing xanthine oxidase to generate an extracellular mixture of ROS *in vitro*[39]. In the presence of this ROS-generating system, the spermatozoa rapidly lose their motility as a consequence of the initiation and propagation of peroxidative damage. If SOD is added to the medium to remove $O_2^{-\bullet}$, motility loss still occurs. However, if catalase is added to the incubation mixture to remove H_2O_2, then lipid peroxidation is

suppressed and sperm motility is fully maintained. The implication of these studies, that H_2O_2 is the major cytotoxic species of ROS as far as spermatozoa are concerned, has been confirmed by experiments in which the direct addition of this oxidant has been shown to influence both the movement of human spermatozoa and their competence for oocyte fusion[38].

Given the damaging nature of H_2O_2 it is obviously important that this oxidant is rapidly removed from spermatozoa before it can initiate lipid peroxidation or DNA damage. The enzymes of the glutathione cycle (glutathione peroxidase and reductase) are responsible for peroxide metabolism in these cells. Under normal circumstances, sufficient NADPH (reduced nicotinamide–adenine dinucleotide phosphate) is generated by the oxidation of glucose through the hexose monophosphate shunt to fuel glutathione reductase and maintain an adequate pool of reduced glutathione (GSH) to counteract the H_2O_2 and lipid peroxides generated as a consequence of sperm metabolism[40]. These reactions can be summarized as follows:

$$\text{Glutathione reductase}$$
$$GSSG + NADPH + H^+ \rightarrow 2GSH + NADP^+$$

$$\text{Glutathione peroxidase}$$
$$2GSH + H_2O_2 \rightarrow GSSG + 2H_2O$$

where GSSG is glutathione disulfide.

It should also be noted that the detoxification of lipid peroxides by glutathione peroxidase requires the concerted action of an additional enzyme in the form of phospholipase A2. This enzyme is required to cleave the lipid peroxide away from the parent phospholipid so that it becomes available for the detoxifying action of glutathione peroxidase.

In addition to these intracellular antioxidants, spermatozoa are also protected by highly specialized extracellular antioxidant enzymes secreted by the male reproductive tract. These enzymes include glutathione peroxidase 5 (GPX5)[41] as well as the extremely large amounts of extracellular SOD present in epididymal and seminal plasma[29].

Indeed, seminal plasma contains more SOD than any other fluid in biology. The world record is held by donkey semen, which contains more than 3000 units of enzyme activity per milliliter[42]. As seen later in this chapter, the antioxidants present in seminal plasma (SOD, albumin, uric acid and vitamin C) become extremely important in protecting spermatozoa from ROS generated by activated leukocytes entering the reproductive tract at points distal to the epididymis, such as the urethra, prostate and seminal vesicles.

EVIDENCE FOR OXIDATIVE STRESS

Given the potential that ROS have for causing cellular damage, it is not surprising that they have been implicated in the etiology of male infertility[22,26]. The evidence for an association between oxidative stress and defective sperm function comes from three major sources. First, there is evidence that many aspects of sperm function including motility and sperm–oocyte fusion are negatively correlated with the lipoperoxidative potential of these cells. This was first suggested in the pioneering studies of Thaddeus Man and colleagues at the University of Cambridge. These authors observed that human spermatozoa were extremely susceptible to the cytotoxic effects of lipid peroxidation, and that severe sperm motility loss was associated with high levels of lipid peroxide generation in the presence of transition metals[29,43]. These studies have subsequently been confirmed and extended in larger cohorts of patients. Thus, the lipoperoxidative potential of freshly prepared spermatozoa (i.e. their capacity to generate lipid peroxides in the presence of a ferrous ion promoter) was found to be highly predictive of their capacity for movement and their ability to exhibit sperm–oocyte fusion[32,44]. Indeed, the tightness of the correlations with sperm movement has suggested that peroxidative damage is one of the major causes of impaired motility[32] (Figure 17.1). Moreover, the lipoperoxidative potential of washed, leukocyte-free sperm

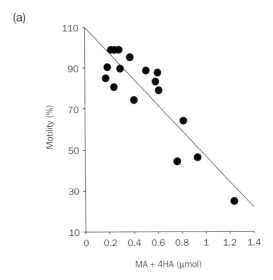

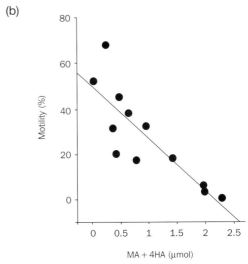

Figure 17.1   Relationship between motility loss observed in populations of human spermatozoa and generation of MA + 4HA in the presence of promoter. (a) Oxidative stress induced by the incubation of spermatozoa for 15 h at 37°C. (b) Oxidative stress induced using a xanthine oxidase free radical-generating system. MA + 4HA represents μmol of malondialdehyde and 4-hydroxy alkenals generated by 2×10^7 spermatozoa during a 2-h incubation with promoter[32]

suspensions was found to be reflective of the quality of sperm movement in the original ejaculate (Figure 17.2). Such findings reinforce the notion that the diagnostic value of lipoperoxidative potential measurements lies in the fact that

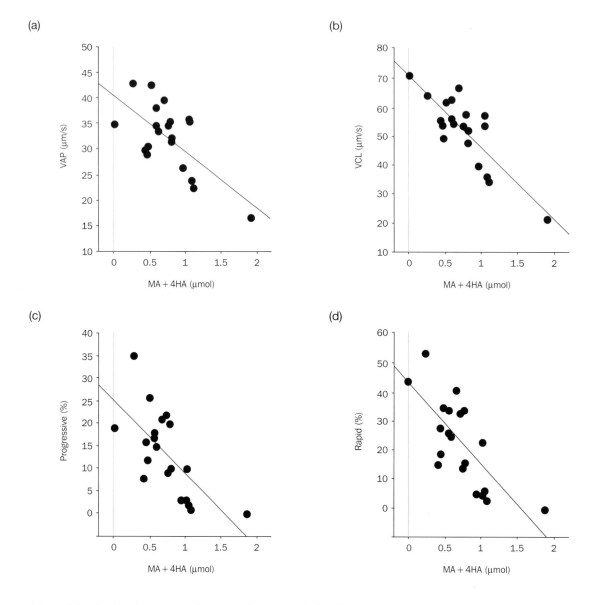

Figure 17.2   Relationships between lipoperoxidation potential of purified sperm suspensions and sperm movement in the original semen samples. (a) VAP (average path velocity); (b) VCL (curvilinear velocity); (c) percentage progressive; and (d) percentage rapid (> 25 μm/s). MA + 4HA represents μmol of malondialdehyde and 4-hydroxy alkenals generated by 2×10^7 spermatozoa during a 2-h incubation with promoter

they give an accurate picture of the accumulated degree of oxidative stress suffered by spermatozoa during their life history[32,45].

Additional evidence for oxidative stress in defective sperm populations comes from the elevated levels of oxidative DNA damage observed in the spermatozoa of infertile men compared with fertile controls[2,27,46]. Positive correlations between sperm DNA damage and the intensity of signals generated in the presence of redox-active probes (luminol and lucigenin) tend to support this view[19,46]. Studies in which defective sperm function has been correlated with the chemiluminescence generated in the presence of such probes also add weight to this argument[22,23,26,47]. In studies involving clinically characterized samples, elevated chemiluminescence signals have been observed in particular groups of patients including those exhibiting oligozoospermia[48], spinal cord injury[49] and varicocele[50]. Significantly elevated chemiluminescence signals have also been observed in patients exhibiting unexplained infertility[22,51].

Of particular clinical importance is a prospective study in which the chemiluminescence signals generated in the presence of luminol were found to correlate with the incidence of spontaneous pregnancy in a large cohort of untreated patients followed up for a maximum of 4 years[52]. Moreover, within this data set there were no significant correlations between fertility and the conventional criteria of semen quality. Thus, such chemiluminescence measurements of redox activity in human sperm suspensions are clearly able to add value to the traditional semen analysis. The importance of such assays has also been emphasized in studies reporting significant inverse correlations between sperm chemiluminescence and the fertilizing potential of these cells in assisted conception cycles[53].

Although these data are suggestive, there are two notes of caution that should be raised in evaluating these associations between chemiluminescence and fertility. First, the biochemical basis of the activities being measured by luminol- or lucigenin-dependent chemiluminescence is still the subject of debate. In the case of lucigenin, a commonly used experimental paradigm is to trigger chemiluminescence in populations of spermatozoa through the addition of an exogenous electron source in the form of NAD(P)H[54]. Assays performed in this manner generate intense chemiluminescence signals with human spermatozoa that are inversely correlated with the functional competence of these cells[47,55]. The chemistry of lucigenin chemiluminescence is complex, but a key event in the biochemical cascade leading to light

generation is the activation of the probe by a one-electron reduction reaction. Such activation can be achieved enzymatically by cytochrome P450 or cytochrome b5 reductase[56].

Once activated, the probe is then thought to react with $O_2^{-\bullet}$ to create an unstable dioxetane that decomposes with the generation of light. However, it has also been proposed that reduced lucigenin can itself effect the one-electron reduction of ground-state oxygen to produce $O_2^{-\bullet}$ and regenerate the parent lucigenin molecule. If the concentration of NAD(P)H and lucigenin in the reaction mixture is sufficiently high, such redox cycling behavior has the potential to generate a large amount of $O_2^{-\bullet}$ as a consequence, rather than a cause, of probe activation. Doubts have been cast on the validity of this reaction scheme[57] and, as a result, we cannot be certain what proportion of the chemiluminescent signal generated in the presence of lucigenin and NAD(P)H can be accounted for by the primary production of $O_2^{-\bullet}$ or the secondary production of this metabolite via the redox cycling of the probe. If the latter explanation is correct, it would suggest the presence of abnormally high levels of reductase activity in the spermatozoa of infertile men[58].

In the case of luminol, the probe must undergo a one-electron oxidation in order to become activated. In many ways, luminol is a more reliable probe than lucigenin, and has been effectively used to record the ROS generated in human semen samples as a consequence of leukocyte contamination[59,60]. However, herein lies the second point of contention with chemiluminescence data generated using human semen: the extent to which the results have been influenced by the presence of contaminating leukocytes.

SOURCES OF OXIDATIVE STRESS

Although most studies in this area have been careful to exclude leukocytospermic specimens containing large numbers of leukocytes (typically $> 1 \times 10^6$/ml), this does not necessarily mean that the data have not been obfuscated as a result of leukocyte contamination. On a cell-for-cell basis, the most common type of leukocyte found in human semen samples, the neutrophil, is 1000-fold more active in generating ROS than a spermatozoon. Concentrations of leukocytes well below the threshold for leukocytospermia exhibit highly significant correlations with ROS generation by washed sperm suspensions, giving r values in the order of 0.8[61]. Despite the highly significant nature of this correlation, it does not mean that spermatozoa are incapable of generating ROS.

Although various publications have variously asserted that the chemiluminescent signals generated by washed human sperm suspensions emanate exclusively from the spermatozoa[62] or contaminating leukocytes[63], the truth is that both sources of ROS are active. Plots of leukocyte numbers against PMA-induced chemiluminescence activity (Figure 17.3) reveal that redox activity can vary over several log orders of magnitude in the absence of detectable leukocyte contamination. However, when leukocytes are present, the chemiluminescence activity is invariably high. In order

to resolve the spermatozoa's contribution to oxidative stress in the ejaculate, it is essential that all traces of leukocyte contamination are removed from the sperm suspension. Protocols have been described for both the efficient detection of leukocyte contamination and the selective removal of these cells using paramagnetic particles coated with anti-CD45, the common leukocyte antigen[64–66]. However, there are very few studies in which these stringent conditions have been met.

Where this has been achieved, the results unequivocally identify defective spermatozoa as a source of redox activity[49]. In a recent study, leukocyte-free sperm suspensions were exposed to the powerful protein kinase C agonist, 12-myristate, 13-acetate phorbol ester (PMA). The results revealed powerful inverse correlations between the chemiluminescence activity recorded and the quality of spermatozoa, particularly their motility[32]. Even more important, such measurements showed very tight correlations with the fundamental quality of the original semen sample in terms of sperm morphology, count and motility (Figure 17.4)[32]. In other words, the measurement

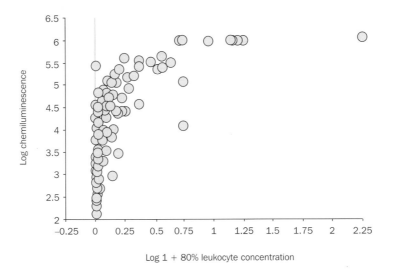

Figure 17.3   Plot of leukocyte concentration against 12-myristate, 13-acetate phorbol ester (PMA)-induced, luminol peroxidase-mediated chemiluminescence. Note the chemiluminescence signal generated by these samples varies over log orders of magnitude in the absence of leukocyte contamination

(a)

(b)

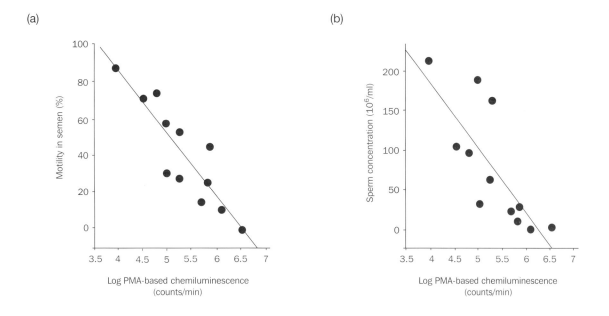

Figure 17.4   Relationships between intensity of the chemiluminescence signal generated by purified leukocyte-free samples in response to 12-myristate, 13-acetate phorbol ester (PMA) in the presence of luminol peroxidase and quality of the original semen samples as reflected by (a) the percentage of motile cells in semen and (b) sperm count in semen[32]

of ROS generation by spermatozoa not only reflects the quality of these cells but also the quality of the underlying spermatogenic process.

Why spermatozoa should vary in their capacity for ROS generation is unknown at the present time. One possibility is that the oxidative stress is being generated by virtue of defects in the sperm mitochondria. Mitochondria are extremely active organelles that are constantly mediating electron transfer reactions through the ETC (electron transport chain) in order to fuel the generation of adenosine triphosphate (ATP). One of the inherent problems with such electron transport activity is that it is leaky, and electrons have a tendency to spill out of the ETC and combine with oxygen to generate $O_2^{-\bullet}$. Aberrant production of ROS by mitochondria is therefore a possible source of oxidative stress in the spermatozoa of infertile men. However, early attempts to address this question failed to find any effect of ETC inhibitors on the chemiluminescence signals generated by suspensions of defective spermatozoa[22].

The caveat with these experiments is that they did not exclude the possibility that the ROS being detected were generated by contaminating leukocytes. Thus, a possible contribution of sperm mitochondria to the generation of ROS by purified human sperm suspensions still requires careful examination.

Another possibility, for which there is considerable evidence, is that the spermatozoa generating high levels of ROS have experienced defective spermiogenesis resulting in morphological defects, particularly in the midpiece region of the cell. During normal spermiogenesis, Sertoli cells actively remove the sperm cytoplasm, just before these cells are released from the germinal epithelium. In most mammals, any residual cytoplasm that remains after spermiogenesis is remodeled into a discrete, spherical, cytoplasmic droplet that slowly migrates down the sperm tail during epididymal transit, prior to its release into the extracellular space. Intriguingly, human spermatozoa have lost this ability to create and shed a cytoplasmic droplet. In these cells, any residual cytoplasm left after spermiation snaps back into the neck region of the spermatozoa and remains there as a ragged appendage that bears witness to the defective testicular origins of the cell. The presence of such excess residual cytoplasm has been correlated with ROS production by several independent groups[67-70]. One suggested mechanism by which such residual cytoplasm might induce ROS production is through the provision of excess substrate to a putative NADPH oxidase on the sperm surface.

ROS production by purified sperm suspensions is highly correlated with the cellular content of cytoplasmic enzymes such as SOD, creatine kinase and glucose-6-phosphate dehydrogenase. Most of these enzymes are simply passengers, confirming the presence of excess residual cytoplasm in sperm populations generating high levels of ROS[67,68]. However, it has been hypothesized that in terms of pathology, the key enzyme is glucose-6-phosphate dehydrogenase[5,67,71]. This enzyme controls the rate of glucose oxidation through the hexose monophosphate shunt, and the latter, in turn, generates the NADPH needed to fuel ROS production by a putative NADPH oxidase enzyme such as Nox 5, a free radical-generating oxidase recently detected in the male germ line[72]. This link between NADPH and ROS generation is reflected in the strong correlation that exists between the glucose-6-phosphate content of purified human sperm suspensions and their capacity to generate a chemiluminescence response to PMA (Figure 17.5). By removing most of the sperm cytoplasm during spermiogenesis, the testes ensure that these cells are only able to generate a limited supply of NADPH, just enough to meet the needs of the protective glutathione cycle and support the ROS-dependent elements of sperm capacitation[73-76]. However, if excess residual cytoplasm is retained because of mistakes during spermiogenesis (Figure 17.6), then there is the potential to generate additional ROS that will, in turn, damage the functional competence of these cells.

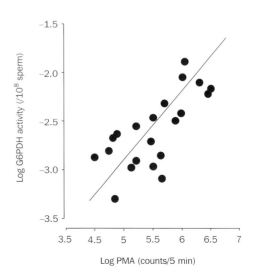

Figure 17.5 Cellular content of glucose-6-phosphate dehydrogenase (G6PDH) and chemiluminescence. The retention of excess residual cytoplasm increases the cellular content of cytoplasmic enzymes such as G6PDH, the presence of which correlates closely with the redox activity exhibited by human spermatozoa in response to 12-myristate, 13-acetate phorbol ester (PMA) provocation in the presence of luminol and peroxidase

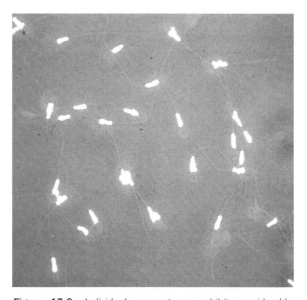

Figure 17.6 Individual spermatozoa exhibit considerable variation in the amount of residual cytoplasm retained following spermiation. Cytoplasm revealed by staining for diaphorase activity[67]

CONSEQUENCES OF OXIDATIVE STRESS

In light of the above, we must conclude that there are two sources of oxidative stress within the ejaculate: leukocytes and defective spermatozoa. The impact of seminal leukocytes will depend on the types of white cell present, their site of entry into the male reproductive tract and their state of activation. All of the information currently available indicates that the major leukocyte species is the neutrophil, and these cells are present in the ejaculate in an activated state[61,62]. Where these cells enter the male reproductive tract is generally unresolved, but has a direct bearing on the pathological consequences of leukocytic infiltration. If the leukocytes gain entry at points distal to the origin of the vas deferens, as a consequence of secondary sexual gland infection for example, then their direct impact on sperm function may be limited, because at the moment of ejaculation the spermatozoa will be protected by the powerful antioxidants in seminal plasma[61]. Conversely, if the neutrophils entered the male reproductive tract at the level of the rete testes or epididymis, then there would be every opportunity for these cells to induce oxidative damage in the spermatozoa.

Free radical-generating leukocytes also have ample opportunity to attack spermatozoa in washed preparations, where the gametes are deprived of the protective effects of seminal plasma. Indeed, apart from albumin and possibly phenol red, most *in vitro* fertilization (IVF) media are devoid of protective antioxidants. Some media are even supplemented with transition metals such as iron and copper, and, in this way, may actually stimulate peroxidative damage in spermatozoa[77]. Whenever activated leukocytes are present in washed sperm suspensions, the fertilizing capacity of the spermatozoa is suppressed[62]. These results have clear implications for the practice of IVF therapy, and it comes as no surprise that negative associations have been observed between leukocyte contamination of washed sperm preparations and fertilization rates in assisted conception cycles[65,66].

The second source(s) of ROS in human ejaculates are the spermatozoa themselves[49,68,69]. Such intracellular free radical generation is associated with the disruption of all aspects of sperm function, including their motility, their capacity for acrosomal exocytosis, their ability to fuse with the vitelline membrane of the oocyte and the integrity of their DNA[6,27]. As indicated above, excess free radical generation is normally associated with defects in spermiogenesis, leading to the retention of excess residual cytoplasm in the midpiece of these cells. It is also possible that excess ROS generation by spermatozoa is driven by the redox cycling of xenobiotics present in the environment, or deficiencies in the mitochondrial ETC[6]. Whether such ROS-generating spermatozoa can also damage the functional competence of other spermatozoa in the immediate vicinity is still an open question. If defective spermatozoa actively generate free radicals from the moment they leave the testes, then the opportunities for collateral damage to other cells in the same sperm population might be considerable.

CONCLUSIONS

In summary, oxidative stress is one of the major causes of defective sperm function. Free radical attacks on these cells damage the DNA in the sperm nucleus and induce lipid peroxidation in the sperm plasma membrane. As a consequence of these changes, the spermatozoa lose their capacity for fertilization and their ability to support normal embryonic development[6]. The origins of oxidative stress include leukocytic infiltration, excess free radical generation by the spermatozoa and defects in the antioxidant protection provided to these cells during their sojourn in the male reproductive tract. Further research in this area should help to advance our understanding of the origins of oxidative stress in the male reproductive tract, and assist in the development of rational approaches towards the prevention and treatment of this condition.

REFERENCES

1. Palermo G, et al. Pregnancies after intracytoplasmic injection of single spermatozoon into an oocyte. Lancet 1992; 340: 17

2. Irvine DS, et al. DNA Integrity in human spermatozoa: relationships with semen quality. J Androl 2000; 21: 33

3. Sawyer DE, et al. Analysis of gene-specific DNA damage and single-strand DNA breaks induced by pro-oxidant treatment of human spermatozoa in vitro. Mutat Res 2003; 529: 21

4. Lewis SEM, Aitken RJ. Sperm DNA damage, fertilization and pregnancy. Cell Tissue Res 2005; in press

5. Aitken RJ. The human spermatozoon – a cell in crisis? The Amoroso Lecture. J Reprod Fertil 1999; 115: 1

6. Aitken RJ. Founders' Lecture. Human spermatozoa: fruits of creation, seeds of doubt. Reprod Fertil Dev 2004; 16: 655

7. Aitken RJ, Krausz CG. Oxidative stress, DNA damage and the Y chromosome. Reproduction 2001; 122: 497

8. Sakkas D, et al. Sperm nuclear DNA damage and altered chromatin structure: effect on fertilization and embryo development. Hum Reprod 1998; 13: 11

9. Duran EH, et al. Sperm DNA quality predicts intrauterine insemination outcome: a prospective cohort study. Hum Reprod 2002; 17: 3122

10. Morris ID, et al. The spectrum of DNA damage in human sperm assessed by single cell gel electrophoresis (comet assay) and its relationship to fertilization and embryo development. Hum Reprod 2002; 17: 990

11. Carrell DT, et al. Elevated sperm chromosome aneuploidy and apoptosis in patients with unexplained recurrent pregnancy loss. Obstet Gynecol 2003; 101: 1229

12. Loft S, et al. Oxidative DNA damage in human sperm influences time to pregnancy. Hum Reprod 2003; 18: 1265

13. Saleh RA, et al. Negative effects of increased sperm DNA damage in relation to seminal oxidative stress in men with idiopathic and male factor infertility. Fertil Steril 2003; 79 (Suppl 3): 1597

14. Bungum M, et al. The predictive value of sperm chromatin structure assay (SCSA) parameters for the outcome of intrauterine insemination, IVF and ICSI. Hum Reprod 2004; 19: 1401

15. Virro MR, Larson-Cook KL, Evenson DP. Sperm chromatin structure assay parameters are related to fertilization, blastocyst development, and ongoing pregnancy in in vitro fertilization and intracytoplasmic sperm injection cycles. Fertil Steril 2004; 81: 1289

16. Sakkas D, Mariethoz E, St John JC. Abnormal sperm parameters in humans are indicative of an abortive apoptotic mechanism linked to the fas-mediated pathway. Exp Cell Res 1999; 251: 350

17. Sakkas D, et al. Origin of DNA damage in ejaculated human spermatozoa. Rev Reprod 1999; 4: 31

18. Sakkas D, et al. Nature of DNA damage in ejaculated human spermatozoa and the possible involvement of apoptosis. Biol Reprod 2002; 66: 1061

19. Barroso G, Morshedi M, Oehninger S. Analysis of DNA fragmentation, plasma membrane translocation of phosphatidylserine and oxidative stress in human spermatozoa. Hum Reprod 2000; 15: 1338

20. Sakkas D, et al. Relationship between the presence of endogenous nicks and sperm chromatin packaging in maturing and fertilizing mouse spermatozoa. Biol Reprod 1995; 52: 1149

21. Manicardi GC, et al. Presence of endogenous nicks in DNA of ejaculated human spermatozoa and its relationship to chromomycin A(3) accessibility. Biol Reprod 1995; 52: 864

22. Aitken RJ, Clarkson JS. Cellular basis of defective sperm function and its association with the genesis of reactive oxygen species by human spermatozoa. The Walpole Lecture. J Reprod Fertil 1987; 83: 459

23. Aitken RJ, Fisher H. Reactive oxygen species generation and human spermatozoa, the balance of benefit and risk. Bioessays 1994; 16: 259

24. Aitken RJ, Krausz CG. Oxidative stress, DNA damage and the Y chromosome. Reproduction 2001; 122: 497

25. Aitken RJ, Koopman P, Lewis SE. Seeds of concern. Nature 2004; 432: 48

26. Sharma RK, Agarwal A. Role of reactive oxygen species in male infertility. Urology 1996; 48: 835

27. Henkel R, et al. Effect of reactive oxygen species produced by spermatozoa and leukocytes on sperm functions in non-leukocytospermic patients. Fertil Steril 2005; 83: 635

28. Halliwell B, Gutteridge JMC. Free Radicals in Biology and Medicine. New York: Oxford University Press, 1999

29. Jones R, Mann T, Sherins RJ. Peroxidative breakdown of phospholipids in human spermatozoa: spermicidal effects of fatty acid peroxides and protective action of seminal plasma. Fertil Steril 1979; 31: 531

30. Kwenang A, et al. Iron, ferritin and copper in seminal plasma. Hum Reprod 1987; 2: 387

31. Aitken RJ, Harkiss D, Buckingham DW. Analysis of lipid peroxidation mechanisms in human spermatozoa. Mol Reprod Dev 1993; 35: 302

32. Gomez E, Irvine DS, Aitken RJ. Evaluation of a spectrophotometric assay for the measurement of malondialdehyde and 4-hydroxyalkenals in human spermatozoa: relationships with semen quality and sperm function. Int J Androl 1998; 21: 81

33. Aitken RJ, Clarkson JS, Fishel S. Generation of reactive oxygen species, lipid peroxidation and human sperm function. Biol Reprod 1989; 40: 183

34. Suleiman SA, et al. Lipid peroxidation and human sperm motility: protective role of vitamin E. J Androl 1996; 17: 530

35. Rhemrev JP, et al. Quantification of the nonenzymatic fast and slow TRAP in a postaddition assay in human seminal plasma and the antioxidant contributions of various seminal compounds. J Androl 2000; 21: 913

36. van Overveld FW, et al. Tyrosine as important contributor to the antioxidant capacity of seminal plasma. Chem Biol Interact 2000; 127: 151

37. Alvarez JG, et al. Spontaneous lipid peroxidation and production of hydrogen peroxide and superoxide in human spermatozoa. J Androl 1987; 8: 338

38. Aitken RJ, et al. Relative impact of oxidative stress on the functional competence and genomic integrity of human spermatozoa. Biol Reprod 1998; 59: 1037

39. Aitken RJ, Buckingham D, Harkiss D. Use of a xanthine oxidase oxidant generating system to investigate the cytotoxic effects of reactive oxygen species on human spermatozoa. J Reprod Fertil 1992; 97: 441

40. Storey BT, Alvarez JG, Thompson KA. Human sperm glutathione reductase activity in situ reveals limitation in the glutathione antioxidant defense system due to supply of NADPH. Mol Reprod Dev 1998; 49: 400

41. Vernet P, et al. In vitro expression of a mouse tissue specific glutathione-peroxidase-like protein lacking the selenocysteine can protect stably transfected mammalian cells against oxidative damage. Biochem Cell Biol 1996; 74: 125

42. Mennella MRF, Jones R. Properties of spermatozoal superoxide dismutase and lack of involvement of superoxides in metal-ion-catalysed lipid-peroxidation reactions in semen. Biochem J 1980; 191: 289

43. Jones R, Mann T, Sherins RJ. Adverse effects of peroxidized lipid on human spermatozoa. Proc R Soc Lond B 1978; 201: 413

44. Aitken RJ, Harkiss D, Buckingham D. Relationship between iron-catalysed lipid peroxidation potential and human sperm function. J Reprod Fertil 1993; 98: 257

45. Kodama H, et al. Increased deoxyribonucleic acid damage in the spermatozoa of infertile male patients. Fertil Steril 1997; 65: 519

46. Henkel R, et al. DNA fragmentation of spermatozoa and assisted reproduction technology. Reprod Biomed Online 2003; 7: 477

47. Aitken RJ, et al. Multiple forms of redox activity in populations of human spermatozoa. Mol Hum Reprod 2003; 9: 645

48. Aitken RJ, et al. Differential contribution of leucocytes and spermatozoa to the high levels of reactive oxygen species recorded in the ejaculates of oligozoospermic patients. J Reprod Fertil 1992; 94: 451

49. De Lamirande E, et al. Increased reactive oxygen species formation in semen of patients with spinal cord injury. Fertil Steril 1995; 63: 637

50. Hendin BN, et al. Varicocele is associated with elevated spermatozoal reactive oxygen species production and diminished seminal plasma antioxidant capacity. J Urol 1999; 161: 1831

51. Pasqualotto FF, et al. Oxidative stress in normospermic men undergoing infertility evaluation. J Androl 2001; 22: 316

52. Aitken RJ, Irvine DS, Wu FC. Prospective analysis of sperm–oocyte fusion and reactive oxygen species generation as criteria for the diagnosis of infertility. Am J Obstet Gynecol 1991; 164: 542

53. Zorn B, Vidmar G, Meden-Vrtovec H. Seminal reactive oxygen species as predictors of fertilization, embryo quality and pregnancy rates after conventional in vitro fertilization and intracytoplasmic sperm injection. Int J Androl 2003; 26: 279

54. Aitken RJ, et al. Reactive oxygen species generation by human spermatozoa is induced by exogenous NADPH and inhibited by the flavoprotein inhibitors diphenylene iodonium and quinacrine. Mol Reprod Dev 1997; 47: 468

55. Said TM, et al. Impact of sperm morphology on DNA damage caused by oxidative stress induced by beta nicotinamide adenine dinucleotide phosphate. Fertil Steril 2005; 83: 95

56. Baker MA, et al. Identification of cytochrome P450-reductase as the enzyme responsible for NADPH-dependent lucigenin and tetrazolium salt reduction in rat epididymal sperm preparations. Biol Reprod 2004; 71: 307

57. Afanasíev IB, Ostrachovich EA, Korkina LG. Lucigenin is a mediator of cytochrome C reduction but

not of superoxide anion production. Arch Biochem Biophys 1999; 366: 267

58. Aitken RJ, Baker MA, O'Bryan MK. Shedding light on chemiluminescence: the application of chemiluminescence in diagnostic andrology. J Androl 2004; 25: 455

59. Aitken RJ, West K. Relationship between reactive oxygen species generation and leucocyte infiltration in fractions isolated from the human ejaculate on Percoll gradients. Int J Androl 1990; 13: 433

60. Aitken RJ, et al. Analysis of sperm movement in relation to the oxidative stress created by leukocytes in washed sperm preparations and seminal plasma. Hum Reprod 1995; 10: 2061

61. Aitken RJ, West K, Buckingham D. Leukocyte infiltration into the human ejaculate and its association with semen quality, oxidative stress and sperm function. J Androl 1994; 15: 343

62. Allamaneni SS, et al. Characterization of oxidative stress status by evaluation of reactive oxygen species levels in whole semen and isolated spermatozoa. Fertil Steril 2005; 83: 800

63. Williams AC, Ford WC. Relationship between reactive oxygen species production and lipid peroxidation in human sperm suspensions and their association with sperm function. Fertil Steril 2005; 83: 929

64. Aitken RJ, et al. On the use of paramagnetic beads and ferrofluids to assess and eliminate the leukocytic contribution to oxygen radical generation by human sperm suspensions. Am J Reprod Immunol 1996; 35: 541

65. Krausz C, et al. Stimulation of oxidant generation by human sperm suspensions using phorbol esters and formyl peptides: relationships with motility and fertilization in vitro. Fertil Steril 1994; 62: 599

66. Krausz C, et al. Analysis of the interaction between N-formylmethionyl-leucyl phenylalanine and human sperm suspensions, development of a technique for monitoring the contamination of human semen samples with leucocytes. Fertil Steril 1992; 57: 1317

67. Gomez E, et al. Development of an image analysis system to monitor the retention of residual cytoplasm by human spermatozoa: correlation with biochemical markers of the cytoplasmic space, oxidative stress and sperm function. J Androl 1996; 17: 276

68. Gil-Guzman E, et al. Differential production of reactive oxygen species by subsets of human spermatozoa at different stages of maturation. Hum Reprod 2001; 16: 1922

69. Ollero M, et al. Characterization of subsets of human spermatozoa at different stages of maturation: implications in the diagnosis and treatment of male infertility. Hum Reprod 2001; 16: 1912

70. Zini A, et al. Human sperm NADH and NADPH diaphorase cytochemistry: correlation with sperm motility. Urology 1998; 51: 464

71. Aitken RJ. A free radical theory of male infertility. Reprod Fertil Dev 1994; 6: 19

72. Banfi B, et al. A Ca(2+)-activated NADPH oxidase in testis, spleen, and lymph nodes. J Biol Chem 2001; 276: 37594

73. de Lamirande E, Gagnon C. Human sperm hyperactivation and capacitation as parts of an oxidative process. Free Radic Biol Med 1993; 14: 157

74. de Lamirande E, Gagnon C. Capacitation-associated production of superoxide anion by human spermatozoa. Free Radic Biol Med 1995; 18: 487

75. Aitken RJ, et al. A novel signal transduction cascade in capacitating human spermatozoa characterised by a redox-regulated, cAMP-mediated induction of tyrosine phosphorylation. J Cell Sci 1998; 111: 645

76. Aitken RJ, et al. Redox regulation of tyrosine phosphorylation in human spermatozoa and its role in the control of human sperm function. J Cell Sci 1995; 108: 2017

77. Gomez E, Aitken J. Impact of in vitro fertilization culture media on peroxidative damage to human spermatozoa. Fertil Steril 1992; 65: 880

18

How do we define male subfertility and what is the prevalence in the general population?

T Igno Siebert, F Haynes van der Merwe, Thinus F Kruger, Willem Ombelet

INTRODUCTION

Several semen parameters are used to discriminate the fertile male from the subfertile male. The most widely used parameters are sperm concentration, motility, progressive motility and sperm morphology. Of these parameters, sperm morphology is the single indicator most widely debated in the literature. A large number of classification systems have been used to describe the factors that constitute a morphologically normal/abnormal spermatozoon. The most widely accepted classification systems for sperm morphology are the World Health Organization (WHO) criteria of 1987 and 1992[1,2] and the Tygerberg strict criteria, now also used by the WHO since 1999[3-6].

Although there is a positive correlation between normal semen parameters and male fertility potential, the threshold values for fertility/subfertility according to WHO criteria[1,2] are of little clinical value in discriminating between the fertile and the subfertile male[7-11]. If these criteria were to be applied, a great number of fertile males (partners having had pregnancies shortly before, after or at the time of a spermiogram) would be classified as subfertile. The predictive values of sperm morphology using strict criteria in *in vitro* fertilization (IVF) and intrauterine insemination (IUI) have been reviewed recently and proved to be useful[12,13].

Much less has been published on the use of this criterion regarding *in vivo* fertility.

In this chapter, we evaluate the classification systems for semen parameters after review of the literature published in English on semen parameters and *in vivo* fertility potential. We also use data from the literature to establish fertility/subfertility thresholds for semen parameters according to the WHO 1999 guidelines[3-6]. These thresholds should be of clinical value and useful when assessing male fertility potential for *in vivo* conditions, in order to identify those males with a significantly reduced chance of achieving success under these conditions.

WHO CRITERIA OF 1987 AND 1992 AND MALE FERTILITY POTENTIAL

The semen analysis is used in clinical practice to assess male fertility potential. To be of clinical value, the methods used should be standardized, and threshold values for fertility/subfertility should be calculated for the different parameters used in the standard semen analysis.

Because there are so many different methods for semen evaluation, it would be difficult to standardize the methods used in its analysis. This applies especially to the assessment of sperm morphology. The two classification systems most widely accepted are the WHO[1,2] and the Tygerberg strict criteria[3–6]. Various methodological problems concerning sperm morphology have been identified. The variants among different methods of morphology assessment have been reported by Ombelet et al.[14–16] and others[17,18], and they recommend standardization of semen analysis methodologies. Some authors recommend that laboratories should adopt the accepted standards, such as those proposed by the WHO[17,18]. Another problem identified is the variation in intra- and interindividual and interlaboratory sperm morphology assessment[18,19]. This problem can be addressed by using the Tygerberg strict criteria, as Menkveld et al. showed that comparable and reliable results between and within observers could be obtained when using this method[19]. Franken et al. delivered dedicated work on continuous quality-control programs for strict sperm morphology assessment, and demonstrated that consistent readings could be achieved; they hence stressed the need for global quality-control measurements in andrology laboratories[20,21]. Cooper et al.[18] also urged the standardization of such quality-control programs and that quality control centers should reach agreement with each other.

Previous WHO thresholds of 50% and 30% for sperm morphology were empirical values and not based on any clinical data. Several authors found these values to be of little or no clinical value[7,9,10]. These studies did, however, find a positive correlation between a high proportion of morphologically normal sperm and an increased likelihood of fertility and/or pregnancy. Other studies have confirmed this correlation[22–25].

Van Zyl et al.[25] were the first to show a faster than linear decline in fertilization rate when the proportion of normal forms dropped to less than 4%. Eggert-Kruse et al.[23] found a higher in vivo pregnancy rate for higher percentage normal forms at thresholds of 4, 7 and 14% using strict criteria for morphology assessment. Zinaman et al.[26] confirmed the value of sperm morphology (strict criteria) by demonstrating a definite decline in pregnancy rate in vivo when the normal morphology dropped below 8% and sperm concentration below 30×10^6/ml. In a study performed by Slama et al.[27], measuring the association between time to pregnancy and semen parameters, it was found that the proportion of morphologically normal sperm influenced the time to pregnancy up to a threshold value of 19%. This value is somewhat higher than that calculated in other studies.

THE USE OF SEMEN PARAMETERS IN IVF AND IUI PROGRAMS

The percentage of normal sperm morphology (strict criteria) has a positive predictive value in IVF and IUI programs. Normal sperm morphology thresholds produced positive predictive values for IVF success when using the 5% and 14% thresholds, respectively, with the overall fertilization rate and overall pregnancy rate significantly higher in the group with normal morphology ≥5% as compared with the <5% group[12]. A meta-analysis of data from IUI programs showed a higher pregnancy rate per cycle in the group with normal sperm morphology ≥5%. In the group with normal sperm morphology <5%, other semen parameters predicted IUI success[13]. In the IUI meta-analysis, motility[28], total motile sperm count[29] and concentration[30] also played a role in some of the studies evaluated, while others[31] stated that sperm morphology alone was enough to predict the prognosis. Because of the high cost of assisted reproduction, males with good or reasonable fertility potential under in vivo conditions should be identified on the basis of semen quality. Conversely, males with a poor fertility potential should be identified, and introduced to assisted reproduction programs.

FERTILITY/SUBFERTILITY THRESHOLDS FOR SPERM MORPHOLOGY USING TYGERBERG STRICT CRITERIA, SPERM CONCENTRATION AND SPERM MOTILITY/PROGRESSIVE MOTILITY

In an effort to establish fertility/subfertility thresholds for the aforementioned parameters, we identified four articles in the published literature. It is our opinion that these articles constitute a representative sample of published studies of the predictive value of sperm morphology, sperm concentration and motility/progressive motility for *in vivo* fertility/subfertility. These articles compared the different semen parameters of a fertile and a subfertile group. They used either classification and regression tree (CART) analysis or receiver operating characteristic (ROC) curve analysis to estimate thresholds for the various semen parameters. The ROC curve was also used to assess the diagnostic accuracy of the different parameters

and their ability to classify subjects into fertile and subfertile groups.

Using ROC curve analysis, Ombelet *et al.*[32] calculated the following thresholds: proportion normal morphology 10%, proportion normal motility 45% and normal sperm concentration 34×10^6/ml. Sperm morphology was shown to be the parameter with the highest prediction power (area under the curve (AUC) 78%). Much lower thresholds were calculated using the 10th centile of the fertile population, these thresholds being 5% for normal morphology, 28% for motility and 14.3×10^6/ml for sperm concentration (Tables 18.1 and 18.2)[32].

Günalp *et al.*[33] also calculated thresholds using ROC curve analysis. These thresholds were: proportion normal morphology 10%, proportion normal motility 52%, proportion progressive motility 42% and sperm concentration 34×10^6/ml. The two parameters that performed best were progressive motility (AUC 70.7%) and

Table 18.1 Thresholds: fertile vs. subfertile populations studied

Authors	Normal morphology (%)	Motility (%)	Progressive motility (%)	Concentration ($\times 10^6$/ml)
Guzick et al.[35] (2001)	9	32	—	13.5
Menkveld et al.[34] (2001)	4	45	—	20
Günalp et al.[33] (2001)	10	52	42	34
Ombelet et al.[32] (1997)	10	45	—	34

Table 18.2 Possible lower thresholds for the general population to distinguish between subfertile and fertile men based on the assumed incidences of subfertile males in their populations

Authors	Normal morphology (%)	Motility (%)	Progressive motility (%)	Concentration ($\times 10^6$/ml)
Menkveld et al.[34] (2001)	3	20	—	20
Günalp et al.[33] (2001)	5	30	14	9
Ombelet et al.[32] (1997)	5	28	—	14.3

morphology (AUC 69.7%). Assuming 50% prevalence of subfertility in the population, the authors used the positive predictive value as an indicator to calculate a lower threshold for each parameter. Values of 5% for proportion normal morphology, 30% for proportion normal motility, 14% for proportion progressive motility and 9×10^6/ml for sperm concentration were calculated (Tables 18.1 and 18.2)[33].

In the most recent article of the four, Menkveld et al.[34] found much lower thresholds than the others. Using ROC curve analysis, the following thresholds were calculated: 4% for normal morphology and 45% for normal motility. Again, morphology showed good predictive value with an AUC of 78.2%. Although a threshold for sperm concentration was not calculated (a sperm concentration less than 20×10^6/ml was used as inclusion criterion), the authors proposed that the cut-off value of 20×10^6/ml could be used with confidence, based on the resultant lower 10th centile of the fertile population. Adjusted cut-off points calculated on the assumption of 50% prevalence of male subfertility were as follows: 3% for proportion normal morphology and 20% for proportion normal motility (Tables 18.1 and 18.2)[34].

In the fourth article by Guzick et al.[35], the authors used CART analysis and calculated two thresholds for each semen parameter which allowed designation into three groups, namely normal (fertile), borderline and abnormal (subfertile). The normal (fertile) group had values greater than 12% for morphology, greater than 63% for motility and higher than 48×10^6/ml for sperm concentration. The abnormal (subfertile) group had values lower than 9% for morphology, lower than 32% for motility and lower than 13.5×10^6/ml for sperm concentration.

In these four articles, the predictive power of the different parameters was calculated as the AUC, using the ROC curve. The AUC for sperm morphology ranged from 66 to 78.2%, confirming the high predictive power of this parameter. In fact, it had the best performance among the different semen parameters in two articles[32,35]. The thresholds calculated in these two articles were 10% and 9%, respectively, while Günalp et al.[33] calculated a threshold of 12% using sensitivity and specificity to analyze their data, and the fourth study calculated a 4% predictive cut-off value. Although sensitivity and specificity for the values are relatively high, the positive predictive values are not. This will therefore result in classifying fertile males as subfertile, probably leading to a degree of anxiety as well as unnecessary and costly infertility treatment. A second and much lower threshold was calculated in three of the four articles. Ombelet et al.[32] calculated this much lower threshold by using the 10th centile of the fertile population, while Günalp et al.[33] screened the population with the positive predictive value as indicator, and Menkveld et al.[34] assumed a 50% prevalence of subfertility in their study population. The lower threshold ranged from 3 to 5% (Table 18.2). These lower thresholds have a much higher positive predictive value than the higher thresholds, with a negative predictive value not much lower.

We suggest that the lower threshold should be used to identify males with the lowest potential for a pregnancy under in vivo conditions. Values above the lower threshold should be regarded as normal. These findings are in keeping with previous publications by Coetzee et al.[12] (IVF data) and Van Waart et al.[13] (IUI data), which reported a significantly lower chance of successful pregnancy in males with normal morphology below their calculated thresholds.

The higher threshold values for percentage motile sperm as calculated in the four articles (using ROC curve or CART analysis) ranged from 32 to 52%, while the lower threshold values ranged from 20 to 30%. Motility also had a high predictive power, with an AUC of between 59 and 79.1%. Günalp et al.[33] calculated thresholds for progressive motility: a higher threshold of 42%, using the ROC curve, and a lower threshold of 14%, with the positive predictive value as indicator. In this study, progressive motility proved to be a marginally better predictor of sub-fertility than sperm morphology, with AUC values of 70.7 and 69.7%, respectively[33]. Montanaro Gauci et al.[28] found percentage motility to be a significant predictor of IUI outcome. The pregnancy rate was almost three times higher in the group with motility > 50% as compared with the group with motility < 50%.

The higher threshold values for sperm concentrations calculated by Ombelet et al.[32], Günalp et al.[33] and Guzick et al.[35] ranged from 13.5 to 34×10^6/ml, while the lower threshold values ranged from 9 to 14.3×10^6/ml. An AUC value of between 55.5 and 69.4% served as confirmation of the predictive power of this parameter. Although Menkveld et al.[34] did not calculate a threshold value for sperm concentration (because values of less than 20×10^6/ml served as inclusion criteria in their study), they suggested a threshold value of 20×10^6/ml to be used with confidence, because it did not influence the results from their fertile population. The clinical value of motility and sperm concentration serves as confirmation of findings reported in numerous other publications[7,8,11,22–24].

Although the various parameters had good predictive power, independent of each other, the clinical value of semen analysis was increased when the parameters were used in combination. Ombelet et al.[32] found that differences between the fertile and subfertile populations only became significant when two or all three semen parameters were combined. Bartoov et al.[36] concluded that fertility potential is dependent on a combination of different semen characteristics. Eggert-Kruse et al.[23] found a significant correlation between the three parameters reviewed in their study. Although the different semen parameters demonstrate good individual predictive power, the clinical value of the semen analysis increases when the parameters are used in combination. We therefore suggest that no parameter should be used in isolation when assessing male fertility potential. The lower thresholds as discussed in this chapter have a much higher positive predictive value and a

high negative predictive value. Therefore, we suggest that these lower thresholds should be used in identifying the subfertile male.

As suggested by the WHO in 1999, each group should develop their own thresholds, based on the population they are working in. It seems as if the sperm morphology threshold of 0–4% normal forms indicates a higher risk group for subfertility, and fits the IVF and IUI data calculated previously[12,13]. The four articles discussed above[32–35] showed the same trends, and can serve as guidelines to distinguish fertile from subfertile males.

As far as concentration and motility are concerned, the thresholds are not clear, but a concentration lower than 10^6/ml and a motility lower than 30% seem to fit the general data[32–35]. However, more, preferably multicenter, studies are needed to set definitive thresholds.

SEMEN PROFILE OF THE GENERAL POPULATION: PARTNERS OF WOMEN WITH CHRONIC ANOVULATION

In general, there is quite a poor level of understanding and evidence regarding the semen analysis profile of the general population. Many male populations have been proposed to mirror the general population in terms of semen analysis. Using donors in a semen-donation program for normality is certainly not the best option, since this population is positively biased for fertility. Army recruits are biased by age. Husbands of tubal-factor patients can be biased by a positive history of infection (tubal factor due to pelvic infection) or a good fertility history (women with tubal sterilization). Therefore, we believe that possibly the best reference group for studying the semen profile in a general population includes partners of women who have been diagnosed with chronic anovulation/PCOS (polycystic ovarian syndrome) (maximum of three menstrual periods per year). We would thus like to propose employing the lower thresholds to indicate patients with subfertility, and, by using the cohort of anovulatory women, we obtain a reflection of the semen profile in a general population.

Two different studies, one retrospective and one prospective, evaluating the semen analysis of partners of women presenting with anovulation were selected.

Retrospective study of partners of women presenting with chronic anovulation (> 35 days) at Tygerberg Fertility Clinic

Included in this study were all male partners of patients diagnosed as anovulatory at the Tygerberg Fertility Clinic. Methods used to examine the semen were according to WHO guidelines[6], and for sperm morphology Tygerberg strict criteria were used[3,4,6]. The laboratory personnel initially evaluated all slides, and each slide was then evaluated by one observer (TFK) according to strict criteria. Sixty-two samples were eventually selected and included in the study (Table 18.3).

Prospective study of partners of women presenting with PCOS at Tygerberg Fertility Clinic

Tygerberg Fertility Clinic conducted a study in patients with PCOS. The patients were diagnosed with PCOS according to the recent Rotterdam consensus statement[37]. The aim of this study was to establish factors influencing ovulation induction in this group.

The semen of the partners of all these women was examined. Methods used to examine the semen were according to WHO guidelines[6], and for sperm morphology Tygerberg strict criteria were used[3,4,6]. The laboratory personnel initially evaluated all slides, and all P-pattern morphology slides were re-evaluated by one observer (TFK) (Table 18.4). The thresholds used for subfertility were those suggested by Van der Merwe et al.[38] in their recent review: 0–4% normal forms, < 30% motility, < 10^6/ml, outlined in the first section of this chapter.

Table 18.3 Retrospective study of partners of women presenting with chronic anovulation (> 35 days) at Tygerberg Fertility Clinic (< 10⁶/ml cut-off)

	Patients n	%
Normozoospermia	29	46.7
Sperm abnormality		
Single-parameter defect		
azoospermia	3	4.8
oligozoospermia (O)	3	4.8
asthenozoospermia (A)	—	0
teratozoospermia (T)	16	25.8
polyzoospermia (P)	2	3.2
immunological factor (I)	1	1.6
Double-parameter defect		
OA	—	0
OT	4	6.5
AT	—	0
TP	1	1.6
TI	1	1.6
Triple-parameter defect		
OAT	2	3.2

Threshold values used: concentration < 10⁶/ml, motility < 30%, morphology < 4% normal forms

DISCUSSION

In the two studies (Table 18.3, retrospective; Table 18.4, prospective) ±50% of patients had a normal semen analysis. The most common single abnormality was that of teratozoospermia (25.8% retrospective, 27.8% prospective). Azoospermia occurred in 1.4–4.8% of patients, with triple-parameter defects found in only 1.4–3.2% of cases (Tables 18.3 and 18.4).

The thresholds as calculated above were used in a group of anovulatory women. These thresholds reflect the prevalence of male factor infertility in the general population. It is interesting to note that in both the retrospective and prospective studies, the prevalence of teratozoospermia (< 4%

Table 18.4 Prospective study of partners of women presenting with polycystic ovarian syndrome (PCOS) at Tygerberg Fertility Clinic (< 10⁶/ml cut-off)		
	Patients	
	n	*%*
Normozoospermia	41	56.9
Sperm abnormality		
Single-parameter defect		
azoospermia	1	1.4
oligozoospermia (O)	1	1.4
asthenozoospermia (A)	—	0
teratozoospermia (T)	20	27.8
polyzoospermia (P)	3	4.2
immunological factor (I)	—	0
Double-parameter defect		
OA	—	0
OT	1	1.4
AT	—	0
TP	3	4.2
TI	1	1.4
OP	—	0
Triple-parameter defect		
OAT	1	1.4

normal morphology) was 25.8–27.8%, making it the most common defect in this group. About 50% of all male patients had normal semen parameters in these two studies using the suggested thresholds as calculated based on the four articles discussed[32–35,38].

It is important to note that in PCOS patients the clinician needs to take into consideration that not only anovulation, but also, in up to 50% of these patients, the male factor needs attention, to assist in achieving a successful outcome in these couples. These lower thresholds are not absolute, but provide a continuum guiding the clinician to respond to the semen analysis. The golden rule is to repeat a semen analysis 4 weeks after the first (abnormal) evaluation to ensure that the correct approach will be followed. If the result is again abnormal, a thorough physical examination should be performed and the necessary treatment offered. In the case of PCOS, the female factor (anovulation) should obviously be corrected, starting, as first-line approach, with weight loss in women with a body mass index >25. Although 50% of these patients had a male factor according to the definition used, it is also important to note that only ±5% of these factors were serious (azoospermia and the triple-parameter defects), with 7–9.7% with a double defect.

To our knowledge, this is the first attempt to use the specific suggested lower thresholds to define prevalence of the subfertile male in the general population by using an anovulatory group of women. These thresholds will guide the clinician towards a more directive management where indicated.

REFERENCES

1. World Health Organization. WHO Laboratory Manual for the Examination of Human Semen and Sperm–Cervical Mucus Interaction, 2nd edn. Cambridge: Cambridge University Press, 1987
2. World Health Organization. WHO Laboratory Manual for the Examination of Human Semen and Sperm–Cervical Mucus Interaction, 3rd edn. Cambridge: Cambridge University Press, 1992
3. Kruger TF, et al. Predictive value of abnormal sperm morphology in in vitro fertilization. Fertil Steril 1988; 49: 112
4. Kruger TF, et al. Sperm morphologic features as a prognostic factor in in vitro fertilization. Fertil Steril 1986; 46: 1118
5. Menkveld R, et al. The evaluation of morphological characteristics of human spermatozoa according to stricter criteria. Hum Reprod 1990; 5: 586
6. World Health Organization. WHO Laboratory Manual for the Examination of Human Semen and Sperm–Cervical Mucus Interaction, 4th edn. Cambridge: Cambridge University Press, 1999
7. Barratt CL, et al. Clinical value of sperm morphology for in-vivo fertility: comparison between World Health Organization criteria of 1987 and 1992. Hum Reprod 1995; 10: 587
8. Ayala C, Steinberger E, Smith DP. The influence of semen analysis parameters on the fertility potential of infertile couples. J Androl 1996; 17: 718

9. Blonde JP, et al. Relation between semen quality and fertility: a population-based study of 430 first-pregnancy planners. Lancet 1998; 352: 1172

10. Chia SE, Tay SK, Lim ST. What constitutes a normal seminal analysis? Semen parameters of 243 fertile men. Hum Reprod 1998; 13: 3394

11. Chia SE, Lim ST, Tay SK, et al. Factors associated with male fertility: a case–control study of 218 infertile and 240 fertile men. Br J Obstet Gynaecol 2000; 107: 55

12. Coetzee K, Kruger TF, Lombard CJ. Predictive value of normal sperm morphology: a structured literature review. Hum Reprod Update 1998; 4: 73

13. Van Waart J, et al. Predictive value of normal sperm morphology in intrauterine insemination (IUI): a structured literature review. Hum Reprod Update 2001; 7: 495

14. Ombelet W, et al. Results of a questionnaire on sperm morphology assessment. Hum Reprod 1997; 12: 1015

15. Ombelet W, Wouters E, Boels L. Sperm morphology assessment: diagnostic potential and comparative analysis of strict or WHO criteria in a fertile and a sub-fertile population. Int J Androl 1997; 20: 367

16. Ombelet W, et al. Multicenter study on reproducibility of sperm morphology assessments. Arch Androl 1998; 41: 103

17. Keel BA, et al. Lack of standardization in performance of the semen analysis among laboratories in the United States. Fertil Steril 2002; 78: 603

18. Cooper TG, et al. Semen analysis and external quality control schemes for semen analysis need global standardization. Int J Androl 2002; 25: 306

19. Menkveld R, et al. The evaluation of morphological characteristics of human spermatozoa according to stricter criteria. Hum Reprod 1990; 5: 586

20. Franken DR, et al. The development of a continuous quality control programme for strict sperm morphology among sub-Saharan African laboratories. Hum Reprod 2000; 15: 667

21. Franken DR, Barendsen R, Kruger TF. A continuous quality control program for strict sperm morphology. Fertil Steril 2000; 74: 721

22. Holland-Moritz H, Krause W. Semen analysis and fertility prognosis in andrological patients. Int J Androl 1992; 15: 473

23. Eggert-Kruse W, et al. Sperm morphology assessment using strict criteria and male fertility under in-vivo conditions of conception. Hum Reprod 1996; 11: 139

24. Dunphy BC, Neal LM, Cooke ID. The clinical value of conventional semen analysis. Fertil Steril 1989; 51: 324

25. Van Zyl JA, Kotze TJ, Menkveld R. Predictive value of spermatozoa morphology in natural fertilization. In Acosta AA, et al., eds. Human Spermatozoa in Assisted Reproduction. Baltimore: Williams & Wilkins, 1990: 319

26. Zinaman MJ, et al. Semen quality and human fertility: a prospective study with healthy couples. J Androl 2000; 21: 145

27. Slama R, et al. Time to pregnancy and semen parameters: a cross-sectional study among fertile couples from four European cities. Hum Reprod 2002; 17: 503

28. Montanaro Gauci M, et al. Stepwise regression analysis to study male and female factors impacting on pregnancy rate in an intrauterine insemination programme. Andrologia 2001; 33: 135

29. Cohlen BJ, et al. Controlled ovarian hyperstimulation and intrauterine insemination for treating male subfertility: a controlled study. Hum Reprod 1998; 13: 1153

30. Ombelet W, et al. Intrauterine insemination after ovarian stimulation with clomiphene citrate: predictive potential of inseminating motile count and sperm morphology. Hum Reprod 1997; 12: 1458

31. Lindheim S, et al. Abnormal sperm morphology is highly predictive of pregnancy outcome during controlled ovarian hyperstimulation and intrauterine insemination. J Assist Reprod Genet 1996; 13: 569

32. Ombelet W, et al. Semen parameters in a fertile versus sub-fertile population: a need for change in the interpretation of semen testing. Hum Reprod 1997; 12: 987

33. Günalp S, et al. A study of semen parameters with emphasis on sperm morphology in a fertile population: an attempt to develop clinical thresholds. Hum Reprod 2001; 16: 110

34. Menkveld R, et al. Semen parameters, including WHO and strict criteria morphology, in a fertile and infertile population: an effort towards standardization of in vivo thresholds. Hum Reprod 2001; 16: 1165

35. Guzick DS, et al. Sperm morphology, motility, and concentration in fertile and infertile men. N Engl J Med 2001; 345: 1388

36. Bartoov B, et al. Estimating fertility potential via semen analysis data. Hum Reprod 1993; 8: 65

37. The Rotterdam ESHRE/ASRM-sponsored PCOS consensus workshop group. Revised 2003 consensus on diagnostic criteria and long-term health risks related to polycystic ovary syndrome (PCOS). Hum Reprod 2004; 19: 41

38. Van der Merwe FH, et al. The use of semen parameters to identify the subfertile male in the general population. Gynecol Obstet Invest 2005; 59: 86

19

DNA fragmentation and its influence on fertilization and pregnancy outcome

Ralf Henkel

INTRODUCTION

Male subfertility is the reason for the unfulfilled wish for children in approximately 50% of involuntary childless couples. In Germany alone, the number of childless partnerships amounts to 1.5–2.0 million, of which about 200 000 couples (10–13%) seek help by assisted reproduction yearly. In 2002, approximately 40 000 children were born in Germany after employing any form of assisted reproductive technologies (ART); 12 000 children were born after *in vitro* fertilization, constituting 1.6% of all births. The high incidence of male factor infertility mandates a complete andrological consultation in all male partners of couples consulting for infertility. Apart from the light microscopic determination of sperm count and morphological malformations, evaluation of functional sperm parameters has become a powerful tool in andrology laboratories. Some of these assays determine biochemical parameters, such as α-glucosidase[1,2] or the polymorphonuclear granulocyte (PMN) elastase[3,4], which have been found to be important for sperm function. Most, however, determine biological functions of spermatozoa (i.e. motility, membrane integrity, morphology, zona binding, acrosome reaction, acrosin activity, oolemma binding, chromatin condensation or DNA integrity) (Figure 19.1), and consequently the sperm cells' capability to fertilize oocytes. All of these parameters have repeatedly shown a significant relationship to both fertilization and pregnancy, *in vitro* and *in vivo*.

Over recent years, the interest of scientists and clinicians has focused on the role of sperm DNA fragmentation in fertility, as this parameter may have a serious impact on fertilization and pregnancy. By employing ART, abnormal, defective spermatozoa, normally restrained by physiological selection barriers, namely the cervical mucus, uterine environment, cumulus oophorus, zona pellucida or the oolemma, are enabled to enter the oocyte. This is of particular importance in intracytoplasmic sperm injection (ICSI), as this method of assisted reproduction bypasses all barriers, with the effect that a genetically damaged spermatozoon may fertilize an oocyte, which in turn may have an impact on the health and wellbeing of the offspring[5–8]. Depending on the degree of DNA damage, embryo development can be affected and hence this may result in embryonic death[9–11]. The damage may even be transferred to the offspring, causing disease. In this respect, reports of increased chromosomal abnormalities, minor or major birth defects or childhood cancer point out the increased risks for babies born after ICSI[6,8,12–15].

Sperm DNA damage can be caused by various factors such as (1) apoptosis[16,17], (2) improper DNA packaging and ligation during

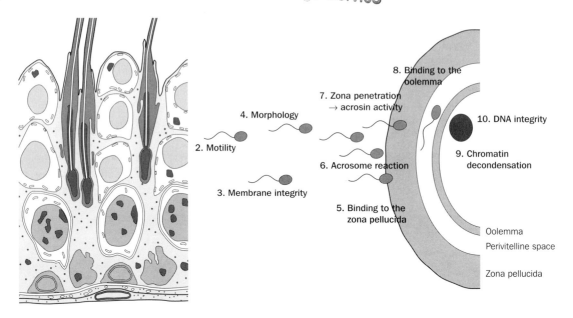

Figure 19.1   Schematic depiction of functional parameters of spermatozoa. Note that the acquisition of capacitation is reflected by the sperm's ability to undergo the acrosome reaction and hyperactivation. In addition, chromatin decondensation must follow proper condensation of sperm DNA material during spermatogenesis and subsequent sperm maturation in the epididymis

spermatogenesis and sperm maturation[18] or (3) oxidative stress[19–21], and is an important issue in assisted reproduction. Thus, it plays an imperative role in the counseling of patients. This chapter focuses on these different aspects of sperm DNA and their influence on fertilization and pregnancy outcome.

APOPTOSIS

Apoptosis is the controlled disassembly of cells from within[22], and is characterized by condensation and fragmentation of the chromatin, compaction of cytoplasmic organelles, reduced mitochondrial transmembrane potential[23], mitochondrial release of cytochrome c[24], production of reactive oxygen species (ROS)[25], dilatation of the endoplasmic reticulum and a decrease in cell volume[26]. This process is also called 'programmed cell death', and is very different from necrosis. It does

not involve any inflammatory response during the phagocytotic elimination of so-called apoptotic bodies[27], from which was derived the term 'apoptosis'. The word 'apoptosis' comes from the Greek 'to fall away from', and refers to the falling of leaves in autumn from deciduous trees[22]. Healthy organisms use this programmed cell death mechanism to maintain a fine balance between life and death. When cells fail to keep this balance and do not fulfill their destiny, become renegade and resist the elimination process, as in some autoimmune diseases or in cancer, such cells grow out of control, which eventually has disastrous effects for the organism. Therefore, this phenomenon plays an essential role in a broad variety of physiological processes during fetal development and in adult tissues. The physiological role of apoptosis is crucial as a homeostatic process during spermatogenesis, and consequently, aberrations of this process can be detrimental for fertility.

The molecular mechanism of apoptosis involves intimate changes of the plasma membrane, which normally shows an asymmetric assembly with an accumulation of phosphatidylethanolamine and the negatively charged phospholipid phosphatidylserine (PS) in the inner leaflet, and sphingomyelin and phosphatidylcholine in the outer leaflet. As a very early sign of apoptosis, PS, normally transferred by an amino phospholipid translocase (flippase) from the outer leaflet to the inner leaflet of the plasma membrane, is translocated in the opposite direction. This translocation of PS to the outer leaflet of the plasma membrane results in its exposure on the external membrane surface[28,29]. Depending on the availability of Ca^{2+}, PS has high affinity to annexin V, a phospholipid-binding protein of about 35 kDa[30].

Another signaling system that is closely involved in the process of apoptosis is the Fas/Fas ligand (FasL; CD95L) system[31]. Fas (CD95; APO-1) is a type I transmembrane receptor protein that belongs to the tumor necrosis factor/nerve growth factor receptor family and transmits the apoptotic signal[32–34]. This molecule contains an intracellular death domain, which is responsible for the activation of multiple intracellular signaling pathways after the binding of FasL to Fas[35]. FasL, on the other hand, is a type II tumor necrosis factor-related transmembrane protein[36]. The Fas system is involved in immune regulation, including the maintenance of peripheral T and B cell tolerance[37], cell-mediated cytotoxicity[38] and the control of immune-privileged sites[39]. Because of this general involvement of the Fas/FasL system in mammalian organisms, the tissue distribution of Fas mRNA is ubiquitous, and particularly high concentrations are found in thymus, spleen and non-lymphoid tissues such as the liver[40]. In contrast, FasL mRNA expression is more restricted to lymphoid organs and the testis, with localization to the Sertoli cells[36].

Intimately involved in the deliberate disassembly of cells into so-called apoptotic bodies are 'cytosolic aspartate-specific proteases' (caspases)[41].

To date, 14 different caspases have been described in the human[42]. Initially, these highly specific enzymes are synthesized as inactive proenzymes of about 30–50 kDa that are activated by proteolytic processing, resulting in two subunits of about 20 kDa and 10 kDa. Functionally, caspases are divided into two functional subgroups, initiating caspases (caspase-6, -8, -9, -10) and effector caspases (caspase-2, -3, -7), which are responsible for the final disassembly of cells and thus apoptotic cell death. A central role in the cascade of apoptotic events is played by caspase-3, which irreversibly activates specific DNases that degrade the DNA[43] leading to DNA fragmentation[44], which can be detected by means of different test systems. Reportedly, caspase-3 is strongly implicated in different pathologies[45].

Although quite a number of pathways have been cited for apoptotic caspase activation and cell death, stronger evidence has been provided only for two (for review see references 46 and 47). In vertebrates, these pathways are (1) the death receptor pathway (extrinsic pathway) and (2) the mitochondrial pathway (intrinsic pathway). In the extrinsic pathway, death receptors of the tumor necrosis factor family, including Fas, transmit the signal via the Fas-associated death domain (FADD) and trigger activation of caspase-8 (initiating caspase), which in turn activates the executing caspase-3. In contrast, in the intrinsic pathway, the executing caspase-3 is activated by caspase-9 (initiating caspase). Caspase-9 is activated following the binding of its death-fold caspase recruitment domain (CARD) to the CARD of apoptotic protease-activating factor-1 (APAF-1), which is present in the cytosol of living cells. APAF-1, in turn, is activated by cytochrome c, which is released from the mitochondria due to permeabilization of the mitochondrial outer membrane following apoptosis-inducing signals. A variety of proapoptotic (BH1, BH2, BH3, Bax, Bak, Bok) and antiapoptotic regulator proteins (Bcl-2, Bcl-xL, A1, Bcl-w, Mcl-1) of the Bcl-2 family orchestrate the whole system[48,49].

Impact of early markers of apoptosis in male germ cells on fertilization and pregnancy

Spermatogenesis is a highly dynamic process, in which undifferentiated diploid spermatogonial stem cells develop and differentiate through mitotic and meiotic cell divisions into spermatozoa that can be released from the germinal epithelium into the lumen of the seminiferous tubules, in a process called spermiation. The process of spermatogenesis can be divided into two phases, the first (first 'wave' of spermatogenesis) being initiated just after birth (in the human between birth and 6 months of age) and characterized by the differentiation of gonocytes into spermatogonia[50]. This first wave of spermatogenesis is accompanied by a massive surge of germ cell apoptosis in the testis[51]. As Sertoli cells can only support a limited number of germ cells[52], this adjustment of the number of germ cells to the number of supporting Sertoli cells is an important step for the normal progression of spermatogenesis in the adult[53].

The second phase of spermatogenesis starts with puberty, which is characterized by increased gonadotropin and androgen levels as well as by a continuous progression of spermatocyte development and the onset of meiotic divisions, resulting in haploid spermatids and eventually in fully differentiated spermatozoa. In order to achieve a stable ratio between Sertoli cells and pre- and post-meiotic germ cells on the one hand, and germ cell renewal on the other, as well as to ensure the quality control of spermatogenesis as a whole[54], this process requires a fine balance, for which apoptosis appears to be the regulatory mechanism. In the human, the daily production of germ cells amounts to 200×10^6, of which up to 75% die spontaneously before release and final maturation to differentiated, functional spermatozoa[55,56]. While spermatogonia and round spermatids show the classical morphological and biochemical features of apoptosis, elongated spermatids do not display the characteristic morphological changes, although DNA fragmentation can be determined,

and a translocation of phosphatidylserine has taken place in some cells. This might be due to initiation of the specific chromatin condensation and morphogenesis of spermatozoa. Finally, during spermiation, spermatozoa are released into the lumen of the seminiferous tubules, and the residual cytoplasm is removed by a nuclear-independent apoptotic process and phagocytosed by the Sertoli cells[57].

Since Sertoli cells express FasL and Fas has been localized on mature spermatozoa[17,58–61], the Fas/FasL system appears to be involved in the regulation of spermatogenesis with regard to the limiting number of sperm cells that can be supported by the Sertoli cell[31,51]. Thus, these germ cells earmarked for apoptosis might be phagocytosed by Sertoli cells. For spermatocytes and spermatids, Pentikäinen et al.[62] demonstrated Fas-mediated, caspase-regulated apoptosis. However, Fas-positive spermatozoa are also present in the ejaculate, and the question arose of how these spermatozoa appear in the ejaculate. Based on this observation, Sakkas et al.[58] suggested a hypothesis according to which these earmarked spermatozoa escape apoptosis because of (1) non-functional Fas or (2) too high a number of earmarked spermatozoa available for FasL on Sertoli cells. This hypothesis has been called 'abortive apoptosis'. However, the molecular mechanism of how Fas-positive sperm escape apoptotic elimination is unknown. Furthermore, there is controversial evidence as to the presence of Fas receptors or Fas-mediated responses in human ejaculated spermatozoa, casting doubts about this hypothesis[60,63].

Currently, there is no consensus about the percentage of Fas-positive sperm in the human ejaculate. Whereas Castro et al.[63] did not find substantial amounts of Fas present in ejaculated spermatozoa of both normozoospermic and non-normozoospermic men, and Taylor et al.[60] did not document a response to Fas ligand in terms of caspase activation or the induction of DNA fragmentation, Sakkas et al.[17] and Henkel et al.[59] found means of 9.7% and 19.8% Fas-positive sperm with maxima of 47.3% and 78%, respectively. While

Sakkas et al.[17] reported higher incidences of Fas positivity in men with compromised semen parameters, McVicar et al.[61] could demonstrate Fas only in the sperm of infertile men. On the other hand, it also appears that Fas positivity of ejaculated human spermatozoa is related neither to DNA damage as detected by means of the comet assay[61], nor to fertilization or pregnancy[59]. Thus, it seems that Fas expression in ejaculated human sperm does not contribute to male infertility. In addition, DNA fragmentation as determined by the TUNEL (terminal deoxynucleotide transferase-mediated dUDP nick-end labeling) assay and apoptotic markers such as Fas do not always exist in unison[17], and neither FasL, nor hydrogen peroxide, significantly increased caspase activity in human spermatozoa[60]. On the other hand, as mentioned above, Castro et al.[63] did not find substantial amounts of Fas present on ejaculated human spermatozoa of both normozoospermic and non-normozoospermic subjects and therefore did not support the 'abortive apoptosis' hypothesis. Recent data of Lachaud et al.[64] suggest that ejaculated healthy human spermatozoa are even incapable of initiating apoptosis.

However, since another early marker of apoptosis, the externalization of PS, identified by means of annexin V binding, and DNA fragmentation as a late marker of programmed cell death can be detected in spermatozoa of almost every ejaculate[59,65–68], the death of sperm might not involve the classical apoptotic pathways, because caspases seem not to be employed[69]. On the other hand, caspases (caspase-1, -3, -8, -9) of the main pathways of apoptosis are present in human spermatozoa and can become activated[68,70], which in turn would then support the apoptosis theory. In order to explain this discrepancy for the survival of immature spermatozoa, Cayli et al.[71] hypothesized that caspase-3 is activated in these earmarked spermatozoa. Nevertheless, protection against apoptotic cell death is provided by expression of the antiapoptotic regulator protein Bcl-xL and is inferred from the presence of the heat shock protein HspA2, which has also been described as an inhibitor of apoptosis[72].

With respect to annexin V binding to ejaculated human spermatozoa, data reported by different working groups are not conclusive. In a pilot study consisting of 102 patients visiting the infertility clinic, Oosterhuis et al.[67] found that 20% of ejaculated spermatozoa were apoptotic as determined by annexin V binding. Moreover, there was an inverse relationship between PS externalization and sperm concentration and motility. These authors concluded that this test would be a reliable approach for testing the functional viability of human spermatozoa. On the other hand, Henkel et al.[59] did not find a significant relationship of annexin V binding test results to either fertilization in vitro or pregnancy, although there was a significant correlation between Fas expression and PS externalization. However, Henkel et al.[59] also found that about one-fifth of ejaculated spermatozoa presented externalized phosphatidylserine. At this point, some questions arise, including: what is the origin of these earmarked sperm and what causes PS externalization?

As discussed before, some authors attribute early signs of apoptosis such as Fas expression or externalization of PS to 'abortive apoptosis' in the testis, and believe that these sperm simply escape cell death. Recent research, however, has demonstrated that the translocation of PS from the inner to the outer leaflet of the sperm plasma membrane also takes place after incubation in capacitating media. In the light of this, PS externalization appears to be an important and physiological event in the process of capacitation in ejaculated spermatozoa[73,74] that is not related to apoptosis. Moreover, PS translocation in bicarbonate-triggered human spermatozoa has been shown to be caspase-independent. Likewise, mitochondrial degeneration or DNA fragmentation could not be observed[75]. Muratori et al.[76], however, oppose this view and favor the abortive apoptosis theory.

In the context of the loss of plasma membrane asymmetry, it is also important to mention the impact of cryopreservation on the highly susceptible sperm plasma membrane. It is well known that cryopreservation significantly compromises sperm motility and fertilizing ability. Disturbance of membrane asymmetry with the externalization of PS is one of the various effects that the freezing–thawing process exerts on living cells[66]. Recent research has provided evidence that this increase in the percentage of annexin V-positive spermatozoa after the freezing–thawing procedure does not result in higher rates of sperm DNA fragmentation[77,78]. However, cryopreservation was associated with significant activation of caspases-3, -8 and -9 as well as disruption of the mitochondrial membrane potential[78]. Therefore, the annexin V binding test appears to be a valuable parameter for predicting the quality of cryopreserved human sperm[79].

Impact of DNA fragmentation on fertilization and pregnancy

Although the early markers of apoptosis in human spermatozoa, especially ejaculated spermatozoa, are very much debated with regard to their impact on male fertility, the effect of the late marker of programmed cell death, DNA fragmentation, seems to be rather clear. Today, there is no doubt that sperm DNA damage not only may compromise fertilization and the onset of pregnancy, but has detrimental effects on the health of the offspring[5–8,12–15].

Repeatedly and unequivocally, this negative impact of sperm DNA damage has been shown for intrauterine insemination (IUI)[80] and *in vitro* fertilization (IVF)[59,65,81,82]. Data obtained by Twigg *et al.*[5] and Henkel *et al.*[20,59] even suggest that spermatozoa with fragmented DNA are still able to fertilize an oocyte, but, at the time when the paternal genome is switched on, further development stops, resulting in a failed pregnancy. Even in natural conception, oxidative sperm DNA damage has a negative impact on human fertility and on the time to pregnancy[83,84]. However, for intracytoplasmic sperm injection (ICSI),

contradictory results have been reported. While a number of authors from different working groups[20,85–87] have shown a significant influence of damaged sperm DNA on fertilization and pregnancy, some others[88–90] have not seen any effect.

If there is an effect of sperm DNA damage on fertilization, it seems quite plausible that fragmented DNA is a reason for poor embryo quality, poor blastocyst development and even early embryo death[11,91,92]. Janny and Ménézó[93] found a strong relationship between cleavage and blastocyst formation rate, and Shoukir *et al.*[94] revealed a lower blastocyst formation rate after ICSI, compared with IVF. In a very recent report by Greco *et al.*[95], the authors demonstrated significantly higher percentages of DNA damage in ejaculated spermatozoa than in testicular sperm, and concluded, in the light of the severe damage that can be caused, that it is actually safer to use testicular sperm for ICSI. An investigation of the fertilization and pregnancy rates showed significantly higher pregnancy and implantation rates when testicular sperm were used for ICSI, whereas ICSI with ejaculated spermatozoa resulted in only one pregnancy, which aborted spontaneously. Thus, the authors suggest ICSI with testicular spermatozoa as a therapeutic option in men with high levels of sperm DNA fragmentation in ejaculated spermatozoa.

Although the evidence for a detrimental impact of sperm DNA fragmentation on the outcome of assisted reproduction is overwhelming, the reasons for the oxidative damage of the male genome are still unclear. Apoptosis appears to be one explanation, and has legitimacy where the early stages of spermatogenesis are concerned. With regard to the appearance of so-called apoptotic spermatozoa in the ejaculate, especially the origin of sperm DNA damage, the 'abortive apoptosis' hypothesis is still questionable. Therefore, alternative hypotheses that can explain sperm DNA fragmentation are discussed in the following section of this chapter.

IMPROPER DNA PACKAGING AND LIGATION DURING SPERMATOGENESIS AND SPERM MATURATION

The second hypothesis that explains the origin of fragmented DNA in spermatozoa arises from animal experiments showing that endogenous nicks are normally present at late stages of spermatogenesis (step-12–13 spermatids) in rats and mice. It appears that the presence of these endogenous nicks is highest during the transition from round to elongated spermatids. At the time when chromatin packaging is completed, these nicks disappear completely[18,96–99]. Therefore, they are thought to have physiological and functional importance during sperm chromatin condensation. McPherson and Longo[18] postulated that chromatin packaging during spermiogenesis requires the endogenous nuclease topoisomerase II to create and ligate nicks in order to facilitate protamination. Topoisomerase II plays a major role in linking DNA replication to chromosome condensation, and interplays with condensin, a large protein complex that has crucial functions in mitotic chromosome assembly and organization[100,101]. This enzyme has also been identified in human seminiferous tubules[102]. The proposed mechanism of action during spermiogenesis is thought to be the transient introduction of DNA double-strand breaks that allows passage of a double helix through the cut with subsequent resealing of the strand break[103]. This would then result in the relief of torsional stress and supports chromatin rearrangement during the displacement of histones by protamines[18,100,104]. Consequently, endogenous nicks (DNA fragmentation) in ejaculated sperm are indicative of the incomplete maturation of spermatozoa during spermiogenesis, resulting in disturbed chromatin condensation, which in turn is due to underprotamination[105–107].

OXIDATIVE STRESS

Finally, the third hypothesis on the origin of sperm DNA fragmentation describes oxidative stress as a causal factor for sperm DNA damage. Since oxidative stress seems to play a pivotal role in reproduction[108,109], not only in female[110–112] but also in male reproductive physiology and pathology[113–117], this field of research has attracted the particular interest of scientists during the past 20 years. In an ejaculate, ROS can be produced either by leukocytes or by the spermatozoa themselves.

Influence of leukocyte-derived ROS on sperm DNA fragmentation

Genital tract inflammation and an increased number of leukocytes in the ejaculate have been repeatedly associated with male subfertility and infertility[114,118–120]. This clinical picture is seen in about 10–20% of infertile men[3]. Although there are also contradictory reports stating that seminal plasma leukocytes have no influence on sperm fertilizing capacity *in vitro* or even exert a favorable effect on sperm function[121–123], most groups support a detrimental effect of leukocytes on male fertility. Unfortunately, the current cut-off value for leukocytospermia ($> 1.0 \times 10^6$ leukocytes/ml)[3] is empirical[124], and gives only an approximate classification. Thus, the observation of leukocytospermia is not a reliable indicator of an asymptomatic urogenital tract infection[125]. Moreover, there is also no common agreement about how leukocytes should be detected.

The World Health Organization (WHO)[3] recommends two different methods, namely the peroxidase method and immunofluorescence with monoclonal antibodies, which actually give different results. Villegas *et al.*[126] compared the peroxidase method recommended by the WHO[3] with both counting of round cells and immunofluorescent detection of CD15-positve (granulocytes), CD45-positive (for all leukocytes) and CD68-positive cells (macrophages). The methods correlated significantly, but on different levels. It also appeared that the more specific immunofluorescent techniques correlated better with each other than with the histochemical method. In particular, the number of detected peroxidase-positive cells was significantly lower than that identified by immunofluorescence. These enormous differences reflect the difficulties of an exact determination of the number of leukocytes in semen and a reliable cut-off value, which is important for diagnosis and especially for prediction of the success of assisted reproduction.

Leukocytes secrete cytokines that have been shown to be negatively correlated with fertility[127] and semen quality[128] as well as PMN elastase[129] and ROS[130]. Apart from PMN elastase, which is known to provoke cell deterioration[131], ROS can directly damage biological membranes by inducing a process called lipid peroxidation. Because of the extraordinarily high content of polyunsaturated fatty acids in the plasma membrane, spermatozoa are extremely susceptible to oxidative stress[132], impairing membrane function and resulting in the loss of motility and reduced penetration rates in the sperm penetration assay[115,133] or even death of the spermatozoa.

Lopes et al.[134] and Irvine et al.[135] showed that sperm DNA fragmentation could be induced by ROS, and more recently, Alvarez et al.[136] demonstrated that sperm DNA integrity was even significantly impaired in leukocytospermic semen samples. This finding is of particular importance, as sperm DNA fragmentation is a reason for fertilization and pregnancy failure in IUI, IVF and ICSI. With respect to ROS, one has to distinguish where the ROS originate, from external sources such as leukocytes that are present in almost any ejaculate[118] and produce up to 1000 times more ROS than spermatozoa[137], or from the spermatozoa themselves[138], as they are physiologically produced in any living cell during respiration.

Although ROS have been shown to induce apoptosis in both somatic cells[139,140] and maturing spermatozoa[105], indicating an indirect mechanism of action of oxidative stress caused by ROS leading to DNA fragmentation, there is also evidence suggesting a rather direct mechanism of action[21,141,142]. Data that support this theory arise from studies that have shown increased levels of

specific forms of oxidative damage, such as 8-hydroxydeoxyguanosine in sperm DNA[134,143]. Interestingly, spermatozoa from infertile men are generally more susceptible to DNA fragmentation by hydrogen peroxide (H_2O_2)[144,145], and a protective effect against DNA damage can be provided by antioxidants such as vitamin C, vitamin E, glutathione or hypotaurine[146,147]. Furthermore, this direct effect of ROS can also be explained by the fact that oxidants produced by leukocytes have an extremely high oxidative potential, with half-lives in the nanosecond ($OH^\bullet$; hydroxyl radicals) to millisecond range (O_2^-; superoxide anion). Additionally, H_2O_2 is persistent and can even penetrate plasma membranes, while other ROS including superoxide (O_2^-) or the hydroxyl radical ($OH^\bullet$) are non-membrane-permeable. At this point, it should also be noted that leukocyte-mediated sperm damage gains importance when spermatozoa are separated in vitro and when the seminal plasma, which contains scavengers for ROS[148], is being eliminated.

Pasqualotto et al.[149] demonstrated that infertile patients not only had elevated ROS levels but also had reduced levels of antioxidant capacity. This observation supports the concept that the balance between ROS generation and antioxidant capacity in the semen plays a critical role in the pathophysiology of genital tract inflammation and its impact on sperm function and fertilization/pregnancy[150]. Likewise, recent studies have suggested that the numbers of leukocytes present in the ejaculate that are still regarded as normal (leukocytospermia: more than 1×10^6/ml ejaculate) might be too high[21,120]. As numbers of leukocytes even much lower than 1×10^6/ml in the ejaculate and low amounts of ROS are harmful to sperm DNA integrity[21,151], a causality between leukocytes in the ejaculate and DNA fragmentation should not be neglected.

Influence of sperm-derived ROS

Besides the leukocyte-mediated effect of oxidants on sperm DNA fragmentation, the sperm cell's own ROS production, however, should not be neglected. During spermatogenesis, Sertoli cell function can be affected and consequently result in poor morphogenesis of the sperm. It is also well known that poor morphology, especially excess residual cytoplasm, significantly affects sperm fertilizing potential[152]. Spermatozoa that have such cytoplasmic residues have a higher content of cytoplasmic enzymes, e.g. glucose-6-phosphate dehydrogenase[138], which are thought to stimulate the generation of ROS in spermatozoa[138,153]. The clinical importance of this is underlined by the considerably stronger correlation of the percentage of ROS-producing spermatozoa with sperm DNA fragmentation than that of leukocyte-derived ROS-production in the ejaculate, found in a recent study by Henkel et al.[20]. Thus, this finding supports the idea of Muratori et al.[154] about an involvement of endogenously produced ROS as cause for sperm DNA fragmentation.

CONCLUSIONS

During recent years, sperm DNA fragmentation has been recognized as a major contributing factor to male infertility that cannot be accurately determined with the current semen analysis techniques according to WHO standards. As sperm DNA damage is an important cause of fertilization and pregnancy failure, and even a possible cause of early embryonic death or offspring disease such as childhood cancer, assessment of this parameter should be a component of the extended andrology laboratory diagnosis. The causes of sperm DNA damage appear to be multifactorial, and a firm conclusion about pathogenic mechanisms cannot yet be drawn. However, three putative hypotheses, namely (1) 'abortive apoptosis', (2) improper DNA packaging and ligation during spermatogenesis and (3) oxidative stress, are discussed in this chapter, and there is good evidence to support each one of them. For the last hypothesis, two sources of ROS seem to be of importance, leukocytes and spermatozoa. To date, however, it

appears that more than one of these causes may be responsible for sperm DNA fragmentation. Therefore, in order to improve pregnancy rates and to prevent early childhood disease, more research is necessary to investigate this important sperm functional parameter.

REFERENCES

1. Jochum M, Pabst W, Schill W-B. Granulocyte elastase as a sensitive diagnostic parameter of silent male genital tract inflammation. Andrologia 1986; 18: 413
2. Viljoen MH, et al. Alpha-glucosidase activity and sperm motility. Andrologia 1990; 22: 205
3. World Health Organization. WHO Laboratory Manual for the Examination of Human Semen and Sperm–Cervical Mucus Interaction, 4th edn. Cambridge: Cambridge University Press, 1999
4. Zorn B, et al. Semen polymorphonuclear neutrophil leukocyte elastase as a diagnostic and prognostic marker of genital tract inflammation – a review. Clin Chem Lab Med 2003; 41: 2
5. Twigg JP, Irvine DS, Aitken RJ. Oxidative damage of DNA in human spermatozoa does not preclude pronucleus formation at intracytoplasmic sperm injection. Hum Reprod 1998; 13: 1864
6. Aitken RJ, Krausz C. Oxidative stress, DNA damage and the Y chromosome. Reproduction 2001; 122: 497
7. Alvarez JG. DNA fragmentation in human spermatozoa: significance in the diagnosis and treatment of infertility. Minerva Ginecol 2003; 55: 233
8. Aitken RJ, Sawyer D. The human spermatozoon – not waving but drowning. Adv Exp Med Biol 2003; 518: 85
9. Qiu J, Hales BF, Robaire B. Damage to rat spermatozoal DNA after chronic cyclophosphamide exposure. Biol Reprod 1995; 53: 1465
10. Qiu J, Hales BF, Robaire B. Effects of chronic low-dose cyclophosphamide exposure on the nuclei of rat spermatozoa. Biol Reprod 1995; 52: 33
11. Seli E, et al. Extent of nuclear DNA damage in ejaculated spermatozoa impacts on blastocyst development after in vitro fertilization. Fertil Steril 2004; 82: 378
12. In't Veld P, et al. Sex chromosomal abnormalities and intracytoplasmic sperm injection. Lancet 1995; 346: 773

13. Kurinczuk JJ, Bower C. Birth defects in infants conceived by intracytoplasmic sperm injection: an alternative interpretation. Br Med J 1997; 315: 1260

14. Ji BT, et al. Paternal cigarette smoking and the risk of childhood cancer among offspring of non-smoking mothers. J Natl Cancer Inst 1997; 89: 238

15. Aitken RJ, et al. Relative impact of oxidative stress on the functional competence and genomic integrity of human spermatozoa. Biol Reprod 1998; 59: 1037

16. Sakkas D, et al. Origin of DNA damage in ejaculated human spermatozoa. Rev Reprod 1999; 4: 31

17. Sakkas D, et al. Nature of DNA damage in ejaculated human spermatozoa and the possible involvement of apoptosis. Biol Reprod 2002; 66: 1061

18. McPherson SMG, Longo FJ. Localization of DNAse I-hypersensitive regions during rat spermatogenesis: stage dependent patterns and unique sensitivity of elongating spermatids. Mol Reprod Dev 1992; 31: 268

19. Agarwal A, Saleh RA. Role of oxidants in male infertility: rationale, significance and treatment. Urol Clin North Am 2002; 29: 817

20. Henkel R, et al. DNA fragmentation of spermatozoa and ART. Reprod Biomed Online 2003; 7: 477

21. Henkel R, et al. Effect of reactive oxygen species produced by spermatozoa and leukocytes on sperm functions in non-leukocytospermic patients. Fertil Steril 2005; 83: 635

22. Kerr JF, Wyllie AH, Currie AR. Apoptosis: a basic biological phenomenon with wide-ranging implications in tissue kinetics. Br J Cancer 1972; 26: 239

23. Luo X, et al. Bid, a Bcl2 interacting protein, mediates cytochrome c release from mitochondria in response to activation of cell surface death receptors. Cell 1998; 94: 481

24. Bossy-Wetzel E, Newmeyer DD, Green DR. Mitochondrial cytochrome c release in apoptosis occurs upstream of DEVD-specific caspase activation and independently of mitochondrial transmembrane depolarization. EMBO J 1998; 17: 37

25. Whittington K, et al. Reactive oxygen species (ROS) production and the outcome of diagnostic tests of sperm function. Int J Androl 1999; 22: 236

26. Arends M, Wyllie A. Apoptosis: mechanism and roles in pathology. Int Rev Exp Pathol 1991; 32: 223

27. Wyllie AH. Glucocorticoid-induced thymocyte apoptosis is associated with endogenous endonuclease activation. Nature 1980; 284: 555

28. Martin SJ, et al. Early redistribution of plasma membrane phosphatidylserine is a general feature of apoptosis regardless of the initiating stimulus: inhibition by overexpression of Bcl-2 and Abl. J Exp Med 1995; 182: 1545

29. Vermes I, Haanen C, Reutelingsperger CPM. A novel assay for apoptosis: flow cytometric detection of phosphatidylserine expression on early apoptotic cells using fluorescence labelled annexin V. J Immunol Meth 1995; 180: 39

30. Van Heerde WL, Degroot PG, Reutelingsperger CPM. The complexity of the phospholipid binding protein annexin V. Thromb Haemost 1995; 73: 172

31. Lee J, et al. The Fas system is a key regulator of germ cell apoptosis in the testis. Endocrinology 1997; 138: 2081

32. Watanabe-Fukunaga R, et al. The cDNA structure, expression, and chromosomal assignment of the mouse Fas antigen. J Immunol 1992; 148: 1274

33. Krammer PH, et al. Regulation of apoptosis in the immune system. Curr Opin Immunol 1994; 6: 279

34. Schulze-Osthoff K, et al. Cell nucleus and DNA fragmentation are not required for apoptosis. J Cell Biol 1994; 127: 15

35. Nagata S, Golstein P. The Fas death factor. Science 1995; 267: 1449

36. Suda T, et al. Molecular cloning and expression of the Fas ligand, a novel member of the tumor necrosis factor family. Cell 1993; 75: 1169

37. Nagata S, Suda T. Fas and Fas ligand: lpr and gld mutations. Immunol Today 1995; 16: 39

38. Rouvier E, Luciani MF, Golstein P. Fas involvement in Ca(2+)-independent T cell-mediated cytotoxicity. J Exp Med 1993; 177: 195

39. Griffith TS, et al. Fas ligand-induced apoptosis as a mechanism of immune privilege. Science 1995; 270: 1189

40. French LE, et al. Fas and Fas ligand in embryos and adult mice: ligand expression in several immune-privileged tissues and coexpression in adult tissues characterized by apoptotic cell turnover. J Cell Biol 1996; 133: 335

41. Thornberry NA, Lazebnik Y. Caspases: enemies within. Science 1998; 281: 1312

42. Nicholson DW. Caspase structure, proteolytic substrates, and function during apoptotic cell death. Cell Death Differ 1999; 6: 1028

43. Earnshaw WC, Martins LM, Kaufmann SH. Mammalian caspases: structure, activation, substrates, and functions during apoptosis. Annu Rev Biochem 1999; 68: 383

44. Steller H. Mechanisms and genes of cellular suicide. Science 1995; 267: 1445

45. Reed JC. Apoptosis-regulating proteins as targets for drug discovery. Trends Mol Med 2001; 7: 314

46. Reed JC. Mechanisms of apoptosis. Am J Pathol 2000; 157: 1415

47. Green DR. Overview: apoptotic signaling pathways in the immune system. Immunol Rev 2003; 193: 5

48. Wei MC, et al. Proapoptotic BAX and BAK: a requisite gateway to mitochondrial dysfunction and death. Science 2001; 292: 727

49. Kuwana T, et al. Bid, Bax, and lipids cooperate to form supramolecular openings in the outer mitochondrial membrane. Cell 2002; 111: 331

50. Print CG, Loveland KL. Germ cell suicide: new insights into apoptosis during spermatogenesis. BioEssays 2000; 22: 423

51. Rodriguez I, et al. An early and massive wave of germinal cell apoptosis is required for the development of functional spermatogenesis. EMBO J 1997; 16: 2262

52. Russell LD, Peterson RN. Determination of the elongate spermatid–Sertoli cell ratio in various mammals. J Reprod Fertil 1984; 70: 635

53. Orth JM, Gunsalus GL, Lamperti AA. Evidence from Sertoli cell-depleted rats indicates that spermatid number in adults depends on numbers of Sertoli cells produced during perinatal development. Endocrinol 1988; 122: 787

54. Braun RE. Every sperm is sacred – or is it? Nat Genet 1998; 18: 202

55. Huckins C. The morphology and kinetics of spermatogonial degeneration in normal adult rat: an analysis using a simplified classification of the germinal epithelium. Anat Rec 1978; 190: 905

56. Blanco-Rodriguez J. A matter of death and life: the significance of germ cell death during spermatogenesis. Int J Androl 1998; 21: 236

57. Blanco-Rodriguez J, Martinez-Garcia C. Apoptosis is physiologically restricted to a specialized cytoplasmic compartment in rat spermatids. Biol Reprod 1999; 61: 1541

58. Sakkas D, Mariethoz E, St. John JC. Abnormal sperm parameters in humans are indicative of an abortive apoptotic mechanism linked to the Fas-mediated pathway. Exp Cell Res 1999; 251: 350

59. Henkel R, et al. Influence of deoxyribonucleic acid damage on fertilization and pregnancy. Fertil Steril 2004; 81: 965

60. Taylor SL, et al. Somatic cell apoptosis markers and pathways in human ejaculated sperm: potential utility as indicators of sperm quality. Mol Hum Reprod 2004; 10: 825

61. McVicar CM, et al. Incidence of Fas positivity and deoxyribonucleic acid double-stranded breaks in human ejaculated sperm. Fertil Steril 2004; 81 (Suppl 1): 767

62. Pentikäinen V, Erkkilä K, Dunkel L. Fas regulates germ cell apoptosis in the human testis in vitro. Am J Physiol Endocrinol Metab 1999; 276: E310

63. Castro A, et al. Absence of Fas protein detection by flow cytometry in human spermatozoa. Fertil Steril 2004; 81: 1019

64. Lachaud C, et al. Apoptosis and necrosis in human ejaculated spermatozoa. Hum Reprod 2004; 19: 607

65. Sun JG, Jurisicova A, Casper RF. Detection of deoxyribonucleic acid fragmentation in human sperm: correlation with fertilization in vitro. Biol Reprod 1997; 56: 602

66. Glander HJ, Schaller J. Binding of annexin V to plasma membranes of human spermatozoa: a rapid assay for detection of membrane changes after cryostorage. Mol Hum Reprod 1999; 5: 109

67. Oosterhuis GJ, et al. Measuring apoptosis in human spermatozoa: a biological assay for semen quality? Fertil Steril 2000; 74: 245

68. Weng SL, et al. Caspase activity and apoptotic markers in ejaculated human sperm. Mol Hum Reprod 2002; 8: 984

69. Weil M, Jacobson MD, Raff MC. Are caspases involved in the death of cells with a transcriptionally inactive nucleus? Sperm and chicken erythrocytes. J Cell Sci 1998; 111: 2707

70. Paasch U, et al. Activation pattern of caspases in human spermatozoa. Fertil Steril 2004; 81: 802

71. Cayli S, et al. Cellular maturity and apoptosis in human sperm: creatine kinase, caspase-3 and Bcl-XL levels in mature and diminished maturity sperm. Mol Hum Reprod 2004; 10: 365

72. Li CY, et al. Heat shock protein 70 inhibits apoptosis downstream of cytochrome c release and upstream of caspase-3 activation. J Biol Chem 2000; 275: 25665

73. Gadella BM, Harrison RAP. Capacitation induces cyclic adenosine 3′,5′-monophosphate-dependent, but apoptosis-unrelated, exposure of aminophospholipids at the apical head plasma membrane of boar sperm cells. Biol Reprod 2002; 67: 340

74. Kotwicka M, Jendraszak M, Warchol JB. Plasma membrane translocation of phosphatidylserine in human spermatozoa. Folia Histochem Cytobiol 2002; 40: 111

75. de Vries KJ, et al. Caspase-independent exposure of aminophospholipids and tyrosine phosphorylation

in bicarbonate responsive. Biol Reprod 2003; 68: 2122

76. Muratori M, et al. AnnexinV binding and merocyanine staining fail to detect human sperm capacitation. J Androl 2004; 25: 797

77. Duru NK, et al. Cryopreservation–thawing of fractionated human spermatozoa is associated with membrane phosphatidylserine externalization and not DNA fragmentation. J Androl 2001; 22: 646

78. Paasch U, et al. Cryopreservation and thawing is associated with varying extent of activation of apoptotic machinery in subsets of human spermatozoa. Biol Reprod 2004; 71: 1828

79. Sion B, et al. Annexin V binding to plasma membrane predicts the quality of human cryopreserved spermatozoa. Int J Androl 2004; 27: 108

80. Duran EH, et al. Sperm DNA quality predicts intrauterine insemination outcome: a prospective cohort study. Hum Reprod 2002; 17: 3122

81. Host E, Lindenberg S, Smidt-Jensen S. DNA strand breaks in human spermatozoa: correlation with fertilization in vitro in oligozoospermic men and in men with unexplained infertility. Acta Obstet Gynecol Scand 2000; 79: 189

82. Morris ID, et al. The spectrum of DNA damage in human sperm assessed by single cell gel electrophoresis (Comet assay) and its relationship to fertilization and embryo development. Hum Reprod 2002; 17: 990

83. Spano M, et al. Sperm chromatin damage impairs human fertility. Fertil Steril 2000; 73: 43

84. Loft S, et al. Oxidative DNA damage in human sperm influences time to pregnancy. Hum Reprod 2003; 18: 1265

85. Lopes S, et al. Sperm deoxyribonucleic acid fragmentation is increased in poor-quality semen samples and correlates with failed fertilization in intracytoplasmic sperm injection. Fertil Steril 1998; 69: 528

86. Lewis SEM, et al. An algorithm to predict pregnancy in assisted reproduction. Hum Reprod 2004; 19: 1385

87. Tesarik J, Greco E, Mendoza C. Late, but not early, paternal effect on human embryo development is related to sperm DNA fragmentation. Hum Reprod 2004; 19: 611

88. Host E, Lindenberg S, Smidt-Jensen S. The role of DNA strand breaks in human spermatozoa used for IVF and ICSI. Acta Obstet Gynecol Scand 2000; 79: 559

89. Bungum M, et al. The predictive value of sperm chromatin structure assay (SCSA) parameters for the outcome of intrauterine insemination, IVF and ICSI. Hum Reprod 2004; 19: 1401

90. Gandini L, et al. Full-term pregnancies achieved with ICSI despite high levels of sperm chromatin damage. Hum Reprod 2004; 19: 1409

91. Jurisicova A, Varmuza S, Casper RF. Programmed cell death and human embryo fragmentation. Mol Hum Reprod 1996; 2: 93

92. Tomsu M, Sharma V, Miller D. Embryo quality and IVF treatment outcomes may correlate with different sperm comet assay parameters. Hum Reprod 2002; 17: 1856

93. Janny L, Ménézó YJR. Evidence for a strong paternal effect on human preimplantation embryo development and blastocyst formation. Mol Reprod Dev 1994; 38: 36

94. Shoukir Y, et al. Blastocyst development from supernumerary embryos after intracytoplasmic sperm injection: a paternal influence? Hum Reprod 1998; 13: 1632

95. Greco E, et al. Efficient treatment of infertility due to sperm DNA damage by ICSI with testicular spermatozoa. Hum Reprod 2005; 20: 226

96. Ward WS, Coffey DS. DNA packaging and organization in mammalian spermatozoa: comparison with somatic cells. Biol Reprod 1991; 44: 569

97. McPherson SMG, Longo FJ. Nicking of rat spermatid and spermatozoa DNA: possible involvement of DNA topoisomerase II. Dev Biol 1993; 158: 122

98. McPherson SMG, Longo FJ. Chromatin structure–function alterations during mammalian spermatogenesis: DNA nicking and repair in elongating spermatids. Eur J Histochem 1993; 37: 109

99. Sakkas D, et al. Relationship between the presence of endogenous nicks and sperm chromatin packing in maturing and fertilizing mouse spermatozoa. Biol Reprod 1995; 52: 1149

100. Hirano T. The ABCs of SMC proteins: two-armed ATPases for chromosome condensation, cohesion, and repair. Genes Dev 2002; 16: 399

101. Cuvier O, Hirano T. A role of topoisomerase II in linking DNA replication to chromosome condensation. J Cell Biol 2003; 160: 645

102. Sakkas D, et al. Abnormal spermatozoa in the ejaculate: abortive apoptosis and faulty nuclear remodelling during spermatogenesis. Reprod Biomed Online 2003; 7: 428

103. Wang JC, Caron PR, Kim RA. The role of DNA topoisomerases in recombination and genome stability: a double-edged sword? Cell 1990; 62: 403

104. Chen JL, Longo FJ. Expression and localization of DNA topoisomerase II during rat spermatogenesis. Mol Reprod Dev 1996; 45: 61

105. Gorczyca W, et al. Presence of DNA strand breaks and increased sensitivity of DNA in situ to denaturation in abnormal human sperm cells: analogy to apoptosis of somatic cells. Exp Cell Res 1993; 207: 202

106. Manicardi GC, et al. Presence of endogenous nicks in DNA of ejaculated human spermatozoa and its relationship to chromomycin A3 accessibility. Biol Reprod 1995; 52: 864

107. Sailer BL, Jost LK, Evenson DP. Mammalian sperm DNA susceptibility to in situ denaturation associated with the presence of DNA strand breaks as measured by the terminal deoxynucleotidyl transferase assay. J Androl 1995; 16: 80

108. Riley JCM, Behrman HR. Oxygen radicals and reactive oxygen species in reproduction. Proc Soc Exp Biol Med 1991; 198: 781

109. Agarwal A, Saleh RA, Bedaiwy MA. Role of reactive oxygen species in the pathophysiology of human reproduction. Fertil Steril 2003; 79: 829

110. Oyawoye O, et al. Antioxidants and reactive oxygen species in follicular fluid of women undergoing IVF: relationship to outcome. Hum Reprod 2003; 18: 2270

111. Sharma RK, Agarwal A. Role of reactive oxygen species in gynecologic diseases. Reprod Med Biol 2004; 3: 177

112. Glamoclija V, et al. Apoptosis and active caspase-3 expression in human granulosa cells. Fertil Steril 2005; 83: 426

113. Aitken RJ, Clarkson JS. Cellular basis of defective sperm function and its association with the genesis of reactive oxygen species by human spermatozoa. J Reprod Fertil 1987; 81: 459

114. Plante M, de Lamirande E, Gagnon C. Reactive oxygen species released by activated neutrophils, but not by deficient spermatozoa, are sufficient to affect normal sperm motility. Fertil Steril 1994; 62: 387

115. Vigil P, et al. Assessment of sperm function in fertile and infertile men. Andrologia 1994; 26: 55

116. Whittington K, et al. Reactive oxygen species (ROS) production and the outcome of diagnostic tests of sperm function. Int J Androl 1999; 22: 236

117. Koksal IT, et al. Potential role of reactive oxygen species on testicular pathology associated with infertility. Asian J Androl 2003; 2: 95

118. Wolff H. The biologic significance of white blood cells in semen. Fertil Steril 1995; 63: 1143

119. Ochsendorf FR. Infections in the male genital tract and reactive oxygen species. Hum Reprod Update 1999; 5: 399

120. Sharma RK, et al. Relationship between seminal white blood cell counts and oxidative stress in men treated at an infertility clinic. J Androl 2001; 22: 575

121. Tomlinson MJ, et al. Round cells and sperm fertilizing capacity: the presence of immature germ cells but not seminal leukocytes are associated with reduced success of in vitro fertilization. Fertil Steril 1992; 58: 1257

122. Tomlinson MJ, Barratt CL, Cooke ID. Prospective study of leukocytes and leukocyte subpopulations in semen suggests they are not a cause of male infertility. Fertil Steril 1993; 60: 1069

123. Kaleli S, et al. Does leukocytospermia associate with poor semen parameters and sperm functions in male infertility?: The role of different seminal leukocyte concentrations. Eur J Obstet Gynecol Reprod Biol 2000; 89: 185

124. Aitken RJ, Baker HW. Seminal leukocytes: passengers, terrorists or good samaritans? Hum Reprod 1995; 10: 1736

125. Barratt CLR, Bolton AE, Cooke ID. Functional significance of white blood cells in the male and the female reproductive tract. Hum Reprod 1990; 5: 639

126. Villegas J, et al. Indirect immunofluorescence using monoclonal antibodies for the detection of leukocytospermia: comparison with peroxidase staining. Andrologia 2002; 34: 69

127. Hill JA, Cohen J, Anderson DJ. The effects of lymphokines and monokines on sperm fertilizing ability in the zona-free hamster egg penetration test. Am J Obstet Gynecol 1989; 160: 1154

128. Eggert-Kruse W, et al. Relationship of seminal plasma interleukin (IL)-8 and IL-6 with semen quality. Hum Reprod 2001; 16: 517

129. Schill W-B, et al. Biochemical aspects of semen analysis. In Hedon B, Bringer J, Mares P, eds. Fertility and Sterility. A Current Overview. New York: Parthenon Publishing, 1995, 303

130. Aitken RJ, West KM. Analysis of the relationship between reactive oxygen species production and leukocyte infiltration in fractions of human semen separated on Percoll gradients. Int J Androl 1990; 13: 433

131. Hautamaki RD, et al. Requirement for macrophage elastase for cigarette smoke-induced emphysema in mice. Science 1997; 277: 2002

132. Aitken RJ, Clarkson JS, Fishel S. Generation of reactive oxygen species, lipid peroxidation, and human sperm function. Biol Reprod 1989; 40: 183

133. Aitken RJ, Clarkson JS. Significance of reactive oxygen species and antioxidants in defining the efficacy of sperm preparation techniques. J Androl 1988; 9: 367

134. Lopes S, et al. Reactive oxygen species: potential cause for DNA fragmentation in human spermatozoa. Hum Reprod 1998; 13: 896

135. Irvine DS, et al. DNA integrity in human spermatozoa: relationships with semen quality. J Androl 2000; 21: 33

136. Alvarez JG, et al. Increased DNA damage in sperm from leukocytospermic semen samples as determined by the sperm chromatin structure assay. Fertil Steril 2002; 78: 319

137. de Lamirande E, Gagnon C. Capacitation-associated production of superoxide anion by human spermatozoa. Free Radic Biol Med 1995; 18: 487

138. Gomez E, et al. Development of an image analysis system to monitor the retention of residual cytoplasm by human spermatozoa: correlation with biochemical markers of the cytoplasmic space, oxidative stress, and sperm function. J Androl 1996; 17: 276

139. Ratan RR, Murphy TH, Baraban JM. Oxidative stress induces apoptosis in embryonic cortical neurons. J Neurochem 1994; 62: 376

140. Huang C, et al. Hydrogen peroxide-induced apoptosis in human hepatoma cells is mediated by CD95(APO-1/Fas) receptor/ligand system and may involve activation of wild-type p53. Mol Biol Rep 2000; 27: 1

141. Saleh RA, et al. Leukocytospermia is associated with increased reactive oxygen species production by human spermatozoa. Fertil Steril 2002; 78: 1215

142. Moustafa MH, et al. Relationship between ROS production, apoptosis and DNA denaturation in spermatozoa from patients examined for infertility. Hum Reprod 2004; 19: 129

143. Shen H, Ong C. Detection of oxidative DNA damage in human sperm and its association with sperm function and male infertility. Free Radic Biol Med 2000; 28: 529

144. Hughes CM, et al. A comparison of baseline and induced DNA damage in human spermatozoa from fertile and infertile men, using a modified comet assay. Mol Hum Reprod 1996; 2: 613

145. Hughes CM, et al. The effects of antioxidant supplementation during Percoll preparation on human sperm DNA integrity. Hum Reprod 1998; 13: 1240

146. Donnelly ET, McClure N, Lewis SEM. The effect of ascorbate and alpha-tocopherol supplementation in vitro on DNA integrity and hydrogen peroxide-induced DNA damage in human spermatozoa. Mutagenesis 1999; 14: 505

147. Donnelly ET, McClure N, Lewis SEM. Glutathione and hypotaurine in vitro: effects on human sperm motility, DNA integrity and production of reactive oxygen species. Mutagenesis 2000; 15: 61

148. Iwasaki A, Gagnon C. Formation of reactive oxygen species in spermatozoa of infertile patients. Fertil Steril 1992; 57: 409

149. Pasqualotto FF, et al. Relationship between oxidative stress, semen characteristics, and clinical diagnosis in men undergoing infertility investigation. Fertil Steril 2000; 73: 459

150. Sikka SC. Relative impact of oxidative stress on male reproductive function. Curr Med Chem 2001; 8: 851

151. Zorn B, Virant-Klun I, Meden-Vrtovec H. Semen granulocyte elastase: its relevance for the diagnosis and prognosis of silent genital tract inflammation. Hum Reprod 2000; 15: 1978

152. Keating J, et al. Investigation of the association between the presence of cytoplasmic residues on the human sperm midpiece and defective sperm function. J Reprod Fertil 1997; 110: 71

153. Aitken RJ, et al. Reactive oxygen species generation by human spermatozoa is induced by exogenous NADPH and inhibited by the flavoprotein inhibitors diphenylene iodonium and quinacrine. Mol Reprod Dev 1997; 47: 468

154. Muratori M, et al. Spontaneous DNA fragmentation in swim-up selected human spermatozoa during long term incubation. J Androl 2003; 24: 253

20

The impact of the paternal factor on embryo quality and development: the embryologist's point of view

Marie-Lena Windt

INTRODUCTION

The ultimate goal of assisted reproduction is to achieve a singleton, ongoing pregnancy and the birth of a healthy baby. The need to characterize embryos with optimal implantation potential is obvious, and a variety of characteristics during embryo developmental stages *in vitro* (from one cell to the blastocyst) have been proposed as markers for embryo quality and viability. Identification of the embryo destined for implantation can improve success rates and, at the same time, by transferring fewer embryos, ensure that multiple pregnancies are avoided[1,2].

Embryo selection is traditionally performed using *embryo morphology* and *cleavage rate* as guides[2-4].

Methods of selection include *pronuclear morphology*[5-14]; *oocyte and pronuclei polarity* and cleavage symmetry[1,5,6-9,12,15]; *early cleavage* to the 2-cell stage[16-29]; and extended *blastocyst culture*[9,15,30-36]. Several studies suggest that a combination of all the methods should be implemented[37] to give a graduated embryo score (GES)[38], a cumulative embryo score (CES) or a mean score of transferred embryos (MSTE)[39].

Alternatively, the detection of certain *metabolites* in embryo culture medium has also received some attention in the past few years. The most promising of these are increased levels of *platelet-activating factor* (PAF)[40] and *soluble human leukocyte antigen-G* (sHLA-G)[41,42]. The presence of these molecules has been associated with increased pregnancy rates, but more in-depth studies are needed to establish their true significance.

Although poor culture conditions can negatively influence embryo implantation potential, the origin of these embryo viability and pregnancy-associated factors is mainly accredited to the oocyte. Less pronounced, but certainly also a contributing factor to embryo viability and implantation potential, is the role of the fertilizing spermatozoon. In a recent review by Tesarik[43], paternal effects on cell division of the human preimplantation embryo are discussed.

SPERMATOZOA, EMBRYO MORPHOLOGY AND EMBRYO SELECTION METHODS

Embryo culture metabolites

Platelet-activating factor

Increased PAF concentrations in embryo culture medium (day-3 embryos) were significantly associated with patients who became pregnant compared with those who did not become pregnant in a study by Roudebush et al.[40]. A cut-off value of 45 pmol/l/per embryo PAF was predictive of a pregnancy. The authors suggested that PAF can act as an autocrine stimulator of embryo development, and showed that the addition of PAF to embryo culture medium can promote embryo development in the mouse[44,45].

Paternal effect   Of interest is that PAF is also found in human spermatozoa[46], and has been positively correlated with seminal parameters and pregnancy outcomes. In some primate species the spermatozoal PAF content is significantly increased during the mating season. Enhanced embryo development was also reported when oocytes were fertilized with PAF-treated spermatozoa[46]. Although the exact mechanism of PAF in sperm function, embryo development and pregnancy is uncertain, it seems to have an important influence on reproduction.

Soluble human leukocyte antigen-G

HLA-G is a non-classical type-1 human leukocyte antigen that has been associated with embryo cleavage rate and implantation potential. In a study by Sher et al.[42], a significant, positive predictive value of 71% for pregnancy was found when at least one HLA-G-positive embryo was transferred, with a significant negative predictive value of 85% when only HLA-G-negative embryos were transferred. The role of HLA-G in implantation is thought to be the prevention of allorecognition by maternal cytotoxic killer cells.

In a similar study by Noci et al.[41], the detection of HLA-G was not correlated with embryo morphology (number of blastomeres, blastomere irregularity and embryo fragmentation), but when no HLA-G was detected in the supernatants of transferred embryos, also no pregnancy resulted. It was found, however, that pregnancies occurred only when HLA-G was detectable in the embryo culture medium.

Paternal effect   The role of the sperm cell in the production of HLA-G is uncertain, and there is no evidence that a paternal factor is involved in this embryo viability marker.

Pre-embryo and embryo characteristics

Pronuclear-stage morphology

Criteria for the evaluation of pronucleate (PN, also used to denote pronucleus, pronuclei) embryo morphology (18 hours postinsemination) were defined by Tesarik and Greco[5], and the so-called 0-pattern PN zygotes were significantly correlated with better embryo morphology, less multinucleation and higher implantation potential. The 0-pattern PN can be summarized as follows: nucleolar precursor bodies (NPBs) never differ by more than three; the number of NPBs is never less than three; NPBs are polarized when there are fewer than seven but never polarized when there are more than seven in at least one pronucleus; the distribution of NPBs is either polarized or non-polarized in both pronuclei[2].

Similar studies evaluating the role of PN scoring showed a good correlation with early cleavage, embryo morphology, blastocyst rate and implantation rate[12–14,47,48].

The incorporation of PN scoring into embryo selection for transfer is therefore a valuable addition.

Paternal effect   The possible role of the sperm cell in the formation of a good-quality pronucleate embryo was investigated by Demirel et al.[49]. They used two sperm cell sources, i.e. ejaculated sperm cells (ES) and testicular sperm cells (TS) in intracytoplasmic sperm injection (ICSI) cycles. It was thought that differences in nuclear DNA packing, concentration of oocyte-activating sperm factors and sperm cell maturity between ES and TS might influence fertilization and PN morphology. Their results showed, however, that there was no difference between ES and TS in terms of PN morphology.

A similar study by Rossi-Ferragut et al.[50] showed, however, that ICSI with ES of non-male-factor patients resulted in significantly more 0-pattern PN compared with ICSI with oligozoospermia and TS patients. The TS patients were also divided into two groups, i.e. epididymal and testicular. Significantly more 0-pattern PN were found in the epididymal group. The results suggested that sperm quality may influence PN morphology and that some paternally associated factor could play a role in the chromosomal quality of the embryo.

In a study by Tesarik et al.[51], sibling oocytes were treated (ICSI) with different semen samples. Certain samples showed consistently poorer PN morphology compared with others, and the authors concluded that this impaired developmental potential could be attributed exclusively to the fertilizing spermatozoon and not the oocyte. Interestingly, fertilization rates for the sperm donors were not different. The poor PN morphology was also apparent in the resulting poorer-quality day-2 and -3 morphology of embryos for the different sperm donors. The authors hypothesized as to the underlying mechanisms involved, and mentioned that early transcriptional failure of the male PN could be the cause of paternally derived developmental impairment. However, it could also be caused by epigenetic sperm factors responsible for oocyte activation or by a defective aster-assembling action of the sperm centrosome. The authors concluded that the sperm factor causing poor PN morphology is not related to any of the other semen parameters, and also not to its fertilizing ability with ICSI.

In a recent study and a review, also by Tesarik et al.[43,52], donor oocytes were treated with ICSI with different semen samples from patients sharing sibling oocytes. Insemination with specific semen samples resulted consistently in significantly poorer PN morphology (10.5%) and poorer implantation rates (3.3%) when compared with control patients (with sibling oocytes) having 0-pattern PN (66.2%) and good implantation rates (36.7%). DNA fragmentation (terminal deoxynucleotide transferase-mediated dUTP nick-end labeling (TUNEL) positive) in both

groups of semen samples were, however, not significantly different (8.9% vs. 8.7%). These patients were thought to have an early paternal factor influencing embryo quality and implantation rates, even before the activation of embryonic genome expression. The early paternal effect may be caused by abnormalities of the sperm centriole or of the sperm-derived oocyte activating factor.

A late paternal factor was also identified in the same study in another subset of patients. When compared with a control group with sibling oocytes, the incidence of 0-pattern PN morphology was the same, but DNA fragmentation in the two groups (27.6% vs. 8.3%) as well as the implantation rate (0% vs. 37.5%) was significantly different. This result showed that repeated assisted reproductive technologies (ART) failures without apparent impairment of zygote and embryo morphology often present with spermatozoa with a high percentage of fragmented DNA.

The authors[43,52] concluded that there is a possibility of the existence of two distinct pathologies, i.e. an early as well as a late paternal effect, influencing ART outcome.

Early-dividing embryos

This approach (early cleavage to the 2-cell stage 25–27 hours postinsemination) was first reported by Shoukir et al.[16] and Sakkas et al.[17]. Since then, several other studies have confirmed their results, and all studies consistently show the value of early division as a marker for embryo viability[18–29].

The marker 'early-dividing embryos' (EDE) was positively correlated with increased pregnancy rates in all the above-mentioned studies except the study of Çiray et al.[27], but implantation rates were significantly increased. EDE was also positively correlated with most other embryo viability markers, such as 0-pattern PN zygotes[21,49], good-quality cleavage-stage embryos[17,20,22,24,26–29], mononucleation[24] and blastocyst rates[22,28,29].

A study by Van Montfoort et al.[28] showed also that early-cleavage status was an independent predictor for both pregnancy outcome and blastocyst development. This was also true for ICSI patients in the study of Lundin et al.[20].

The results from our own program[29] were similar to the above reported studies. The clinical and ongoing pregnancy rates in cases where EDE were transferred were significantly higher than when only late-dividing embryos (LDE) were available for transfer. Statistical evaluation, also taking into account the total number of embryos transferred, showed EDE to be significantly favorable for pregnancy outcome.

Paternal effect The reason for early cleavage according to Shoukir et al.[16] is not obvious, and can possibly be attributed to intrinsic factors within the oocyte or embryo. Sakkas et al.[17] proposed that HLA-G could possibly be involved in this regard. They also reported that the incidence of early cleavage was not different in males with different semen parameters[17].

In the study by Lundin et al.[20], it was speculated that early-cleaving embryos develop from oocytes with appropriate cytoplasmic and nuclear maturity, but they also considered the contribution of the paternal factor (spermatozoa) to be of possible importance. Spermatozoa introduce the centrioles, controlling the first mitotic division of the oocyte into the embryo, and may therefore be a factor in early cleavage[20,27].

The role of the fertilizing spermatozoon in early cleavage was also discussed by Fenwick et al.[22] and Wharf et al.[26]. Both groups hypothesized that the ability of oocytes to undergo the first cleavage may be due to differences in the ability of individual spermatozoa to stimulate calcium transients, since the transition of the fertilized oocyte to a 2-cell embryo depends on the sperm-induced free calcium concentration. It could, however, also be possible that oocyte maturity plays a role, and that less mature oocytes do not have the capability to respond to the sperm-induced stimulus.

Finally, chromosome abnormalities in either the fertilizing spermatozoon or the oocyte may also influence the incidence of early cleavage[26].

Cleavage-stage embryo quality

Embryo *cleavage rate* (number of blastomeres at a specified time) has been shown to be significantly associated with implantation efficacy[3,4]. Transfer of day-2 embryos that were at the 4- or 5-cell stage and day-3 embryos that were at least at the 7-cell stage yielded significantly higher implantation rates. However, 70% of embryos cleaving too fast (> 8 cells on day 3) have been shown to be chromosomally abnormal[53,54].

The most commonly used method for *embryo selection for transfer* is *cleavage-stage embryo morphology*[2,55]. The factors taken into account when assessing embryo morphology are blastomere size and symmetry, as well as the degree of blastomere fragmentation. *Multinucleation* of blastomeres (especially at the 2- and 4-cell stage) is also considered a very important factor in the viability of the embryo[56]. Multinucleation is often associated with embryos showing poor-quality blastocysts and asymmetric blastomeres[56,57], and embryos with evenly sized, symmetric blastomeres were shown to have the highest viability[2,58]. Also, the degree (> 15%) and pattern (large fragments associated with blastomeres) of fragmentation have a significant negative impact on pregnancy rates and blastocyst formation, according to Alikani et al.[59].

Many *in vitro* fertilization (IVF) laboratories have recently implemented prolonged culture to the *blastocyst stage* on day 5 or 6 in an attempt to allow better embryo selection, and, by doing so, a decrease in the multiple pregnancy rate. At this stage of development, the embryonic genome has been expressed, and the paternal genetic factors that are thought to have an influence on embryo viability may have made their impact. The selection of genetically normal embryos is envisioned using extended blastocyst culture, and therefore increased pregnancy rates should result. Although controversy about the benefit of blastocyst culture still exists, the majority of studies show no difference in pregnancy outcome for blastocyst transfer compared with day-3 embryo transfer[2,35]. There seems to be a good correlation between blastocyst rate and PN morphology, early division and good cleavage-stage morphology[60], but Rubio et al.[61] reported that blastocyst culture does not exclude chromosomally abnormal embryos.

It was shown, however, that blastocyst transfer resulted in increased implantation rates and decreased multiple pregnancy rates[2], and it will remain one of the preferred selection methods in many laboratories.

Paternal effect

Cleavage rate A significant *sperm morphology* (strict criteria) effect on embryo cleavage rate was found in a study by Salumets et al.[62]. Other semen parameters had no effect on embryo cleavage rate. In the same study[62], the oocyte was shown to have a significant impact on both embryo cleavage rate and morphology[63].

It is suggested that since some studies show a correlation between sperm cell morphology and DNA damage or poor sperm packaging[64], this could be the factor responsible for the correlation between poor sperm morphology and embryo cleavage rate. Also mentioned as a possible reason are centrosome defects in morphologically abnormal spermatozoa[62].

The significant effect of very low sperm cell concentration (*cryptozoospermia*) on cleavage rate was shown by Strassburger et al.[65]. Significantly fewer embryos reached the 4-cell stage on day 2 compared with other patient groups with higher sperm cell concentrations.

Embryo morphology The majority of studies that investigated the role of a paternal factor in embryo development used embryo morphology as the measured outcome. These studies concentrated mainly on the effect of semen parameters (especially sperm cell morphology) and DNA status of the spermatozoa on embryo morphology.

Cohen et al.[66] and Parinaud et al.[67] reported that *poor sperm cell morphology* resulted in poor embryo quality in their systems. Embryo quality was influenced by semen quality and especially by sperm head abnormalities, suggesting an

important role of the male gamete in the early stages of embryogenesis[67]. In a review, Grow and Oehninger[68] also speculated that higher incidences of head abnormalities lead to embryos with a lower pregnancy potential.

The majority of studies, however, reported that *normal sperm cell morphology* had no significant effect on embryo morphology. The study by Salumets et al.[62] evaluating sperm morphology (unprepared semen) using the Tygerberg strict criteria showed no significant effect on embryo morphology (although cleavage rate was significantly affected: see previous paragraph). The same results were reported by Host et al.[69], using both the strict criteria and the World Health Organization (WHO) criteria for sperm cell morphology: no correlation between sperm cell morphology and embryo morphology. De Vos et al.[70] concluded that individual sperm morphology assessed at the moment of ICSI correlated well with fertilization outcome, but did not affect embryo development. Unpublished results from our own laboratory (Kellerman and Windt, 2004) also failed to show any correlation between strict-criteria sperm cell morphology (P, G and N patterns) and embryo quality on days 2 and 3 for both ICSI and IVF patients.

Similar results were reported by Moilanen et al.[71] and Miller and Smith[72], where embryo morphology was not influenced by any *semen parameter*, using an ICSI group of patients as the poor-quality sperm parameter group and an IVF group as a good-quality sperm parameter group. This result was also apparent in the study by Sakkas et al.[73], where embryo score was not different for IVF compared with ICSI in an oocyte-sharing model. The authors stressed, however, that in some patients, poor-quality embryos were persistent and could not be explained by an oocyte factor. In these patients a paternal effect, other than the classical semen parameters, could not be excluded. They hypothesized on other possible causes such as anomalies at the nuclear level, defective centrosomes and oxidative stress. Virant-Klun et al.[74] also reported that classical *semen parameters* did not correlate with embryo quality or arrested embryo development.

A study by Katsoff *et al.*[75] showed that IVF with spermatozoa with a low score in the *hypoosmotic swelling test* (HOS), a test that examines the functional integrity of the sperm cell membrane, significantly decreased pregnancy rates (50% vs. 0%), but had no effect on fertilization rate or embryo quality (morphology). Embryo viability was thought to be influenced by a paternal factor associated with the sperm membrane, which is transferred to and impairs the oocyte membrane as well.

The possible role of *reactive oxygen species* (ROS) originating from sperm cells during long (20 hours) and short (2 hours) IVF incubation was investigated by Kattera *et al.*[76]. The short incubation time had a significant positive effect on embryo quality and ongoing pregnancy rates. This result could be explained by the shorter exposure to defective or dead spermatozoa in the 2-hour incubation group. Defective spermatozoa may generate ROS, and increased ROS levels are known to have adverse effects especially on pregnancy outcome. Also of interest was the fact that the 2-hour incubation group had reduced levels of estradiol (E_2) and progesterone (P_4) in the day-1 culture medium. These hormones might have had a direct toxic effect on the 20-hour incubation group, where cumulus cells, releasing the hormones, were also present for the 20-hour period. A clear paternal effect on embryo quality could therefore not be established.

The study of Strassburger *et al.*[65] showed a significant negative effect of very low concentrations of spermatozoa (*cryptozoospermia*) on embryo quality. They concluded that a genetic etiology or damaged sperm cell DNA could be responsible, since a high incidence of DNA fragmentation coincides with sperm samples with poor quality.

The *centrosome* of the embryo is paternally inherited, and serves as a microtubule-organizing center during fertilization, and is also responsible for formation of the sperm aster and consequent movement towards each other of the male and female pronuclei. It is therefore essential and critical for oocyte fertilization and embryo development.

The sperm centrioles were implicated to be the reason for poor-quality embryos and implantation failure in a case study reported by Obasaju *et al.*[77]. Embryos resulting after numerous IVF cycles with the husband's spermatozoa were of poor quality, and preimplantation genetic diagnosis (PGD) revealed chaotic mosaicism in the majority of the embryos. Transfer resulted in an early abortion, a biochemical pregnancy and several failed pregnancies. A consecutive cycle with donor spermatozoa showed not only normal embryos (PGD) but also a successful pregnancy. Due to the diagnosis of chaotic mosaicism, abnormal centriole function rather than chromosomal abnormality was indicated. Another reported study[78] that implicated the sperm cell centrosome in fertilization and embryo development showed that ICSI with sperm heads alone had no effect on embryo quality, but resulted in decreased fertilization rates and cell stage compared with ICSI with whole spermatozoa.

The role of genetic or *chromosomal* abnormalities in sperm cells and their effect on embryo quality have been the subject of many publications. In some studies, the possible negative effect of a *chromosomally abnormal sperm* cell involved in the fertilization process and its effect on embryo quality could only be assumed.

In a study by Stalf *et al.*[79], ICSI embryos had a significantly lower score compared with IVF embryos, and this outcome was thought to be because of an andrological factor possibly caused by genetic or chromosomal disturbances. This was also the assumption for better embryo quality with fresh versus frozen testicular spermatozoa after ICSI in a study by Aoki *et al.*[80]. The authors attributed the poorer embryo morphology with frozen testicular spermatozoa to possible increased *DNA damage* caused by the freezing process. Vernaeve *et al.*[81] compared the outcomes of ICSI using obstructive and non-obstructive testicular spermatozoa and found no significant difference in embryo quality between the two groups, irrespective of the fact that both fertilization and implantation rates were significantly lower in the non-obstructive group. The possible explanation for this pregnancy result was increased chromosomal aneuploidy in testicular spermatozoa from men with non-obstructive azoospermia.

In many other studies, genetic and chromosomal sperm cell abnormalities have been detected and studied and in some cases correlated with poor embryo quality. Van Golde et al.[82] conducted a study comparing outcomes in patients with and without microdeletion in the azoospermic factor (AZFc) region of the Y chromosome. The authors showed a significant decrease in fertilization rate and embryo quality in patients with the microdeletion. It was hypothesized that the reduced sperm quality or function could be related to the presence of the deletion. Pregnancy and take-home baby rates were, however, not different in the two groups, and interestingly, only female babies were born to couples with the microdeletion.

Saleh et al.[83] reported that an increase of spermatozoa with abnormal chromatin structure or DNA damage (expressed as DNA fragmentation index, DFI) correlated negatively with ICSI and IVF fertilization rates, embryo quality and overall pregnancy rates. Since seminal ROS values in the same study also correlated negatively with fertilization rates and embryo quality, the authors speculated that the damage to sperm nuclear DNA might be ROS-induced. Similar results were reported by Virant-Klun et al.[74], using the acridine orange (AO) test to detect abnormal single-stranded DNA in spermatozoa. When single-stranded DNA was increased in ICSI patients, a significant increase in heavily fragmented and arrested embryos was observed. Although fertilization rates were also negatively affected, no correlation between single-stranded DNA, pregnancy rate and live birth rates could be established, except in cases where 0% single-stranded DNA was detected. The observation of increased numbers of arrested embryos at the 2–6-cell stage in the high single-stranded DNA group was thought

to be related to the switch from the maternal to the embryonic genome. Increased single-stranded sperm DNA was also predictive for pregnancy loss, and might therefore have been related to reduced embryo quality in this group of patients.

The results from a study conducted by Tomsu et al.[84] showed that sperm DNA damage could be the underlying etiology for repeated cases with unexplained poor embryo quality and pregnancy failure. Using the comet assay, where a higher mean head density (MHD) correlates with normal double-stranded DNA, it was shown that couples with good-quality embryos had significantly better MHD compared with couples with poorer embryo quality (in the unexplained subfertility group). This result suggested the presence of a hidden anomaly causing the poor embryo quality.

Conversely, Benchaib et al.[85], Gandini et al.[86] and Greco et al.[87] reported no correlation between embryo quality and sperm DNA abnormalities.

In the study by Benchaib et al.[85], sperm DNA fragmentation (TUNEL) showed no effect on embryo quality (days 2 and 3). Fertilization rates in both ICSI and IVF were also not influenced by DNA fragmentation, but in patients where a pregnancy was obtained after ICSI, sperm DNA fragmentation was significantly decreased. The authors suggested that the effect of sperm DNA fragmentation has an impact only after the 6–8-cell embryo stage, especially in ICSI where no natural selection of the fertilizing sperm cell takes place. Gandini et al.[86] used the sperm chromatin structure assay (SCSA) and DFI in a study of IVF and ICSI patients, and failed to show any correlation between damaged sperm DNA and embryo quality on day 2 in pregnant and non-pregnant couples. The authors concluded that the DFI has no clear predictive value for ICSI fertilization rate, embryo quality and pregnancy.

Finally, in a very recent study by Greco et al.[87], sperm DNA fragmentation was also not correlated with embryo morphology and fertilization in ICSI patients. In this study, testicular and ejaculated spermatozoa from the same patients were analyzed for DNA fragmentation (TUNEL) and used for

ICSI fertilization in consecutive cycles. Testicular spermatozoa had significantly lower DNA fragmentation compared with ejaculated spermatozoa from the same male. Although embryo morphology and fertilization were not different after ICSI with testicular and ejaculated spermatozoa, the use of testicular spermatozoa significantly increased the pregnancy rate. This study suggested that in male patients with increased DNA damage of ejaculated spermatozoa, the percentage of DNA damage is much lower in the testis. It also indicated the presence of a late paternal effect, i.e. spermatozoa with DNA damage can fertilize oocytes and even give rise to good-morphology embryos, which then fail to implant or develop into a viable pregnancy.

Multinucleation   The possible influence of a paternal factor on the incidence of multinucleation was shown to be insignificant in a study conducted by Van Royen et al.[56]. The authors concluded that the incidence of multinucleation was positively correlated with certain stimulation protocols (short stimulation, high follicle stimulating hormone (FSH) dose and high number of oocytes retrieved), and therefore could be associated with a developmental failure of the oocyte[56].

Blastocyst development   The role of a paternal factor in blastocyst development potential was first reported by Janny and Menezo[88], who showed that good semen parameters were correlated with good blastocyst development.

Since the development of defined sequential media, blastocyst culture and transfer have become popular. Sakkas et al.[89] suggested that this method may provide a non-invasive means to eliminate abnormal embryos that could be attributed to a possible paternal effect. Banerjee et al.[90], however, reported that blastocyst transfer does not prevent the inheritance of abnormal chromosomes since the development of the fertilized oocyte to the blastocyst is generally independent of the paternal genotype, and reflects mainly the macromolecular and enzymatic competence of the oocyte. The authors mentioned, nevertheless, that

in certain circumstances abnormal paternal chromosomes might have an impact on the normal development of blastocysts.

Shoukir et al.[91] reported that only sperm motility could be related to increased blastocyst development. Other semen parameters (morphology and concentration) did not affect blastocyst development. These authors also found a significantly lower blastocyst development rate in ICSI compared with IVF patients, and attributed this result to the poorer semen parameters and therefore to a paternal effect in the ICSI group. The possible effect of sperm motility on blastocyst development can be explained in terms of a possible sperm centrosome defect, according to the authors. Semen samples with poor motility often present with increased centriolar defects, and if a defective sperm centriole is introduced into an oocyte, abnormal development may result. Poor blastocyst development may therefore occur after mitotic spindle disturbances are introduced by a spermatozoon with a sperm motility defect. The authors concluded that spermatozoa that have the ability to fertilize may not be able to contribute to normal blastocyst development.

Miller and Smith[72] reported similar results. Compared to IVF, significantly more ICSI embryos arrested at the 5–8-cell stage failed to develop into blastocysts and were of poor blastocyst quality. Poor semen parameters (especially sperm morphology (strict criteria) and motility) were also correlated with decreased blastocyst development and quality. Arrest at the 5–8-cell stage coincides with activation of the paternal genome, and implicates a paternal factor. The authors also suggested that good sperm motility might indicate adequate metabolic viability and a lower incidence of centriolar defects.

The effect of ROS on day-4 morula and blastocyst formation was studied by Zorn et al.[92]. A negative association between ROS levels and blastocyst development was found in ICSI patients, but pregnancy rates were not affected.

Spermatozoa with a high incidence of nuclear DNA damage (strand breaks in DNA (TUNEL)) were negatively correlated with blastocyst development in IVF and ICSI, but pregnancy rates were not significantly affected, in a study reported by Seli *et al.*[93]. The authors hypothesized that this effect could be attributed to the fact that at the blastocyst stage the embryonic genome has become activated and transcriptional activity has started, and the paternal genome might therefore play a significant role in the embryo, i.e. blastocyst development.

CONCLUSIONS

This review emphasizes the fact that, in many cases, the influence of a paternal effect on embryo quality at different stages of development is not known. Many studies have reported contradictory results, and this might be because many different detection and analysis methods have been implemented, but, more important, because embryo quality is determined by a multitude of factors, only one of which might be the fertilizing spermatozoon.

Based on the available literature discussed, it is clear that the sperm cell plays an important role in the fate of the developing embryo and the outcome of ART.

Although many studies are focused on embryo selection methods, especially since single embryo transfer has become a necessity in many countries, methods for selection of the genetically normal spermatozoon with the potential to contribute to normal embryo development with the highest potential of implantation are under current investigation.

REFERENCES

1. Boiso I. Fundamentals of human embryonic growth in vitro and the selection of high quality embryos. Reprod Biomed Online 2002; 5: 328
2. Balaban B, Urman B. Embryo culture as a diagnostic tool. Reprod Biomed Online 2003; 6: 671
3. Gerris J, et al. Prevention of twin pregnancy after in vitro fertilization or intracytoplasmic sperm injection based on strict embryo criteria: a prospective randomized trail. Hum Reprod 1999; 14: 2581
4. Van Royen E, et al. Characterization of a top quality embryo, a step towards single-embryo transfer. Hum Reprod 1999; 14: 2345
5. Tesarik J, Greco E. The probability of abnormal preimplantation development can be predicted by a single static observation on pronuclear stage morphology. Hum Reprod 1999; 14: 1318
6. Scott LA, Smith S. The successful use of pronuclear embryo transfers the day following oocyte retrieval. Hum Reprod 1998; 13: 1003
7. Payne D, et al. Preliminary observations on polar body extrusion and pronuclear formation in human oocytes using time-lapse video cinematography. Hum Reprod 1997; 12: 532
8. Edwards RG, Beard HK. Oocyte polarity and cell determination in early mammalian embryos. Mol Hum Reprod 1997; 3: 863
9. Edwards RG, Beard HK. Blastocyst stage transfer: pitfalls and benefits. Is the success of human IVF more a matter of genetics and evolution than growing blastocysts? Hum Reprod 1999; 14: 1
10. Scott L, et al. The morphology of human pronuclear embryos is positively related to blastocyst development and implantation. Hum Reprod 2000; 15: 2394
11. Tesarik J, et al. Embryos with high implantation potential after intracytoplasmic sperm injection can be recognized by a simple non-invasive examination of pronuclear morphology. Hum Reprod 2000; 15: 1396
12. Ludwig M, et al. Clinical use of a pronuclear stage score following intracytoplasmic sperm injection: impact on pregnancy rates under the conditions of the German embryo protection law. Hum Reprod 2000; 15: 325
13. Salumets A, et al. The predictive value of pronuclear morphology of zygotes in the assessment of human embryo quality. Hum Reprod 2002; 16: 2177
14. Scott L. Pronuclear scoring as a predictor of embryo development. Reprod Biomed Online 2003; 6: 201
15. Behr B. Blastocyst stage transfer: pitfalls and benefits. Blastocyst culture and transfer. Hum Reprod 1999; 14: 5
16. Shoukir Y, et al. Early cleavage of in vitro fertilized human embryos to the 2-cell stage: a novel indicator of embryo quality and viability. Hum Reprod 1997; 12: 1531

17. Sakkas D, et al. Early cleavage of human embryos to the two-cell stage after intracytoplasmic sperm injection as an indicator of embryo viability. Hum Reprod 1998; 13: 182

18. Sakkas D, et al. Assessment of early cleaving in vitro fertilized human embryos at the 2-cell stage before transfer improves embryo selection. Fertil Steril 2001; 76: 1150

19. Bos-Mikich A, Mattos ALG, Ferrari AN. Early cleavage of human embryos: an effective method for predicting successful IVF/ICSI outcome. Hum Reprod 2001; 16: 2658

20. Lundin K, Bergh K, Hardarson T. Early embryo cleavage is a strong indicator of embryo quality in human IVF. Hum Reprod 2001; 16: 2652

21. Petersen CG, et al. Embryo selection by the first cleavage parameter between 25 and 27 hours after ICSI. J Assist Reprod Genet 2001; 18: 209

22. Fenwick J, et al. Time from insemination to first cleavage predicts developmental competence of human preimplantation embryos in vitro. Hum Reprod 2002; 17: 407

23. Isiklar A, et al. Early cleavage of human embryos to the two-cell stage. A simple effective indicator of implantation and pregnancy in intracytoplasmic sperm injection. J Reprod Med 2002; 47: 540

24. Salumets A, et al. Early cleavage predicts the viability of human embryos in elective single transfer procedures. Hum Reprod 2003; 18: 821

25. Tsai YC, et al. Clinical value of early cleavage embryo. Int J Gynecol Obstet 2002; 76: 293

26. Wharf E, et al. Early embryo development is an indicator of implantation potential. Reprod Biomed Online 2003; 8: 212

27. Çiray N, Ulug U, Bahçeci M. Transfer of early-cleaved embryos increases implantation rate in patients undergoing ovarian stimulation and ICSI–embryo transfer. Reprod Biomed Online 2004; 8: 219

28. Van Montfoort APA, et al. Early cleavage is a valuable addition to existing embryo selection parameters: a study using single embryo transfers. Hum Reprod 2004; 19: 2103

29. Windt M-L, et al. Comparative analysis of pregnancy rates after the transfer of early dividing embryos versus slower dividing embryos. Hum Reprod 2004; 19: 1155

30. Gardner DK, et al. A prospective randomised trial of blastocyst culture and transfer in in-vitro fertilization. Hum Reprod 1998; 13: 3434

31. Gardner DK, Lane M, Schoolcraft WB. Physiology and culture of the human blastocyst. J Reprod Immunol 2002; 55: 85

32. Tsirigotis M. Blastocyst stage transfer: pitfalls and benefits. Too soon to abandon current practice? Hum Reprod 1998; 13: 3285

33. Jones GM, Trounson AO. Blastocyst stage transfer: pitfalls and benefits. The benefit of extended culture. Hum Reprod 1999; 14: 1405

34. Sakkas D. Blastocyst stage transfer: pitfalls and benefits. The use of blastocyst culture to avoid inheritance of an abnormal paternal genome after ICSI. Hum Reprod 1999; 14: 4

35. Kolibianakis EM, Devroey P. Blastocyst culture: facts and fiction. Reprod Biomed Online 2002; 5: 285

36. Blake D, et al. Cleavage stage versus blastocyst stage transfer in assisted conception (Cochrane Review). In The Cochrane Library, Issue 2. Oxford: Update Software, 2003

37. De Placido G, et al. High outcome predictability after IVF using a combined score for zygote and embryo morphology and growth rate. Hum Reprod 2001; 9: 2402

38. Fisch JD, et al. The graduated embryo score (GES) predicts blastocyst formation and pregnancy rate from cleavage stage embryos. Hum Reprod 2001; 9: 1970

39. Terriou P, et al. Embryo score is a better predictor of pregnancy than the number of transferred embryos or female age. Fertil Steril 2001; 75: 525

40. Roudebush WE, et al. Embryonic platelet-activating factor: an indicator of embryo viability. Hum Reprod 2002; 17: 1306

41. Noci I, et al. Embryonic soluble HLA-G as a marker of developmental potential in embryos. Hum Reprod 2005; 20: 138

42. Sher G, et al. Expression of sHLA-G in supernatants of individually cultured 46-h embryos: a potentially valuable indicator of 'embryo competency' and IVF outcome. Reprod Biomed Online 2004; 9: 74

43. Tesarik J. Paternal effects on cell division in the human preimplantation embryo. Reprod Biomed Online 2005; 10: 370

44. Roudebush WE, Duralia DR, Butler WJ. Effect of platelet activating factor (PAF) on preimplantation mouse B6D2F1/J embryo formation. Am J Reprod Immunol 1996; 35: 272

45. Roudebush WE, et al. Exposure of preimplantation embryos to platelet activating factor increases birth rate. J Assist Reprod Genet 2004; 21: 297

46. Roudebush WE, et al. The significance of platelet-activating factor and fertility in the male primate: a review. J Med Primatol 2005; 24: 20

47. Balaban B, et al. The effect of pronuclear morphology on embryo quality and blastocyst transfer outcome. Hum Reprod 2001; 16: 2357

48. Scott L. Embryological strategies for overcoming recurrent assisted reproductive technology treatment failure. Hum Fertil (Camb) 2002; 5: 206

49. Demirel LC, et al. The impact of the source of spermatozoa used for ICSI on pronuclear morphology. Hum Reprod 2001; 16: 2327

50. Rossi-Ferragut LM, et al. Pronuclear and morphological features as a cumulative score to select embryos in ICSI (intracytoplasmic sperm injection) cycles according to sperm origin. J Assist Reprod Genet 2003; 20: 1

51. Tesarik J, Greco E, Mendoza C. Paternal effects during the first cell cycle of human preimplantation development after ICSI. Hum Reprod 2002; 17: 184

52. Tesarik J, Greco E, Mendoza C. Late, but not early, paternal effect on human embryo development is related to sperm DNA fragmentation. Hum Reprod 2004; 19: 611

53. Harper J, et al. Detection of fertilization in embryos with accelerated cleavage by fluorescence in situ hybridization. Hum Reprod 1994; 9: 1733

54. Magli M, et al. Incidence of chromosomal abnormalities from a morphologically normal cohort of embryos in poor-prognosis patients. J Assist Reprod Genet 1998; 15: 297

55. Veeck L. Atlas of the Human Oocyte and Early Conceptus. Baltimore: Williams & Wilkins, 1991; 2

56. Van Royen E, et al. Multinucleation in cleavage stage embryos. Hum Reprod 2003; 18: 1062

57. Harderson T, et al. Human embryos with unevenly sized blastomeres have lower pregnancy and implantation rates: indications for aneuploidy and multinucleation. Hum Reprod 2001; 16: 313

58. Racowsky C. Day 3 and day 5 morphological predictors of embryo viability. Reprod Biomed Online 2003; 6: 323

59. Alikani M, et al. Human embryo fragmentation in vitro and its implications for pregnancy and implantation. Fertil Steril 1999; 71: 836

60. Balaban B, et al. Blastocyst quality affects the success of blastocyst stage embryo transfer. Fertil Steril 2000; 74: 282

61. Rubio C, et al. Clinical experience employing co-culture of human embryos with autologous human endometrial epithelial cells. Hum Reprod 2000; 15: 31

62. Salumets A, et al. Influence of oocytes and spermatozoa on early embryonic development. Fertil Steril 2002; 78: 1082

63. Loutradis D, et al. Oocyte morphology correlates with embryo quality and pregnancy rate after intracytoplasmic sperm injection. Fertil Steril 1999; 72: 240

64. Tomlinson MJ. Interrelationships between seminal parameters and sperm nuclear DNA damage before and after density gradient centrifugation: implications for assisted conception. Hum Reprod 2001; 16: 2160

65. Strassburger D, et al. Very low sperm count affects the result of intracytoplasmic sperm injection. J Assist Reprod Genet 2000; 17: 431

66. Cohen J, et al. Partial zona dissection or subzonal sperm insertion: microsurgical fertilization alternatives based on evaluation of sperm and embryo morphology. Fertil Steril 1991; 56: 696

67. Parinaud J, et al. Influence of sperm parameters on embryo quality. Fertil Steril 1993; 60: 888

68. Grow D, Oehninger S. Strict criteria for the evaluation of human sperm morphology and its impact on assisted reproduction. Andrologia 1995; 27: 325

69. Host E, et al. Sperm morphology and IVF: embryo quality in relation to sperm morphology following the WHO and Kruger's strict criteria. Acta Obstet Gynecol Scand 1999; 78: 526

70. De Vos A, et al. Influence of individual sperm morphology on fertilization, embryo morphology, and pregnancy outcome of intracytoplasmic sperm injection. Fertil Steril 2003; 79: 42

71. Moilanen JM, et al. Fertilization, embryo quality, and cryosurvival in in vitro fertilization and intracytoplasmic sperm injection cycles. J Assist Reprod Genet 1999; 16: 17

72. Miller JE, Smith TT. The effect of intracytoplasmic sperm injection and semen parameters on blastocyst development in vitro. Hum Reprod 2001; 16: 918

73. Sakkas D, et al. Use of egg-share model to investigate the paternal influence on fertilization and embryo development after in vitro fertilization and incytoplasmic sperm injection. Fertil Steril 2004; 82: 74

74. Virant-Klun I, Tomazevic T, Meden-Vrtovec H. Sperm single-stranded DNA, detected by acridine orange staining, reduces fertilization and quality of ICSI-derived embryos. J Assist Reprod Genet 2002; 19: 319

75. Katsoff D, Check ML, Check JH. Evidence that sperm with low hypoosmotic swelling scores cause embryo implantation defects. Arch Androl 2000; 44: 227

76. Kattera S, Chen C. Short coincubation of gametes in in vitro fertilization improves implantation and pregnancy rates: a prospective, randomized, controlled study. Fertil Steril 2003; 80: 1017

77. Obasaju M, et al. Sperm quality may adversely affect the chromosome constitution of embryos that result

from intracytoplasmic sperm injection. Fertil Steril 1999; 72: 1113

78. Johnson JE, et al. Expectations for oocyte fertilization and embryo cleavage after whole sperm versus sperm head intracytoplasmic sperm injection. Fertil Steril 2004; 82: 1412

79. Stalf T, et al. Different cumulative pregnancy rates in patients with repeated IVF- or ICSI cycles: possible influence of a male factor. Andrologia 1999; 31: 149

80. Aoki VW, et al. Improved in vitro fertilization embryo quality and pregnancy rates with intracytoplasmic sperm injection of sperm from fresh testicular biopsy samples. Fertil Steril 2004; 82: 1532

81. Vernaeve V, et al. Intracytoplasmic sperm injection with testicular spermatozoa is less successful in men with nonobstructive azoospermia than in men with obstructive azoospermia. Fertil Steril 2003; 79: 529

82. Van Golde RJ, et al. Decreased fertilization rate and embryo quality after ICSI in oligozoospermic men with microdeletions in the azoospermia factor c region of the Y chromosome. Hum Reprod 2001; 16: 289

83. Saleh RA, et al. Negative effects of increased sperm DNA damage in relation to seminal oxidative stress in men with idiopathic and male infertility. Fertil Steril 2003; 79: 1597

84. Tomsu M, Sharma V, Miller D. Embryo quality and IVF treatment outcomes may correlate with different sperm comet assay parameters. Hum Reprod 2002; 17: 1856

85. Benchaib M, et al. Sperm DNA fragmentation decreases the pregnancy rate in an assisted reproductive technique. Hum Reprod 2003; 18: 1023

86. Gandini L, et al. Full-term pregnancies achieved with ICSI despite high levels of sperm chromatin damage. Hum Reprod 2004; 19: 1409

87. Greco E, et al. Efficient treatment of infertility due to sperm DNA damage by ICSI with testicular spermatozoa. Hum Reprod 2005; 20: 226

88. Janny L, Menezo YJR. Evidence for a strong paternal effect on human preimplantation embryo development and blastocyst formation. Mol Reprod Dev 1994; 38: 36

89. Sakkas D. The use of blastocyst culture to avoid inheritance of an abnormal paternal genome. Hum Reprod 1999; 14: 4

90. Banerjee S, et al. Does blastocyst culture eliminate paternal chromosome defects and select good embryos? Hum Reprod 2000; 15: 2455

91. Shoukir Y, et al. Blastocyst development from supernumerary embryos after intracytoplasmic sperm injection: a paternal influence? Hum Reprod 1998; 13: 1632

92. Zorn B, Vidmar G, Meden-Vrtovec H. Seminal reactive oxygen species as predictors of fertilization, embryo quality and pregnancy rates after conventional in vitro fertilization and intracytoplasmic sperm injection. Int J Androl 2003; 26: 279

93. Seli E, et al. Extent of nuclear DNA damage in ejaculated spermatozoa impacts on blastocyst development after in vitro fertilization. Fertil Steril 2004; 82: 378

Section 3

Therapeutic alternatives for male infertility

21

Clinical management of male infertility

Murat Arslan, Sergio Oehninger, Thinus F Kruger

INTRODUCTION

It is estimated that male subfertility is present in up to 40–50% of infertile couples, alone or in combination with female factors[1,2]. There has been extensive progress in the diagnosis and treatment of male factor infertility since the inception of assisted reproductive technologies (ART). Moreover, the advent of intracytoplasmic sperm injection (ICSI) has resulted in a dramatically increased likelihood of pregnancy in couples suffering from most causes of male infertility. Fundamental advances have been made in the genetics of male disorders. Nevertheless, and at the same time, we are now witnessing a steady state in the development of assays that can be predictive of sperm functional capacities, both under *in vivo* and *in vitro* conditions.

Therefore, it is evident now, as it was a few years ago, that more research is needed to establish the causes and pathogenic mechanisms involved in male disorders leading to abnormal sperm function. The correct approach for male infertility evaluation should include a rational program composed of careful evaluation of the patient's history, a complete physical examination, laboratory tests of basic/extended semen analysis and a urological, endocrinological and genetic work-up, as appropriate.

A comprehensive semen analysis following the World Health Organization (WHO) guidelines[3] is fundamental at the primary-care level to make a rational initial diagnosis and to select the appropriate clinical management. Collection and analysis of the semen must be undertaken by properly standardized procedures in appropriately qualified and accredited laboratories[4]. The 'basic' semen evaluation should include: (1) assessment of physical semen characteristics (volume, liquefaction, appearance, consistency, pH and agglutination); (2) evaluation of sperm concentration, grading of motility and analysis of morphological characteristics (using strict criteria)[5]; (3) determination of sperm vitality (viability), testing for sperm auto-antibodies (using the mixed antiglobulin test and/or the direct immunobead test), presence of leukospermia and immature sperm cells; and (4) bacteriological studies. The identification and separation of the motile sperm fraction is also an integral part of the initial semen evaluation[6–8].

Clinicians and scientists are still searching for semen parameter thresholds in the so-called 'normal fertile populations' in order to be able to define fertility, subfertility and infertility more accurately. Recent publications have appropriately readdressed these issues as part of both European and American studies[9,10]. In a recent publication[11], van der Merwe *et al.*, reassessed fertility/subfertility thresholds for normal basic sperm parameters by a thorough, structured review of the current literature. Results demonstrated new and lower threshold levels for fertility/subfertility. These cut-off values included a sperm concentration < 15 million/ml, progressive motility < 30% and < 5% normal morphology. These thresholds also fit data from the *in vitro* fertilization (IVF)[12] and intrauterine insemination (IUI)[13] settings.

There are multiple structural and biochemical sperm alterations that are present in subfertile men. Anatomically, they can be divided into: *membrane alterations* (that can be assessed by tests of resistance to osmotic changes, translocation of phosphatidylserine and others), *nuclear aberrations* (abnormal chromatin condensation, retention of histones and presence of DNA fragmentation), *cytoplasmic lesions* (excessive generation of reactive oxygen species, loss of mitochondrial membrane potential and retention of cytoplasm – with excessive creatine kinase content or the presence of active caspases) and *flagellar disturbances* (disturbances of the microtubules and fibrous sheath). Some of these alterations are indicative of immaturity, the presence of an apoptosis phenotype, infection-necrosis or other unknown causes[14–24].

Attention has shifted to the examination of sperm nuclear abnormalities. Currently, various tests are available for the detection of chromatin/DNA defects, including aniline blue staining[25], acridine orange[26], the sperm chromatin structure assay (SCSA)[27], the assessment of DNA fragmentation[16,28,29] and fluorescence *in situ* hybridization (FISH) for aneuploidy[30].

Notwithstanding their occurrence and correlation with clinical outcomes, it is not clear how these abnormalities directly influence sperm function, particularly gamete transportation, fertilization and contribution to embryogenesis. Furthermore, most such assays are still experimental, and more research is needed to validate their results in the clinical setting and to determine their true capacity to predict male fertility potential.

On the other hand, there are other specific and critical sperm functional capacities that can be more reliably examined *in vitro*. These functions include: motility, competence to achieve capacitation, zona pellucida binding and the acrosome reaction. The assessment of these features is what is typically considered as sperm functional testing.

The extended semen analysis should include the preferential examination of these essential sperm functional attributes. These assays have been categorized into: (1) tests that examine defective sperm function indirectly through the use of biochemical means (i.e. measurement of the generation of reactive oxygen species or evidence of peroxidative damage, measurement of enzyme activities such as creatine phosphokinase and others); (2) bioassays of gamete interaction (i.e. the heterologous zona-free hamster-oocyte test and homologous sperm–zona pellucida binding assays) and induced acrosome-reaction scoring; and (3) computer-aided sperm motion analysis (CASA) for the evaluation of sperm motion characteristics[3,31–41].

We reported an objective, outcome-based examination of the validity of the currently available assays based upon the results obtained from 2906 subjects evaluated in 34 published and prospectively designed, controlled studies. The aim was carried out through a meta-analytical approach that examined the predictive value of four categories of sperm functional assays (computer-aided sperm motion analysis or CASA, induced acrosome-reaction testing, sperm penetration assay or SPA and sperm–zona pellucida binding assays) for IVF outcome[42].

Results of this meta-analysis demonstrated a high predictive power of the sperm–zona pellucida binding and induced acrosome-reaction assays for fertilization outcome under *in vitro* conditions[42]. On the other hand, the findings indicated a poor clinical value of the SPA as predictor of fertilization, and a real need for standardization and further investigation of the potential clinical utility of CASA systems. Although this study provided objective evidence based on which clinical management and future research may be directed, the analysis also pointed out limitations of the current tests and a need for the standardization of present methodologies and the development of novel technologies.

Typically, male infertility presents clinically as an abnormal basic or extended semen analysis. Abnormalities in sperm indices may occur as an isolated parameter or as a combination of various parameters. Oligozoospermia and teratozoospermia are the most frequently observed isolated defects in our clinical practices, but more frequently, various degrees of oligoasthenoteratozoospermia (OAT) are present[43]. Here, it is our aim to examine the causes and clinical management of the various single and multiple sperm defects.

ISOLATED SPERM ABNORMALITIES

Decreased sperm concentration (azo-/oligozoospermia)

Pathologies classified as 'decreased sperm concentration' range from mild oligospermia (< 15 million sperm/ml)[11] to azoospermia (no sperm in the ejaculate). On a simplistic basis, the clinically known causative entities can be subdivided into those of pretesticular, testicular and post-testicular origin.

A variety of endocrinopathies that disrupt the hypothalamic–pituitary–testicular axis constitute pretesticular etiologies of oligozoospermia. These endocrinopathies might be congenital (Kallmann's syndrome) or acquired (prolactinoma, other hypothalamic–pituitary tumors and pathologies), and require the measurement of serum prolactin levels together with follicle stimulating hormone (FSH), luteinizing hormone (LH) and testosterone for differential diagnosis in a patient with decreased sperm concentration. Further evaluation with assessment of other pituitary hormones (thyroid stimulating hormone (TSH), growth hormone, cortisol) and intracranial imaging

systems (computed tomography (CT), magnetic resonance imaging (MRI)) is crucial in cases of hypogonadotropic hypogonadism.

Six to 24 months of treatment in patients with idiopathic hypogonadotropic hypogonadism, either with gonadotropins or pulsatile gonadotropin-releasing hormone (GnRH), frequently results in sperm indices sufficient for fertility in these patients[44,45]. Patients with a diagnosis of prolactinoma respond rapidly to antidopaminergic agents[46]. Because of their impressive therapeutic effects in patients with prolactinoma, these agents have also been tried in idiopathic oligoasthenozoospermia to improve sperm parameters. However, it has recently been shown in a meta-analysis that although they decrease serum prolactin levels further within the normal range, they are not helpful in improving sperm indices or fertility[47].

Post-testicular etiologies resulting in reduced or absent sperm output include a variety of obstructive lesions of the genital tract (inflammatory-infectious, congenital or iatrogenic, such as vasectomy) and ejaculatory disorders, particularly retrograde ejaculation. Retrograde ejaculation should be suspected in any case of azoospermia with low seminal volume, and might be congenital, acquired (prostatic and bladder-neck surgery, diabetes mellitus, inguinal lymph node excision) or idiopathic in origin[48].

Testicular causes include hypospermatogenesis due to a reduction in the number of germ cells[49], incomplete/complete maturation arrest of germinal cell differentiation[50,51] and germinal cell aplasia[52,53]. These entities are characterized by disturbances of spermatogenesis and/or an aberrant apoptotic process occurring during mitosis, meiosis and/or spermiogenesis/spermiation. Some of these pathologies are end results or the sequelae of viral infections, iatrogenic agents (chemo- and radiotherapy) and varicocele, as well as disturbances secondary to genetic/chromosomal/environmental aberrations[15,54,55]. Nonetheless, it is our experience that in almost all such cases oligozoospermia is associated with moderate to severe degrees of astheno- and teratozoospermia (see below).

Decreased sperm motility (asthenozoospermia)

Asthenozoospermia is defined as the presence of progressive motility <30%[11]. Its origin can be iatrogenic, structural, functional, genetic or environmental. Possible causes of isolated asthenozoospermia include: iatrogenic reasons (improper handling of the semen sample), anti-sperm antibodies, infections, partial axonemal defects, sperm-tail fibrous sheath defects and poor development of the outer dense fibers, the presence of fewer mitochondria in the midpiece or even aplasia, sperm centriole dysfunction, carboxymethyl transferase enzyme deficiency and epididymal pathologies (typically associated with inflammation-infection)[56–62].

The autosomal recessive-inherited immotile cilia syndrome[63] and sperm mitochondrial DNA mutations[64–67] have been identified as two gene-related causes of isolated sperm motility disorders. Recently, Baccetti et al.[68], reported a patient with severe isolated asthenozoospermia characterized by an absence of the fibrous sheath in the principal-piece region of the tail in the whole sperm population, which strongly suggests a genetic origin.

In patients with documented asthenozoospermia, the diagnosis work-up should emphasize repeated semen analyses in order to exclude inappropriate handling of the specimen as the cause. Repeated semen and urine cultures together with immunological tests should also be performed. Structural analysis of the sperm tail (flagellum) under transmission electron microscopy is the method of choice for diagnosis of immotile cilia syndrome in suspected patients with isolated severe asthenozoospermia.

It is worth mentioning that for isolated asthenozoospermia, many different sperm preparation techniques, with or without *in vitro* motility enhancers, have been tried. These agents have included pentoxifylline, 2-deoxyadenosine, kallikrein, platelet-activating factor and some antioxidants[69,70]. Although different levels of improvement have been reported with these agents, none of them has truly gained acceptance for routine use in clinical practice.

Decreased normal morphology (teratozoospermia)

The importance of sperm morphology in male factor infertility has been demonstrated in multiple reports[5,12,71–76] even though there is no complete uniformity in the definition of normal sperm morphology and teratozoospermia[3,71,77,78]. After the introduction and validation of strict criteria by Kruger et al.[5], sperm morphology gained acceptance as the most important sperm parameter in the prediction of IVF outcome[72,79]. Later on, many studies demonstrated good correlation between sperm morphology and sperm functional tests such as zona pellucida binding assays[34,80–83] and the zona-free hamster-oocyte penetration assay[84,85]. Poor morphology also correlates with abnormal sperm calcium influx[86] and an abnormal acrosome reaction[87]. Its prognostic value has also been validated in IUI cycles[3,88–90].

On the other hand, the pathophysiology of teratozoospermia is not completely understood. Numerical and structural chromosomal defects have been claimed in its pathogenesis. Investigations of spermatozoa from somatically normal men during meiosis using the FISH technique resulted in findings of a higher percentage of disomy, trisomy or tetrasomy for chromosome 1[91], chromosome 7[92], chromosome 8[93], chromosome 13[94,95], chromosome 18[92,93,96], chromosome 21[94] and the sex chromosomes[91–93,95,96]. Importantly, these abnormalities occurred mostly in populations with combined defects of sperm parameters (OAT) and infertility. The authors of these studies proposed that the effects of factors that impair sperm indices during gametogenesis extend to the cytogenetic constitution of spermatozoa. Conversely, some other studies could not find any correlation between sperm chromosomal abnormality and fertility[97–99].

Harkonen et al.[92] focused on isolated teratozoospermia and demonstrated higher frequencies of disomies 7, 18, YY and XY and diploidy in patients having < 10% normal morphology. Calogero et al.[93] found higher incidences of disomies 8, 18, X and Y in patients with isolated teratozoospermia and OAT, compared with men with normozoospermia. These authors suggested that teratozoospermia might be the critical sperm parameter associated with aneuploidy. The same group also showed an increase in sperm aneuploidy rate in patients with OAT, particularly in the presence of an elevated percentage of spermatozoa with enlarged heads[100].

On the other hand, Gole et al.[101] found a higher incidence of sex chromosomal disomy in patients with OAT compared with teratozoospermic patients. Recently, Burrello et al.[102] reported a higher aneuploidy rate for spermatozoa with abnormal head shapes from OAT patients, compared with normally shaped spermatozoa from normal men. Their results showed that normal morphology in patients with OAT does not rule out the presence of aneuploidy in selected sperm for ICSI. These results weaken the possibility of a direct causal relationship between isolated teratozoospermia and sperm chromosomal abnormalities. However, there is consensus in the literature that infertile men and/or men with poor sperm indices carry a higher frequency of aneuploidy in their spermatozoa. More studies are needed to identify the effects of different chromosomal aberrations on different sperm parameters/functions.

There is also substantial evidence in the literature supporting that deregulation of specific genes might play a role in the appearance of morphological abnormalities in ejaculated spermatozoa. It has been shown in a mouse model that *azh* mutations (abnormal spermatozoon head shape) on chromosome 4 might cause specific structural changes in the sperm head[103,104]. Adham et al.[105] showed the development of sperm head abnormalities in mice containing *Tnp2* (transition protein 2) gene disruption, which takes part in the nuclear organization of spermatozoa. Xu et al.[106] also demonstrated that male mice lacking a regulatory protein in the process of spermatogenesis (protein casein kinase 2 α, Csnk2a) due to Csnk2a gene disruption performed by transgenesis were infertile, with globozoospermia (acrosomeless sperm). In addition, the altered expression and arrangement of some cytoskeletal proteins (calicin, protein 4.1) has been associated with aberrant morphological changes during spermiogenesis[107,108]. Recently, Milatiner et al.[109] demonstrated a correlation between the severity of teratozoospermia in infertile men and changes in the nucleotide structure of the androgen receptor gene.

COMBINED SPERM ABNORMALITIES: OLIGOASTHENOTERATOZOOSPERMIA

As mentioned above, OAT is the most common clinical presentation of male infertility. It is typically the reflection of abnormal (testicular) spermatogenesis but it can also be due to post-testicular etiologies. Approximately half of clinical cases, however, still remain idiopathic.

There are numerous known spermatogenesis defects leading to OAT[20,54,110–114]. They include: germ cell anomalies (depletion, aberrant apoptosis, defective differentiation), mitotic and meiotic defects and alterations of spermiogenesis/spermiation. Aberrant apoptosis has been observed at the primary spermatocyte and spermatid levels[115,116] and also in Sertoli cells[117]. Arrest or quantitatively abnormal spermatogenesis at any stage may result in oligozoospermia. Meiotic alterations and spermiogenesis defects are probably associated with teratozoospermia.

The concept of sperm immaturity has gained acceptance. Retention of cytoplasm (including retention of organelles and enzymes participating in metabolism, apoptosis and other functions that become exaggerated) is probably the result of an abnormal Sertoli cell–late spermatid interaction, leading to the release of dysmorphic, dyskinetic and dysfunctional spermatozoa[15,19–21,23,118,119] (Figure 21.1). Abnormalities of sperm release from the seminiferous tubules (or spermiation) are also probably present in some cases. Epididymal dysfunctions or pathologies can also influence sperm membrane domain constitution and may induce morphogenic/dysfunctional changes[120].

CLINICAL MANAGEMENT

The treatment plan should be constructed based upon complete identification of both male and female factors (Figure 21.2). In the presence of pure male infertility (no identifiable female factors), therapy may be: (1) medical (endocrine such as in hypogonadism or hyperprolactinemia, antibiotics in case of infection); (2) urological (surgical or non-surgical treatments, such as conventional, microsurgical or laparoscopic surgery, including correction of varicocele, epididymo- and vasovasostomy and modern approaches for ejaculatory disorders); and/or (3) low- or high-complexity assisted reproductive technologies (ART). The severity of male subfertility and some important prognostic risk factors in the female (e.g. age, duration of infertility, presence of endometriosis and other pathologies) may accelerate the indication for ART.

It is our opinion that, at the present time, there is no clinical role for the 'empirical' use of medical treatments of normogonadotropic subfertile men with idiopathic OAT. In the absence of a defined medical indication, there are no evidence-based data to support the use of gonadotropins, anti-estrogens, antioxidants, multivitamins or other unproven therapies.

Currently recommended ART options include: 'low-complexity' IUI therapy, 'standard' IVF and embryo transfer, and IVF augmented with ICSI. If the female partner is aged < 35 years, typically 4–6 cycles of IUI using the husband's sperm in combination with controlled ovarian hyperstimulation are recommended as a simple (low-complexity) ART approach, particularly if > 1 million motile sperm can be recovered[90,121].

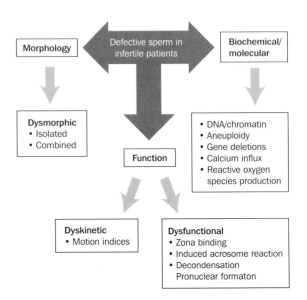

Figure 21.1 Abnormal spermatozoa in subfertile men. Identification of anomalies including decreased sperm output, dysmorphic sperm, dyskinetic sperm, sperm dysfunctions and molecular–cellular lesions

Preliminary data suggest that in order to increase cost-efficiency and loss of valuable time, IUI should not be performed if the total motile recoverable fraction is low, if the hemizona index (HZI) is < 31%[122], if the calcium ionophore-induced acrosome reaction is ≤ 22[123], if the zona pellucida-induced acrosome reaction is < 16%[87] and/or if the proportion of sperm depicting DNA fragmentation is > 12%[124].

Patients with a motile sperm fraction of < 5 million motile spermatozoa following swim-up or gradient centrifugation, but with mild to moderate teratozoospermia (in the range 4–14% normal forms by strict criteria), may be offered 'standard' IVF therapy. In those cases, good fertilization and pregnancy rates are achieved with an increase in the sperm insemination concentration[125,126]. However, nowadays, these patients are offered ICSI in an effort to eliminate any risk of low or failed fertilization, or a combination of IVF and ICSI (in sibling oocytes) in the group with sperm morphology > 14% normal forms, dependent on the individual IVF unit.

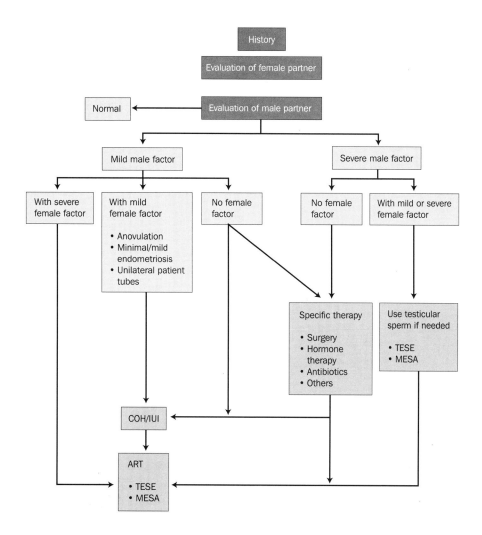

Figure 21.2   Algorithm for clinical management of the subfertile man. COH, controlled ovarian hyperstimulation; IUI, intrauterine insemination; ART, assisted reproductive technologies; IVF, *in vitro* fertilization; ICSI, intracytoplasmic sperm injection; TESE, testicular sperm extraction; MESA, microsurgical epididymal sperm aspiration

In our programs, patients are selected for ICSI according to the following indications[7,127]:

- Poor sperm parameters (i.e. $< 5 \times 10^6$ total spermatozoa with adequate progressive motility after separation and/or severe teratozoospermia with $< 4\%$ normal forms in the presence of a borderline to low total motile fraction);

- Poor functional abilities, including a defective sperm–zona pellucida binding capacity with a

hemizona assay index $< 30\%$[82,128] and/or a low ($< 16\%$) zona pellucida-induced acrosome reaction or ZIAR[87,129,130];

- Previous failed fertilization in IVF;

- Failure of IUI therapy in cases presenting with moderately abnormal sperm parameters ($5–10 \times 10^6$ total spermatozoa with adequate progressive motility after separation or morphology in the range of 5–14%), and also including the presence of antisperm antibodies;

- Presence of obstructive or non-obstructive azoospermia, where ICSI is combined with sperm extraction from the testes or the epididymis[7,127,131–134].

- In the presence of severe oligoasthenoteratozoospermia or if the outcome of sperm function testing indicates a significant impairment of fertilizing capacity, couples should be immediately directed to ICSI. This approach is probably more cost-effective and will avoid loss of valuable time, particularly in women > 35 years.

Based on currently available data, we estimate that ICSI should be indicated when male infertility is properly diagnosed based upon a state-of-the-art extended evaluation of the male partner, and also in cases with previous failed fertilization. Published prospective, randomized studies have demonstrated that it is not beneficial to perform ICSI in non-male infertility or unexplained infertility cases. Altogether, there are no data to suggest that ICSI should be performed in all cases of *in vitro* conception (reviewed in references 135 and 136). Consequently, to perform ICSI in all cases on a purely pragmatic basis appears to be a significant departure from principles of evidence-based medicine.

Greco *et al.*[137] recently reported that ICSI with testicular spermatozoa provides the first-line ART option for men with high levels of DNA damage in ejaculated sperm. Nonetheless, more studies are needed clinically to validate methods of assessing DNA damage and the impact of DNA abnormalities on clinical outcomes.

Sperm cryopreservation represents a valuable therapeutic option in the management of male infertility. Current indications include: (1) mandatory use in artificial insemination programs with donor semen; (2) patient's convenience (i.e. partner's absence where IUI is performed in the presence of normal sperm parameters); (3) preservation of reproductive capacity in men with various types of neoplasias before undergoing radical surgery and/or radio-chemotherapy[138]; (4) aiding in the management of infertile men undergoing vasectomy reversal (vasovasostomy) or epididymovasostomy, when 'banking' may provide a future sperm source for possible use in IUI or ICSI therapies; and (5) because of the outstanding success with ICSI, even infertile men with different degrees of oligoasthenoteratozoospermia can now be offered the use of cryopreserved–thawed spermatozoa for assisted fertilization. Today, this applies not only to ejaculated but also to testicular and epididymal spermatozoa recovered for the purpose of ICSI[139,140].

Interesting and challenging concepts to be applied to future treatment modalities of male infertility are germ cell transplantation and *in vitro* spermatogenesis[141,143]. Further progress in the identification of spermatogonial stem cells and techniques of germ cell transplantation[144], in addition to the optimization of culture systems for *in vitro* spermatogenesis[145], may give new options to patients with azoospermia.

REFERENCES

1. Irvine DS. Declining sperm quality: a review of facts and hypotheses. Baillieres Clin Obstet Gynaecol 1997; 11: 655

2. Centers for Disease Control and Prevention. 2000 Assisted Reproductive Technology Success Rates. National Summary and Fertility Clinic Reports. Atlanta: CDC, US Department of Health and Human Services, 2002

3. World Health Organization. WHO Laboratory Manual for the Examination of Human Semen and Sperm–Cervical Mucus Interaction, 4th edn. Cambridge: Cambridge University Press, 1999: 4

4. De Jonge C. Commentary: forging a partnership between total quality management and the andrology laboratory. J Androl 2000; 21: 203

5. Kruger TF, et al. Sperm morphologic features as a prognostic factor in in vitro fertilization. Fertil Steril 1986; 46: 1118

6. Oehninger S. An update on the laboratory assessment of male fertility. Hum Reprod 1995; 10 (Suppl 1): 38

7. Oehninger S. Clinical and laboratory management of male infertility: an opinion on its current status. J Androl 2000; 21: 814

8. Mortimer D. Sperm preparation methods. J Androl 2000; 21: 357

9. Ombelet W, et al. Semen parameters in a fertile versus subfertile population: a need for change in the interpretation of semen testing. Hum Reprod 1997; 12: 987

10. Zinaman MJ, et al. Semen quality and human fertility: a prospective study with healthy couples. J Androl 2000; 21: 145

11. van der Merwe FH, et al. The use of semen parameters to identify the subfertile male in the general population. Gynecol Obstet Invest 2005; 59: 86

12. Coetzee K, Kruger TF, Lombard CJ. Predictive value of normal sperm morphology: a structured literature review. Hum Reprod 1998; 4: 73

13. Van Waart J, et al. Predictive value of normal sperm morphology in intrauterine insemination (IUI): a structured literature review. Hum Reprod 2001; 7: 495

14. Baccetti B, Collodel G, Piomboni P. Apoptosis in human ejaculated sperm cells (notulae seminologicae 9). J Submicrosc Cytol Pathol 1996; 28: 587

15. Baccetti B, et al. Recent advances in human sperm pathology. Contraception 2002; 65: 283

16. Barroso G, Morshedi M, Oehninger S. Analysis of DNA fragmentation, plasma membrane translocation of phosphatidylserine and oxidative stress in human spermatozoa. Hum Reprod 2000; 15: 1338

17. Ergur AR, et al. Sperm maturity and treatment choice of in vitro fertilization (IVF) or intracytoplasmic sperm injection: diminished sperm HspA2 chaperone levels predict IVF failure. Fertil Steril 2002; 77: 910

18. Marchetti C, et al. Study of mitochondrial membrane potential, reactive oxygen species, DNA fragmentation and cell viability by flow cytometry in human sperm. Hum Reprod 2002; 17: 1257

19. Weng SL, et al. Caspase activity and apoptotic markers in ejaculated human sperm. Mol Hum Reprod 2002; 8: 984

20. Oehninger S, et al. Presence and significance of somatic cell apoptosis markers in human ejaculated spermatozoa. Reprod Biomed Online 2003; 7: 469

21. Taylor SL, et al. Somatic cell apoptosis markers and pathways in human ejaculated sperm: potential utility as indicators of sperm quality. Mol Hum Reprod 2004; 10: 825

22. Aitken RJ, Baker MA. Oxidative stress and male reproductive biology. Reprod Fertil Dev 2004; 16: 581

23. Huszar G, et al. Semen characteristics after overnight shipping: preservation of sperm concentrations, HspA2 ratios, CK activity, cytoplasmic retention, chromatin maturity, DNA integrity, and sperm shape. J Androl 2004; 25: 593

24. Cayli S, et al. Cellular maturity and apoptosis in human sperm: creatine kinase, caspase-3 and Bcl-XL levels in mature and diminished maturity sperm. Mol Hum Reprod 2004; 10: 365

25. Hoffmann N, Hilscher B. Use of aniline blue to assess chromatin condensation in morphologically normal spermatozoa in normal and infertile men. Hum Reprod 1991; 6: 979

26. Tejada RI, et al. A test for the practical evaluation of male fertility by acridine orange (AO) fluorescence. Fertil Steril 1984; 42: 87

27. Evenson DP, et al. Utility of the sperm chromatin structure assay as a diagnostic and prognostic tool in the human fertility clinic. Hum Reprod 1999; 14: 1039

28. Aitken RJ, et al. Relative impact of oxidative stress on the functional competence and genomic integrity of human spermatozoa. Biol Reprod 1998; 59: 1037

29. Sakkas D, et al. Origin of DNA damage in ejaculated human spermatozoa. Rev Reprod 1999; 4: 31

30. Pfeffer J, et al. Aneuploidy frequencies in semen fractions from ten oligoasthenoteratozoospermic patients donating sperm for intracytoplasmic sperm injection. Fertil Steril 1999; 72: 472

31. Yanagimachi R, Yanagimachi H, Rogers BJ. The use of zona-free animal ova as a test-system for the assessment of the fertilizing capacity of human spermatozoa. Biol Reprod 1976; 15: 471

32. Cross NL, Lambert H, Samuels S. Sperm binding activity of the zona pellucida of immature mouse oocytes. Cell Biol Int Rep 1986; 10: 545

33. Burkman LJ, et al. The hemizona assay (HZA): development of a diagnostic test for the binding of human spermatozoa to the human hemizona pellucida to predict fertilization potential. Fertil Steril 1988; 49: 688

34. Liu DY, et al. A human sperm–zona pellucida binding test using oocytes that failed to fertilize in vitro. Fertil Steril 1988; 50: 782

35. Aitken RJ, Clarkson JS, Fishel S. Generation of reactive oxygen species, lipid peroxidation, and human sperm function. Biol Reprod 1989; 41: 183

36. Aitken RJ, et al. Analysis of the relationship between defective sperm function and the generation of reactive oxygen species in cases of oligozoospermia. J Androl 1989; 10: 214

37. Aitken RJ, Irvine DS, Wu FC. Prospective analysis of sperm–oocyte fusion and reactive oxygen species generation as criteria for the diagnosis of infertility. Am J Obstet Gynecol 1991; 164: 542

38. World Health Organization. WHO Laboratory Manual for the Examination of Human Semen and Sperm–Cervical Mucus Interaction, 3rd edn. Cambridge: Cambridge University Press, 1992: 23

39. Huszar G, Vigue L, Morshedi M. Sperm creatine phosphokinase M-isoform ratios and fertilizing potential of men: a blinded study of 84 couples treated with in vitro fertilization. Fertil Steril 1992; 57: 882

40. Huszar G, Vigue L. Correlation between the rate of lipid peroxidation and cellular maturity as measured by creatine kinase activity in human spermatozoa. J Androl 1994; 15: 71

41. ESHRE Andrology Special Interest Group. Consensus Workshop on Advanced Diagnostic Andrology Techniques. Hum Reprod 1996; 11: 1463

42. Oehninger S, et al. Sperm function assays and their predictive value for fertilization outcome in IVF therapy: a meta-analysis. Hum Reprod Update 2000; 6: 160

43. Oehninger S. Pathophysiology of oligoasthenoteratozoospermia: are we improving in the diagnosis? Reprod Biomed Online 2003; 7: 433

44. Burris AS, et al. A low sperm concentration does not preclude fertility in men with isolated hypogonadotropic hypogonadism after gonadotropin therapy. Fertil Steril 1988; 50: 343

45. Burgues S, Calderon MD. Subcutaneous self-administration of highly purified follicle stimulating hormone and human chorionic gonadotrophin for the treatment of male hypogonadotrophic hypogonadism. Spanish Collaborative Group on Male Hypogonadotropic Hypogonadism. Hum Reprod 1997; 12: 980

46. De Rosa M, et al. Hyperprolactinemia in men: clinical and biochemical features and response to treatment. Endocrine 2003; 20: 75

47. Vandekerckhove P, et al. Bromocriptine for idiopathic oligo/asthenospermia. Cochrane Database Syst Rev 2000; (2): CD000152

48. Yavetz H, et al. Retrograde ejaculation. Hum Reprod 1994; 9: 381

49. Wong TW, Straus FH, Warner NE. Testicular biopsy in the study of male infertility. Arch Pathol 1973; 95: 151

50. Aumuller G, Fuhrmann W, Krause W. Spermatogenetic arrest with inhibition of acrosome and sperm tail development. Andrologia 1987; 19: 9

51. de Rooij DG, de Boer P. Specific arrests of spermatogenesis in genetically modified and mutant mice. Cytogenet Genome Res 2003; 103: 267

52. Levin HS. Testicular biopsy in the study of male infertility: its current usefulness, histologic techniques, and prospects for the future. Hum Pathol 1979; 10: 569

53. Nakamoto T, et al. Impaired spermatogenesis and male fertility defects in CIZ/Nmp4-disrupted mice. Genes Cells 2004; 9: 575

54. De Kretser DM, et al. Expanding our understanding of spermatogenesis: the future genetic tests for infertility. Int J Androl 2000; 23 (Suppl 2): 30

55. Aitken RJ, Sawyer D. The human spermatozoon – not waving but drowning. Adv Exp Med Biol 2003; 518: 85

56. Marchini M, et al. Etiology of severe asthenozoospermia and fertility prognosis. A screening of 5216 semen analyses. Andrologia 1991; 23: 115

57. Courtade M, et al. Clinical characteristics and light and transmission electron microscopic sperm defects of infertile men with persistent unexplained asthenozoospermia. Fertil Steril 1998; 70: 297

58. Gopalkrishnan K, et al. Severe asthenozoospermia: a structural and functional study. Int J Androl 1995; 18 (Suppl 1): 67

59. Mundy AJ, Ryder TA, Edmonds DK. Asthenozoospermia and the human sperm mid-piece. Hum Reprod 1995; 10: 116

60. Nagy ZP. Sperm centriole disfunction and sperm immotility. Mol Cell Endocrinol 2000; 166: 59

61. Gagnon C, et al. Deficiency of protein-carboxyl methylase in immotile spermatozoa of infertile men. N Engl J Med 1982; 306: 821

62. Kao SH, et al. Sperm mitochondrial DNA depletion in men with asthenospermia. Fertil Steril 2004; 82: 66

63. Afzelius BA, Camner P, Mossberg B. Acquired ciliary defects compared to those seen in the immotile-cilia syndrome. Eur J Respir Dis Suppl 1983; 127: 5

64. Kao S, Chao HT, Wei YH. Mitochondrial deoxyribonucleic acid 4977-bp deletion is associated with

diminished fertility and motility of human sperm. Biol Reprod 1995; 52: 729

65. Kao SH, Chao HT, Wei YH. Multiple deletions of mitochondrial DNA are associated with the decline of motility and fertility of human spermatozoa. Mol Hum Reprod 1998; 4: 657

66. Ruiz-Pesini E, et al. Human mtDNA haplogroups associated with high or reduced spermatozoa motility. Am J Hum Genet 2000; 67: 682

67. Rovio AT, et al. Mutations at the mitochondrial DNA polymerase (POLG) locus associated with male infertility. Nat Genet 2001; 29: 261

68. Baccetti B, et al. An ultrastructural and immunocytochemical study of a rare genetic sperm tail defect that causes infertility in humans. Fertil Steril 2004; 82: 463

69. Henkel RR, Schill WB. Sperm preparation for ART. Reprod Biol Endocrinol 2003; 1: 108

70. Morshedi M, et al. Efficacy and pregnancy outcome of two methods of semen preparation for intra-uterine insemination: a prospective randomized study. Fertil Steril 2003; 79 (Suppl 3): 1625

71. Kruger TF, et al. Predictive value of abnormal sperm morphology in in vitro fertilization. Fertil Steril 1988; 49: 112

72. Menkveld R, et al. The evaluation of morphological characteristics of human spermatozoa according to stricter criteria. Hum Reprod 1990; 5: 586

73. Ombelet W, et al. Teratozoospermia and in-vitro fertilization: a randomized prospective study. Hum Reprod 1994; 9: 1479

74. Grow DR, et al. Sperm morphology as diagnosed by strict criteria: probing the impact of teratozoospermia on fertilization rate and pregnancy outcome in a large in vitro fertilization population. Fertil Steril 1994; 62: 559

75. Oehninger S, Kruger T. The diagnosis of male infertility by semen quality. Clinical significance of sperm morphology assessment. Hum Reprod 1995; 10: 1037

76. Kruger TF, Coetzee K. The role of sperm morphology in assisted reproduction. Hum Reprod Update 1999; 5: 172

77. Liakatas J, Williams AE, Hargreave TB. Scoring sperm morphology using the scanning electron microscope. Fertil Steril 1982; 38: 227

78. Baker HW, Clarke GN. Sperm morphology: consistency of assessment of the same sperm by different observers. Clin Reprod Fertil 1987; 5: 37

79. Liu DY, Baker HW. Relationships between human sperm acrosin, acrosomes, morphology and fertilization in vitro. Hum Reprod 1990; 5: 298

80. Franken DR, et al. Hemizona assay and teratozoospermia: increasing sperm insemination concentrations to enhance zona pellucida binding. Fertil Steril 1990; 54: 497

81. Oehninger S, et al. Prediction of fertilization in vitro with human gametes: is there a litmus test? Am J Obstet Gynecol 1992; 167: 1760

82. Oehninger S, et al. Clinical significance of human sperm–zona pellucida binding. Fertil Steril 1997; 67: 1121

83. Liu DY, et al. Human sperm–zona pellucida binding, sperm characteristics and in-vitro fertilization. Hum Reprod 1989; 4: 696

84. Kruger TF, et al. Abnormal sperm morphology and other semen parameters related to the outcome of the hamster oocyte human sperm penetration assay. Int J Androl 1988; 11: 107

85. Vazquez-Levin MH, et al. The relationship between critical evaluation of sperm morphology and the TYB-optimized zona free hamster oocyte sperm penetration assay. Int J Androl 1999; 22: 329

86. Oehninger S, et al. Defective calcium influx and acrosome reaction (spontaneous and progesterone-induced) in spermatozoa of infertile men with severe teratozoospermia. Fertil Steril 1994; 61: 349

87. Bastiaan HS, et al. Relationship between zona pellucida-induced acrosome reaction, sperm morphology, sperm–zona pellucida binding, and in vitro fertilization. Fertil Steril 2003; 79: 49

88. Toner JP, et al. Value of sperm morphology assessed by strict criteria for prediction of the outcome of artificial (intrauterine) insemination. Andrologia 1995; 27: 143

89. Spiessens C, et al. Isolated teratozoospermia and intrauterine insemination. Fertil Steril 2003; 80: 1185

90. Duran HE, et al. Intrauterine insemination: a systematic review on determinants of success. Hum Reprod Update 2002; 8: 373

91. Moosani N, et al. Chromosomal analysis of sperm from men with idiopathic infertility using sperm karyotyping and fluorescence in situ hybridization. Fertil Steril 1995; 64: 811

92. Harkonen K, Suominen J, Lahdetie J. Aneuploidy in spermatozoa of infertile men with teratozoospermia. Int J Androl 2001; 24: 197

93. Calogero AE, et al. Aneuploidy rate in spermatozoa of selected men with abnormal semen parameters. Hum Reprod 2001; 16: 1172

94. McInnes B, et al. Abnormalities for chromosomes 13 and 21 detected in spermatozoa from infertile men. Hum Reprod 1998; 13: 2787

95. Templado C, et al. Aneuploid spermatozoa in infertile men: teratozoospermia. Mol Reprod Dev 2002; 61: 200

96. Lewis-Jones I, et al. Sperm chromosomal abnormalities are linked to sperm morphologic deformities. Fertil Steril 2003; 79: 212

97. Miharu N, Best RG, Young SR. Numerical chromosome abnormalities in spermatozoa of fertile and infertile men detected by fluorescence in situ hybridization. Hum Genet 1994; 93: 502

98. Guttenbach M, et al. Incidence of diploid and disomic sperm nuclei in 45 infertile men. Hum Reprod 1997; 12: 468

99. Celik-Ozenci C, et al. Sperm selection for ICSI: shape properties do not predict the absence or presence of numerical chromosomal aberrations. Hum Reprod 2004; 19: 2052

100. Vicari E, et al. Absolute polymorphic teratozoospermia in patients with oligo-asthenozoospermia is associated with an elevated sperm aneuploidy rate. J Androl 2003; 24: 598

101. Gole LA, et al. Does sperm morphology play a significant role in increased sex chromosomal disomy? A comparison between patients with teratozoospermia and OAT by FISH. J Androl 2001; 22: 759

102. Burrello N, et al. Morphologically normal spermatozoa of patients with secretory oligo-astheno-teratozoospermia have an increased aneuploidy rate. Hum Reprod 2004; 19: 2298

103. Meistrich ML, Trostle-Weige PK, Womack JE. Mapping of the azh locus to mouse chromosome 4. J Hered 1992; 83: 56

104. Mendoza-Lujambio I, et al. The Hook1 gene is non-functional in the abnormal spermatozoon head shape (azh) mutant mouse. Hum Mol Genet 2002; 11: 1647

105. Adham IM, et al. Teratozoospermia in mice lacking the transition protein 2 (Tnp2). Mol Hum Reprod 2001; 7: 513

106. Xu X, et al. Globozoospermia in mice lacking the casein kinase II alpha' catalytic subunit. Nat Genet 1999; 23: 118

107. von Bulow M, et al. Molecular nature of calicin, a major basic protein of the mammalian sperm head cytoskeleton. Exp Cell Res 1995; 219: 407

108. Rousseaux-Prevost R, et al. Abnormal expression of protein 4.1 in spermatozoa of infertile men with teratospermia. Lancet 1994; 343: 764

109. Milatiner D, et al. Associations between androgen receptor CAG repeat length and sperm morphology. Hum Reprod 2004; 19: 1426

110. Martin-du Pan RC, Campana A. Physiopathology of spermatogenic arrest. Fertil Steril 1993; 60: 937

111. Tesarik J, et al. In-vitro effects of FSH and testosterone withdrawal on caspase activation and DNA fragmentation in different cell types of human seminiferous epithelium. Hum Reprod 2002; 17: 1811

112. Matzuk MM, Lamb DJ. Genetic dissection of mammalian fertility pathways. Nat Med 2002; 8(Suppl): S33

113. Maduro MR, et al. Microsatellite instability and defects in mismatch repair proteins: a new aetiology for Sertoli cell-only syndrome. Mol Hum Reprod 2003; 9: 61

114. Casella R, et al. Androgen receptor gene polyglutamine length is associated with testicular histology in infertile patients. J Urol 2003; 169: 224

115. Lin WW, et al. Apoptotic frequency is increased in spermatogenic maturation arrest and hypospermatogenic states. J Urol 1997; 158: 1791

116. Lin WW, et al. Demonstration of testicular apoptosis in human male infertility states using a DNA laddering technique. Int Urol Nephrol 1999; 31: 361

117. Tesarik J, et al. Caspase-dependent and -independent DNA fragmentation in Sertoli and germ cells from men with primary testicular failure: relationship with histological diagnosis. Hum Reprod 2004; 19: 254

118. Aitken RJ, et al. Reactive oxygen species generation by human spermatozoa is induced by exogenous NADPH and inhibited by the flavoprotein inhibitors diphenylene iodonium and quinacrine. Mol Reprod Dev 1997; 47: 468

119. Gergely A, et al. Morphometric assessment of mature and diminished-maturity human spermatozoa: sperm regions that reflect differences in maturity. Hum Reprod 1999; 14: 2007

120. Vernet P, Aitken RJ, Drevet JR. Antioxidant strategies in the epididymis. Mol Cell Endocrinol 2004; 216: 31

121. Ombelet W, et al. Semen quality and intrauterine insemination. Reprod Biomed Online 2003; 7: 485

122. Arslan M, et al. Predictive value of sperm–zona pellucida binding capacity under hemizona assay conditions for pregnancy outcome in intrauterine insemination therapy. Hum Reprod 2005; in press

123. Katsuki T, et al. Prediction of outcomes of assisted reproduction treatment using the calcium ionophore-induced acrosome reaction. Hum Reprod 2005; 20: 469

124. Duran EH, et al. Sperm DNA quality predicts intrauterine insemination outcome: a prospective cohort study. Hum Reprod 2002; 17: 3122

125. Oehninger S, et al. Corrective measures and pregnancy outcome in in vitro fertilization in patients with severe sperm morphology abnormalities. Fertil Steril 1988; 50: 283

126. Oehninger S, et al. A comparative analysis of embryo implantation potential in patients with severe teratozoospermia undergoing in-vitro fertilization with a high insemination concentration or intracytoplasmic sperm injection. Hum Reprod 1996; 11: 1086

127. Oehninger S. Place of intracytoplasmic sperm injection in management of male infertility. Lancet 2001; 357: 2068

128. Oehninger S, Franken D, Kruger T. Approaching the next millennium: how should we manage andrology diagnosis in the intracytoplasmic sperm injection era? Fertil Steril 1997; 67: 434

129. Liu de Y, Baker HW. Disordered zona pellucida-induced acrosome reaction and failure of in vitro fertilization in patients with unexplained infertility. Fertil Steril 2003; 79: 74

130. Liu de Y, Garrett C, Baker HW. Clinical application of sperm–oocyte interaction tests in in vitro fertilization – embryo transfer and intracytoplasmic sperm injection programs. Fertil Steril 2004; 82: 1251

131. Silber SJ, et al. High fertilization and pregnancy rate after intracytoplasmic sperm injection with spermatozoa obtained from testicle biopsy. Hum Reprod 1995; 10: 148

132. Palermo GD, et al. Fertilization and pregnancy outcome with intracytoplasmic sperm injection for azoospermic men. Hum Reprod 1999; 14: 741

133. Tournaye H. Surgical sperm recovery for intracytoplasmic sperm injection: which method is to be preferred? Hum Reprod 1999; 14 (Suppl 1): 71

134. Monzó A, et al. Outcome of intracytoplasmic sperm injection in azoospermic patients: stressing the liaison between the urologist and reproductive medicine specialist. Urology 2001; 58: 69

135. Ola B, et al. Should ICSI be the treatment of choice for all cases of in-vitro conception? Considerations of fertilization and embryo development, cost effectiveness and safety. Hum Reprod 2001; 16: 2485

136. Oehninger S, Gosden RG. Should ICSI be the treatment of choice for all cases of in-vitro conception? No, not in light of the scientific data. Hum Reprod 2002; 17: 2237

137. Greco E, et al. Efficient treatment of infertility due to sperm DNA damage by ICSI with testicular spermatozoa. Hum Reprod 2005; 20: 226

138. Oehninger S. Strategies for fertility preservation in female and male cancer survivors. J Soc Gynecol Invest 2005; 12: 222

139. Tournaye H. Use of testicular sperm for the treatment of male infertility. Baillieres Clin Obstet Gynaecol 1997; 11: 753

140. Oehninger S, et al. Assessment of sperm cryodamage and strategies to improve outcome. Mol Cell Endocrinol 2000; 169: 3

141. Brinster RL, Zimmermann JW. Spermatogenesis following male germ-cell transplantation. Proc Natl Acad Sci USA 1994; 91: 11298

142. Tesarik J, et al. Pharmacological concentrations of follicle-stimulating hormone and testosterone improve the efficacy of in vitro germ cell differentiation in men with maturation arrest. Fertil Steril 2002; 77: 245

143. Tanaka A, et al. Completion of meiosis in human primary spermatocytes through in vitro coculture with Vero cells. Fertil Steril 2003; 79 (Suppl 1): 795

144. Cozzolino DJ, Lamb DJ. Germ cell transplantation: a potential treatment of severe testicular failure. Curr Urol Rep 2000; 1: 262

145. Tesarik J. Overcoming maturation arrest by in vitro spermatogenesis: search for the optimal culture system. Fertil Steril 2004; 81: 1417

22

Urological interventions for the treatment of male infertility

Victor M Brugh, Donald F Lynch Jr

INTRODUCTION

In the United States and Europe, 20% of couples either are unable to conceive, or have fewer children than they would like to have. In 50% of these cases, problems with the male partner are either the primary difficulty or an important contributor to the couple's inability to achieve a pregnancy. The urologist is often the first specialist that the man will see regarding his infertility.

In the past two decades, major advances in assisted reproduction have made it possible for couples who previously could never have achieved pregnancy to have the families they desire. With the evolution of new treatments, the role of the urologist as an integral part of the assisted reproduction team has expanded. This chapter describes non-surgical evaluation and treatment as well as several fertility-related surgical procedures that the urologist can be expected to provide.

VARICOCELE

Varicoceles are the most common correctable cause of male infertility. A varicocele is comprised of dilated internal spermatic veins which course along the spermatic cord with the vasal and cremasteric veins, often producing a characteristic 'bag of worms' mass in the scrotum. Varicoceles occur in about 15% of the general population, but are found in up to 35% of men being evaluated for primary infertility and up to 80% of men with secondary infertility[1]. They may be completely asymptomatic or may be associated with scrotal pain, often brought on by physical exertion or prolonged standing.

Varicoceles are thought to be caused by incompetent venous valves in the spermatic veins. They are most common on the left side, but frequently occur bilaterally. Several studies in both animals and humans have shown that varicoceles are associated with a progressive and time-dependent deterioration in testicular function. One theory holds that the impaired venous drainage disrupts heat regulation in the scrotum and cord, and the resulting elevated testicular temperature results in diminished spermatogenesis. The build-up of toxic substances in the testis from decreased venous drainage may also contribute to faulty sperm production[2]. Characteristically, the semen analysis demonstrates a decrease not only in total sperm count and motility but also in the numbers of normal sperm as measured by strict criteria.

VARICOCELE REPAIR

There are several surgical approaches for the repair of varicoceles using retroperitoneal, inguinal and subinguinal approaches. Open retroperitoneal varicocele repair (Palomo procedure) usually involves a small muscle-splitting incision at the level of the internal inguinal ring, with exposure of the internal spermatic vein or veins retroperitoneally near the left ureter[3]. At this level the testicular artery is usually separated from the internal spermatic vein, and often only one or two veins are present. The retroperitoneal approach may also be managed laparoscopically, with the surgeon mobilizing the internal spermatic vein and ligating it close to its drainage into the left renal vein[4]. Either procedure is quick, well-tolerated and easily performed on an outpatient basis by an experienced surgeon. However, disadvantages include a high incidence (15%) of recurrence, thought to be due to small parallel collaterals which may not be evident at the time of initial surgery, as well as postoperative hydrocele, which may develop in up to a third of patients[5].

In the inguinal approach (Ivanissevich procedure), a 3–4-cm incision is made in the groin, and the spermatic cord is mobilized over a Penrose drain. Using loupe lenses or an operating microscope, the branches of the testicular artery and the major lymphatic channels are carefully identified and spared, while the veins are systematically ligated and divided. Some surgeons will also mobilize the testis and ligate and divide the gubernacular veins and external spermatic perforators[6,7].

With the subinguinal approach, the incision is made just below the external inguinal ring, and the spermatic cord is mobilized over a section of Penrose drain. The testis can be mobilized through the incision, and the internal spermatic perforators and gubernacular veins are ligated and divided. Using magnification, and taking care to spare the lymphatics and the branches of the testicular artery, the veins are carefully ligated and divided[8].

Varicocelectomy results in a significant improvement in semen quality in 60–80% of patients, with spontaneous pregnancy rates ranging from 20 to 60% being reported. There have been few randomized trials assessing the results of varicocelectomy, but Madgar et al. reported that 71% of men treated with varicocelectomy achieved spontaneous pregnancy, compared with 10% of men randomized to no treatment in a prospective trial[9]. In addition to improvements in sperm count, motility and pregnancy rates, substantial improvements in sperm strict morphology[10–12], the sperm penetration assay and seminal reactive oxygen species have recently been described following varicocele repair[13]. Return of sperm to the ejaculate has been reported for some azoospermic men following varicocele repair[14].

ENDOCRINOPATHIES

The hormonal milieu of the testis plays a critical role in spermatogenesis. The cornerstone of hormonal control lies in the hypothalamic–pituitary–gonadal (HPG) axis. The hypothalamus is the center of the HPG axis as it receives input from many regions within the brain, as well as feedback in the form of steroid and protein hormones from both the gonads and adrenal glands. The hypothalamus releases gonadotropin-releasing hormone (GnRH) from the preoptic and arcuate nuclei as the end result of its integrative function. GnRH, in turn, is secreted in a pulsatile fashion into the portal hypophyseal vasculature, which feeds the anterior pituitary. GnRH stimulates the release of luteinizing hormone (LH) and follicle stimulating hormone (FSH) from the anterior pituitary gland. LH release is modulated by the feedback of androgens at both the pituitary and hypothalamic levels. The release of FSH appears to be regulated by the negative feedback of inhibin from the Sertoli cells of the testis. In the testis, LH stimulates testosterone production by the Leydig cells, whereas FSH is crucial to the initiation and maintenance of spermatogenesis. Both LH and FSH are necessary for quantitatively normal spermatogenesis. Feedback within this axis is essential for normal function and it occurs at multiple levels, allowing for precise regulation of hormonal activity. Abnormalities anywhere in the HPG axis have the potential for a negative impact on fertility in the male, and may include abnormal hormone production or receptor function at any level in the HPG axis. In general, endocrine defects leading to male infertility can be initially evaluated by assaying testosterone, LH, FSH, prolactin and estradiol.

Disorders of production or secretion of GnRH

Disorders resulting in abnormal synthesis and release of GnRH and subsequent low levels of FSH and LH without an anatomical cause are termed idiopathic hypogonadotropic hypogonadism (IHH). Without adequate levels of gonadotropins, androgen production and spermatogenesis fails.

Kallmann's syndrome is a deficiency in GnRH secretion from the hypothalamus, and is the most common X-linked disorder in male infertility, occurring in approximately 1 in 10 000 to 1 in 60 000 live births[15,16]. Kallmann's syndrome results from a mutation in the *Ka1* gene (Xp22.3). Phenotypic characteristics of these patients include: tall stature, anosmia, firm prepubertal-size testes and small penis. Due to the lack of FSH and LH stimulation of the testis, spermatogenesis is absent as is testosterone production, and some patients will present due to failure of pubertal initiation.

Fertility can be achieved in many IHH patients with hormone replacement[17]. GnRH can be given exogenously via an infusion pump with 90-minute pulses, or twice daily subcutaneous injections. The more common treatment approach for IHH involves starting hormone replacement with human chorionic gonadotropin (hCG) (2000 IU subcutaneously three times a week). Treatment with hCG will initiate spermatogenesis, although completion of spermatogenesis often requires the addition of FSH either as human menopausal gonadotropin (hMG) or recombinant FSH (37.5–75 IU intramuscularly three times a week)

3–6 months after initiation of hCG. Other defects in GnRH secretion or the GnRH receptor lead to IHH that can also be treated with replacement of FSH and hCG.

Disorders of pituitary function

LH and FSH are released from the pituitary under the influence of the pulsatile stimulation of GnRH. Pituitary masses can interfere with the release of gonadotropins either via direct compression of the portal system or by decreased FSH/LH secretion, resulting in hypogonadotropic hypogonadism. In patients with decreased testosterone levels in the setting of low LH, one must consider a pituitary adenoma, and magnetic resonance imaging (MRI) of the head is essential.

Hyperprolactinemia can also be seen in association with adenomas of the pituitary. Hyperprolactinemia may also be caused by the selective serotonin reuptake inhibitors (SSRIs), which have become widely prescribed for numerous mental-health conditions. Elevated prolactin interferes with the normal pulsatile release of GnRH, and thus can itself be a cause of hypogonadism with subsequent sexual dysfunction and infertility. Surgery, radiation and medical treatment have all been used as effective treatment, with cabergoline (Dostinex®) and bromocriptine (Parlodel®) as the mainstays of medical therapy. In general, evaluation of the pituitary with MRI is only warranted when symptoms and/or routine hormone studies suggest pituitary disease.

Mutations resulting in biologically inactive FSH or LH are due to abnormalities in FSH or LH structure, or FSH or LH receptor activity. These abnormalities result in a spectrum of disease from complete virilization failure to less severe hypogonadism[18–20].

Disorders of testosterone synthesis and function

Androgen synthesis and metabolism is a complex, stepwise process, and mutations in the enzymes involved in this biosynthesis will influence male reproductive function. Five enzymes are required for the synthesis of testosterone from cholesterol. Mutations in these enzymes lead to congenital adrenal hyperplasia, resulting in phenotypes ranging from incomplete virilization to completely feminized genitalia with cryptorchid testes[22]. Testosterone is metabolized to dihydrotestosterone (DHT) by 5α-reductase in the external genitalia and prostate. Mutations in the 5α-reductase gene lead to incomplete development of the external genitalia[21], and infertility follows due to the inability to deliver sperm effectively.

Testosterone and DHT diffuse freely into all cells, although they can be delivered to the nucleus only by androgen receptors in order to effect cellular activity. Defects in the androgen receptor gene (AR) defunctionalize this receptor, and may cause a wide range of internal and external virilization abnormalities known as androgen-insensitivity syndromes (Reifenstein's syndrome, testicular feminization, Lub's syndrome and Rosewater's syndrome)[22]. Another form of androgen insensitivity is due to the expansion of a polyglutamine tract within the AR transactivation domain, and is associated with an adult-onset motor neuron disease. Spinal and bulbar muscular atrophy (SMBA) or Kennedy's disease is an X-linked genetic disease. These patients have progressive weakness in the proximal spinal and bulbar muscles with associated gynecomastia, testicular atrophy and spermatogenic impairment that begin during midlife[23].

Today, testosterone replacement with different gels, patches and injection therapies has become quite common. More frequently than ever, reproductive-aged patients who have been evaluated for low energy levels, poor libido or erectile dysfunction are started on testosterone replacement. Other men will use anabolic steroids for professional or amateur body-building. It is well understood that the administration of exogenous androgen causes a suppression of endogenous testosterone production. The absence of adequate intratesticular levels of testosterone leads to the

failure of spermatogenesis and subsequent azoospermia. The extent and reversibility of the detrimental effect of steroids on spermatogenesis are variable. Spermatogenesis will return in 6 months to 1 year after discontinuation of exogenous testosterone in many men[24]. If normal endogenous testosterone production does not return, some men may be successfully treated with hCG and hMG to restart testicular testosterone production and spermatogenesis[25].

Other hormonal therapies exist for the treatment of men with idiopathic oligospermia, including the use of aromatase inhibitors and antiestrogens. Testosterone is metabolized to estradiol by aromatase. This conversion may be blocked by aromatase inhibitors such as testolactone (steroidal aromatase inhibitor) or anastrozole and letrozole (non-steroidal aromatase inhibitors). Early studies using testolactone for the treatment of idiopathic oligospermia had mixed results, and one randomized placebo-controlled double-blind crossover study showed no advantage of testolactone over placebo[26]. Recent investigations have revealed a subpopulation of men with poor sperm concentration and motility who have decreased testosterone/estradiol ratios. In these patients, treatment with aromatase inhibitors, anastrozole and letrozole, has resulted in statistically significant increases in sperm concentration and motility[27].

Circulating estradiol causes feedback inhibition of the secretion of GnRH. Antiestrogens such as clomiphene citrate and tamoxifen citrate block feedback inhibition of estrogen at the level of the hypothalamus, and lead to increased secretion of LH and FSH. The overall effect of these medications is the increased production of testosterone and possibly increased spermatogenesis. There are many uncontrolled studies revealing improved semen parameters for men with idiopathic oligospermia using clomiphene citrate. However, in a review of ten randomized controlled studies using clomiphene or tamoxifen, increases in testosterone levels were seen, but ultimate pregnancy rates were similar in the treatment and placebo arms[28]. Finally, a small proportion of men treated with clomiphene citrate will experience worsening semen parameters[29].

CRYPTORCHIDISM AND ORCHIOPEXY

Although up to 5% of male infants may exhibit testicular maldescent at birth, the incidence of cryptorchidism at 1 year of age is 0.8%[30,31]. Spontaneous descent of the testis does not occur after 6–9 months, and attempts to treat cryptorchidism with hormonal manipulation have been disappointing. Over the past three decades, the ideal age for surgical intervention has declined from just before puberty to about 1 year. After that time, structural changes suggesting deterioration have been identified in the cryptorchid testis, and evidence suggests that, left alone, such testes progress to be reproductively non-functional by puberty, with Sertoli-cell-only findings in 70%. Intervention at around 1 year of age is also favorable from both anesthetic risk and psychological perspectives[32].

Boys born with cryptorchidism are known to be at increased risk of developing testicular malignancy. Orchiopexy does not alter this risk, but does bring the testis to a position where it can be more easily examined. Men with a history of testicular maldescent should undergo testis biopsy to assess for carcinoma *in situ* at the time of a testicular intervention for infertility.

A variety of surgical procedures have been described for the correction of testicular maldescent. Bevan described the principles for a successful orchiopexy: adequate mobilization of the spermatic cord, repair of the associated hernia and satisfactory placement and fixation of the testis in the scrotum[33]. While the majority of maldescended testes will lie within the inguinal canal or just within the internal inguinal ring, some may be intra-abdominal or frankly ectopic, located anywhere from the suprapubic tissues to the perineum[34].

In a standard orchiopexy, an inguinal incision is carried down to the inguinal canal, which is opened, taking care to avoid injury to the ilioinguinal nerve. The spermatic cord is identified, gently separated from the floor of the canal and retracted with a vessel loop. With proximal traction on the cord, the testis is identified and its abnormal gubernacular attachments divided. It is then carefully mobilized to the level of the internal inguinal ring. At this point it is separated from the accompanying hernia. Taking care to protect the vas deferens, the sac is ligated and excised. Dissection of the cord is continued up into the retroperitoneal space until a sufficient length of spermatic cord is obtained, to allow placement of the testis in the scrotum without tension. The testis is then secured with permanent suture in a scrotal 'dartos pouch' developed between the skin and the dartos fascia. The scrotal skin and the inguinal incision are then closed with fine Vicryl® or Monocryl® suture[35].

When the testis is high in the canal, at the level of the internal ring, or just within the ring in the retroperitoneal space, transection of the testicular artery and mobilization of the testis as described by Fowler and Stephens may be required[36]. Laparoscopic techniques have also been employed, and microvascular autotransplantation may be indicated in some difficult cases[37].

DISORDERS OF EJACULATION AND DUCTAL OBSTRUCTION

Patients with dysfunctional ejaculation and obstructive disorders are unique in that many will have normal spermatogenesis, and the cause of infertility lies only in the inability to deliver sperm to the vaginal vault. Therefore, some of these couples have multiple treatment options, including medical (for some men with ejaculatory dysfunction) or surgical either by reconstruction or testicular sperm extraction in conjunction with *in vitro* fertilization/intracytoplasmic sperm injection (IVF/ICSI).

Ejaculatory dysfunction

Ejaculation consists of the coordinated deposition of semen into the prostatic urethra (emission), closure of the bladder neck and contraction of the periurethral and pelvic floor muscles causing expulsion of the semen through the urethra (ejaculation). The process of ejaculation is dependent on central and peripheral nervous-system control. Emission is controlled by sympathetic neurons originating from T10–L3 that travel through the paravertebral sympathetic ganglia. Ejaculation requires somatic motor innervation from S2–4, and continues through the pudendal nerves to the bladder neck and pelvic floor musculature.

Abnormalities of ejaculation can result from lack of emission or ejaculation and retrograde ejaculation. Failure of emission or ejaculation can be caused by excision of a portion of the sympathetic chain or pelvic nerves during retroperitoneal lymph node dissection for testicular cancer, or other retroperitoneal, abdominal or pelvic surgery. Retrograde ejaculation is caused by incomplete closure of the bladder neck during ejaculation. Diabetes mellitus causes peripheral nervous system injury, resulting in possible retrograde ejaculation or anejaculation. Central nervous system lesions, such as spinal cord injury and myelodysplasia, can also cause ejaculatory dysfunction. Finally, some medications will affect ejaculation, such as α-blockers (causing retrograde ejaculation), antidepressants, antipsychotics and some antihypertensives (causing anorgasmia or retarded ejaculation). Anatomical causes of ejaculatory dysfunction include obstruction of the ejaculatory ducts, and prior surgery on the bladder neck (YV-plasty of the bladder neck, transurethral incision or resection of the prostate) leading to retrograde ejaculation.

Treatment of ejaculatory disorders may be medical or surgical. Neurological causes of failure of emission or ejaculation and retrograde ejaculation can be treated with sympathomimetic agents that will enhance emission and close the bladder neck. These medications include imipramine hydrochloride and pseudoephedrine hydrochloride. Overall, medical therapy for ejaculatory dysfunction is successful in 50% of cases[38]. If conversion from retrograde to antegrade ejaculation fails or if an anejaculatory male is converted to retrograde ejaculation, functional sperm may be retrieved from the bladder and used for intrauterine insemination or IVF cycles. In order to attain viable sperm in a post-ejaculate urine specimen, the urine pH must be raised to 7.5 or higher with alkalinizing agents such as sodium bicarbonate or potassium citrate. Other techniques to attain semen from men with ejaculatory dysfunction include vibratory stimulation and electroejaculation. Vibratory stimulation requires the use of a vibrator to induce ejaculation, and requires an intact reflex arc within the thoracolumbar spinal cord[39]. The best predictors of success using this technique include reflex hip flexion when the soles of the feet are scratched[40] and an intact bulbocavernosus reflex[41]. Vibratory stimulation leads to successful ejaculation in up to 83% of spinal cord-injured males in some studies[42].

Men who fail both medical therapy and vibratory stimulation may proceed to electroejaculation. Electroejaculation requires general anesthesia in the incomplete paraplegic male and in men with anejaculation secondary to retroperitoneal lymph node dissection. This procedure causes electrical stimulation of ejaculation using a rectal probe, and is almost uniformly successful. The most significant risk of electroejaculation is triggering autonomic dysreflexia in the spinal cord-injury patient. Nowadays, for men who fail therapies to induce ejaculation, men who do not desire these techniques and couples with a female factor requiring IVF, epididymal or testicular sperm extraction with IVF/ICSI is the recommended treatment option.

OBSTRUCTION

Obstruction of the excretory ductal system can occur along the ejaculatory ducts, vas deferens or epididymis. History, physical examination, semen parameters and radiological studies can be used to identify the location of the obstruction. Vasal obstruction is most commonly caused by vasectomy, but may also be caused by scrotal, inguinal (such as hernia repair) or pelvic surgery. Scrotal surgery, such as prior spermatocelectomy, orchiopexy or hydrocelectomy, may result in epididymal obstruction. Also, recurrent bouts of epididymitis may lead to epididymal obstruction. On physical examination, the absence of the vas deferens will be found in patients with congenital bilateral absence of the vas deferens (CBAVD), and dilated epididymides indicates possible obstruction.

VASECTOMY

Vasectomy is a popular form of permanent birth control in the United States, with some half a million men undergoing the procedure each year. It is largely successful, with reported failure rates of only 0.1–0.3%, if the vas stumps are ligated and cauterized. Although some initial studies have suggested a possible link between vasectomy and cardiac death, more recent studies have shown no such association. Additionally, concerns about a possible increased risk of prostatic adenocarcinoma and testicular tumors in vasectomized men in early studies are now felt to be the result of statistical selection bias. Epidemiological studies are continuing, but at present there is no convincing evidence of increased tumor risk to suggest that a change in the clinical practice of vasectomy is indicated[43].

Vasectomy technique

Conventional vasectomy

The vas should be isolated from the other spermatic cord structures by palpation, and the skin of the scrotum overlying it and the tissues around it infiltrated with 0.2% lidocaine without epinephrine. The vas is fixated to the scrotal skin with a towel clip, and a 4–7-mm incision made over it. The vas is identified and carefully dissected away from the vasal and spermatic cord vessels. The vas is then ligated or doubly clipped distally and proximally isolating a 5-mm segment of vas. This segment is then excised, and the cut ends of the vas fulgurated to seal the vasal lumens. Alternatively, the vas can be ligated with silk or Vicryl suture and then fulgurated. The scrotal skin incision is then closed with 4-0 Vicryl suture. An identical procedure is then performed on the contralateral side.

'No-scalpel' technique

An alternative technique developed in China uses a special clamp designed to grasp the vas and fixate it to the scrotal skin. A specially modified dissecting curved hemostat is then used to puncture the skin and create an opening large enough to mobilize a segment of vas. A large enough portion of the vas is teased out through the puncture so that it can be ligated and divided or fulgurated. The stumps are returned to the scrotum. The puncture site is usually small enough not to require sutures, and bleeding and manipulation of the tissues are minimized, resulting in less discomfort and return to normal activity almost immediately[44].

Postoperative evaluation of the semen is performed 4–6 weeks following the vasectomy, and again 4–6 weeks later. The presence of persistent sperm in the semen beyond 3 months suggests that the procedure has failed and should be repeated.

Vasectomy reversal

Vasovasostomy

Some 2–6% of men who have undergone vasectomy will subsequently request a reversal. Additionally, damage to the vasa deferentia in the groin from hernia repairs and other procedures may occur. Some reports suggest that injuries to the vas from pediatric hernia repairs may be 1–2%[45].

Change in marital status, with the desire on the part of the new couple to have children of their own, constitutes the largest group of men requesting reversal. There are several procedures in widespread use.

Modified single-layer vasovasostomy With the patient anesthetized in the supine position, the sites of the vasectomy are identified by palpation. Using either a midline scrotal incision or bilateral upper scrotal incisions – depending on the level of the previous vasectomy – the testis is mobilized and removed from the hemiscrotum and wrapped in a moist sponge, and the vas site is mobilized and exposed. The scarred tissues surrounding the vas site and the sperm granuloma, if present, are resected. The microscope is then positioned, and the abdominal vas stump examined. The lumen may require gentle dilatation with lacrimal duct probes to allow insertion of a 27-gauge pediatric intracath. A small amount of saline is then gently injected to assure patency of that segment of the vas.

The lumen of the testicular segment is then examined for fluid, which may range from thin and watery to somewhat thick and pasty in consistency. A touch prep of distal vasal fluid is done, and the fluid examined under the microscope for the presence of sperm. If no fluid is encountered, additional vas is excised, and the examination is repeated. In some instances, if no fluid or sperm are seen, vasoepididymostomy may be indicated. Testicular biopsy, if indicated, can be done easily at this point.

Once the vas segments have been prepared and checked for patency, they are aligned in a vas clip, and a posterior serosal suture of 8-0 nylon is placed. Four through-and-through sutures of 9-0 nylon are then placed 90° apart, through the serosa, into the lumen, and back through the opposite lumen and out. These are secured with square knots assuring good alignment of the vasal lumens. Occasionally, if the structures or lumens are large, additional through-and-through sutures may be required.

Once the vasal ends are aligned and the through-and-through sutures are secured, 4–6 serosal sutures are then placed to assure a watertight anastomosis. The vasa are further anchored to the surrounding cord structures with sutures of 4-0 chromic, and the testis is then returned to the scrotum. The contralateral vasovasostomy is performed in a similar manner. Following completion of both vasal reanastomoses, the scrotum is closed in layers without drains[46].

Two-layer vasovasostomy ('Microdot' technique) Initial exposure and preparation of the vas is as described for the modified one-layer procedure. Once the vasa are mobilized and their ends prepared, 6–8 microdots are placed on the muscularis in radial fashion around the lumen using a microtip marking-pen. The vas is then stabilized with the cut ends closely approximated using a vas clip. Double-armed 10-0 nylon sutures are then placed through the lumens, exiting through the microdots. Three or four such sutures are placed in the anterior aspect of the vas, and then two serosal sutures of 8-0 nylon are placed to secure further the anterior anastomosis. The clip and vas are then rotated 180°, and three or four additional 10-0 nylon sutures are placed to finish the mucosal anastomosis. Three or four additional 8-0 nylon serosal sutures complete the vasal anastomosis. The use of double-armed mucosal sutures reduces the risk of 'back walling'. The vasal sheath is secured with 4-0 or 5-0 chromic or Vicryl suture, and the scrotum is then closed as described above. Drains are placed only if extensive dissection has taken place.

Although both techniques have their advocates, results are similar, with return of sperm to the ejaculate in 80–90% of cases, and pregnancy rates of 50–65%[46,47]. Even if counts do not reach 'normal' levels, sperm are made readily available for intrauterine insemination (IUI) or ICSI procedures.

Vasoepididymostomy In instances where the distal epididymis is obstructed, vasoepididymostomy above the level of obstruction should be performed. Once the testis and vas have been mobilized, and epididymal obstruction confirmed, examination of the epididymis with the operating microscope will usually reveal dilated epididymal tubules. Occasionally the site of epididymal obstruction can be identified. It is essential to assure that the proximal segment of vas can reach the epididymis to allow a tension-free anastomosis. Mobilizing the globus minor and isthmus of the epididymis from the vas can result in additional length.

The tunic covering the epididymis is opened, and a dilated loop of epididymal tubule is gently mobilized with microscissors. A small incision is made in one of the proximal tubules, and fluid is obtained and examined under the microscope for the presence of normal-appearing sperm. A tension-free end-to-side anastomosis using 9-0 or 10-0 nylon is then completed, usually with four or five sutures. The serosa of the vas is secured to the fibrous tunic of the epididymis. Additional anchoring sutures of 8-0 or 9-0 nylon are placed to secure the vasal serosa to the epididymal tunic just above the anastomosis, taking care not to place these too deep and risk injuring or occluding the epididymis.

The testis is then returned to the scrotum and the scrotum closed, usually with no drain. In several series, return of sperm to the ejaculate ranged from around 60 to 85%, with pregnancy rates of 30–45%[48].

VASOVASOSTOMY VERSUS ICSI

The choice of a vasovasostomy or ICSI will depend on several factors, including the health status of the couple, the maternal age and the length of time since the vasectomy. For the younger couple who aspire to have more than one child together, vasovasostomy will likely be the more acceptable option. If successful, it will be significantly less expensive per pregnancy than ICSI. This would assume that the fertility status of

the woman is normal and that she is not approaching the menopause[49].

For couples where the female is in her mid- or late 30s or early 40s, a narrowing window of opportunity for pregnancy before the onset of premenopausal status may make ICSI the preferred option. For couples in whom there is a history of significant adverse factors or where gynecological disease is present – endocrine issues, endometriosis, anatomical abnormalities, prior surgery or pelvic inflammation – ICSI, with TESA or microsurgical epididymal sperm aspiration (MESA) as required, will likely provide more assurance of pregnancy than vasovasostomy[49,50].

For younger couples or selected older couples where a vasovasostomy has failed, repeat vasovasostomy or vasoepididymostomy has a reasonable success rate and may be less expensive than ICSI[50,51]. As ICSI delivery rates have continued to improve, however, this difference is diminishing.

OTHER SITES OF OBSTRUCTION

Semen analysis will vary with the site of obstruction. Complete ejaculatory duct obstruction (EDO) will result in a low-volume, acidic, fructose-negative ejaculate. Obstruction of the vasa or epididymides will result in a normal-volume, basic, fructose-positive ejaculate. Men with obstruction as the only cause for their infertility will have normal testosterone and FSH. Radiographic studies are necessary when obstruction of the ejaculatory ducts is suspected. Transrectal ultrasound (TRUS) will support the diagnosis of EDO by identifying dilated ejaculatory ducts and seminal vesicles as well as cystic masses and stones causing obstruction. A transrectal aspirate of dilated seminal vesicles during TRUS that reveals numerous sperm provides additional evidence that EDO is present. The absence or presence of hypoplastic seminal vesicles on TRUS is confirmatory of CBAVD. If vasal occlusion is suspected, a vasogram during scrotal exploration will confirm the diagnosis and identify the site of obstruction. Threading a 1-0 nylon suture through the abdominal vas at the time of vasography will determine the exact distance from the vasostomy to the site of obstruction. The treatment of choice for EDO is transurethral resection of the ejaculatory ducts (TURED). Approximately half of the men undergoing this procedure for EDO will have an improvement of their semen parameters, and half of the men who improve will achieve a subsequent pregnancy[52]. Men with vasal obstruction or obstruction at the epididymis are candidates for microsurgical reconstruction to allow natural conception, or MESA for sperm retrieval to be used with IVF/ICSI.

Congenital bilateral absence of the vas deferens

Congenital bilateral absence of the vas deferens (CBAVD) is the most frequently found congenital obstruction of the extratesticular ductal system, affecting 1–2% of infertile men. CBAVD is part of the phenotypic spectrum of cystic fibrosis (CF), an autosomal recessive disease, of which 1/25 Caucasians are carriers[53]. CF is caused by a genetic mutation of the cystic fibrosis transmembrane conductance regulator gene (CFTR). The CFTR gene is large (250 000 base pairs), and to date more than 1000 CFTR mutations have been identified. Characteristics of men with CBAVD include absence of the vas deferens, hypoplastic, non-functional seminal vesicles and ejaculatory ducts, and an epididymal remnant, frequently composed of only the caput region that is firm and distended[54]. Spermatogenesis is not impaired in these patients; therefore, sperm may be harvested from the epididymis with MESA or from the testis (TESA) for use in ICSI, allowing affected couples to achieve a pregnancy. Men with CBAVD and their wives should be screened for CFTR mutations and referred to genetic counseling prior to sperm retrieval.

Routine analysis of the CFTR gene is available from most genetic laboratories. Only about 30 mutations, of the possible 1000, are regularly screened for in the clinical diagnostic laboratory, so a specific mutation may be present that will not be identified. Therefore, the absence of a mutation in these limited assays will not guarantee that an offspring will not be born with cystic fibrosis if the wife is also a carrier. In addition to the 1000 known mutations in this gene, there is a polymorphism in intron 8 (non-coding region) that quantitatively influences the production of the CFTR gene product. The alleles of this polymorphic region of thymidines in intron 8 of the CFTR gene contain five (5T), seven (7T) or nine (9T) thymidines. The 5T allele results in the least efficient processing of CFTR mRNA. 5T mutations lead to a lower amount of protein production and increased severity of the observed phenotype[54].

To assess this most common polymorphism (5T), a separate analysis must be ordered; however, this test is not routinely run in all clinical laboratories performing routine cystic fibrosis gene analysis, reinforcing the limits associated with a negative result. Due to the many variable mutations and difficulty identifying all possible mutations in a single patient, all patients with CBAVD are now thought to have a genetic form of cystic fibrosis[54]. Men with idiopathic epididymal obstruction have also been found to have an increased incidence of CF mutations. These men should also undergo CF testing prior to reconstruction or MESA/TESA. Finally, patients presenting with unilateral absence of the vas deferens are also considered at risk and should undergo analysis of the CFTR gene, although unilateral absence of the vas deferens in a patient with a contralateral solitary kidney may represent a different congenital anomaly.

TESTIS BIOPSY

Biopsy of the testis is performed for diagnostic purposes, and also to obtain tubular tissue for the extraction of sperm for ICSI. It is usually an office procedure, performed under cord block with supplemental local anesthesia. Diagnostic biopsies may be done as a needle biopsy, using a spring-loaded biopsy needle such as that used for prostate biopsy.

When larger amounts of tubular tissue are required, the biopsy is performed as an open technique. The spermatic cord is blocked with 2% lidocaine or 0.5% bupivacaine, and the skin overlying the testis is also infiltrated with local anesthetic. A 4-0 Vicryl stay suture is placed medially into the scrotal skin, and a 1.5-cm transverse incision is carried down to open the scrotum and expose the tunica albuginea of the testis. A second 4-0 Vicryl stay suture is placed into the medial tunica albuginea, and a 4–5-mm incision made in the tunica. Usually, spermatic tubular tissue will bulge out, and a small (0.1 ml) volume of that tissue is excised with microscissors and placed on saline-soaked filter paper, or placed in holding medium, for evaluation by the embryologist. Once satisfactory sperm have been identified in the sample, the tunica is closed by running the 4-0 Vicryl stay suture, and the skin of the scrotum is also closed with 4-0 Vicryl skin stay suture[55].

Men with obstructive azoospermia who undergo testicular sperm extraction for ICSI should always be offered the possibility to cryopreserve testicular tissue for future use.

FUTURE DIRECTIONS: SPERMATOGONIAL STEM CELL TRANSPLANTATION

Spermatogenesis is the cornerstone of male fertility, and can be affected by many factors. Chemotherapy and radiotherapy halt spermatogenesis temporarily or permanently, and recovery may take years. With the current success of chemotherapy and radiotherapy for many malignancies, fertility after treatment has become a major concern. Males have the option of cryopreservation of semen, pre-therapy. While pre-emptive treatment for possible male infertility is helpful for many men, semen cryopreservation is not an option for prepubertal males or men with severely compromised semen parameters as a result of their illness, does not allow natural conception and allows only a limited number of attempts at pregnancy using assisted reproduction. Accordingly, novel methods are currently under development aimed at rejuvenation of spermatogenesis after toxic insult. Advances have been made in spermatogonial stem cell transplantation which allow sterile mice to be transplanted with donor spermatogonial stem cells, and donor-derived spermatogenesis is subsequently seen.

Brinster and colleagues first described successful spermatogonial stem cell transplantation in 1994[56,57]. Initially, a heterogeneous mixture of donor-mouse testis cells was collected from mice carrying the *Escherichia coli* β-galactosidase gene (LacZ). Expression of this gene allows the identification of successful recovery of transplanted donor-mouse spermatogenesis. The donor testis cells were microinjected into the seminiferous tubules of sterile mice (either Sertoli cell-only variants or busulfan-treated mice). Donor germ cells migrate through the luminal compartment to the base of the seminiferous epithelium. After allowing recipient mice to recover, donor-derived spermatogenesis can be identified after 1 month, and complete sperm production is present at 3 months[58]. Transplant techniques have been improved, with microinjection into the rete testes and efferent ductules, which are found to lead to more efficient transplantation into the seminiferous tubules. Also, conditions of low testosterone have been found to increase the efficiency of transplantation[59], and using cryptorchid donors has enhanced the spermatogonial stem cell population in the transplanted cells[60].

For men with malignancies who are interested in preserving their fertility, spermatogonial stem cell transplantation will allow the harvest of spermatogonial stem cells pre-therapy. These cells can be cryopreserved for use after the patient has completed his therapy and is rendered disease-free.

Transplantation of the spermatogonial stem cells will reinstate spermatogenesis and fertility. The current focus of research in this field is to identify markers to allow isolation of the spermatogonial stem cells. The spermatogonial stem cells will have to be isolated from potentially contaminating cancer cells prior to cryopreservation, to avoid recurrence of the original cancer through transplantation of the stem cells after therapy. Ultimately, this technique will allow prepubertal males as well as those with impaired spermatogenesis to preserve their fertility prior to cancer treatment, and will permit couples limitless attempts at conception after spermatogenesis has been reinstituted. Nevertheless, these techniques should still be considered as experimental in the human[61].

REFERENCES

1. Poland ML, et al. Variation of semen measures within normal men. Fertil Steril 1985; 44: 396

2. Gorelick J, Goldstein M. Loss of fertility in men with varicocoele. Fertil Steril 1993; 59: 613

3. Palomo A. Radical cure of varicocoele by a new technique: a preliminary report. J Urol 1949; 61: 604

4. Hagood PG, et al. Laparoscopic varicocoelectomy: a preliminary report of a new technique. J Urol 1992; 147: 73

5. Szabo R, Kessler R. Hydrocoele following internal spermatic vein ligation: a retrospective study and review of the literature. J Urol 1984; 132: 924

6. Ivanissevich O. Left varicocoele due to reflux. Experience with 44709 cases in 42 years. J Int Coll Surg 1960; 34: 742

7. Goldstein M, et al. Microsurgical inguinal varicocoelectomy with the delivery of the testis: an artery and lymphatic-sparing technique. J Urol 1992; 148: 1808

8. Marmar JL, DeBenedictis TJ, Praiss D. The management of varicocoeles by microdissection of the spermatic cord at the external inguinal ring. Fertil Steril 1985; 43: 583

9. Madgar I, et al. Controlled trial of high spermatic vein ligation for varicocele in infertile men. Fertil Steril 1995; 63: 120

10. Kibar Y, Seckin B, Erduran D. The effects of subinguinal varicocelectomy on Kruger morphology and semen parameters. J Urol 2002; 168: 1071

11. Schatte EC, et al. Varicocelectomy improves sperm strict morphology and motility. J Urol 1998; 160: 1338

12. Vazquez-Levin MH, et al., Response of routine semen analysis and critical assessment of sperm morphology by Kruger classification to therapeutic varicocelectomy. J Urol 1997; 158: 1804

13. Mostafa T, et al. Varicocelectomy reduces reactive oxygen species levels and increases antioxidant activity of seminal plasma from infertile men with varicocele. Int J Androl 2001; 24: 261

14. Kadioglu A, et al. Microsurgical inguinal varicocele repair in azoospermic men. Urology 2001; 57: 328

15. Franco B, et al. A gene deleted in Kallmann's syndrome shares homology with neural cell adhesion and axonal path-finding molecules. Nature 1991; 353: 529

16. Bick D, et al. Brief report: intragenic deletion of the KALIG-1 gene in Kallmann's syndrome. N Engl J Med 1992; 326: 1752

17. Sigman M, La HS. Evaluation of the subfertile male. In Lipshultz LI, Howards SS, eds. Infertility in the Male, 3rd edn. St Louis: Mosby, 1997: 173

18. Weiss J, et al. Hypogonadism caused by a single amino acid substitution in the beta subunit of luteinizing hormone. N Engl J Med 1992; 326: 179

19. Wu SM, et al. Luteinizing hormone receptor mutations in disorders of sexual development and cancer. Front Biosci 2000; 5: D343

20. Simoni M, et al. Mutational analysis of the follicle-stimulating hormone (FSH) receptor in normal and infertile men: identification and characterization of two discrete FSH receptor isoforms. J Clin Endocrinol Metab 1999; 84: 751

21. Griffin JE. Androgen resistance – the clinical and molecular spectrum. N Engl J Med 1992; 326: 611

22. Quigley CA, et al. Androgen receptor defects: historical, clinical, and molecular perspectives. Endocr Rev 1995; 16: 271

23. Casella R, et al. Significance of the polyglutamine tract polymorphism in the androgen receptor. Urology 2001; 58: 651

24. Gazvani MR, et al. Conservative management of azoospermia following steroid abuse. Hum Reprod 1997; 12: 1706

25. Menon DK. Successful treatment of anabolic-steroid-induced azoospermia with human chorionic gonadotropin and human menopausal gonadotropin. Fertil Steril 2003; 79(Suppl 3): 1659

26. Clark R, Sherins R. Treatment of men with idiopathic oligozoospermic infertility using the aromatase

inhibitor, testolactone: results of a double-blinded, randomized placebo-controlled trial with cross over. J Androl 1989; 10: 69

27. Pavlovich CP, et al. Evidence of a treatable endocrinopathy in infertile men. J Urol 2001; 165: 837

28. Vandekerckhove P, Lilford R, Vail A, et al. Clomiphene or tamoxifen for idiopathic oligo/asthenospermia. Cochrane Database Syst Rev 2003; (2): CD000151

29. Gilbaugh JH III, Lipshultz, LI. Nonsurgical treatment of male infertility. Urol Clin North Am 1994; 21: 531

30. Villumsen AL, Zachau-Christiansen B. Spontaneous alterations in position of the testes. Arch Dis Child 1966; 41: 198

31. Lynch DF, Brock WA, Kaplan GW. Orchiopexy: experiences at 2 centers. Urology 1982; 19: 507

32. Leissner J, et al. The undescended testis: considerations and impact on fertility. Br J Urol Int 1999; 83: 885

33. Bevan AD. The surgical treatment of undescended testicle: a further contribution. JAMA 1903; 41: 718

34. Kleinteich B, et al. Kongenitole Hodendiptopien. Stuttgart: George Thieme, 1979

35. Lattimer JK. Scrotal pouch technique for orchiopexy. J Urol 1957; 78: 628

36. Fowler R, Stephens FD. The role of testicular vascular anatomy in the salvage of high undescended testes. Aust NZ J Surg 1959; 29: 92

37. Frey P, Bianchi A. Microvascular autotransplantation of intra-abdominal testes. Prog Pediatr Surg 1989; 23: 115

38. Kamischke A, Nieschlag E. Treatment of retrograde ejaculation and anejaculation. Hum Reprod Update 1999; 5: 448

39. Shaban SFE, et al. Treatment of abnormalities of ejaculation. In Lipschultz LI, Howards SS, eds. Infertility in the Male, 3rd edn. St Louis: Mosby, 1997: 423

40. Brindley GS. Reflex ejaculation under vibratory stimulation in paraplegic men. Paraplegia. 1981;19:299-302

41. Bird VG, et al. Reflexes and somatic responses as predictors of ejaculation by penile vibratory stimulation in men with spinal cord injury. Spinal Cord 2001; 39: 514

42. Sonksen J, Biering-Sorensen F, Kristensen JK. Ejaculation induced by penile vibratory stimulation in men with spinal cord injuries. The importance of the vibratory amplitude. Paraplegia 1994; 32: 651

43. Giovannucci E, et al. A prostate cohort study of vasectomy and prostate cancer in US men. JAMA 1993; 269: 873.

44. Li S, et al. The no-scalpel vasectomy. J Urol 1991; 145: 341

45. Belker AM, et al. Results of 1469 microsurgical vasectomy reversals by the Vasovasostomy Study Group. J Urol 1991; 145: 505

46. Silber SJ. Microscopic vasectomy reversal. Fertil Steril 1977; 28: 1191

47. Owen ER. Microsurgical vasovasostomy: a reliable vasectomy reversal. Aust NZ J Surg 1977; 47: 305

48. Thomas AJ. Vasoepididymostomy. Atlas Urol Clin North Am 1999; 7: 65

49. Pavlovich CP, Schlegel PN. Fertility options after vasectomy: a cost-effectiveness analysis. Fertil Steril 1997; 67: 133

50. Callahan TL, et al. The economic impact of multiple gestation pregnancies and the contribution of assisted reproduction techniques to their incidence. N Engl J Med 1994; 331: 244

51. Donovan JF, et al. Comparison of microscopic epididymal sperm aspiration and intracytoplasmic sperm injection/in-vitro fertilization with repeat microscopic reconstruction following vasectomy. Hum Reprod 1998; 13: 387

52. Schlegel P. Management of ejaculatory duct obstruction. In, Lipschultz LI, Howards SS, eds. Infertility in the Male 3rd edn. St Louis: Mosby, 1997: 385

53. Quinzii C, Castellani C. The cystic fibrosis transmembrane regulator gene and male infertility. J Endocrinol Invest 2000; 23: 684

54. Daudin M, et al. Congenital bilateral absence of the vas deferens: clinical characteristics, biological parameters, cystic fibrosis transmembrane conductance regulator gene mutations, and implications for genetic counseling. Fertil Steril 2000; 74: 1164

55. Sigman M. Testis biopsy. Atlas Urol Clin North Am 1999; 7: 21

56. Brinster RL, Zimmerman JW. Spermatogenesis following male germ cell transplantation. Proc Natl Acad Sci USA 1994; 91: 11298

57. Brinster RL, Avarbock MR, Germline transmission of donor haplotype following spermatogonial transplantation. Proc Natl Acad Sci USA 1994; 91: 11303

58. Nagano M, Avarbock MR, Brinster RL. Pattern and kinetics of mouse donor spermatogonial stem cell colonization in recipient testes. Biol Reprod 1999; 60: 1429

59. Ogawa T, Dobinski I, Avarbock MR, Brinster RL. Leuprolide, a gonadotropin-releasing hormone

agonist, enhances colonization after spermatogonial transplantation into mouse testes. Tissue Cell 1998; 30: 583

60. Shinohara T, Avarbock MR, Brinster RL. Functional analysis of spermatogonial stem cells in steel and cryptorchid infertile mouse models. Dev Biol 2000; 220: 401

61. Oehninger S. Strategies for fertility preservation in female and male cancer survivors. J Soc Gynecol Invest 2005; 12: 222

23

Medical treatment of male infertility

Gerhard Haidl

INTRODUCTION

Although the modern techniques of assisted reproduction play an important role in the treatment of severe male fertility disorders, these methods cannot be applied in every infertile couple. Based on exact diagnostic measures, conservative medical treatment modalities can be administered alone or, on occasion, in combination with surgical procedures and the simplest form of artificial reproduction, namely intrauterine insemination. Before initiating any treatment, the correct diagnosis has to be established. Moreover, it should be considered that, frequently, several factors contribute to disturbed male fertility, and different degrees of severity of male fertility disorders may exist. In some patients, a harmful influence can be eradicated and spermatogenesis can be restored. In others, the damage may be irreparable due to the severity of the condition. In light of these considerations, current treatment options for male fertility disorders are discussed in this chapter, taking into account that recommendations for medical treatment for male infertility are indicated in specific conditions, but in others their use has been predominantly empirical.

SPECIFIC TREATMENT

Hormone replacement

Gonadotropins

The only generally accepted causal treatment in andrology is hormonal substitution in patients with hypogonadotropic hypogonadism. Well-established treatment regimens with human gonadotropins and with highly purified and recombinant follicle stimulating hormone (FSH) exist and are used to substitute patients with low levels of gonadotropins. Recombinant luteinizing hormone (LH) and human chorionic gonadotropin (hCG) are meanwhile also available; clinical studies with recombinant hCG have demonstrated effectiveness, whereas recombinant LH is not suitable for use in hormonal substitution therapy in the male, owing to its short half-life.

Alternatively, gonadotropin-releasing hormone (GnRH) can be used. If pregnancy is not desired, treatment is with testosterone only. The usual dosage of hCG is 1000–2500 IU, two to three times per week, intramuscularly (IM) or subcutaneously (SC). Human menopausal gonadotropin (hMG), IM or SC, or highly purified or recombinant FSH, at the dose of 75, 100 or 150 IU, SC, three times per week, is used in patients with hypogonadotropic hypogonadism attempting to have children. If the hypogonadotropic hypogonadism has not been treated for a long period with gonadotropins or the patient has received only testosterone before, initial monotherapy with hCG for stimulation of their own testosterone production is recommended for 4–6 weeks, adding hMG thereafter. In more than 90% of patients, the onset of spermatogenesis can be observed. On average it takes approximately 6–9 months before spermatozoa appear in the ejaculate; however, in individual patients this period can be much longer[1–3].

GnRH

GnRH can be administered as an alternative to combined hCG/hMG or FSH treatment. Pulsatile subcutaneous administration of approximately 50 ng GnRH/kg body weight every 2 hours has been recommended. Indications for such treatment are tertiary hypogonadotropic hypogonadism (e.g. Kallmann's syndrome) or idiopathic hypogonadotropic hypogonadism. Following this treatment, normal serum testosterone levels as well as an increase in testicular volume can be achieved. However, normal semen parameters are only rarely obtained. In patients with disturbed spermatogenesis and elevated FSH levels, GnRH as well as the combination of hCG and hMG are not effective[1,3,4].

Androgens

Androgens are used for the correction of testosterone deficiency in patients with hypogonadism. Testosterone deficiency can be substituted by IM testosterone enanthate 250 mg every 3–4 weeks, or by testosterone undecanoate 1000 mg, IM, injected at 12-week intervals, which allows serum testosterone levels in the normal range, in contrast to supraphysiological levels within the first days after the injection of testosterone enanthate. Oral administration of testosterone undecanoate,

120–160 mg daily, can be associated with absorption problems. Preparations for cutaneous application are also available. First, a trans-scrotal patch was developed, consisting of a film containing 10 or 15 mg of natural testosterone. Although testosterone levels could be achieved resembling the normal diurnal variations of serum testosterone, this kind of testosterone patch is meanwhile no longer available due to lack of acceptance and also new developments. Transdermal delivery systems placed on non-scrotal skin also result in physiological serum levels.

The enhancers used in patches to facilitate absorption cause skin irritation in a high percentage of patients, frequently leading to termination of this mode of testosterone application. Moreover, testosterone patches are impractical and unacceptable for certain patients, such as manual workers or patients living in hot climates. The latest development in androgen replacement therapy is a gel preparation containing 25 or 50 mg testosterone in 2.5 or 5 g gel. Studies have shown good clinical effects and tolerability. Furthermore, testosterone can be applied subdermally by the use of pellets and microcapsules, and via the buccal mucosa. Although testosterone can be used effectively in the treatment of hypogonadotropic hypogonadism (although not to initiate spermatogenesis), its use in the treatment of idiopathic male infertility has not been demonstrated to increase pregnancy rates in controlled studies[5]. However, recently, significant improvements of sperm quality as well as pregnancy rates have been reported after combination treatment with tamoxifen and testosterone undecanoate (see below).

Treatment of emission and ejaculatory disturbances

Apart from hormone replacement therapy in patients with hormonal deficiencies, effective treatment is available for patients with emission and ejaculatory failures. In patients with retrograde ejaculation or transport aspermia secondary to emission failure, for example as a result of retroperitoneal lymphadenectomy or diabetes mellitus, α-sympathomimetic and anticholinergic therapy is often helpful. Medical treatment of retrograde ejaculation not only offers the patient the possibility of conceiving offspring naturally, but is also the less invasive method compared with electrovibratory stimulation, sperm recovery from urine and surgical procedures, and should therefore be considered the first choice for such patients.

The drug most commonly recommended for the treatment of retrograde ejaculation is imipramine[6]. In addition, the combination of chlorpheniramine, phenylpropanolamine and midodrine can be used[7,8]. Particularly in cases of retrograde ejaculation in diabetic patients, good experience has been reported with brompheniramine[9]. Recently, the successful treatment of retrograde ejaculation with amezinium 10 mg orally has been reported[10]. Recommended dosages are midodrine 5–15 mg intravenously or (where no longer available in this preparation) orally (drops), applied immediately before ejaculation as a single dose; for longer use, oral imipramine 25–75 mg or brompheniramine 8 mg three times daily; amezinium 10 mg orally; and chlorpheniramine and phenylpropanalamine: 50 mg/day orally. The duration of therapy is individually determined.

Anti-infectious treatment

Antibacterial agents are used for the treatment of male adnexitis (prostatitis and vesiculitis) according to sensitivity tests. Depending on the micro-biological findings, the following agents are mostly used: doxycycline 200 mg/day, tetracycline 1.5–2 g/day, fluoroquinolones (ofloxacin, norfloxacin, ciprofloxacin, levofloxacin, etc. 0.5–1 g/day), cotrimoxacole (sulfamethoxacole 800 mg, trimethoprim 160 mg) or macrolides, e.g. erythromycin 1.5–2 g/day. These drugs are administered for 2–3 weeks. The aims of therapy in male accessory-gland infection include reduction or eradication of micro-organisms in prostatic secretions and seminal fluid, normalization of inflammatory parameters such as leukocytes and biochemical markers such as granulocyte elastase and improvement of sperm parameters. However, most studies of this subject have concluded that antibacterial therapy is effective in reducing infectious influences and should therefore be administered in patients with genital tract infection, but that it does not necessarily improve conception rates[11].

EMPIRICAL TREATMENT

Antiestrogens

Whereas the treatment options discussed so far refer to indications in specific diagnoses, the major part of male fertility disturbances are classified as idiopathic. Therefore, causal treatment is not possible in these cases, and as a consequence, empirical methods have been applied. However, empirical treatments are not necessarily ineffective. The World Health Organization (WHO) recommends treatment with antiestrogens – preferably tamoxifen – for idiopathic oligozoospermia[12], and guidelines published by the European Association of Urology (EAU) also recommend tamoxifen treatment – with limitations – as the only available option for idiopathic fertility disorders[13] (Table 23.1).

If serum FSH is not elevated, tamoxifen can be given in a dose of 20 mg per day. Several double-blind, placebo-controlled studies demonstrated a significant increase in sperm concentration, and indicated the probability of conception to be increased, although no significant effect was found in meta-analysis[14]. Recently, a double-blind, placebo-controlled study which used combined androgen and antiestrogen therapy involved 121 infertile men, each of whom received either placebo or tamoxifen 20 mg and testosterone undecanoate 120 mg for 6 months. A significant improvement of semen quality as well as a significant increase in pregnancy rates (33.9% vs.

Table 23.1 European Association of Urology (EAU) guidelines for conservative treatment of idiopathic oligoasthenoteratozoospermia (OAT) syndrome

Hormonal treatment	EAU	Non-hormonal treatment	EAU
GnRH	Not recommended	Kallikrein	(Recommended only in clinical research studies)
hCG/hMG	Not recommended	Bromocriptine	not recommended
Recombinant FSH	Not recommended	Antioxidants	(Recommended only in clinical research studies)
Androgens	Not recommended	α-Blockers	Not recommended
Antiestrogens	Recommended with limitations	Corticosteroids	Not recommended

GnRH, gonadotropin-releasing hormone; hCG, human chorionic gonadotropin; hMG, human menopausal gonadotropin; FSH, follicle stimulating hormone

10.3%) was shown after combined treatment with tamoxifen and testosterone undecanoate, thus confirming a previous study demonstrating a superior effect of combined antiestrogen–androgen therapy compared with each compound alone or placebo[15,16].

Therefore, treatment with tamoxifen can be considered to be appropriate in some patients with idiopathic oligozoospermia, particularly when sperm morphology and motility are not severely impaired; further studies are needed, especially confirming a potential additional effect of testosterone undecanoate. Clomiphene citrate is not recommended because of its intrinsic estrogenic effects and its lower effectiveness with regard to an improvement of semen quality and pregnancy rates, compared with tamoxifen[12].

Aromatase inhibitors

Treatment with testosterone aromatase inhibitors, which block the conversion of testosterone to estradiol and that of androstendione to estrone, gave controversial results in older studies. More recently, it was shown that in men with severe fertility disorders and a low testosterone/estradiol ratio, significant increases of sperm count and motility as well as a correction of hormonal abnormality could be achieved after treatment with the aromatase inhibitor testolactone, 50–100 mg twice daily. However, there was only a small study group, lacking a control group. Similar changes were observed after treatment with the more selective aromatase inhibitor anastrazole 1 mg/day. On the basis of these experiences, aromatase inhibitors could be administered to patients with subnormal testosterone and high estradiol levels to increase testicular testosterone levels, and, thus, possibly spermatogenic activity[17,18]. However, as in other areas of medical treatment of male infertility, larger and randomized controlled studies are needed to confirm efficacy.

Purified/recombinant FSH

Purified FSH has also been used in men with severely impaired fertility. Several authors have shown that disturbed sperm substructures and sperm functions improved after daily treatment with 75–150 IU pure FSH for at least 2 months. No significant changes in ejaculate quality could be observed; however, in men who previously failed to fertilize in an *in vitro* fertilization (IVF) program, fertilization rates increased dramatically[19].

Moreover, higher implantation rates after intracytoplasmic sperm injection (ICSI) could be achieved[19–21]. This observation was confirmed in a recent study in 44 couples with at least two failed IVF or intrauterine insemination (IUI) trials, the male partners showing idiopathic oligoasthenozoospermia. Before ICSI treatment, 24 of them received highly purified FSH, 150 IU for 3 months; the control group of 20 patients was not treated. Transmission electron microscopy after treatment revealed a significant improvement in sperm quality, and the pregnancy rate after ICSI was 33% in the treated group and 20% in the controls, indicating a positive role of FSH therapy before ICSI[22]. In a further study, a significant improvement of sperm parameters as well as an improvement of hypospermatogenesis, as shown by cytological analysis after testicular fine-needle aspiration, was reported in patients with idiopathic oligozoospermia (sperm count < 10^6/ml, normal plasma FSH and inhibin B levels) after treatment with recombinant FSH 100 IU on alternate days for 3 months[23].

Although the use of recombinant FSH needs to be confirmed by studies, a recent communication has provided more evidence to support its use following a prospective, controlled and randomized clincial study. Foresta *et al.* reported that treatment of male idiopathic infertility improved sperm concentrations and pregnancies in a subgroup of men with idiopathic oligospermia showing normal FSH and inhibin levels and without spermatogenesis arrest[24].

Antioxidants

Leukocytes in semen and, to a lesser extent, immature spermatozoa generate reactive oxygen species (ROS) that damage sperm membranes and DNA. Increased lipid peroxidation results in decreased membrane fluidity, which causes low sperm motility and impairment of important functions such as the acrosome reaction. Damage of sperm DNA may result in lower fertilization and pregnancy rates, and possibly genetic disturbances if such

spermatozoa are used for ICSI[25]. Antioxidant treatment may reduce the oxidative damage and may increase the fertilizing capacity of spermatozoa.

Agents with antioxidative properties are tocopherol (vitamin E), ascorbic acid (vitamin C), acetylcysteine and glutathione[26]. Moreover, pentoxifylline has been shown to exhibit antioxidative functions[27]. Most studies have been carried out with tocopherol. Tocopherol is a fat-soluble vitamin, approved for the treatment of decreased vitality and vitamin deficiency. In andrological indications, the action of tocopherol is a protective effect on lipid peroxidation in sperm membranes via the scavenging of free oxygen radicals. Suggested andrological indications for tocopherol (daily dose 300–600 mg) are asthenozoospermia and sperm dysfunction, including an abnormal acrosome reaction[11]. Increased sperm motility has been observed in a double-blind, randomized, placebo-controlled study in 87 men who received tocopherol 100 mg three times daily for 6 months[28]. Furthermore, an open study has demonstrated a positive effect of tocopherol on fertilization rates in an IVF program[29]. Improved sperm function (sperm–zona pellucida binding capacity) has also been achieved in a double-blind, placebo-controlled crossover study in 30 healthy men who had increased concentrations of ROS in the seminal plasma and were given tocopherol 600 mg/day for 3 months[30].

These optimistic results could not be confirmed in a further controlled study in patients with asthenozoospermia or moderate oligoasthenozoospermia who received high dose ascorbic acid and tocopherol. No changes of semen parameters occurred, and no pregnancies were initiated[31]. The treatment of men with oligozoospermia with acetylcysteine and retinol (vitamin A) plus tocopherol and essential fatty acids led to improved sperm numbers, a reduction of ROS and an increase of the acrosome reaction[32]. Antagonizing the generation and effects of ROS by means of antioxidant treatment seems to be a promising approach, perhaps most suitable as follow-up/complementary treatment after/to conventional treatment according to the WHO, i.e. embolization of the internal spermatic vein(s) in varicocele, antibiotic treatment in male accessory-gland infection, antiestrogen treatment of men with idiopathic oligozoospermia, etc.[12].

A double-blind study in which infertile men were given 3 months of either natural astaxanthin or placebo, after they had received conventional treatment as mentioned above, demonstrated a significant decrease of ROS and an increase of linear progressive motility of spermatozoa. Also, the attachment of spermatozoa to zona-free hamster oocytes was increased in treated cases, compared with controls, as well as the percentage of oocyte penetration. After 3 months, the pregnancy rate was 23% in the treated group and 3.6% in the controls[25]. Well-conducted multicenter trials should confirm this very promising approach.

Carnitines

Free L-carnitine is necessary in mitochondrial β-oxidation of long-chain fatty acids. Fatty acids must undergo activation to enter the mitochondria. They are bound to coenzyme A (CoA), thus forming acyl-CoA, and use L-carnitine to cross the internal mitochondrial membrane. After transport of acyl-carnitine into the mitochondria, the acyl group is transferred to the mitochondrial CoA; β-oxidation with the product adenosine triphosphate leads to the formation of acetyl-CoA. Carnitine also protects the cell membrane and DNA against damage induced by ROS[33]. The highest levels of L-carnitine in the human body are found in the epididymal fluid, where its concentration is 2000 times higher than in the blood serum.

As L-carnitine has been shown to stimulate human sperm motility *in vitro* and is reduced in the seminal plasma of men with oligoasthenozoospermia, L-carnitine and L-acetyl-carnitine have been proposed and used as possible treatments in selected forms of oligoasthenoteratozoospermia. A clear effect could not be demonstrated previously by controlled studies. A recently published placebo-controlled double-blind randomized study using a combination of L-carnitine (2 g/day) and L-acetyl-carnitine (1 g/day) for 6 months in 60 patients with asthenozoospermia showed a significant increase of sperm motility, especially in men with lower baseline levels[34]. The rationale for treatment with L-carnitines may be the same as for treatment with antioxidants. Future studies examining pregnancy rate as the outcome of treatment are needed.

Mast cell blockers

The idea of treating male fertility disturbances with mast cell blockers is based on the observation of elevated numbers of mast cells in the testicular tissue of infertile men[35]. An increase of mast cells in close contact with the seminiferous tubules indicates a relationship between mast cell proliferation and a dysfunction of the blood–testis barrier. The use of mast cell stabilizers, which inhibit the release of histamine and other vasoactive substances from mast cells, for treatment of idiopathic fertility disorders in the male has repeatedly been recommended. In a previous study, 17 men with idiopathic normogonadotropic oligozoospermia and 22 men with idiopathic asthenozoospermia received ketotifen 1 mg twice daily for 3 months. A moderate but statistically significant improvement of sperm count and motility was observed; the pregnancy rate, however, was in the range of spontaneous conceptions[36].

Later on, a placebo-controlled randomized single-blind study was conducted in 50 men with normal gonadotropin levels and sperm counts below 5 million/ml, who received the mast cell blocker tranilast 300 mg/day for 3 months. The treatment group showed significantly higher values of sperm density, motility and total motile sperm count compared with the placebo group. Moreover, the pregnancy rate in the mast cell stabilizer group was 28.6%, versus 0% in the placebo group[37]. Smaller uncontrolled studies with ebastine resulted in an improvement of sperm quality and pregnancy rates as well[38]. As these studies are already 5 and 10 years old, respectively, and no further confirmation about the efficacy of such a treatment has been reported, one has to be cautious in the interpretation of these results. Nevertheless, the approach with mast cell blockers seems logical; therefore, studies with defined selection criteria are needed, perhaps considering the concentration of mast cell products such as tryptase or interleukin-6 in the seminal plasma.

Phosphodiesterase inhibitors

In vivo and *in vitro* investigations have shown that pentoxifylline, a methylxanthine derivative, can increase both the motility and the number of spermatozoa. The suggested mode of action is that pentoxifylline interferes with the metabolism of cyclic adenosine monophosphate (cAMP) by inhibiting phosphodiesterase and thereby increasing sperm cAMP. The recommended oral dose is 400–600 mg three times daily for 3–6 months[11]. In a review paper summarizing reports of the treatment of idiopathic male-factor infertility by oral administration of pentoxifylline, it was concluded that the reported results were conflicting, and that the published data do not support a beneficial role for the systemic use of pentoxifylline in idiopathic male infertility[39]. As this is the case with many of the other drugs used for the treatment of male infertility, prospective studies are needed, based on suitable selection criteria.

Because of its antioxidant and radical scavenging properties, pentoxifylline may be useful for indications discussed in the above section. Recently, the effect of another phosphodiesterase inhibitor, sildenafil, a drug used for the treatment of erectile dysfunction, was investigated. The administration of 50 mg sildenafil 1 hour before ejaculation as well as the *in vitro* addition of 8-bromo-cyclic guanosine monophosphate (cGMP) to the ejaculate resulted in an increase of sperm motility and of the binding rate to the zona pellucida, supporting a potential role of phosphodiesterase inhibitors for sperm motility[40].

Zinc salts

Controlled studies showing beneficial effects of zinc administration, which is widely used in male infertility, are rare[41]. Recently, a significant increase in total normal sperm count was observed in a group of subfertile men as well as in fertile men after combined treatment with zinc sulfate and folic acid for 26 weeks[42]. Nevertheless, a beneficial effect on the outcome in terms of pregnancy rate remains to be established.

Kallidinogenase

Together with the renin–angiotensin system, the kallikrein–kinin system is involved in the paracrine regulation of testicular functions, particularly at the level of the Sertoli cell, where the occurrence of significant amounts of kallidinogenase has been demonstrated. Kallidinogenase was also observed to be localized within epithelial cells of the epididymis[43]. Therefore, it has been looked upon as a possible modulator and mediator of spermatogenesis, and has been used for more than a decade in patients with idiopathic oligoasthenozoospermia[44]. After previous reports of its beneficial effects, two double-blind studies failed to demonstrate any positive results in patients with idiopathic oligoasthenozoospermia[45]. Prolongation of the license was not applied for in Germany in 2001, but the drug is still available in some countries. There are some promising new results in basic research[46]; possibly future and more precise studies will discover better defined indications for this drug. The EAU recommends its use only in clinical research studies (see Table 23.1).

α-Adrenoceptor antagonists

Treatment of patients with idiopathic moderate oligozoospermia (sperm count between 5 and 20 million/ml) with the α-adrenoceptor antagonist bunazosin, 2 mg/day for 6 months, resulted in a pregnancy rate of 26%, compared with 6.7% in the placebo group. Moreover, the α-adrenoceptor antagonist group showed higher levels of sperm density and total motile sperm count[47]. However, the number of patients enrolled in this study was rather small ($n = 34$), and hence this kind of treatment cannot be generally recommended until it has been confirmed in larger trials. A positive effect on sperm transport and storage in the testis and epididymis is assumed based on the mode of action of α-adrenoceptor antagonists[47].

Immunosuppressive treatment

Corticosteroids at various dosages have been recommended for the treatment of antisperm antibodies by several authors[48,49]. However, the majority of experts have questioned the effectiveness of corticosteroids in patients with antisperm antibodies and recommended IVF or ICSI, the latter being considered as the method of choice[50–52]. The addition of glucocorticoid treatment to artificial reproductive technologies has been reported to be ineffective[53,54]. In contrast, higher success rates of ICSI were reported more recently in patients with obstructive azoospermia when prednisolone was administered preoperatively[55]. Similarly, others reported higher fertilization rates during IVF in patients with antisperm antibodies and immunosuppressive therapy, compared with IVF alone[56]. Therefore, the treatment of antisperm antibodies with corticosteroids cannot be generally recommended, but could be considered in patients with antisperm antibodies and previously failed fertilization and pregnancy in IVF or ICSI, or in patients who are unable or unwilling to undergo ICSI treatment. Further indications for corticosteroid treatment are silent inflammatory conditions of the testis, which, however, can so far only be diagnosed by testicular biopsy and histological examination[57]. For the prevention of fertility following acute forms of orchitis, for example mumps orchitis, interferon-α has been recommended[58].

Antiphlogistic treatment

Chronic torpid inflammation of the testis and the male genital tract can be a major cause of severe impairment of sperm quality, particularly when the testis and/or epididymis are involved. Such conditions are difficult to diagnose, because clinical symptoms are frequently absent. In addition to the number of peroxidase-positive cells in the ejaculate, markers of inflammation such as granulocyte elastase or interleukin-6 can be helpful to establish the diagnosis[59]. Non-steroidal antiphlogistic treatment with or without antibacterials is recommended to prevent local occlusions and the induction of local immunological phenomena[60]. As such inflammatory influences are frequently accompanied by elevated levels of ROS, antiphlogistic treatment can help to reduce ROS and their harmful effects on sperm motility and, in particular, DNA integrity[61]. Correction of a disturbed epididymal outlet can lead to higher sperm numbers after anti-inflammtory treatment.

Although no prospective controlled studies exist so far, several authors have reported preliminary experience with diclofenac or indomethacin[60,62,63]. The treatment of ten patients with severe oligozoospermia and ten patients with azoospermia in whom partial epididymal obstruction secondary to inflammatory processes were assumed resulted in an improvement of the sperm count in 13 out of 20 patients, including six previously azoospermic patients. Treatment was carried out with 100 mg diclofenac daily for 3 weeks[64]. A similar case was reported more recently. Using such an antiphlogistic treatment, testicular sperm extraction (TESE) could be avoided and patients could be referred for ICSI using ejaculated spermatozoa[65]. Significantly increased sperm motility and viability were also observed after antiphlogistic treatment with nimesulide 2×100 mg daily for 2 months, followed by carnitines for 2 months in patients with prostatovesiculoepididymitis and elevated leukocyte concentrations in the seminal fluid[66]. Future studies should elucidate this promising approach, including the development of suitable diagnostic selection criteria, in particular for inflammatory reactions in the testis. So far, the recommended dosage for diclofenac is 50 mg, twice daily for 3–6 weeks[11].

CONCLUSIONS

Controlled, randomized, prospective studies are lacking for most of the treatment regimens discussed in this chapter. Despite this problem, the experience of many experts for many years cannot be neglected. The fact that controlled studies according to the criteria of evidence-based medicine are not available in sufficient numbers does not necessarily mean that all the previously recommended treatment regimens are ineffective. For the time being, one can conclude that causal factors of disturbed male fertility, such as inflammatory processes, should be eliminated and/or life-style habits such as smoking be avoided. For the large group of idiopathic male infertility, treatment with tamoxifen, potentially in combination with androgens, can be suggested, and recommendations can also be made for complementary antioxidant treatment[12,25]. Both treatment modalities should be confirmed by further studies, not least because of the potential side-effects of androgen therapy. A promising treatment option for the future may be the antiphlogistic approach, and studies of this subject are already under way. Patients with more severe male fertility disorders should be referred to methods of assisted reproduction. No time should be wasted on frustrating treatment trials in patients with a poor fertility prognosis, and in any case early cooperation between the andrologist and the gynecologist should be striven for.

REFERENCES

1. Büchter D, et al. Pulsatile GnRH or human chorionic gonadotropin/human menopausal gonadotropin as effective treatment for men with hypogonadotrophic hypogonadism: a review of 42 cases. Eur J Endocrinol 1998; 139: 298

2. Kliesch S, Behre HM, Nieschlag E. Recombinant human follicle-stimulating hormone for induction of spermatogenesis in a hypogonadotropic male. Fertil Steril 1995; 63: 1326

3. Schopohl J, et al. Comparison of gonadotropin-releasing hormone and gonadotropin therapy in male patients with idiopathic hypothalamic hypogonadism. Fertil Steril 1991; 56: 1143

4. Knuth UA, et al. Treatment of severe oligospermia with human chorionic gonadotropin/human menopausal gonadotropin: a placebo-controlled, double blind trial. J Clin Endocrinol Metab 1987; 65: 1081

5. Nieschlag E, Behre HM. Clinical uses of testosterone in hypogonadism and other conditions. In Nieschlag E, Behre HM, eds. Testosterone. Action Deficiency Substitution, 3rd edn. Cambridge: Cambridge University Press, 2004: 375

6. Ochsenkühn R, Kamischke A, Nieschlag E. Imipramine for successful treatment of retrograde ejaculation caused by retroperitoneal surgery. Hum Reprod 1999; 22: 173

7. Kamischke A, Nieschlag E. Update on medical treatment of ejaculatory disorders. Rev Int J Androl 2002; 25: 333

8. Köhn FM, Schill W-B. The alpha-sympathomimetic drug midodrin as a tool for diagnosis and treatment of sperm transport disturbances. Andrologia 1994; 26: 283

9. Schill W-B. Pregnancy after brompheniramine treatment of a diabetic with incomplete emission failure. Arch Androl 1990; 25: 101

10. Ichiyanagi O, et al. Successful treatment of retrograde ejaculation with amezinium. Arch Androl 2003; 49: 215

11. Haidl G. Management strategies for male factor infertility. Drugs 2002; 62: 1741

12. Rowe PJ, et al. WHO Manual for the Standardized Investigation, Diagnosis and Management of the Infertile Male. Cambridge: Cambridge University Press, 2000

13. Weidner W, et al.; EAU Working Group on Male Infertility. EAU guidelines on male infertility. Eur Urol 2002; 42: 313

14. Liu PY, Handelsman DJ. The present and future state of hormonal treatment for male infertility. Hum Reprod Update 2003; 9: 9

15. Adamopoulos DA, et al. The combination of testosterone undecanoate with tamoxifen citrate enhances

the effects of each agent given independently on seminal parameters in men with oligozoospermia. Fertil Steril 1997; 67: 756

16. Adamopoulos DA, et al. Effectiveness of combined tamoxifen citrate and testosterone undecanoate treatment in men with idiopathic oligozoospermia. Fertil Steril 2003; 80: 914

17. Pavlovich CP, et al. Evidence of a treatable endocrinopathy in infertile men. J Urol 2001; 165: 837

18. Raman JD, Schlegel PN. Aromatase inhibitors for male infertility. J Urol 2002; 167: 624

19. Acosta AA, Khalifa E, Oehninger S. Pure human follicle stimulating hormone has a role in the treatment of severe male infertility by assisted reproduction: Norfolk's total experience. Hum Reprod 1992; 7: 1067

20. Ashkenazi J, et al. The role of purified follicle stimulating hormone therapy in the male partner before intracytoplasmic sperm injection. Fertil Steril 1999; 72: 670

21. Ben-Rafael Z, et al. Follicle-stimulating hormone treatment for men with idiopathic oligoteratoasthenozoospermia before in vitro fertilization: the impact on sperm microstructure and fertilization potential. Fertil Steril 2000; 73: 24

22. Baccetti B, et al. Effect of follicle-stimulating hormone on sperm quality and pregnancy rate. Asian J Androl 2004; 6: 133

23. Foresta C, et al. Use of recombinant follicle-stimulating hormone in the treatment of male factor infertility. Fertil Steril 2002; 77: 238

24. Foresta C, et al. Treatment of male idiopathic infertility with recombinant human follicle-stimulating hormone: a prospective, controlled, randomized clinical study. Fertil Steril 2005; 84: 654

25. Comhaire F, et al. Factors affecting male fertility. In De Vriese SR, Christophe AB, eds. Male Fertility and Lipid Metabolism. Champaign, IL: AOCS Press, 2003: 1

26. Lenzi A, et al. Placebo controlled, double-blind, cross-over trial of glutathione therapy in male infertility. Hum Reprod 1993; 8: 1657

27. Bhat VB, Madyastha KM. Antioxidant and radical scavenging properties of 8-oxo derivatives of xanthine drugs pentoxifylline and lysofylline. Biochem Biophys Res Commun 2001; 288: 1212

28. Suleiman SA, et al. Lipid peroxidation and human sperm motility: protective role of vitamin E. J Androl 1996; 17: 530

29. Geva E, et al. The effect of antioxidant treatment on human spermatozoa and fertilization rate in an in vitro fertilization program. Fertil Steril 1996; 66: 430

30. Kessopoulou E, et al. A double-blind randomized placebo cross-over controlled trial using antioxidant vitamin E to treat reactive oxygen species associated with male infertility. Fertil Steril 1995; 64: 825

31. Rolf C, et al. Antioxidant treatment of patients with asthenozoospermia or moderate oligoasthenozoospermia with high-dose vitamin C and vitamin E: a randomized, placebo-controlled, double-blind study. Hum Reprod 1999; 14: 1028

32. Comhaire F, et al. The effects of combined conventional treatment, oral antioxidants and essential fatty acids on sperm biology in subfertile men. Prostaglandins Leukot Essent Fatty Acids 2000; 63: 159

33. Jeulin C, Lewin LM. Role of free L-carnitine and acetyl-carnitine in post-gonadal maturation of mammalian spermatozoa. Hum Reprod Update 1996; 2: 87

34. Lenzi A, et al. A placebo-controlled double-blind randomized trial of the use of combined L-carnitine and L-acetyl-carnitine treatment in men with asthenozoospermia. Fertil Steril 2004; 81: 1578

35. Maseki Y, et al. Mastocytosis occurring in the testes from patients with idiopathic male infertility. Fertil Steril 1981; 36: 814

36. Schill W-B, Schneider J, Ring J. The use of ketotifen, a mast cell blocker, for treatment of oligo- and asthenozoospermia. Andrologia 1986; 18: 570

37. Yamamoto M, Hibi H, Miyake K. New treatment of idiopathic severe oligozoospermia with mast cell blocker: results of a single-blind study. Fertil Steril 1995; 64: 1221

38. Matsuki S, Sasagawa I, Suzuki Y, et al. The use of ebastine, a mast cell blocker, for treatment of oligozoospermia. Arch Androl 2000; 44: 129

39. Tournaye H, van Steirteghem AC, Devroey P. Pentoxifylline in idiopathic male-factor infertility: a review of its therapeutic efficacy after oral administration. Hum Reprod 1994; 9: 996

40. Du Plessis SS, de Jongh PS, Franken DR. Effect of acute in vivo sildenafil and in vitro 8-bromo-cGMP treatments on semen parameters and sperm function. Fertil Steril 2004; 81: 1026

41. Kynaston HG, et al. Changes in seminal quality following oral zinc therapy. Andrologia 1988; 20: 21

42. Wong WY, et al. Effects of folic acid and zinc sulfate on male factor subfertility: a double-blind, randomized, placebo-controlled trial. Fertil Steril 2002; 77: 491

43. Saitoh S, Kumamoto Y, Ohno K. Studies of kallikrein–kinin system in human male sexual organs. Jpn J Fertil Steril 1985; 30: 276

44. Schill W-B. Treatment of idiopathic oligozoospermia by kallikrein: results of a double-blind study. Arch Androl 1975; 2: 163

45. Keck C, et al. Ineffectiveness of kallikrein in treatment of idiopathic male infertility: a double-blind, randomized placebo-controlled study. Hum Reprod 1994; 9: 325

46. Monsees TK, et al. Tissue kallikrein and bradykinin B2 receptors in the reproductive tract of the male rat. Andrologia 2003; 35: 24

47. Yamamoto M, Hibi H, Mijake K. Comparison of the effectiveness of placebo and alpha-blocker therapy for treatment of idiopathic oligozoospermia. Fertil Steril 1995; 63: 396

48. Hendry WF, et al. Comparison of prednisolone and placebo in subfertile men with antibodies to spermatozoa. Lancet 1990; 335: 85

49. Shulman S. Steroids and male immunological infertility. Hum Reprod 1996; 11: 1585

50. Bals-Pratsch M, et al. Cyclic corticosteroid immunosuppression is unsuccessful in the treatment of sperm antibody related male infertility: a controlled study. Hum Reprod 1992; 7: 99

51. Lahteenmaki A, Reima I, Hovatta O. Treatment of severe male immunological infertility by intracytoplasmic sperm injection. Hum Reprod 1995; 10: 2824

52. Lombardo F, et al. Antisperm immunity in natural and assisted reproduction. Hum Reprod Update 2001; 7: 450

53. Grigoriou O, et al. Corticosteroid treatment does not improve the results of intrauterine insemination in male subfertility caused by antisperm antobodies. Eur J Obstet Gynecol Reprod Biol 1996; 65: 227

54. Lahteenmaki A, Rasanen M, Hovatto O. Low-dose prednisolone does not improve the outcome of in-vitro fertilization in male immunological infertility. Hum Reprod 1995; 10: 3124

55. Shin D, et al. Indications for corticosteroid immunosuppression prior to epididymal sperm retrieval. Int J Fertil Womens Med 1998; 43: 165

56. Ulcova-Gallova Z, et al. Effect of corticosteroids on sperm antibody concentration in different biological fluids and on pregnancy outcome in immunologic infertility. Zentralbl Gynaekol 2000; 122: 495

57. Schuppe H-C, et al. Inflammatory reactions in testicular biopsies of infertile men. Andrologia 2005; 37: 188

58. Erpenbach KH. Systemic treatment with interferon-alpha 2B: an effective treatment to prevent sterility after bilateral mumps orchitis. J Urol 1991; 146: 54

59. Kopa Z, et al. The role of granulocyte-elastase and interleukin 6 in the diagnosis of male genital tract inflammation. Andrologia 2005; 37: 188

60. Haidl G. Macrophages in semen are indicative of chronic epididymal infection. Arch Androl 1990; 25: 5

61. Alvarez JG, et al. Increased DNA damage in sperm from leukocytospermic semen samples as determined by the sperm chromatin structure assay. Fertil Steril 2002; 78: 319

62. Barkay J, et al. The prostaglandin inhibitor effect of antiinflammatory drugs in the therapy of male infertility. Fertil Steril 1984; 42: 406

63. Moskovitz B, et al. Effects of diclofenac sodium (Voltaren) on spermatogenesis of infertile oligospermic patients. Eur Urol 1988; 14: 395

64. Martin-Du Pan R, Bischof P, de Boccard G, Campana A. Is diclofenac helpful in the diagnosis of partial epididymal obstruction? Hum Reprod 1997; 12: 396

65. Montag M, et al. Recovery of ejaculated spermatozoa for intracytoplasmic sperm injection after antiinflammatory treatment of an azoospermic patient with genital tract infection: a case report. Andrologia 1999; 31: 179

66. Vicari E, Calogero AE. Antioxidant treatment with carnitines is effective in infertile patients with prostatovesiculoepididymitis and elevated seminal leukocyte concentrations after treatment with nonsteroidal anti-inflammatory compounds. Fertil Steril 2002; 78: 1203

24

Male tract infections: diagnosis and treatment

Frank H Comhaire, Ahmed MA Mahmoud

INTRODUCTION

Urinary tract infections are common in men[1], and clinicians working with infertility frequently encounter patients with these diseases. Infections include either cystourethritis, caused by trivial urinary bacteria or by sexually transmitted pathogens, or prostatovesiculoepididymitis, affecting fertility.

The possible relationship between infection and infertility has been the subject of controversy since the second half of the 1970s[2], and several therapeutic trials have been initiated since then. The criteria for infection-associated infertility have been laid down in the World Health Organization (WHO) manuals[3,4], and several studies of the pathogenesis of reproductive disturbance in infected men have been published in the past decade.

An understanding of the link between infection of the 'accessory sex glands' and reduced male fertility has been scientifically acquired and diagnostic tools are available, but the results of antibiotic treatment in terms of fertility remain disappointing. The last is probably due to the irreversibility of functional damage caused by chronic infection/inflammation. Therefore, prevention, early diagnosis and adequate treatment of infections of the male tract, both trivial and sexually transmitted, are of pivotal importance.

DEFINITION OF THE DISEASE

The diagnosis of male accessory-gland infection (MAGI) is given when the semen classification is azoospermia or abnormal spermatozoa and this is considered to result from present or past infection of the accessory sex glands, or inflammatory disease of the urogenital tract[4].

The term male accessory-gland infection does not refer to an organ-specific disease. It does not distinguish between acute disease and chronic or recurrent infection, between inflammation and infection, nor between organ-specific diseases such as prostatitis or epididymitis. The term MAGI is too vague, and should probably be replaced by more specific terminology.

ETIOLOGY AND PHYSIOPATHOLOGY

Infection of the accessory sex glands includes epididymitis, vesiculitis and/or prostatitis, which are caused either by pathogens transmitted by sexual contact or by so-called trivial urological pathogens. Among the former, *Chlamydia trachomatis* is the most common pathogen[5], but gonococcus may also occur. The urological pathogens commonly identified are *Escherichia coli, Streptococcus* group D, *Proteus* species and *Klebsiella* species. The role of coagulase-negative staphylococcus is uncertain[6], while *Staphylococcus aureus* is usually a laboratory contaminant[7].

Infection causes inflammation, characterized by classical symptoms such as pain, swelling and impaired function. The last is responsible for the deficient secretion of minerals, enzymes and fluids that are needed for optimal function and transport of the spermatozoa. The abnormal biochemical composition of the seminal plasma results in decreased seminal volume, abnormal viscosity and liquefaction, abnormal pH and impaired functional capacity of the spermatozoa. This is typically expressed as poor motility, in many occasions associated with attached antisperm antibodies of the immunoglobulin G (IgG) and/or IgA class, causing immunological infertility.

Infection/inflammation increases the number of peroxidase-positive white blood cells (pus cells), generating reactive oxygen species that change the lipid composition of the sperm membrane[8], reducing its fluidity and fusogenic capacity with impaired acrosome reactivity and ability to fuse with the oolemma[9]. Reactive oxygen species induce oxidative damage to sperm DNA, with excessive production of, for example, 8-hydroxy-2-deoxyguanosine, and mutagenesis[10]. The last is also related to a decreased monthly conception rate among first-pregnancy planners[11].

Also, inflammation increases the production of a number of cytokines such as interleukin-1 (α and β)[12], interleukin-6[12] and -8 and tumor necrosis factor, which further impair sperm function and fertilizing capacity[13,14]. Chronic inflammation of the epididymis may cause (partial) obstruction of the sperm passage with oligo- or azoospermia[15], and rupture of the 'blood–testis barrier' from back-pressure induces antisperm antibodies[16].

DIAGNOSIS AND DIFFERENTIAL DIAGNOSIS

The diagnosis is accepted if patients with abnormal semen quality, i.e. oligo- and/or astheno- and/or teratozoospermia, or azoospermia, have combined abnormalities under the following categories[4,17]:

- A history of urinary infection, epididymitis, sexually transmitted disease, and/or physical signs: thickened or tender epididymis, thickened vas deferens, abnormal digital rectal examination;

- Abnormal urine after prostatic massage and/or detection of *C. trachomatis* in the urine;

- Ejaculate abnormalities:
  - Elevated number of peroxidase-positive white blood cells;
  - Culture with significant growth of pathogenic bacteria;
  - Abnormal viscosity and/or abnormal biochemical composition and/or high levels of inflammatory markers or highly elevated reactive oxygen species.

The diagnosis requires either two signs from different categories, or at least two ejaculate signs in each of two subsequent semen samples. If bacteria are detected, they should be identical in urine and in semen, or in the two semen samples. Measurement of interleukin-6 in seminal plasma[18], or of elastase[19], may serve as a biochemical marker of an inflammatory reaction, or white blood cell infiltration.

Male accessory sex-gland infection may be combined with other diseases such as varicocele[20], in which case as few as 300 000 white blood cells may cause complementary damage[21], an immunological factor[22] or sexual or ejaculatory dysfunction. These diseases require adequate management *per se*, and they may interfere with fertility outcome after treatment of the infection. On the other hand, other factors, such as a high proportion of abnormal spermatozoa, chemical or environmental toxins, including toxins for example from tobacco smoke, and viral infections, can provoke immunobiological reactions similar to those seen in infection-induced inflammation. In addition, male accessory-gland infection reduces couple fertility due to effects on the female partner[23].

CLINICAL AND LABORATORY FINDINGS

History-taking commonly reveals one or several episodes of dysuria and/or pollakiuria, which may have disappeared spontaneously or after short treatment with an antibiotic or urinary antiseptic. However, the patient may be unaware of any urinary symptoms in the past[24]. Sometimes, the patient mentions recurrent episodes of intrascrotal pain with a dull feeling being exacerbated by soft pressure. Ejaculatory symptoms may occur, such as reduced ejaculation force or volume, painful sensation during or immediately after ejaculation or blood-staining of the ejaculate (hematospermia)[25]. Finally, sexual complaints may include decreased libido and orgasmic sensation or erectile dysfunction[26].

Clinical examination should focus on careful palpation of the scrotal content, particularly the epididymides and vasa deferentia. Any swelling or nodularity should be noted, as well as pain during soft pressure. Digital rectal examination can be performed, but transabdominal and particularly transrectal echography may reveal more relevant information[27].

Blood analysis may suggest signs of infection, such as an increased number of white blood cells, increased sedimentation rate or abnormal globulin proportions upon protein electrophoresis. Specific tests for circulating antibodies against *Chlamydia* should be included into the routine investigation for male infertility, and the indirect mixed antiglobulin reaction (SpermMar® test; Fertipro, Beernem, Belgium) detects antisperm antibodies of the IgG class in the serum.

Urine analysis may reveal bacterial infection or an increased number of white blood cells, but analysis of the urine obtained after prostate massage should be more relevant[28,29]. The detection of *C. trachomatis* uses nucleic acid amplification methods in urine, which is not applicable, however, in semen[30]. The absence of urinary abnormalities does not exclude male accessory-gland infection, particularly epididymitis.

Semen analysis is of pivotal importance to the diagnosis. Semen must be collected following particular instructions, avoiding contamination with cells and bacteria from the skin or urethra[31]. When semen culture is performed for the counting and identification of bacteria, preparatory dilution of the sample is required, reducing the bacteriostatic capacity of seminal plasma, and the prostate fluid in particular[17].

The number of 'round cells' must be counted, and these must be differentiated into peroxidase-negative cells, mostly spermatogenetic cells, and peroxidase-positive (white blood) cells[31]. Also, it is mandatory to perform biochemical analysis of the seminal plasma to measure the markers of secretion of the sex glands, including for example, α-glucosidase for the epididymides (Episcreen®; Fertipro), citric acid or γ-glutamyl transferase (or calcium or zinc) for the prostate and, possibly, fructose for the seminal vesicles. Finally, the presence of antisperm antibodies on spermatozoa must be traced by means of, for example, the direct mixed antiglobulin tests for both IgG and IgA[31].

TREATMENT

Treatment of the infection should be the same as for urinary tract infections, but must be given for a longer period of time. However, abnormal secretion of the prostate results in an alkaline environment in this gland, meaning that antibiotics such as doxycycline are not concentrated and therefore inefficient[32]. The third-generation quinolones, pefloxacin[33], ofloxacin, ciprofloxacin[34] and levofloxacin[35], are concentrated in both an alkaline and an acidic milieu, and therefore penetrate well into the diseased prostate and the seminal vesicles[33]. In the case of *Streptococcus* infection, the quinolones are ineffective, and treatment with amoxicillin, macrolides[36,37] or cephalosporins may be indicated. Certain authors advocate frequent ejaculation to increase the success rate of antibiotic treatment[38].

Commonly, bacterial infestation can be successfully eradicated, but it may recur with the same or a different pathogen. It may be necessary to add a second, longer-term treatment with another antibiotic. Whereas bacteria can usually be eliminated from the genitourinary tract, white blood cells may persist for several months, and functional impairment of the accessory glands is commonly irreversible. This implies that the processes impairing the fertilizing capacity of spermatozoa remain active, and that fertility is not restored.

In general, the success rate of antibiotic treatment of a male accessory-gland infection in terms of spontaneous conception is poor, and not significantly better than that of placebo. Treatment aiming at the elimination of pathogens is, however, indicated for reasons of 'good medical practice', and in order to reduce the risk of future complications, including prostate cancer[39].

Because oxygen damage caused by excessive numbers of white blood cells to the sperm membrane and, most of all, DNA may persist after antibiotic treatment, intrauterine insemination and *in vitro* fertilization may yield poor results. *In vitro* fertilization and intracytoplasmic sperm injection may generate good numbers of pre-embryos, but may fail in creating an ongoing pregnancy[40]. Complementary treatment with food supplements containing antioxidants may be required[41], and treatment similar to that of idiopathic oligozoospermia may be warranted[42].

PROGNOSIS AND PREVENTION

Depending on the localization of the infection/inflammation, the prognosis after treatment is variable. Whereas the effects of prostatitis and vesiculitis are less important and treatment yields favorable results regarding fertility, (chronic) epididymitis usually causes irreversible damage to the quality and fertilizing capacity of spermatozoa[43]. Also, immunological infertility, resulting from rupture of the blood–testis barrier, is irreversible.

In view of the poor prognosis regarding the restoration of fertility, prevention of infectious disease is of primordial importance. Prevention of sexually transmitted disease, and its immediate treatment in positive cases, will reduce the risk of infertility in a later stage. In particular, recurrent infections with *Chlamydia* have been documented to cause disastrous effects that were irreversible[44]. Men who smoke run a 4–5-times higher risk of prostatitis and subsequent spread of infection to the other accessory sex glands. In addition, tobacco-smoking causes surplus amounts of oxygen radicals and toxic damage to the spermatozoa. Avoiding tobacco is, therefore, the most important factor in the prevention of male accessory-gland infection by common urological pathogens. Any episode of urinary complaints suggestive for infection in the male must be treated adequately, in particular using quinolones, in order to avoid pathogens being harbored in the prostate gland.

REFERENCES

1. Cates W, Farley TM, Rowe PJ. Worldwide patterns of infertility: is Africa different? Lancet 1985; 2: 596

2. Henry-Suchet J, Steg A, Constantin A. Infection et Fécondité. Paris: Masson, 1977

3. Rowe PJ, et al. WHO Manual for the Standardized Investigation and Diagnosis of the Infertile Couple, 1st edn. Cambridge: Cambridge University Press, 1993

4. Rowe PJ, et al. WHO Manual for the Standardized Investigation, Diagnosis and Management of the Infertile Male, 1st edn. Cambridge: Cambridge University Press, 2000

5. Keck C, et al. Seminal tract infections: impact on male fertility and treatment options. Hum Reprod Update 1998; 4: 891

6. Huwe P, et al. Influence of different uropathogenic microorganisms on human sperm motility

parameters in an in vitro experiment. Andrologia 1998; 30 (Suppl 1): 55

7. Rodin DM, Larone D, Goldstein M. Relationship between semen cultures, leukospermia, and semen analysis in men undergoing fertility evaluation. Fertil Steril 2003; 79 (Suppl 3): 1555

8. Zalata AA, et al. White blood cells cause oxidative damage to the fatty acid composition of phospholipids of human spermatozoa. Int J Androl 1998; 21: 154

9. Comhaire FH, et al. Mechanisms and effects of male genital tract infection on sperm quality and fertilizing potential: the andrologist's viewpoint. Hum Reprod Update 1999; 5: 393

10. Chen CS, et al. Hydroxyl radical-induced decline in motility and increase in lipid peroxidation and DNA modification in human sperm. Biochem Mol Biol Int 1997; 43: 291

11. Loft S, et al. Oxidative DNA damage in human sperm influences time to pregnancy. Hum Reprod 2003; 18: 1265

12. Depuydt C, et al. Mechanisms of sperm deficiency in male accessory gland infection. Andrologia 30 1998; 29(Suppl 1): 30

13. Depuydt C, et al. The relation between reactive oxygen species and cytokines in andrological patients with or without male accessory gland infection. J Androl 1996; 17: 699

14. Gruschwitz MS, Brezinschek R, Brezinschek HP. Cytokine levels in the seminal plasma of infertile males. J Androl 1996; 17: 158

15. Dohle GR, et al. Subtotal obstruction of the male reproductive tract. Urol Res 2003; 31: 22

16. Hendry WF. Clinical significance of unilateral testicular obstruction in subfertile males. Br J Urol 1986; 58: 709

17. Comhaire F, Verschraegen G, Vermeulen L. Diagnosis of accessory gland infection and its possible role in male infertility. Int J Androl 1980; 3: 32

18. Paulis G, et al. Evaluation of the cytokines in genital secretions of patients with chronic prostatitis. Arch Ital Urol Androl 2003; 75: 179

19. Ludwig M, et al. Chronic prostatitis/chronic pelvic pain syndrome: seminal markers of inflammation. World J Urol 2003; 21: 82

20. Vicari E, et al. Varicocele and coincidental abacterial prostato-vesiculitis: negative role about the sperm output. Arch Ital Urol Androl 2003; 75: 35

21. Everaert K, et al. Chronic prostatitis and male accessory gland infection – is there an impact on male infertility (diagnosis and therapy)? Andrologia 2003; 35: 325

22. Witkin SS, Kligman I, Bongiovanni AM. Relationship between an asymptomatic male genital tract exposure to Chlamydia trachomatis and an autoimmune response to spermatozoa. Hum Reprod 1995; 10: 2952

23. Eggert-Kruse W, et al. Chlamydial serology in 1303 asymptomatic subfertile couples. Hum Reprod 1997; 12: 1464

24. Drach GW. Prostatitis: man's hidden infection. Urol Clin North Am 1975; 2: 499

25. Yagci C, et al. Efficacy of transrectal ultrasonography in the evaluation of hematospermia. Clin Imaging 2004; 28: 286

26. Liang CZ, et al. Prevalence of sexual dysfunction in Chinese men with chronic prostatitis. Br J Urol Int 2004; 93: 568

27. Horcajada JP, et al. Transrectal prostatic ultrasonography in acute bacterial prostatitis: findings and clinical implications. Scand J Infect Dis 2003; 35: 114

28. Meares EM Jr, Stamey TA. The diagnosis and management of bacterial prostatitis. Br J Urol 1972; 44: 175

29. Fari A, et al. Incidence des états inflammatoires ou infectieux des glandes génitales annexes sur le sperme. In Henry-Suchet J, Steg A, Constantin A, eds. Infection et Fécondité, 1st edn. Paris: Masson, 1977: 43

30. Fredlund H, et al. Molecular genetic methods for diagnosis and characterisation of Chlamydia trachomatis and Neisseria gonorrhoeae: impact on epidemiological surveillance and interventions. APMIS 2004; 112: 771

31. World Health Organization. WHO Laboratory Manual of the Examination of Human Semen and Sperm–Cervical Mucus Interaction, 4th edn. Cambridge: Cambridge University Press, 1999

32. Comhaire FH, Rowe PJ, Farley TM. The effect of doxycycline in infertile couples with male accessory gland infection: a double blind prospective study. Int J Androl 1986; 9: 91

33. Comhaire FH. Concentration of pefloxacine in split ejaculates of patients with chronic male accessory gland infection. J Urol 1987; 138: 828

34. Weidner W, et al. Outcome of antibiotic therapy with ciprofloxacin in chronic bacterial prostatitis. Drugs 1999; 58 (Suppl 2): 103

35. Bundrick W, et al. Levofloxacin versus ciprofloxacin in the treatment of chronic bacterial prostatitis: a randomized double-blind multicenter study. Urology 2003; 62: 537

36. Hooton TM, et al. Erythromycin for persistent or recurrent nongonococcal urethritis. A randomized,

placebo-controlled trial. Ann Intern Med 1990; 113: 21

37. Skerk V, et al. Comparative randomized pilot study of azithromycin and doxycycline efficacy in the treatment of prostate infection caused by Chlamydia trachomatis. Int J Antimicrob Agents 2004; 24: 188

38. Branigan EF, Muller CH. Efficacy of treatment and recurrence rate of leukocytospermia in infertile men with prostatitis. Fertil Steril 1994; 62: 580

39. Roberts RO, et al. Prostatitis as a risk factor for prostate cancer. Epidemiology 2004; 15: 93

40. Zorn B, et al. Seminal elastase-inhibitor complex, a marker of genital tract inflammation, and negative IVF outcome measures: role for a silent inflammation? Int J Androl 2004; 27: 368

41. Comhaire FH, Mahmoud A. The role of food supplements in the treatment of the infertile man. Reprod Biomed Online 2003; 7: 385

42. Comhaire F. Clinical andrology: from evidence-base to ethics. The 'E' quintet in clinical andrology. Hum Reprod 2000; 15: 2067

43. Vicari E. Effectiveness and limits of antimicrobial treatment on seminal leukocyte concentration and related reactive oxygen species production in patients with male accessory gland infection. Hum Reprod 2000; 15: 2536

44. Gonzales GF, et al. Update on the impact of Chlamydia trachomatis infection on male fertility. Andrologia 2004; 36: 1

25

Sperm-washing techniques for the HIV-infected male: rationale and experience

Gary S Nakhuda, Mark V Sauer

INTRODUCTION

It is estimated that the probability for viral transmission to occur from a human immunodeficiency virus (HIV)-seropositive male to an uninfected female is approximately 0.001 per act of unprotected sexual intercourse[1–4]. Although the risk of acquiring infection is low per event, if a couple wishes to conceive, a woman faces considerable risk of infection, given the need for numerous acts of unprotected intercourse that are often required in order to achieve pregnancy. HIV infection is most prevalent in adults of reproductive age, and sexual intercourse is the most common means by which women are infected with HIV.

The introduction of highly active antiretroviral therapy (HAART) has greatly improved the clinical course of this disease, and most compliant patients are now living healthy productive lives[5]. The reasonable desire of HIV-seropositive patients to have children is stymied by the fact that natural conception is not without risk of viral transmission. However, the drive to bear children is strong, and some couples will risk viral transmission in order to conceive unless provided with safer alternatives[6]. Although still considered to be the safest options for beginning a family, adoption or the use of donor sperm is not acceptable to many patients[7].

Albeit not entirely risk-free, assisted reproductive technologies (ART) offer HIV-serodiscordant couples a chance for conception with their own gametes. The principle underlying this intervention is based upon the knowledge that functional sperm can be separated from infectious elements in the semen. While levels of HIV in semen correlate with values in peripheral blood in many instances[8,9], there is also evidence for compartmentalization of seminal HIV, suggesting an independent regulation of viral load in the reproductive tract[10,11]. The sperm, separated from seminal plasma and its cellular components, are believed to be free of virus and when properly prepared can be utilized either *in vivo* using artificial insemination or for *in vitro* techniques with reduced risk for transmitting HIV to the uninfected female.

Since the early work published by Semprini *et al.* in 1992[12], multiple investigators have employed sperm separation methods to treat HIV-serodiscordant couples who wish to bear children. In the current world literature, thousands of ART cycles have been reported in such couples, yielding hundreds of babies without a single documented case of infection in mother or child (Table 25.1)[13–28].

Despite the safe and effective outcomes demonstrated by these methods, and wider

Table 25.1 Summary of published results for HIV-1-serodiscordant couples undergoing assisted reproduction for risk reduction of male to female viral transmission

Study	Cycles (n)	Patients (n)	Pregnancies (n)	Births (n)	Infection
IUI cycles					
Semprini et al., 1997[13]	1954	623	272	242	0
Vernazza et al., 1997[14]	46	16	5	3	0
Brechard et al., 1997[15]	11	—	5	—	0
Marinia et al., 1998[16], 2001[17]	458	233	116	86	0
Tur et al., 1999[18]	155	67	32	—	0
Weigel et al., 2001[19]	143	64	19	14	0
Bujan et al., 2001[20]	62	28	14	2	0
Daudin et al., 2001[21]	93	39	18	—	0
Gilling-Smith et al., 2003[22]	92	36	12	10	0
Delvigne et al., 2003[23]	5	5	4	4	0
Total	3019	1111	497	361	0
IVF–ICSI cycles					
Ohl et al., 2003[24]	54	39	20	14	0
Marina et al., 2003[25]	219	156	92	75	0
Garrido et al., 2004[26]	73	73	29	19	0
Mencaglia et al., 2005[27]	78	35	22	22	0
Sauer et al., 2006[28]	275	135	94	112	0
Total	699	438	257	242	0

IUI, intrauterine insemination; IVF–ICSI, *in vitro* fertilization–intracytoplasmic sperm injection

acceptance of the use of assisted reproduction for HIV-serodiscordance gained over the years, there remain many controversies and challenges. The following review examines the clinical aspects of providing fertility care for HIV-positive men and their uninfected female partners, focusing on the technical facets of sperm processing and options available for treatment.

PATIENT SELECTION

As is true of any elective procedure, patients must initially be properly screened to determine whether they are appropriate candidates for treatment. The basic criteria used in selecting HIV-positive individuals for fertility care ensures that

the patient is healthy and without signs or symptoms of acute or chronic conditions that may indicate deterioration of health. The patient should have a thorough medical evaluation by his primary-care specialist, and demonstrate stable CD4 counts and HIV viral loads over the 6 months prior to beginning fertility treatment. There should be no evidence of acquired immune deficiency syndrome (AIDS)-defining illness. With due respect for the couple's autonomy in deciding to bear children, care providers must consider the risks of a pregnancy when one (or both) of the partners has a life-threatening condition. Unfortunately, even when properly screened, HIV-positive patients may experience rapid deterioration of health and die within a short interval[29].

Female partners should be verified as HIV-negative using a screening enzyme immunoassay (EIA) within 1 month of initiating assisted reproduction. Although these women are undergoing treatment in order to reduce infectious risk, and likely do not have coexisting factors that are associated with infertility, they should still have a thorough reproductive evaluation. Due to the expensive and labor-intensive nature of assisted reproduction, which often involves the use of ovulation induction agents, monitoring of cycles and insemination or *in vitro* fertilization–intracytoplasmic sperm injection (IVF–ICSI) procedures, it is prudent to screen for potential problems that would complicate care prior to beginning treatment. A comprehensive evaluation of the female will allow an optimized approach, improving the likelihood of success while minimizing the number of treatment cycles and thus reducing the exposure to sperm from her HIV-positive partner.

It is important to emphasize that serodiscordant couples must remain committed to safe sexual practices. In the single reported case of presumed HIV transmission to a woman following the intrauterine insemination (IUI) of processed semen, it is possible that the infection was secondary to either unprotected intercourse or condom misuse coincident with her fertility treatment, and not because of the IUI itself[30].

SEMEN AND SPERM AS VECTORS FOR HIV

CD4-positive lymphocytes and macrophages are the principal reservoirs of HIV in the semen. Isolating motile sperm cells from these infected non-motile cells provides an opportunity to use the uninfected spermatozoa of HIV-seropositive men for assisted reproduction. Common techniques known to all andrology laboratories utilizing density-gradient centrifugation, successive sperm washing and swim-up permit separation of the highly

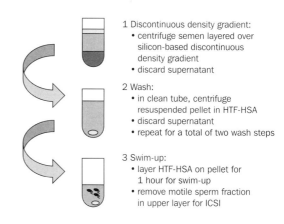

1 Discontinuous density gradient:
• centrifuge semen layered over silicon-based discontinuous density gradient
• discard supernatant

2 Wash:
• in clean tube, centrifuge resuspended pellet in HTF-HSA
• discard supernatant
• repeat for a total of two wash steps

3 Swim-up:
• layer HTF-HSA on pellet for 1 hour for swim-up
• remove motile sperm fraction in upper layer for ICSI

Figure 25.1 Schematic for processing of HIV-positive semen for *in vitro* fertilization–intracytoplasmic sperm injection (IVF–ICSI). HTF-HSA, human tubal fluid–human serum albumin

motile fraction of spermatozoa, believed to be free of HIV proviral DNA or RNA[31] (Figure 25.1).

It remains indeterminate whether or not spermatozoa harbor HIV. The initial debate focused on the presence or absence of the CD4 molecule on spermatozoa, the receptor for which the gp120 glycoprotein of the HIV virus has a primary affinity. In 1987, it was suggested that the CD4 receptor was expressed on human spermatozoa[32]. Subsequently, however, much conflicting evidence using molecular techniques has been presented documenting both the presence[33] and the absence of the CD4 receptor on the sperm surface[34]. Furthermore, morphological evidence based on transmission electron microscopy suggested the presence of HIV viral particles on the surface and in the cytoplasm of spermatozoa[35], while others used the same techniques to demonstrate that viral particles exist in the seminal fluid but not on the sperm themselves[36].

Although the necessary glycoprotein co-receptors for cellular HIV entry, CXCR4 and CCR5, are notably absent from the germ cells of rats and humans[37], an alternative route for the association of HIV with spermatozoa via the galactosyl-alkyl-acylglycerol (GalAAG) glycolipid was suggested[38]. CD4-negative neural cells and colonic epithelium possessing galactosyl ceramide on the cell membrane demonstrated an affinity for gp120[39], and the analogous GalAAG, localized to the equatorial and midpiece regions of the sperm, may present a similar portal[40]. Interestingly, in experiments conducted with human oocytes, direct infection by HIV could not be demonstrated, nor was there evidence of CD4, CCR5 or GalAAG receptors in the zona pellucida or cumulus cells, suggesting that tropism of HIV for germ cells is curiously specific to the male[41].

Compelling evidence exists on both sides of the debate, and a consensus regarding the infectivity of HIV to spermatozoa has yet to be reached. While it appears biologically plausible that individual spermatozoa may be associated with HIV, the clinical importance of this theory in the context of assisted reproduction may be insignificant, considering the lack of viral transmission in current clinical reports using sperm-processing techniques. While further investigation is certainly necessary, patients should continue to be counseled with respect to the theoretical risks, but may be reassured by the clinical evidence thus far published.

FACTORS THAT MAY AFFECT SPERM QUALITY IN HIV-POSITIVE MEN

HIV infection may be detrimental to normal spermatogenesis, as progression of the disease is related to a worsening of sperm parameters. However, healthy HIV-seropositive men do not necessarily have semen analyses that are significantly different from those of non-infected controls[42–44]. Hypogonadism and endocrine disorders are relatively frequent in HIV-positive men, and when present, subsequently affect spermatogenesis[45]. Androgens prescribed to improve well-being and lessen muscle-wasting[46] may iatrogenically induce hypogonadism[47]. It is important that clinicians are aware of these possibilities when evaluating HIV-serodiscordant couples prior to attempting assisted conception. Each step of the 'sperm washing' technique is associated with a considerable reduction in sperm yield[48], and therefore the normalcy of the specimen being processed may influence the treatment plan if a reasonable number of motile sperm cannot be obtained post-processing.

Antiretroviral therapy often involves disruption of nucleic acid synthesis and DNA integration, and therefore may potentially have adverse affects on spermatogenesis. All classes of antiretrovirals have been associated with male sexual dysfunction[49]. At the molecular level, long-term exposure to HAART has been linked with multiple mitochondrial DNA deletions which may affect spermatogenesis at the stem cell level[50]. However, clinical data do not support the detrimental effect of HAART on semen profiles[26] or reproductive capacity using ART such as IVF–ICSI[51]. Discontinuation of antiretroviral medications could promote viral resistance and worsening of disease[52], and therefore should not be advocated with the intent of improving reproductive capacity.

SEMEN PROCESSING

Handling the semen samples of HIV-seropositive men requires facilities dedicated to the processing of infectious agents. A separate class II biological hood, as well as dedicated use incubators and storage tanks, should be devoted solely to specimens obtained from men known to be HIV-positive[53].

Standard sperm 'washing' methods provide a motile fraction of spermatozoa, theoretically free of seminal plasma and CD4-positive cells. Most processing techniques involve a combination of density-gradient centrifugation, resuspension and centrifugation of the sperm pellet, followed by swim-up. An outline of the processing technique used in our laboratory is presented in Table 25.2.

Discontinuous-gradient separation alone resulted in a more marked reduction of the total number of copies of HIV-RNA and proviral DNA than did continuous-gradient. However, 8% of

Table 25.2 Processing protocol for semen samples from HIV-1-positive males for *in vitro* fertilization–intracytoplasmic sperm injection (IVF–ICSI)

All procedures performed in class II biological safety cabinet

Sample transferred from collection container to sterile 15-ml conical centrifuge tube

Discontinuous density gradient:
- 1.5 ml 47% upper fraction layered over 1.5 ml 90% lower fraction (volumes are adjusted according to volume of semen sample)
- 1–2 ml of semen layered on top of upper gradient fraction
- centrifuge at $300\,g \times 10$–20 min
- transfer pellet to clean centrifuge and dilute with 5 ml of modified human tubal fluid (HTF) supplemented with 5% (v/v) human serum albumin (HSA)

Wash 1:
- sample centrifuged 10 min at $300\,g$
- discard supernatant
- resuspend pellet in 3 ml HTF-HSA

Wash 2:
- sample centrifuged 10 min at $300\,g$
- discard supernatant

Swim-up:
- add small volume (0.2–1 ml) HTF-HSA to pellet from wash 2
- allow 45 min for swim-up
- select motile sperm from upper fraction of specimen for ICSI

semen samples obtained from patients with HIV infection still had a detectable viral load after this technique was used alone. When the discontinuous gradient was followed by swim-up, HIV-RNA was reduced to < 1 copy per 10^5 pre-centrifugation copies, and proviral DNA was undetectable using sensitive nested polymerase chain reaction (PCR) techniques[54]. Others, however, found that up to 5% of samples remained positive for HIV after the gradient/swim-up technique[16], and that gradient/swim-up did not provide significantly better viral removal than gradient alone[31].

Comparison of commercial gradient media (Percoll™, Isolate®, PureSperm®, PureCeption™, etc.) showed no differences in their ability to remove HIV-RNA copy numbers when 47%/90% gradients were used[31]. Interestingly, the same study found that Percoll strongly inhibited HIV-RNA detection by a reverse transcriptase (RT)-PCR assay, but not with the NucliSens® assay. The efficiency of removing HIV from semen samples is dose-dependent, depending on the amount of virus present in the original sample, with lower initial viral concentrations resulting in lower post-processing levels[55]. Comparing several techniques for processing HIV-contaminated semen, specimens with $< 10^6$ copies of HIV-RNA became free of virus after processing regardless of the washing technique used[31].

Politch *et al.* recently introduced a novel and simple method to isolate motile sperm from an HIV-positive semen specimen. According to the investigators, a 'double tube gradient' procedure was more effective in removing HIV-RNA than was the popular gradient/swim-up method. This method was also faster, and simpler, and resulted in significantly higher sperm yields[31]. If validated, this promising technique could improve access to safer conception for HIV-serodiscordant couples in areas where more sophisticated laboratory procedures are not available.

Regardless of which method is selected for processing sperm from HIV-positive men, patients cannot be guaranteed that 100% of the virus is removed. Thus, a theoretical risk of infection remains possible. However, a reduction of viral load to undetectable levels, or even 1% of the original viral load, can be achieved using relatively simple methods. This is true even when seminal viral loads are high[31], and should certainly reduce, if not eliminate, the risk of viral transmission, as evidenced by the cumulative clinical data.

VIRAL TESTING OF PROCESSED SPECIMENS

Ultrasensitive viral detection methods such as nested PCR and quantitative nucleic acid sequence-based amplification assays are available to detect HIV-RNA viral loads as low as 10 copies/ml[56]. Multiple investigators have used these methods to validate that semen processing techniques are indeed effective for reducing the viral load of the specimen below the limits of detection[13,54,55,57,58]. What remains uncertain is whether or not post-processing testing is necessary for routine clinical use.

Viral testing of the processed specimen requires additional expense and delays treatment, as immediate analysis of samples with ultrasensitive techniques is not readily available. Post-wash samples need to be cryopreserved until negative results permit their use, at which time the specimen is thawed. Freeze–thaw processing results in additional reductions in sperm yield, which may adversely affect success.

Some investigators insist on the quarantine of processed semen samples from HIV-positive men until they are reassured by results of the ultrasensitive techniques, especially in cases where subjects are known to have poorly controlled infection[59]. While their point is not without merit, we submit that patients without well-controlled disease are not suitable candidates for assisted reproduction, and fertility care should be deferred to such a time that clinical improvement can be demonstrated.

IUI VERSUS ICSI

Intrauterine insemination (IUI) and *in vitro* fertilization with intracytoplasmic sperm injection (IVF–ICSI) are the most commonly chosen techniques used to establish pregnancy in serodiscordant couples. Both methods have advantages and disadvantages.

The largest body of evidence, collected by European groups, suggests that IUI of processed sperm from HIV-positive men is a safe and effective procedure[60]. Compared with IVF–ICSI, IUI is less expensive, technically easier and highly efficient in well-selected patients. However, IUI requires that the female patient has patent

Fallopian tubes, and large numbers of motile sperm must be harvested to be effective (at least $1-2 \times 10^6$/ml). A large number of sperm need to be inseminated, which theoretically presents a higher probability of contamination by viral particles or infected CD4-positive cells, than in the case of IVF–ICSI where only a small number of isolated sperm are used. Further of note, the Centers for Disease Control and Prevention (CDC) do not endorse the use of IUI of processed sperm from HIV-positive men, based on the previously cited case from 1990 where a female seroconverted subsequent to an unsuccessful IUI attempt using a specimen obtained from her HIV-positive husband[30]. Additionally, some jurisdictions in the United States have regulations that prohibit insemination of HIV-infected material, preventing physicians from providing this service in these areas[61].

IVF–ICSI, used in clinical practice to treat male factor infertility since 1992, is an alternative to IUI for HIV-serodiscordant couples. IVF–ICSI is more expensive, is more labor-intensive for the patient and physician, poses inherent risks to the woman since it requires ovarian hyperstimulation with gonadotropins and may be associated with an increased risk of congenital defects[62]. The major theoretical advantage of IVF–ICSI in HIV is the dramatically limited exposure to potentially infective material compared with IUI. Because only a single sperm is injected into a single egg, maternal exposure to non-sperm cells for which HIV has an affinity is virtually eliminated. The immediate and cumulative pregnancy success rates of IVF–ICSI are impressive, with more than 90% of treated young couples achieving conception within three cycles of treatment (Figure 25.2).

Critics contend that viral particles attached to the sperm via the GalAAG receptor may enter the oocyte during fertilization prior to the formation of cleavage-stage embryos[63]. The theoretical implication of these *in vitro* data seems to suggest that HIV could be directly transmitted to the conceptus via ICSI with contaminated sperm. While biologically plausible, an HIV-positive baby has never been born to an HIV-negative mother, and thus the probability of such a situation seems very low. While IUI requires the introduction of several million sperm directly into the female reproductive tract, the ultimate step of the IVF–ICSI procedure involves the transfer of generally only 2–3 embryos. Furthermore, in men with compromised semen parameters or women with non-patent Fallopian tubes, IVF–ICSI is the treatment of choice. Finally, as IVF–ICSI does not involve the direct placement of HIV-positive sperm into the female, in the United States at least, this procedure technically does not violate laws that prohibit insemination treatment of HIV-serodiscordant couples. Therefore, in some centers IVF–ICSI may be more acceptable to practitioners who wish to lessen the risk of possible legal entanglements.

Clearly, both treatments have merits and shortcomings, and neither is entirely optimal for satisfying the needs of every patient. Ideally, the selection of individualized treatment plans by a well-informed patient should occur, thus permitting couples who possess a clear understanding of the risks and benefits of each procedure a role in determining their course of action. Unfortunately, in most regions of the world, financial, political and social factors continue to limit the scope of reproductive options available to HIV-serodiscordant couples.

FOLLOW-UP SURVEILLANCE

Following IUI or IVF–ICSI with samples from HIV-positive men, it is essential to screen closely for viral transmission. In our practice, if the female partner becomes pregnant, surveillance screening for HIV is performed during each trimester. Immediately postpartum, the mother and offspring are tested in the neonatal period, then again at 3 and 6 months using high-sensitivity HIV-RNA or proviral DNA tests. In the event that pregnancy fails to occur, or in cases of spontaneous miscarriage, the female is tested 3 and 6 months later.

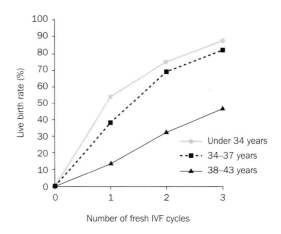

Figure 25.2 Life-table analysis depicting cumulative delivery rates of HIV-serodiscordant couples with successive attempts at *in vitro* fertilization–intracytoplasmic sperm injection (IVF–ICSI) as stratified by the woman's age

Between 1997 and 2005, nearly 275 cycles of IVF–ICSI have been performed in over 135 patients, resulting in more than 100 live births at Columbia University. To date, there has not been a single case of HIV infection in the treated female partner or her offspring (Table 25.3).

CONCLUSIONS

Most of the nearly 40 million people in the world who are currently infected with HIV are of reproductive age[64]. As a result of improvements in the medical management of the disease, many patients are now leading relatively normal and healthy lives, making the prospect of child-bearing a reasonable consideration. For those who are determined to start families, it is important that safe options for conception are available.

Effective sperm processing methods that isolate HIV and its vectors from a useful fraction of motile sperm permit the implementation of techniques such as IUI and IVF–ICSI in order to establish a pregnancy safely. Wider availability of these services will permit more infected

Table 25.3 Outcomes of *in vitro* fertilization–intracytoplasmic sperm injection (IVF–ICSI) in HIV-1-serodiscordant couples at Columbia University. Values are expressed as *n*, % or mean ± SD (range)

Couples initiating IVF–ICSI (*n*)	135	
Total cycles (*n*)	275	
Number of IVF attempts per couple	2 ± 3.2	1–6
Female age (years)	33.7 ± 4.9	21–48
Male age (years)	37.2 ± 5.5	22–49
Years of HIV diagnosis	8.3 ± 5.6	1–20
Viral load (copies/ml)	3171.2 ± 5976.6	51–28 424
CD4 (/mm^3)	585.9 ± 309.5	33–1810
Clinical pregnancies, total (*n*)	111	
Clinical pregnancies per IVF cycle (%)	47.60	
Ongoing/delivered pregnancies per IVF cycle (%)	41.60	
Infants delivered (*n*)	113	

individuals the opportunity to enjoy family life. Perhaps more important from a public-health perspective, utilizing assisted reproduction may lessen the disease burden within the general population by reducing the number of infected partners and offspring.

Providing fertility care to HIV-seropositive individuals is endorsed by the American College of Obstetricians and Gynecologists, and the American Society for Reproductive Medicine[65,66]. In the United States, 18% of 182 fertility clinics reported providing some form of assisted reproduction to HIV-infected couples, although the specific services that were offered at these centers was not described[67].

The extensive European experience seems to reflect greater access to services. While many HIV-serodiscordant couples in developed countries have benefited from ART, the impact of the technologies would be most profound if extended to areas where HIV is highly prevalent. For instance, in sub-Saharan Africa, an area where 64% of the world's HIV/AIDS population resides, the main route of transmission is through heterosexual activity[64]. More than half of the HIV-infected individuals are women, and AIDS is a significant cause of infant mortality and orphaning. Clearly,

any effort that reduces heterosexual transmission of HIV should produce a significant impact in these endemic populations. Future research needs to focus on simple, effective, and inexpensive techniques that could be easily implemented in such regions, so that HIV-serodiscordant couples may bear children without assuming the mortal risks inherent to natural conception.

REFERENCES

1. Downs AM, De Vincenzi I. Probability of heterosexual transmission of HIV: relationship to the number of unprotected sexual contacts. European Study Group in Heterosexual Transmission of HIV. J Acquir Immune Defic Syndr Hum Retrovirol 1996; 11: 388
2. Gray RH, et al. Probability of HIV transmission per coital act in monogamous, heterosexual, HIV-discordant couples in Rakai, Uganda. Lancet 2001; 357: 1149
3. Padian NS, et al. Heterosexual transmission of human immunodeficiency virus (HIV) in northern California: results from a ten-year study. Am J Epidemiol 1997; 146: 350
4. Peterman TA, et al. Risk of human immunodeficiency virus transmission from heterosexual adults with transfusion-associated infections. JAMA 1988; 259: 55

5. Gilling-Smith C, Smith JR, Semprini AE. HIV and infertility: time to treat. There's no justification for denying treatment to parents who are HIV positive. Br Med J 2001; 322: 566

6. Chen JL, et al. Fertility desires and intentions of HIV-positive men and women. Fam Plann Perspect 2001; 33: 144, 165

7. Klein J, et al. Understanding the motivations, concerns, and desires of human immunodeficiency virus 1-serodiscordant couples wishing to have children through assisted reproduction. Obstet Gynecol 2003; 101: 987

8. Ball JK, et al. HIV in semen: determination of proviral and viral titres compared to blood, and quantification of semen leukocyte populations. J Med Virol 1999; 59: 356

9. Gupta P, et al. High viral load in semen of human immunodeficiency virus type 1-infected men at all stages of disease and its reduction by therapy with protease and nonnucleoside reverse transcriptase inhibitors. J Virol 1997; 71: 6271

10. Byrn RA, Kiessling AA. Analysis of human immunodeficiency virus in semen: indications of a genetically distinct virus reservoir. J Reprod Immunol 1998; 41: 161

11. Coombs RW, et al. Association between culturable human immunodeficiency virus type 1 (HIV) in semen and HIV RNA levels in semen and blood: evidence for compartmentalization of HIV between semen and blood. J Infect Dis 1998; 177: 320

12. Semprini AE, et al. Insemination of HIV-negative women with processed semen of HIV-positive partners. Lancet 1992; 340: 1317

13. Semprini AE, Fiore S, Pardi G. Reproductive counselling for HIV-discordant couples. Lancet 1997; 349: 1401

14. Vernazza PL, et al. Quantification of HIV in semen: correlation with antiviral treatment and immune status. Aids 1997; 11: 987

15. Brechard N, et al. Etude de la localisation du VIH dans le sperme. Contracept Fertil Sex 1997; 25: 389

16. Marina S, et al. Human immunodeficiency virus type 1-serodiscordant couples can bear healthy children after undergoing intrauterine insemination. Fertil Steril 1998; 70: 35

17. Marina S. Round Table Discussion. Fourth International Symposium on AIDS and Reproduction, Genoa, 2001

18. Tur RA, et al. Artificial insemination with processed sperm samples from serodiscordant couples for HIV-1. Hum Reprod 1999; 14: 208 (P-133)

19. Weigel MM, et al. Reproductive assistance to HIV-discordant couples – the German approach. Eur J Med Res 2001; 6: 259

20. Bujan L. Reproduction, laboratory, and HIV-1. Fourth International Symposium on AIDS and Reproduction, Genoa, 2001

21. Daudin MPC, Izopet J. Le protocole ANRS 096: prise en charge en assistance medicale a la procreation des couples serodifferents dont l'homme est infecte par le VIH. Reprod Humaine Horm 2001; 14: 365

22. Gilling-Smith CFL, Tamberlin B. Reducing reproductive risks in HIV infected couples: a comprehensive programme of care. Hum Reprod 2003; 18 (Suppl. 1): xviii

23. Delvigne ABP, Manigart Y. Fertility treatment in couples where either or both partners are HIV infected. Hum Reprod 2003; 18: P-405

24. Ohl J, et al. Assisted reproduction techniques for HIV serodiscordant couples: 18 months of experience. Hum Reprod 2003; 18: 1244

25. Marina SSA, et al. Results of 219 IVF-ICSI cycles in serodiscordant couples (seropositive men) to HIV-1. Hum Reprod 2003; 18: P-450

26. Garrido N, et al. Semen characteristics in human immunodeficiency virus (HIV)- and hepatitis C (HCV)-seropositive males: predictors of the success of viral removal after sperm washing. Hum Reprod 2005; 20: 1028

27. Mencaglia L, et al. ICSI for treatment of human immunodeficiency virus and hepatitis C virus-serodiscordant couples with infected male partner. Hum Reprod 2005; 20: 2242

28. Sauer MVNG, et al. IVF-ICSI for the prevention of viral transmission in HIV-1 serodiscordant couples: the experience at Columbia University. ESHRE Annual Meeting, Prague, 2006

29. Nakhuda GS, Pena JE, Sauer MV. Deaths of HIV-positive men in the context of assisted reproduction: five case studies from a single center. AIDS Patient Care STDS 2005; 19: 712

51. Nakhuda G, Pena J, Sauer MV. Antiretroviral therapy does not adversely affect the semen parameters of HIV+ men undergoing IVF-ICSI. American Society for Reproductive Medicine, Annual Meeting, 2004

30. Centers for Disease Control and Prevention. HIV infection and artificial insemination with processed semen. MMWR Morb Mortal Wkly Rep 1990; 39: 249, 255

31. Politch JA, et al. Separation of human immunodeficiency virus type 1 from motile sperm by the double tube gradient method versus other methods. Fertil Steril 2004; 81: 440

32. Ashida ER, Scofield VL. Lymphocyte major histo-compatibility complex-encoded class II structures may act as sperm receptors. Proc Natl Acad Sci USA 1987; 84: 3395

33. Gobert B, et al. CD4-like molecules in human sperm. FEBS Lett 1990; 261: 339

34. Quayle AJ, et al. The case against an association between HIV and sperm: molecular evidence. J Reprod Immunol 1998; 41: 127

35. Baccetti B, et al. HIV particles detected in spermato-zoa of patients with AIDS. J Submicrosc Cytol Pathol 1991; 23: 339

36. Borzy MS, Connell RS, Kiessling AA. Detection of human immunodeficiency virus in cell-free seminal fluid. J Acquir Immune Defic Syndr 1988; 1: 419

37. Habasque C, et al. Study of the HIV receptors CD4, CXCR4, CCR5 and CCR3 in the human and rat testis. Mol Hum Reprod 2002; 8: 419

38. Brogi A, et al. Human sperm and spermatogonia express a galactoglycerolipid which interacts with gp120. J Submicrosc Cytol Pathol 1995; 27: 565

39. Harouse JM, Collman RG, Gonzalez-Scarano F. Human immunodeficiency virus type 1 infection of SK-N-MC cells: domains of gp120 involved in entry into a CD4-negative, galactosyl ceramide/3′ sulfo-galactosyl ceramide-positive cell line. J Virol 1995; 69: 7383

40. Brogi, A, et al. Interaction of human immunodefi-ciency virus type 1 envelope glycoprotein gp120 with a galactoglycerolipid associated with human sperm. AIDS Res Hum Retroviruses 1996; 12: 483

41. Baccetti B, et al. Failure of HIV to infect human oocytes directly. J Acquir Immune Defic Syndr 1999; 21: 355

42. Krieger JN, et al. Fertility parameters in men infected with human immunodeficiency virus. J Infect Dis 1991; 164: 464

43. Muller CH, Coombs RW, Krieger JN. Effects of clinical stage and immunological status on semen analysis results in human immunodeficiency virus type 1-seropositive men. Andrologia 1998; 30 (Suppl 1): 15

44. Politch JA, et al. The effects of disease progression and zidovudine therapy on semen quality in human immunodeficiency virus type 1 seropositive men. Fertil Steril 1994; 61: 922

45. Sellmeyer DE, Grunfeld C. Endocrine and metabolic disturbances in human immunodeficiency virus infection and the acquired immune deficiency syn-drome. Endocr Rev 1996; 17: 518

46. Bhasin S, et al. Testosterone replacement and resist-ance exercise in HIV-infected men with weight loss and low testosterone levels. JAMA 2000; 283: 763

47. Pena JE, Thornton MH, Jr. Sauer MV. Reversible azoospermia: anabolic steroids may profoundly affect human immunodeficiency virus-seropositive men undergoing assisted reproduction. Obstet Gynecol 2003; 101: 1073

48. Evliyaoglu Y, Ciftci U, Bozdemir N. Spermatozoa selection by the swim-up procedure and two-layer percoll gradient centrifugation. Int Urol Nephrol 1996; 28: 409

49. Collazos J, et al. Sexual dysfunction in HIV-infected patients treated with highly active antiretroviral ther-apy. J Acquir Immune Defic Syndr 2002; 31: 322

50. White DJ, et al. Sperm mitochondrial DNA dele-tions as a consequence of long term highly active anti-retroviral therapy. AIDS 2001; 15: 1061

51. Sauer MV. Sperm washing techniques address the fer-tility needs of HIV-seropositive men: a clinical review. Reprod Biomed Online 2005; 10: 135

52. Foli A, et al. Strategies to decrease viral load rebound, and prevent loss of CD4 and onset of resistance dur-ing structured treatment interruptions. Antivir Ther 2004; 9: 123

53. Sauer MV, Chang PL. Establishing a clinical program for human immunodeficiency virus 1-seropositive men to father seronegative children by means of in vitro fertilization with intracytoplasmic sperm injec-tion. Am J Obstet Gynecol 2002; 186: 627

54. Hanabusa H, et al. An evaluation of semen process-ing methods for eliminating HIV. AIDS 2000; 14: 1611

55. Fiore JR, et al. The efficiency of sperm washing in removing human immunodeficiency virus type 1 varies according to the seminal viral load. Fertil Steril 2005; 84: 232

56. Notermans DW, et al. Evaluation of a second-gener-ation nucleic acid sequence-based amplification assay for quantification of HIV type 1 RNA and the use of ultrasensitive protocol adaptations. AIDS Res Hum Retroviruses 2000; 16: 1507

57. Kim LU, et al. Evaluation of sperm washing as a potential method of reducing HIV transmission in HIV-discordant couples wishing to have children. Aids 1999; 13: 645

58. Pasquier C, et al. Sperm washing and virus nucleic acid detection to reduce HIV and hepatitis C virus transmission in serodiscordant couples wishing to have children. AIDS 2000; 14: 2093

59. Leruez-Ville M, et al. Assisted reproduction in HIV-serodifferent couples: the need for viral validation of processed semen. AIDS 2002; 16: 2267
60. Semprini AE, Fiore S. HIV and reproduction. Curr Opin Obstet Gynecol 2004; 16: 257
61. Public Law No. 184 of 1989, 5 May 1989. Annu Rev Popul Law 1989; 16: 53
62. Rimm AA, et al. A meta-analysis of controlled studies comparing major malformation rates in IVF and ICSI infants with naturally conceived children. J Assist Reprod Genet 2004; 21: 437
63. Baccetti B, et al. HIV-particles in spermatozoa of patients with AIDS and their transfer into the oocyte. J Cell Biol 1994; 127: 903
64. UNAIDS. AIDS epidemic update: 2004. Geneva: UNAIDS, 2004
65. The Committee on Ethics of the American College of Obstetricians and Gynecologists. Human immunodeficiency virus: physicians' responsibilities. ACOG Committee Opinion No. 255. Washington, DC: ACOG, 2001
66. Ethics Committee of the American Society for Reproductive Medicine. Human immunodeficiency virus and infertility treatment. Fertil Steril 2004; 82 (Suppl 1): S228
67. Stern JE, et al. Access to services at assisted reproductive technology clinics: a survey of policies and practices. Am J Obstet Gynecol 2001; 184: 591

Treatment of HIV-discordant couples: the Italian experience

Augusto E Semprini, Lital Hollander

SAFER REPRODUCTION OPTIONS FOR HIV-POSITIVE MEN

The Western world discovered human immunodeficiency virus/acquired immune deficiency syndrome (HIV/AIDS) as a disease of gay men and intravenous drug users. However, the growing global HIV epidemic is currently fueled by heterosexual transmission. Although effective antiviral treatment was shown to reduce the sexual and vertical transmission of HIV[1–4], the rates of heterosexual transmission in industrialized countries are on the rise[5–8]. This fact may reflect the delayed detection of heterosexually infected individuals who, not perceiving themselves at risk, refrain from testing and can transmit the infection to their sexual partners. On the other hand, attention to safe-sex practices may diminish in HIV-positive individuals taking highly active antiretroviral treatment (HAART). Also, their HIV-negative sexual partners might perceive HIV infection as less infectious or even less dangerous[9].

In HIV-positive men, HAART increases both quality of life and the duration of disease-free survival, encouraging many to consider parenthood. Be they men or women, people infected by HIV are living longer, most of them are of fertile age and their natural wish for a family and parenthood needs to be addressed with more than the general recommendation to refrain from pregnancy.

This chapter discusses the evidence regarding HIV transmission and safe parenthood in men infected with HIV. Reproductive counseling and the provision of semen washing and assisted reproductive technologies (ART) are the milestones in offering reproductive assistance to these individuals.

EPIDEMIOLOGY OF HIV INFECTION IN EUROPE

According to World Health Organization (WHO)/United Nations Program on HIV/AIDS (UNAIDS) official estimates, by the end of 2004, the number of people living with HIV and AIDS (PLWHA) in Europe was 2 010 000 (estimated range 1.40–2.86 million), with an estimated European prevalence of 0.4% (range 0.2–0.6% in different countries)[10]. Figure 26.1 shows the estimated number of HIV infections per year, by the middle of 2004.

The current epidemiological situation in Europe is characterized by the continuing spread of HIV and rapid growth of the number of people in need of antiretroviral therapy in Eastern Europe. Over one million people affected by the epidemic in the region (according to WHO and UNAIDS estimates) represent a real challenge to

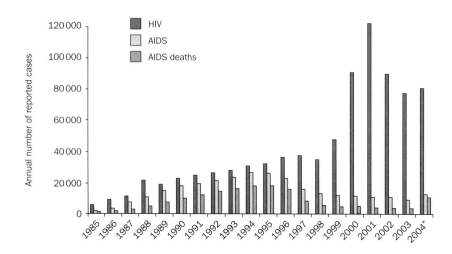

Figure 26.1 Number of yearly HIV infections in Europe[10]. *Preliminary and incomplete data

the social and economic development of countries and to their national security.

This constant increase in the number of people living with HIV/AIDS in Europe is due to both the number of newly registered cases and an increase in the availability of antiretroviral therapy, which prolongs life from the moment of infection. The large majority of HIV infections are observed in young males. This predominance is due to prevalent homosexual transmission in countries such as France, Germany, Scandinavia and Greece, and to a rampant epidemic among intravenous drug users in Italy, Spain and Eastern Europe[10].

However, in recent years the number of women involved in the epidemic has continually increased. In 2003, the proportion of newly registered HIV/AIDS cases attributed to women was 37% in Western Europe and 38% in Eastern Europe, compared with 1999, when the proportion of newly registered women with HIV/AIDS was 31% and 25%, respectively. In some countries of Eastern Europe, such as Russia and Ukraine, the proportion of child-bearing-aged (15–49 years old) women infected through heterosexual contact with an infected male is almost 50%.

Men taking HAART have lower seminal concentrations of HIV, and sexual transmission may be reduced. However, a certain percentage of aviremic men retain viral presence in the semen, and unprotected intercourse to achieve fertilization must be discouraged. HIV-discordant couples for male seropositivity should be informed that sperm washing can remove HIV from the semen, allowing conception without the risk of infection for the seronegative female, and eventually the child.

HETEROSEXUAL SPREAD OF HIV

Recent studies reveal that the heterosexual population is currently most subjected to infection. In a British surveillance study, 1624 young people (aged 15–24 years) were diagnosed with HIV during the period 1997–2001, of whom 55% had been infected heterosexually[11]. Different international studies confirm this increase of heterosexual infections[5–8]. Figure 26.2 shows the trends of transmission for different exposure categories in Western Europe. The effective reduction in transmission among the 'classic' risk groups, namely

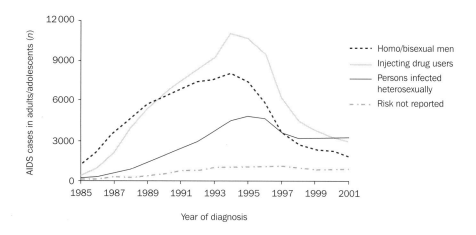

Figure 26.2   HIV transmission by mode of exposure in Western Europe[12]. Data are adjusted for reporting delays

intravenous drug users and men having sex with men, is evident. In contrast, infections due to heterosexual transmission are undergoing a significant increase.

Increased heterosexual infection rates might also depend on the availability of HAART. In a recent study, 40% of seronegative stable heterosexual partners of HIV-positive individuals reported less fear of infection and an increased likelihood to engage in risk behavior[9]. This is particularly dangerous in HIV-discordant couples who wish to conceive, where condom use may be abandoned in favor of unprotected intercourse.

Reasons for the increased risk in heterosexual women are rarely addressed in epidemiological studies investigating rates of infection. However, there is evidence that a proportion of such exposures may be intentional. An Italian study analyzing the population of women requesting HIV tests in two distinct time periods (1985–89 and 1993–97) showed a sharp increase of partners of HIV-1-infected males (from 8.7 to 36.5%) among voluntary testers[13]. A study of 581 seroconverters revealed that 56% of women who seroconverted knew that a sexual partner was HIV-positive[14]. An additional study of the incidence of heterosexual transmission of HIV in women investigated the temporal relationship with pregnancy. In 449 initially HIV-negative women with no history of parenteral drug use, there had been four seroconversions at 30 months of follow-up. Three of these four seroconverters became pregnant, with a pregnancy rate five-fold that of the general population[15]. Hence, there is evidence to suggest that partnership with HIV-positive men, and conception attempts, are among the factors that expose women to HIV transmission.

The advent of HAART and the effects of massive prevention campaigns targeted at 'high-risk' groups may have contributed to this shift in the epidemic. In fact, heterosexual individuals are more likely to consider themselves 'at low risk', and therefore ignore safe-sex recommendations. Voluntary testing is also less frequent in this group. An analysis of over 30 000 AIDS cases reported in Spain in the years 1994–2000 showed an increase of late testers, from 24% in 1994–96 to 35% in 1998–2000. Late testing was independently associated with male sex, residence in provinces with a lower AIDS incidence and absence of a history of drug use or prison stay[16].

THE IMPACT OF HIGHLY ACTIVE ANTIRETROVIRAL TREATMENT ON SEMINAL VIRAL EXCRETION

The administration of effective antiretroviral therapy normally leads to a marked reduction in viral replication, with a several-log reduction in blood HIV-RNA concentrations within weeks. The majority of patients adhering to medication will experience persistent aviremia. An estimated risk of infection per act of unprotected intercourse in heterosexual couples where the man is regularly taking HAART is not available. However, a longitudinal study in 415 HIV-discordant Ugandan couples observed that no seroconversion occurred in couples where the man's viral load was less than 1500 copies/ml, while the probability of transmission per coital act rose to 0.0023 per act at 38 500 copies/ml or more[17]. Support of the evidence that HAART reduces HIV infectivity comes from a study showing a 60% decline in partnership probability of transmission in gay couples in the period 1994–99, during which HAART became widespread[1].

The probability of sexual transmission of HIV in serodiscordant couples does not follow a linear pattern, as some infected individuals are more efficient in transferring the virus (i.e. high transmitters), while some women could be more vulnerable to infection[18]. Male-to-female transmission of HIV is likely to depend on the amount of virus in the semen, but additional factors can determine the chances of infection[19–21]. In fact, various studies suggest that the model assuming constant infectivity appears seriously to underestimate the risk after very few contacts and seriously to overestimate the risk associated with a large number of contacts[22]. In addition, in long-standing couples, low rates of infection per single act of unprotected intercourse should also be corrected for the frequency of intercourse and other covariates, such as adherence to HAART, possible treatment interruptions or undetected viral failure.

In semen, HIV can be found in cell-associated form within seminal leukocytes, and in cell-free form in seminal plasma. Several studies have analyzed the impact of HAART on the presence of HIV-RNA and DNA in the semen of treated individuals. In most patients, the decrease in blood viral load parallels that in seminal plasma. However, a significant proportion of men with low or undetectable HIV viremia still shed substantial amounts of virus in their semen[23,24].

Bujan et al.[24] measured the frequency of virospermia in 67 HIV-positive men who repeatedly donated sperm (as part of their reproductive health treatment). While 73% of men were constantly HIV-negative, 29% showed HIV presence in at least some of the seminal samples, and two (3%) had constant presence. These findings contrast with the recent view that men with undetectable blood viral loads are not infectious, and corroborate previous findings[19] that the model of 'constant infectivity' is inaccurate, and that men are divided into categories of efficient and non-efficient transmitters.

Seminal HIV viral load may change considerably, even in the same individual. In the above study[24] a man who had consistently low plasma viral load showed an asymptomatic elevation of HIV in the semen to highly infectious concentrations (approximately 300 000 copies/ml). Factors associated with the risk of seminal excretion of the virus can be HIV-related, such as CD4 cell count, HIV viremia and type of treatment. However, the highest correlation is shown with seminal characteristics, and mainly with the presence of seminal leukocytes, which increases the risk of secretion four-fold ($p < 0.001$).

These findings are particularly relevant in counseling HIV-discordant couples who may be tempted not to use condoms regularly during intercourse, in the erroneous belief that viral suppression in blood is a guarantee against infection to the seronegative partner, or that a few timed acts of intercourse entail a very limited risk of infection.

REPRODUCTIVE HEALTH SERVICES FOR INDIVIDUALS WITH HIV

The rapid spread of HIV and AIDS has had repercussions in many aspects of people's lives. The discussions around child-bearing and living with HIV are dynamic and complex, making it impossible and even inappropriate to prescribe a unique and ideal approach.

Some contraceptive methods originally designed for fertility regulation are now seen primarily as methods for protecting against infection with HIV and other sexually transmitted diseases. Arguments for use of the condom, for example, now often focus on the prevention of infection as much as, if not more than, the avoidance of unwanted pregnancy. However, HIV sufferers of both sexes may still wish to have children; they may need counseling about the risk of sexual and vertical transmission of HIV.

Knowledge of the integration of HIV and reproductive health services is still limited. Reproductive health programs, particularly comprehensive programs to prevent sexual transmission to HIV-negative partners during conception attempts, and mother-to-child transmission when the woman is HIV-positive, are highly necessary[25]. Health-care providers should anticipate that HIV-positive individuals might require counseling and support to make choices regarding their sexuality and parenthood, and proactively assist them. In addition, reproductive health programs for HIV-positive individuals should provide, or have explicit mechanisms of referral for, antiretroviral treatment to ensure optimal parental health. Hence, links should be created between HIV/AIDS and reproductive health services and, eventually, harm reduction programs.

Service providers in both reproductive and HIV services should adopt a positive attitude towards reproductive health in HIV-positive individuals. Interventions to promote sexual health among HIV-positive people include assistance with identifying and overcoming impediments to safer sexual behavior, education on the potential for HIV transmission to an uninfected partner even when on antiretroviral treatment, information and counseling on sexually transmitted infection (STI) prevention, including the importance of correct and consistent condom use, and the availability of safer reproductive options.

MALE CONDOM

When used consistently and correctly, male latex condoms protect against both female-to-male and male-to-female transmission of HIV, as shown in studies of discordant couples[26]. Furthermore, condoms offer protection against reinfection with HIV; limited evidence suggests that infection with more than one strain of HIV may accelerate the progression of HIV disease[27].

Laboratory studies have demonstrated the impermeability of male latex condoms to infectious agents contained in genital secretions, including the smallest viruses. Male condoms also protect against other STIs, although their effectiveness may be lower in the case of STIs that are also transmitted by mere skin-to-skin contact (such as herpes, human papilloma virus and syphilis)[28].

The use of condoms should be emphasized by providers in all situations where prevention of pregnancy is not a concern, such as during pregnancy, with infertility, after sterilization or in postmenopausal women. Special support should be considered for couples with discordant serostatus. For sexually active individuals with HIV and an HIV-negative partner, protected sex using a condom is the only way to ensure that their sexual partner remains uninfected.

Notwithstanding the ample proof of condom effectiveness, major barriers to increased condom use still exist even in areas with high HIV prevalence. These include negative attitudes towards condoms, limited access and lack of political commitment. Low rates of condom use have been reported even following disclosure of HIV status to sexual partners[29].

NATURAL VERSUS ASSISTED CONCEPTION IN HIV-DISCORDANT COUPLES

The theoretical limited risk of infection per single act of intercourse could motivate HIV-discordant couples to abandon condom use for empirically timed sexual acts aimed at conception. In 1997, a French group reported their follow-up of 96 HIV-discordant couples aiming at conception through unprotected intercourse. Altogether, 104 pregnancies were achieved, with two seroconversions at 7 months of pregnancy, and two postpartum[30]. This rate of infection is approximately eight-fold that reported in studies observing heterosexual transmission in HIV-discordant couples[17], and the reasons for this observation are not fully discussed in the article, although it is mentioned that the couples in whom the woman seroconverted reported inconsistent condom use. The study was conducted between 1986 and 1996, and only 21 men were receiving antiretroviral medication, which, conceivably, was not HAART[30].

The sexual history of HIV-discordant couples requesting reproductive counseling should be carefully considered, as it might offer an indication about their actual risk of sexual transmission. Paradoxically, couples who have always used condoms have a baseline higher risk of transmission, in comparison with couples who have had long periods of unprotected sex without transmitting the infection. Therefore, couples who report consistent condom use since the beginning of their sexual relationship should be warned about the possibility that the man is a potential high transmitter of the infection.

However, such advice must go hand in hand with the ability to offer the couple a safer alternative for conception. Clinicians may erroneously assume that discouraging HIV-discordant couples from the intention to conceive is effective, and that such couples will adhere to condom use. On the contrary, over two-thirds of 104 heterosexual HIV-discordant couples from the California Partners Study II reported unprotected sex with their partner in the previous 6 months[9]. A Swiss multicenter study evaluating fertility intentions and condom use among 114 HIV-positive persons showed that 45% of positive women and 38% of positive men expressed a desire for children, and that consistent condom use was mentioned by no more than 73% of participants[31].

In surveying the post-insemination quality of life and behavior of our former patients we have discovered that approximately half of the couples who failed to conceive through semen washing proceeded to procreating on their own, abandoning condom use on a few timed occasions. After conception, all couples returned to habitual levels of condom use. In contrast, couples who conceived through our methods reported high compliance with safe-sex behavior.

SEMEN WASHING

Semen washing is the term used to describe the three-step seminal processing method involving gradient centrifugation, washing and spontaneous migration, devised approximately 15 years ago in Milan, reported to the *Lancet* in 1992 after the birth of the first ten healthy children from uninfected mothers[32].

The specific semen washing method is a three-step system which first filters the liquefied semen through a gradient, then washes the recovered spermatozoa to eliminate seminal plasma and hyperosmotic gradient media, followed by a modified swim-up method to recover highly motile spermatozoa, free from leukocytes eventually passed through the gradient step (Figure 26.3) . Anderson *et al.* showed that as a result of this procedure, the HIV titer in the motile sperm fraction decreased to less than 0.1% of that in the semen, and that the sperm fraction was not infectious to peripheral blood lymphocytes *in vitro*[33].

No clinical or immunological exclusion criteria were proposed for access to the program, other than the willingness to refrain from unprotected intercourse, as the method was originally

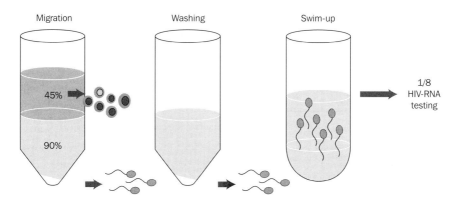

Final dilution: 4×10^6 Volume: 0.3–0.5 ml

Figure 26.3   The sperm washing procedure[32]

conceived as a risk-reduction strategy and therefore most necessary in those individuals who have the highest foreseeable risk of transmission, such as subjects with profound immune deficiency. In fact, HAART, with its known effects on immunological and virological markers, was not available in Italy until 1997. Indeed, all men included in the first 6 years of the program were not taking highly active antiretroviral medication. To date, access to assistance is unrestricted, and this is relevant for patients who do not need pharmacological control of viral replication, who are on structured or other treatment interruptions, who have poor adherence to therapy or who have failed antiretroviral medication.

Similarly, until 1995, when polymerase chain reaction (PCR) assays became available for determination of viral presence in the washed spermatozoa aliquot, nearly 500 cycles of sperm washing and intrauterine insemination (IUI) were conducted. Hence, for a number of years, men with potentially infectious semen were treated without the ability to attest the efficacy of each washing cycle prior to insemination. Yet, no case of seroconversion in the women was observed[34].

Still, all couples who participate in the program of assisted conception through sperm washing are informed that there is a non-zero risk of infection, which must be acknowledged. In order to assess the results, women are requested to undergo HIV-serological testing at 3-monthly intervals for a full year after each assisted-conception cycle.

Since the above, several units in Europe (UK, France, Spain, Germany, Switzerland, Sweden, The Netherlands, Belgium, Denmark and Poland) have started similar programs, and others plan to start them in the future. To improve the state of evidence regarding the safety and efficacy of sperm washing followed by assisted reproductive technologies (ART), the pioneering centers in the field founded CREAThE (Centres for Reproductive Assistance Techniques to HIV couples in Europe), a network comprising all centers currently providing reproductive assistance to couples with HIV and other correlated sexually transmissible infections (i.e. hepatitis C virus (HCV), cytomegalovirus (CMV)).

CREAThE is an open network, and welcomes the addition of new centers offering, or interested in offering, ART services to couples in whom at least one partner is affected by HIV. CREAThE is highly representative of the realities of operating in the field of assisted reproduction. It currently includes 13 active members represented by clinical centers from nine European countries. Recently, the CREAThE centers pooled their treatment data into a joint analysis of safety and efficacy of semen washing. Table 26.1 summarizes the results of this analysis.

To date, over 5000 semen washing procedures, followed by intrauterine insemination or *in vitro* fertilization, have been carried out in Italy. No seroconversion of the mother or birth of an infected child has been reported in any of the above centers.

These remarkable results for the treatment of HIV-discordant couples, with what has been proved to be a safe risk-reduction method, have been followed by numerous communications from notorious experts published in highly distinguished journals. All the above are in accord, not only regarding the opportunity offered by assisted conception methods to HIV-discordant couples, but rather that denying assisted reproduction to couples with HIV is, nowadays, an approach that is unjustifiable from both a scientific and an ethical point of view[35–37].

ASSISTED CONCEPTION WITH SPERM WASHING

Prior to admission to the program, couples must undergo a detailed screening to exclude, or diagnose, infertility factors, and infectious diseases

which may increase the risk of HIV transmission, be transmitted to the infant or compromise the outcome of pregnancy.

As far as infectious screening is concerned, women are requested to undergo a cervical swab for identification of *Chlamydia*, *Ureaplasma* and *Mycoplasma* infections, and a vaginal swab investigating bacterial infections. Blood tests are performed for HIV, hepatitis B virus (HBV), HCV, syphilis, CMV and rubeola antibodies. The gynecological screening includes a Papanicolaou (PAP) test and hysterosalpingography to ascertain tubal patency for women who are candidates for IUI, or alternatively hysteroscopy for women who are candidates for *in vitro* fertilization. The fertility evaluation is completed by hormonal dosings of thyroid stimulating hormone (TSH), luteinizing hormone (LH), follicle stimulating hormone (FSH) and 17β-estradiol during the menstrual phase, and progesterone and prolactin between the 22nd and 24th day of the cycle.

The man's battery of infectious disease tests includes performance of a urethral swab for *Chlamydia*, *Ureaplasma* and *Mycoplasma* and a sperm culture for bacteria. In addition to antibody testing for HBV, HCV, syphilis and CMV, the clinical evaluation includes HIV blood viremia and, for HCV-positive men, HCV viremia, and an evaluation of HIV-related health including

Table 26.1 CREAThE (Centres for Reproductive Assistance Techniques to HIV couples in Europe) retrospective analysis of semen washing and assisted reproductive technologies (ART) cycles performed before 31 December 2002 (unpublished data)

	Couples (n)	Cycles (n)	Pregnancies (n)	Miscarriages (n)	Live births (n)	Ongoing (n)
IUI fresh sperm	1373	3693	524	79	427	59
IUI frozen sperm	142	397	62	13	47	7
IVF–ET/ICSI	254	361	117	17	42	27
ET cryo	16	18	2	0	0	2
Total	1785	4469	705	109	516	95

IUI, intrauterine insemination; IVF–ET, *in vitro* fertilization–embryo transfer; ICSI, intracytoplasmic sperm injection measurements of CD4 and CD8 cell counts, and history of antiretroviral treatment. The male fertility evaluation is mainly based on the characteristics of a baseline spermiogram performed after sperm washing, although hormonal determinations of testosterone, LH, FSH are also performed.

Assisted conception treatment consists of sperm washing, which can be followed either by intrauterine transfer of washed spermatozoa or by *in vitro* fertilization. The indication for resorting to *in vivo* or *in vitro* fertilization should be dictated by the couple's fertility potential, as no evidence is available indicating that *in vitro* fertilization or intracytoplasmic sperm injection (ICSI) could render assisted conception safer than by intrauterine insemination, regardless of HAART. Moreover, ICSI might increase the possibility of transferring viral particles adhering to the external acrosomal membrane within the oocyte's cytoplasm, while this membrane is removed with spontaneous sperm–egg interaction. Finally, the choice of whether sperm washing should be coupled with insemination or *in vitro* fertilization (IVF) must be based on sound clinical evaluation, but also on other factors, such as logistics, the economic resources of the couple and their emotional situation, bearing in mind that the offer of an inaccessible program of assisted conception renders spontaneous conception the only viable option. In consideration of the epidemiology of the HIV epidemic, a highly selective enrollment procedure resulting in the offer of costly procedures to a selected few[38] may exclude the majority of HIV-affected couples in search of a child.

In particular, the indications for the four ART alternatives include:

Intrauterine insemination (IUI) in spontaneous ovulation cycle: indicated in couples in whom both partners are fertile; the woman is less than 35 years old and presents no hormonal imbalance; and the man's seminal sample after the sperm washing procedure has over 1.5 million motile spermatozoa/ml. The chances of conception are 15% per cycle.

IUI with hormonal stimulation of multiple follicular growth: recommended in couples who present a clinical indication for its use; where the woman is over 35 years old; when the couple has undergone three spontaneous cycles with no pregnancy; when the couple lives far away from the center; and when an increase in pregnancy chances is desirable for logistic reasons.

IVF–ET: indicated in the presence of female infertility, including occlusion of the Fallopian tubes, or endometriosis. The man's sample has to have more than 1.5 million spermatozoa/ml. IVF is also used in couples who have undergone repeated inseminations with no pregnancy. In this case as well, the seminal sample of the man must have more than 1.5 million spermatozoa/ml after washing. The chances of conception are 25% per cycle.

IVF–ET/ICSI: indicated in cases of male infertility represented by a reduction of the number of motile spermatozoa to fewer than 1.5 million/ml; by severe reduction in motility; or by conditions characterized by immotile sperm.

FERTILITY IN HIV-DISCORDANT COUPLES

Couples trying for a pregnancy can usually achieve conception within a median of 5.2 months with an average of two acts of intercourse per week, while after 12 months of trying the likelihood of fertilization falls to less than 7% per subsequent year. In HIV-discordant couples, such spontaneous conception attempts are contraindicated due to the implied risk of HIV transmission to the woman.

In the general population, the approximate rate of infertility, defined as an inability to conceive within 1 year of spontaneous trials, is approximately 10%. Comparable data cannot be obtained in HIV-discordant couples because of the risk of sexual transmission of HIV. In the first years of the assisted conception program, couples presented a significantly higher prevalence of infertility factors (Table 26.2), although the prevalence is gradually changing in parallel with the shift in the HIV epidemic from intravenous drug users to the heterosexual population. Nearly 85% of men accessing the program between 1989 and 1995 were former intravenous drug users. In these men the rate of genital tract infections was over 50%, possibly accounting for the 10% prevalence of tubal damage in their female partners. At that time, no antiretroviral medication was available, and the clinical condition of the men was unstable. This highly charged situation could explain the 20% of anovulatory cycles, probably due to high levels of stress in the women.

In the current epidemiological picture, where many men are infected heterosexually, most in satisfactory clinical condition thanks to HAART, the infertility factor distribution is increasingly similar to that of the general population, with the exception of higher percentages of poor seminal counts.

No longitudinal study has unequivocally shown that HIV infection *per se* leads to dyspermia, unless overt wasting or otherwise failing clinical conditions are present. However, HAART has the theoretical possibility of impacting on seminal motility, as mitochondrial toxicity is one of the leading adverse effects of nucleoside antiretrovirals such as inhibitors of inverse transcriptase. Preliminary evidence in this regard has shown a significant reduction in the quantity of mitochondrial RNA in the peripheral blood mononuclear cells of men treated with HAART, suggesting that this might impair sperm motility[39], which would reduce the *in vivo* pregnancy rate with either spontaneous conception or artificial insemination. This effect is likely to be more pronounced in the case of semen washing, as the procedure inevitably selects only the proportion of highly motile spermatozoa.

Therefore, couples in whom any act of intercourse might result in infection, and who are willing to try for a pregnancy on their own, should be counseled on the need to conduct at least a basic fertility evaluation and advised about the

Table 26.2 Frequency of infertility factors in HIV-discordant couples undergoing sperm washing and assisted reproductive technologies (ART) (author's data)

Infertility factor	Prevalence (%)
Male genital tract infections	47
Female genital tract infections	29
< 1.5 million/ml motile spermatozoa	16.5
Hyperprolactinemia	14
Uni- or bilateral tubal damage/obstruction	12
Anovulatory cycles	10
Uterine cavity abnormalities	7
Endometriosis	1.5

protective effect of assisted conception with sperm washing.

CONCLUSIONS

Sperm washing and highly active antiretroviral treatment are the cornerstones in offering men infected with HIV the possibility of responsible, medically controlled procreation. While HAART has an impact on infectious potential by reducing blood, and potentially seminal, viral load, sperm washing effectively reduces the infectiousness of the semen.

In today's reality, where people with HIV lead longer and healthier lives thanks to long-term viral suppression offered by HAART, long-term projects including parenthood become feasible to an ever-larger proportion of infected individuals. In this setting it is both ethically and medically justified to offer them the best viable options for medically controlled conception, also bearing in mind that withdrawing medically assisted reproduction abandons couples to the poor choice between childlessness and spontaneous attempts at conception.

REFERENCES

1. Porco TC, et al. Decline in HIV infectivity following the introduction of highly active antiretroviral therapy. AIDS 2004; 18: 81
2. Shaffer N, et al. Short-course zidovudine for perinatal HIV-1 transmission in Bangkok, Thailand: a randomised controlled trial. Lancet 1999; 353: 773
3. Guay L, et al. Intrapartum and neonatal single-dose of nevirapine compared with zidovudine for prevention of mother-to-child transmission on HIV-1 in Kampala, Uganda: HIVNET 012 randomised trial. Lancet 1999; 354: 795
4. Thorne C Fiore S, Rudin C. Antiretroviral therapy during pregnancy and the risk of an adverse outcome [Comment]. N Engl J Med 2003; 348: 471
5. Cederfjall C, et al. Gender differences in perceived health-related quality of life among patients with HIV infection. AIDS Patient Care STDS 2001; 15: 31
6. CDC. Recommendations of the US Public Health Service Task Force on the use of zidovudine to reduce perinatal transmission of human immunodeficiency virus. MMWR Morb Mortal Wkly Rep 1994; 43: RR-11
7. Hamers EF, Downs AM. HIV in central and eastern Europe. Lancet 2003; 361: 1035
8. Rotily M, et al. Factors related to delayed diagnosis of HIV infection in Southeastern France. EVALVIH group. Int J STD AIDS 2000; 11: 531
9. Van der Straten A, et al. Sexual risk behaviors among heterosexual HIV serodiscordant couples in the era of post-exposure prevention and viral suppressive therapy. AIDS 2000; 14: F47
10. UNAIDS. 2004 Report on the global AIDS epidemic. Executive Summary. Geneva: UNAIDS, 2004
11. Dougan S, et al. Epidemiology of HIV in young people in England, Wales and Northern Ireland. Commun Dis Public Health 2004; 7: 15
12. www.eurohiv.org
13. Giuliani M, et al. Screening for HIV-1 infection targeted to women at a center for sexually transmitted diseases (STD). Comparison between 2 periods of 5 years of work. Minerva Ginecol 2000; 52 (Suppl 1): 34
14. Klevens RM, et al. Knowledge of partner risk and secondary transmission of HIV. Am J Prev Med 2001; 20: 277
15. Chirgwin KD, et al. Incidence and risk factors for heterosexually acquired HIV in an inner-city cohort of women: temporal association with pregnancy. J Acquir Immune Defic Synd Hum Retrovirol 1999; 20: 295
16. Castilla J, et al. Late diagnosis of HIV infection in the era of highly active antiretroviral therapy: consequences for AIDS incidence. AIDS 2002; 16: 1945
17. Gray RH, et al. Probability of HIV-1 transmission per coital act in monogamous, heterosexual, HIV-1-discordant couples in Rakai, Uganda. Lancet 2001; 357: 1149
18. Louria DB, et al. HIV heterosexual transmission: a hypothesis about an additional potential determinant. Int J Infect Dis 2000; 4: 110
19. Chakraborty H, et al. Viral burden in genital secretions determines male-to-female sexual transmission of HIV-1: a probabilistic empiric model. AIDS 2001; 15: 621
20. Mayer KH, Anderson DJ. Heterosexual HIV transmission. Infect Agents Dis 1995; 4: 273
21. Taylor S, Boffito M, Vernazza PL. Antiretroviral therapy to reduce the sexual transmission of HIV [in Process Citation]. J HIV Ther 2003; 8: 55
22. Downs AM, De Vincenzi I. Probability of heterosexual transmission of HIV: relationship to the number of unprotected sexual contacts. European Study Group in Heterosexual Transmission of HIV. J Acquir Immune Defic Syndr Hum Retrovirol 1996; 11: 388
23. Vernazza PL, et al. Potent antiretroviral treatment of HIV-infection results in suppression of the seminal shedding of HIV. The Swiss HIV Cohort Study. AIDS 2000; 14: 117
24. Bujan L, et al. Factors of intermittent HIV-1 excretion in semen and efficiency of sperm processing in obtaining spermatozoa without HIV-1 genomes. AIDS 2004; 18: 757
25. World Health Organization. Progress in Reproductive Health Research, No. 48. Geneva: WHO, 1998
26. Weller S, Davis K. Condom effectiveness in reducing heterosexual HIV transmission. Cochrane Database Syst Rev 2002; (1): CD003255
27. Gottlieb GS, et al. Dual HIV-1 infection associated with rapid disease progression. Lancet 2004; 363: 619
28. World Health Organization. Progress in Reproductive Health Research, No. 59. Geneva: WHO, 2002
29. Norman LR. Predictors of consistent condom use: a hierarchical analysis of adults from Kenya, Tanzania and Trinidad. Int J STD AIDS 2003; 14: 584
30. Mandelbrot L, et al. Natural conception in HIV-negative women with HIV-infected partners. Lancet 1997; 349: 850

31. Panozzo L, et al. High risk behaviour and fertility desires among heterosexual HIV-positive patients with a serodiscordant partner – two challenging issues. Swiss Med Wkly 2003; 133: 124

32. Semprini AE, et al. Insemination of HIV-negative women with processed semen of HIV-positive partners. Lancet 1992; 340: 1317

33. Anderson DJ, et al. Efficacy of conventional semen processing techniques in separation of motile sperm from HIV-1 and HIV-1 host cells. Presented at the 48th Annual Meeting of the American Fertility Society, New Orleans, November 1992; Abstr book: 107, P 213

34. Semprini AE. Semen washing in ART for uninfected women with HIV-positive partners. Presented at the 56th Annual Meeting of the American Society for Reproductive Medicine, San Diego, October 2000

35. Gilling-Smith C, Smith JR, Semprini AE. HIV and infertility: time to treat. There's no justification for denying treatment to parents who are HIV positive. Br Med J 2001; 322: 566

36. Ethics Committee of the American Society for Reproductive Medicine. Human immunodeficiency virus and infertility treatment. Fertil Steril 2002; 77: 218

37. American College of Obstetricians and Gynecologists. ACOG Committee Opinion 255. HIV: Ethical guidelines for obstetricians and gynecologists, April 2001. Washington, DC: ACOG, 2001

38. Peña JE, et al. Providing assisted reproductive care to male haemophiliacs infected with human immunodeficiency virus: preliminary experience. Haemophilia 2003; 9: 309

39. Miro O, et al. Mitochondrial DNA depletion and respiratory chain enzyme deficiencies are present in peripheral blood mononuclear cells of HIV-infected patients with HAART-related lipodystrophy. Antivir Ther 2003; 8: 333

27

Artificial insemination using homologous and donor semen

Willem Ombelet, Martine Nijs

INTRODUCTION

The first documented application of artificial insemination was presented in London in the 1770s by John Hunter. A cloth merchant with severe hypospadias was advised to collect semen in a warmed syringe and inject the sample into the vagina. Sims reported his findings of postcoital tests and 55 inseminations in 1873. Only one pregnancy occurred, but this could be explained by the fact that he believed that ovulation occurred during menstruation.

The rationale behind intrauterine insemination (IUI) with homologous sperm is to bypass the cervical–mucus barrier and to increase the number of motile spermatozoa with a high proportion of normal forms at the site of fertilization[1]. A few decades ago, homologous artificial insemination was performed only in cases of physiological and psychological dysfunction, such as retrograde ejaculation, vaginismus, hypospadias and impotence. With the routine use of postcoital tests, other indications were added, such as hostile cervical mucus and immunological causes with the presence of antispermatozoal antibodies.

The main reason for the renewed interest in IUI is refinement of techniques for the preparation of washed motile spermatozoa associated with the introduction of *in vitro* fertilization (IVF). Washing procedures are necessary to remove prostaglandins, infectious agents and antigenic proteins. Another substantial advantage of these techniques is the removal of non-motile spermatozoa, leukocytes and immature germ cells. This may enhance sperm quality by decreasing the release of lymphokines and/or cytokines and also by a reduction in the formation of free oxygen radicals. The final result is improved fertilizing capacity of the sperm sample *in vitro* and *in vivo*[2].

Despite the extensive literature on the subject of artificial homologous insemination, controversy remains about the effectiveness of this very popular treatment procedure, especially when moderate or severe male subfertility is involved. Contradictory results are observed because most studies are retrospective and vary in (1) comparison of the study group (different groups of male subfertility), (2) use or non-use of different ovarian hyperstimulation regimens, (3) number of inseminations per treatment cycle, (4) timing of ovulation, (5) sites of insemination and (6) methods of sperm preparation.

Nevertheless, there is clear evidence in the literature that IUI can be offered as a first-line treatment in most cases of unexplained, mild and moderate male factor infertility, resulting in acceptable pregnancy rates, before starting more invasive and more expensive techniques of assisted reproduction such as *in vitro* fertilization (IVF) and intracytoplasmic sperm injection (ICSI)[3–5].

The effectiveness of IUI was also reported in a large retrospective analysis of almost 10 000 IUI cycles in which male factor subfertility was associated with a pregnancy rate of 8.2% per cycle in a population with an average female age of 39 years[6].

IUI is much easier to perform, less invasive and less expensive than other methods of assisted reproduction. Moreover, risks are minimal, provided that the incidence of multiple gestations can be reduced to an acceptable level.

ARTIFICIAL INSEMINATION WITH DONOR SEMEN

The first reported artificial insemination with donor semen (AID) was performed by William Pancoast in 1884 to treat a case of 'postgonococcal azoospermia'. Robert Dickinson of New York City should be acknowledged for his contribution towards making this technique acceptable, lawful and legitimate. Despite the growing popularity worldwide, different religions considered this form of non-coital reproduction unacceptable. Nowadays, AID is a successful technique of assisted reproduction, but questions of emotional, religious and legal issues are still important.

In this chapter, we briefly focus on the indications, selection of donors, screening of donors for infectious and genetic diseases, procedure and technical aspects and treatment evaluation.

Indications for AID

Until the introduction of ICSI, AID was the most common treatment of infertility associated with severe oligoasthenoteratozoospermia and azoospermia. Other important indications for AID are genetic disorders, repeated fertilization failure or unsuccessful attempts with IVF. With the introduction of ICSI in 1992[7], even severe male subfertility could be treated successfully, and the number of AID-treated cases dropped significantly all over the world. Nowadays, AID is most commonly used for lesbians and single women, reaching over 50% of all insemination treatments at least in countries where this is ethically and legally permitted. On the other hand, it was reported that although a majority of patients with severe male subfertility could opt for ICSI, AID was still an option for many couples for whom these techniques were either not feasible or not successful. A substantial proportion of patients (33%) did not opt for ICSI[8].

Selection of donors

Different countries have different regulations. A consensus document for donor recruitment remains difficult, but it should consist of at least the following guidelines: (1) counseling must be offered and potential donors must be informed about the use of their gametes, the maximum number of families into which children can be born with their gametes, the legislation and the rules of the center; (2) freely given informed consent is mandatory; (3) the donor must indicate whether he wants to be an anonymous (no information between donor and recipient) or a non-anonymous donor; and (4) reimbursement of donors is possible but it should be limited so that it does not become the primary reason for donation[9]. Governmental bodies such as the European Parliament and Council or the US Food and Drug Administration have produced written directives that set standards of quality and safety for the donation, procurement, testing, processing, preservation, storage and distribution of human reproductive cells.

Screening for donors

Psychological counseling

Psychological counseling must include the evaluation of motivation, assessment of readiness, psychiatric history, fulfillment of the child wish and psychosociological implications of anonymous/non-anonymous sperm donation.

A normal medical history

It is recommended that normal healthy donors without a history of a major (hereditary) disease are recruited. Blood type and rhesus factor are determined. Physical characteristics such as hair and eye color, weight and size are registered.

Screening for infectious disease

All donors must be screened for risk factors and clinical evidence of infectious disease. This screening requires a review of relevant medical records, including a donor medical history interview and physical examination. The screening must specifically address risk factors for, and evidence of, at least: human immunodeficiency virus (HIV), hepatitis B and hepatitis C. Donations from anonymous semen donors must be quarantined until donors are retested and determined eligible at least 6 months after the date of original donation. Those samples in quarantine must be isolated physically or by other effective means while awaiting a decision on their acceptance or rejection.

Screening for genetic disease

A karyotype should always be performed. Donors with major hereditary disease should be rejected, and selective testing should also be performed for recessive genetic diseases that are prevalent according to ethnic origin, such as thalassemia or cystic fibrosis.

Screening for sperm quality

Although the sperm quality of a potential donor should be within the normal limits of motility, concentration and morphology of the World Health Organization (WHO) criteria for sperm normality, the post-thaw quality is also important. A loss of 30% in motility and viability should be taken into account. Moreover, some sperm samples cannot tolerate any freeze–thaw procedure[10]. Therefore, a test thawing of each frozen sample should be performed to ensure good donor quality at the actual time of AID.

Technical aspects of AID

Only frozen and thawed donor semen quarantined for at least 6 months can be used for AID. Before and after quarantine, appropriate tests to avoid the transmission of infectious diseases must be carried out. Accurate records of all donor samples are mandatory, and the regulations linked to the handling and storage of gametes must be clearly defined.

Matching donor and recipient phenotypic characteristics is advisable, if possible. The children born from a single donor should be limited to a low number (mostly ten children in a maximum of five families), not only to avoid the (very low) risk of consanguinity as a consequence of AID, but, more important, for psychological reasons related to the donor.

Treatment evaluation

Each center must strictly record the outcome of all AID cycles, and regional centralization of the data concerning pregnancies should be performed. In cases of anonymous donation, measures should be installed to ensure non-disclosure of data and records. In general, pregnancy outcome results with AID are comparable to those of fresh cycles with homologous semen. Factors influencing the success rate with AID are discussed later in this chapter.

ARTIFICIAL INSEMINATION WITH HOMOLOGOUS SEMEN

Before IUI with homologous semen is applied in daily practice, we must be convinced of the exact value of the technique. Therefore, IUI has to be weighed against expectant management, medical and surgical treatment, timed coitus, IVF and ICSI. This comparison should not only involve success rates but also include a cost–benefit analysis, and analysis of the complication rates of the various treatment options, invasiveness of the techniques and patient compliance.

Effectiveness of IUI

Cervical factor subfertility

In a case of cervical factor subfertility, it seems logical to perform IUI. Bypassing the hostile cervix should increase the probability of conception. The results of a meta-analysis of randomized controlled trials comparing IUI with timed intercourse for couples with cervical factor infertility showed an improved probability of conception for IUI (odds ratio (OR) with 95% confidence interval (CI) 3.6, 2.0–6.5)[11].

Unexplained subfertility

If an infertility work-up is unable to detect a plausible explanation for couples with a history of subfertility of at least 1 year, we use the term 'unexplained infertility'. Because a good explanation for the subfertility is lacking, the treatment is often empirical. A meta-analysis comparing IUI and timed intercourse in natural cycles showed no difference in results; therefore, IUI in natural cycles seems to be ineffective in cases of unexplained infertility. When controlled ovarian hyperstimulation (COH) is used, IUI becomes effective, compared with timed intercourse[11]. Peterson et al.[12] found that three cycles of COH–IUI in couples with unexplained infertility was just as effective as one IVF cycle in achieving pregnancy, but IVF was more expensive.

Male factor subfertility

When a male factor is found in couples with long-standing infertility, expectant treatment seems to be disappointing, with a spontaneous conception rate of only 2% per cycle[13]. Therefore, this strategy is not applicable in clinical practice. For IUI, with or without COH, a pregnancy rate of 10–18% per cycle has been reported[6,14]. In a Cochrane review, Cohlen et al.[15] concluded that IUI is superior to timed intercourse (TI), both in natural cycles and in cycles with COH (natural cycles–IUI vs. TI: OR 2.43, CI 1.54–3.83; COH–IUI vs. TI: OR 2.14, CI 1.30–3.51). According to this review, IUI in natural cycles should be the treatment of choice in cases of moderate to severe male subfertility, providing that an inseminating motile count (IMC) of more than 1 million can be obtained after sperm preparation and in the absence of a triple sperm defect (according to WHO criteria).

Sperm quality and IUI results

In the selection of couples to be treated with IUI or IVF/ICSI, it would be interesting to establish cut-off values of semen parameters above which IUI is a real alternative for IVF/ICSI in male subfertility. According to the literature, the inseminating motile count (IMC) and sperm morphology are the most valuable sperm parameters for predicting IUI outcome[14,16–18]. A trend towards increasing conception rates with increasing IMC was reported, but the cut-off value above which IUI seems to be successful, however, varies[14,18–22] between 0.3 and 20×10^6. A large retrospective analysis in Genk in a selected group of patients with normal ovarian response to clomiphene citrate stimulation showed no significant difference in cumulative ongoing pregnancy rate after three IUI cycles between all patients, providing that the IMC was more than 1 million[16]. Furthermore, in cases with fewer than 1 million motile spermatozoa, IUI remained successful as a first-line option provided that the sperm morphology score was 4% or more (cumulative ongoing pregnancy rate of 21.9% after three IUI cycles).

In a meta-analysis of Van Waart et al.[23], a threshold of $\geq 5\%$ normal forms using strict criteria showed a significant improvement in pregnancy rate. In a large number of studies, 5% normal forms and 1 million motile spermatozoa after sperm preparation are believed to be potential cut-off values to select couples for IUI treatment[16,17,24–31]. For total sperm motility before sperm preparation, cut-off levels between 30 and 50% are reported[14,29,31,32]. Two other parameters influencing the pregnancy rate after IUI are the hypo-osmotic swelling (HOS) test (> 50%, in a study by Tartagni et al.[33]) and sperm DNA fragmentation (< 12%, in a study by Duran et al.[34]).

Cost of ART-related services

Evidence related to the cost and effectiveness of infertility treatment exists, but most studies have focused on in vitro fertilization (IVF). The cost-effectiveness of different interventions should be considered when making decisions about treatment. A number of studies have been performed that focused on the cost-effectiveness of IUI when compared with IVF[3,4,12,35,36].

Published data comparing costs of IVF vs. IUI indicate that the costs of IVF, gamete intrafallopian transfer (GIFT) and zygote intrafallopian transfer (ZIFT) are 4–7 times the cost of a single superovulation/IUI cycle[37–39]. Using meta-analysis, Peterson et al.[12] concluded that the pregnancy rate for three cycles of gonadotropins and IUI in a population group of unexplained infertility was superior to that with IVF or ZIFT and comparable to that with GIFT. In a prospective randomized controlled trial, Goverde et al.[3] concluded that three cycles of IUI offer the same likelihood of a successful pregnancy as does IVF. They concluded that IUI is a more cost-effective approach, not only for unexplained subfertility, but also for moderate male factor subfertility.

This important message was confirmed in another study performed in the UK[4]. In this study the authors complemented existing clinical guidelines by including the cost-effectiveness of various treatment options for infertility in the UK. A series of decision-analytical models were developed to reflect current diagnostic and treatment pathways for the different causes of infertility. According to this study, stimulated IUI for unexplained and moderate male factor infertility is a cost-effective approach. In a systematic review, Garceau et al.[5] also showed that initiating treatment with IUI appears to be more cost-effective than IVF in most cases of unexplained and moderate male subfertility.

Risks and complications of IUI

Severe ovarian hyperstimulation syndrome (OHSS) may complicate all methods of treatment in which gonadotropins are used; however, OHSS seems to be rare after COH–IUI, compared with IVF[40–43]. The incidence of *pelvic inflammatory disease* after intrauterine catheterization and/or transvaginal oocyte aspiration has been estimated to be 0.2% for IVF[41] and 0.01–0.2% for IUI[24,40,43]. The major complication of assisted reproductive technologies (ART) remains, however, the high incidence of *multiple pregnancies*, responsible for considerable mortality, morbidity and costs[44]. In COH–IUI cycles, the prediction of multiple gestation is highly uncertain, especially when gonadotropins are used, and this is despite careful monitoring of the cycle with ultrasonography and serum estradiol determinations. Careful monitoring remains essential, and cancellation of the insemination procedure, 'escape IVF' and follicular aspiration before IUI are reasonable options. Transvaginal ultrasound-guided aspiration of supernumerary ovarian follicles increases both the efficacy and the safety of COH–IUI with gonadotropins[45,46]. This method represents an alternative for conversion of overstimulated cycles to in vitro fertilization ('escape IVF'). Natural-cycle IUI, clomiphene citrate and a minimal-dose regimen with gonadotropins are valuable options to prevent the unacceptably high multiple gestation rates described after ovarian hyperstimulation.

A retrospective analysis of 619 065 pregnancies and 661 065 births between 1993 and 2003 in Flanders (Belgium) showed a multiple gestation rate of 13.3% and 27.8% after artificial insemination and IVF, respectively. Although more than 50% of pregnancies after ART are associated with non-IVF (COH with or without IUI), almost two-thirds of multiple pregnancies after ART are caused by IVF–ICSI. This may be explained by the fact that most centers in Flanders use clomiphene citrate and natural cycles rather than gonadotropins in IUI (Ombelet, unpublished data; questionnaire of the Flemish Society of Obstetrics and Gynecology, 2003).

To our knowledge, only three papers have been published reporting the *obstetric and perinatal outcome* after IUI. According to Nuojua-Huttunen *et al.*[47], and using data obtained from the Finnish Medical Birth Register (MBR), IUI treatment did not increase obstetric or perinatal risks compared with matched spontaneous or IVF pregnancies. Wang *et al.*[48] examined preterm birth in 1015 IUI/AID singleton births compared with 1019 IVF/ICSI and 1019 naturally conceived births. They found that IUI/AID singletons were about 1.5 times more likely to be born preterm than naturally conceived singletons, whereas the IVF/ICSI group were 2.4 times more likely to be born preterm than the naturally conceived group. In a retrospective cohort study, Gaudoin *et al.*[49] described a poorer perinatal outcome for singletons born to subfertile mothers conceived through COH–IUI compared with matched natural conceptions within the Scottish national cohort. This was caused by a higher incidence of premature and low birth-weight infants. They suggested that intrinsic factors in subfertile couples predispose them to having smaller infants. We recently performed a study to investigate differences in perinatal outcome of singleton and twin pregnancies after controlled ovarian hyperstimulation (COH), with or without artificial insemination (AI), compared with pregnancies after natural conception[50].

We analyzed the data from the regional registry of 661 065 births in Flanders (Belgium) during the period 1993–2003. A total of 12 021 singleton and 3108 twin births could be selected. Control subjects were matched for maternal age, parity, fetal sex and year of birth. We found a significantly higher incidence of extreme prematurity (< 32 weeks), very low birth weight (< 1500 g), stillbirths and perinatal death for COH/AI singletons. Twin pregnancies resulting from COH/AI showed a higher rate of neonatal mortality, assisted ventilation and respiratory distress syndrome. According to our results, COH/IUI singleton and twin pregnancies are significantly disadvantaged compared with naturally conceived children, with a higher mortality rate and a higher incidence of low birth weight and prematurity. We also believe that infertility itself predisposes to a worse perinatal outcome compared with naturally conceived babies.

Couple compliance

Since IUI is a simple and non-invasive technique, it can be performed without expensive infrastructure with a good success rate within three or four cycles. It is a safe and easy treatment, with minimal risks and monitoring. These factors are responsible for a high couple compliance for IUI compared with IVF. We previously described a low drop-out rate of 19.6% in a series of 1100 IUI cycles[14]. A much higher drop-out rate and long time interval between treatment cycles for IVF and ICSI has been described before[37]. Table 27.1 gives an overview of the pros and cons of IUI compared with IVF/ICSI.

Treatment strategy in male subfertility: opinion

Figure 27.1 shows the treatment strategy used at the Genk Institute for Fertility Technology. In most cases we start with clomiphene citrate ovarian stimulation, although the cumulative ongoing pregnancy rate is significantly lower compared with follicle stimulating hormone (FSH) and/or luteinizing hormone (LH) stimulation[14], but with the benefit of a low multiple pregnancy rate (less than 7%). Although the cumulative ongoing pregnancy rate after three IUI cycles is comparable to that of only one IVF cycle (25%), more than 90% of our couples agree to follow our protocol, being aware of the better success rate per cycle after IVF. Excellent counseling is mandatory and crucial.

Table 27.1 Overview of the pros and cons of intrauterine insemination (IUI) compared with *in vitro* fertilization (IVF) and intracytoplasmic sperm injection (ICSI). IMC, inseminating motile count; OHSS, ovarian hyperstimulation syndrome; PID, pelvic inflammatory disease; LBW, low birth weight (< 2500 g). Reprinted from an article in *Reproductive Biomedicine Online* by Ombelet *et al.* with permission from Reproductive Healthcare Ltd[51]

Pros	Cons
IUI	
Minimal equipment necessary	⇓ Success rate per cycle
Easy method	⇓ Success if IMC < 1 million
Less invasive	⇓ Success if morphology < 5%
Less expensive	⇑ Risk for LBW, prematurity
Good couple compliance ⇒ low drop-out rate	(risk for antisperm antibodies)
Low risk for OHSS, PID	
Moderate multiple pregnancy rate	
IVF ± ICSI	
Minimal transmission of infection (IVF)	Invasive
High success rate per cycle	⇑ Risk for LBW, prematurity
	High risk for OHSS, PID
	High multiple pregnancy rate
	⇑ Risk for genetic disorders
	Lower couple compliance ⇒ high drop-out rate

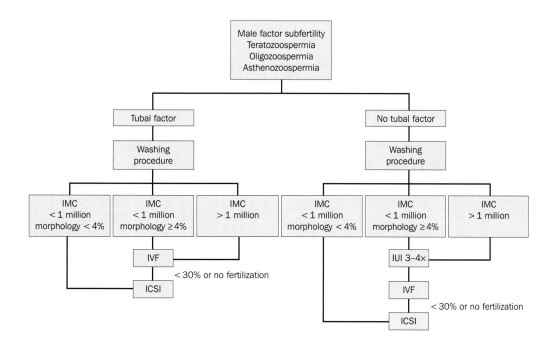

Figure 27.1 Opinion: proposed algorithm of male subfertility treatment at the Genk Institute for Fertility Technology. IMC, inseminating motile count; IVF, *in vitro* fertilization; ICSI, intracytoplasmic sperm injection; IUI, intrauterine insemination. Reprinted from an article in *Reproductive Biomedicine Online* by Ombelet *et al.* with permission from Reproductive Healthcare Ltd[52]

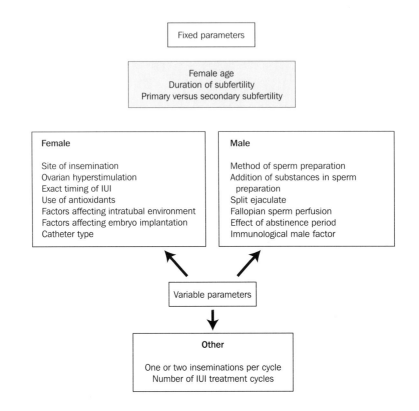

Figure 27.2   Factors influencing the success rate in intrauterine insemination (IUI)

Factors influencing IUI success

Female factors

The duration of subfertility[53], primary or secondary subfertility, endometriosis and the use or non-use of ovarian hyperstimulation are important factors that might influence the success rate of IUI significantly[54]. Other variables might be the site of insemination, the use of antioxidants, factors influencing the intratubal environment and factors influencing embryo implantation (Figure 27.2)[55]. Below the age of 40 years, female age was not predictive of conception rate per cycle after artificial insemination with husband's semen (AIH) treatment[14].

Site of insemination   Artificial insemination can be done intravaginally, intracervically (ICI) or

pericervically using a cap, or be intrauterine (IUI), transcervical intrafallopian (IFI) or directly intraperitoneal (IPI). Most studies consider IUI to be an easy and better way of treatment. In a donor insemination program, Hurd *et al.*[56] reported a significantly better cycle fecundity rate for IUI compared with ICI or IFI. More sperm was found in the peritoneal cavity after IUI when compared with ICI[57]. Studies comparing pregnancy outcomes after IUI versus cervical cap insemination[58] and transuterotubal insemination[59] also favored the intrauterine method. In a large randomized controlled trial, it was shown that among infertile couples, treatment with induction of superovulation and intrauterine insemination was three times as likely to result in pregnancy as was intracervical insemination, and twice as likely to result in pregnancy as was treatment with either superovulation and intracervical insemination or intrauterine insemination alone[60].

Factors influencing oocyte quality and number of oocytes

Natural cycle versus controlled ovarian hyperstimulation (COH) The rationale behind the use of ovarian hyperstimulation in artificial insemination is the increase of the number of oocytes available for fertilization, and to correct subtle unpredictable ovulatory dysfunction[61]. Other advantages of superovulation with human menopausal gonadotropins are the enhanced opportunities for oocyte capture, fertilization and implantation.

On the other hand, in a controlled study, Cohlen *et al.*[62] concluded that in male subfertility cases ovarian stimulation improved the success rate only in moderate cases (IMC > 10 million). Comparing the effects of COH on pregnancy rate after IUI, human menopausal gonadotropin (hMG) stimulation results in a significantly higher monthly fecundability than that with clomiphene citrate treatment[43]. A retrospective study of 1100 IUI procedures in 412 couples showed a pregnancy rate of 17.7% per cycle after hMG stimulation compared with 10% per cycle after clomiphene citrate stimulation, but at the expense of a higher multiple pregnancy rate. This statistical difference was not influenced by the indication for IUI[63]. Considering the risk for multiple pregnancies and ovarian hyperstimulation syndrome (OHSS), a mild COH regimen should be used. Cohlen *et al.*[15] recommend IUI in natural cycles as the treatment of first choice in severe semen defects (IMC > 1 million, no triple semen defect).

Exact timing of IUI Exact timing is probably crucial in IUI treatment cycles. On the other hand, conflicting data are reported in the literature on which methodology is to be used. Combined ultrasound and hormonal monitoring with human chorionic gonadotropin (hCG) induction probably allows the most exact timing but is relatively expensive and time-consuming. Urinary LH-timed IUI is commonly used, but has the disadvantage

that the LH surge can last for up to 2 days before ovulation in some patients. Therefore, its use results in the inaccurate timing of ovulation and insemination[64]. A prospective, randomized crossover study of Zreik *et al.*[65] could not demonstrate an increased pregnancy rate when ultrasound monitoring and hCG were used, compared with urinary LH-timed inseminations. In another study, no benefit was found in waiting for the spontaneous LH surge before administering hCG[66].

To conclude, it seems that being aware of the importance of exact timing is essential in IUI, independent of the method being used.

Perifollicular vascularity of the follicles Chiu and colleagues[67] were the first to report a positive correlation between perifollicular blood flow and pregnancy rate from IVF–embryo transfer (ET) using the power Doppler angiogram. Bhal *et al.*[68] used Doppler imaging to identify those IUI cycles with high-grade perifollicular vascularity, and hence good oxygenation of the follicle with the maturing oocyte. The results again showed a significant correlation between perifollicular blood flow and pregnancy rate (57%) occurring in the group where all follicles had good blood flow, and significantly lower pregnancy rates where there was poor blood flow (11%). Significantly more multiple pregnancies developed when all the follicles exhibited good blood flow at the time of insemination. Monofollicular IUI cycles with poor blood flow are canceled by Bhal *et al.*[69] and Gregory *et al.*[70], since they resulted in no pregnancies in their studies[70].

The use of antioxidants Supplementation of culture media with reactive oxygen species (ROS) scavengers prevents the negative effects of oocyte aging in relation to *in vitro* fertilization, (less cellular fragmentation and development of concepti until the blastocyst stage[71]). Reactive oxygen species generation was also shown to be negatively associated with both the outcome of the sperm–oocyte fusion assay and fertility *in vivo*[72]. Until now, no study has investigated the possible role of antioxidants, for example in culture media or as a dietary supplement, on success rates in IUI cycles.

Factors affecting embryo implantation

Endometrial thickness/polyps   A trilaminar image rather than the exact endometrial thickness and/or Doppler measurement of the spiral and uterine arteries provides a favorable prediction of pregnancy in IUI[73,74]. Treatment should not be canceled because of inadequate endometrial thickness[75]. The use of ethinylestradiol in clomiphene-stimulated cycles[76] looks promising, but requires confirmation. If polyps are present, hysteroscopic polypectomy before IUI is an effective measure to enhance pregnancy results[77].

Which catheter to use   In IVF procedures, many studies have examined the influence of type of catheter and ease of transfer in predicting success after embryo transfer. Ultrasound-guided soft-catheter embryo transfer might improve pregnancy rates in IVF[78,79], although a number of studies did not find any influence on outcome comparing different catheters[80–82]. Lavie *et al.*[83] compared results after IUI using two different catheters. Although one catheter was significantly less traumatic (verified by ultrasound), only a trend towards an increase in the chance of conception was found. According to the results of another prospective randomized study comparing two different catheters, catheter type does not affect the outcome after IUI[84].

Male factors

Laboratory factors: do we need to prepare sperm samples for IUI?   The ejaculate is composed of spermatozoa of different qualities and maturities suspended in the secretions of the epididymis, testis, prostate, seminal vesicles and bulbourethral glands. Cells from the urinary tract and prostate, leukocytes and ROS are also present in the raw semen sample. Preparation and washing will remove ROS and also prostaglandins. These prostaglandins have to be removed since they will cause severe uterine cramps when a raw semen sample is used for IUI[85]. The preparation will concentrate morphologically normal and motile spermatozoa, essential for good results in IUI. Most popular are the swim-up procedures, density gradient centrifugation and the use of Sephadex® columns.

Density gradient centrifugation results in concentrating significantly more spermatozoa that have normal chromatin packaging, reduced levels of chromatin and nuclear DNA anomalies and enhanced rates of nuclear maturity[86–88]. Conflicting data are found on the superiority of any one preparation technique in terms of fecundity[89,90]. This can be explained by the fact that almost all methods of sperm washing and preparation surpass the low threshold number of motile spermatozoa ($> 1 \times 10^6$) needed for conception *in vivo*, with no added benefit of additional sperm. According to a Cochrane review[91], there is insufficient evidence to recommend any specific preparation technique. Large, high-quality, randomized controlled trials, comparing the effectiveness of a gradient and/or swim-up and/or wash and centrifugation technique on clinical outcome are lacking. Results from studies comparing semen parameters may suggest a preference for the gradient technique, but firm conclusions cannot be drawn, and the limitations should be taken into consideration.

Laboratory factors: addition of substances during sperm preparation   Whether the addition of substances such as pentoxifylline, kallikrein, follicular fluid, etc. may improve the results remains unclear and certainly unproven. On the other hand, it is important to recognize that sperm preparation methods may induce damage to spermatozoa by increasing ROS generation by the spermatozoa, and by removing the scavengers from the seminal plasma. Pentoxifylline, a motility stimulator, can also act as a ROS scavenger by reducing the generation of superoxide anion by spermatozoa[92], and may have a clinical role in the treatment of patients susceptible to ROS-induced damage (those with genital infections and smokers). More studies are needed to investigate whether treating spermatozoa with solutions containing antioxidants during sperm preparation can improve pregnancy rates with IUI in selected cases. Two double-blind randomized studies evaluated the effect of platelet-activating factor (PAF) exposure on sperm during semen processing for IUI[93,94]. They demonstrated a significantly higher pregnancy rate for the PAF-treated group in a subpopulation of couples without male factor subfertility.

Use of vaginal misoprostol   In a prospective, placebo-controlled, randomized and double-blind study, Brown *et al.*[95] reported an improved pregnancy rate when the prostaglandin E$_1$ analog misoprostol (400 μg) was placed vaginally at the time of IUI. This finding was confirmed in another prospective study using 200 μg of misoprostol[96]. The rationale behind this observation might be that some seminal constituents (perhaps prostaglandins) have a positive effect on fertility, and due to the sperm preparation these substances are eliminated from the inseminate.

Split ejaculate   The split ejaculate technique concentrates the most viable and motile spermatozoa in the first part of the ejaculate. Several clinicians use this fraction in IUI, although results with IUI using washed spermatozoa are significantly better[97].

Fallopian tube sperm perfusion (large volume of sperm suspension)   In Fallopian tube sperm perfusion (FSP), a large volume of sperm suspension is inseminated in an intrauterine procedure, with excellent results in cases of idiopathic infertility[98,99] and in a donor insemination program[100]. Since semen quality after a freezing–thawing procedure is comparable to that of a subfertile spermiogram, one might expect good results with FSP in male factor subfertility patients. However, we still wait for confirmation on this matter. A meta-analysis done by Trout and Kemmann[101] showed that FSP is only beneficial in cases of unexplained infertility after COH with hMG. Cantineau *et al.*[102] conducted a systematic review

based on a Cochrane review. They found that FSP gives rise to higher pregnancy rates in couples with unexplained subfertility. For other indications, FSP has not been proved more effective, compared with IUI. On the other hand, Biacchiardi *et al.*[103] performed a randomized, prospective, cross-over study and found that after COH, FSP is less effective than IUI in couples with unexplained infertility.

The effect of the abstinence period   Prolonged abstinence time increases ejaculate volume, sperm count, sperm concentration and the total number of motile spermatozoa[104,105], although the effect on sperm concentration is only small for oligozoospermic men[106]. In a prospective study we performed in Genk, abstinence did not influence pH, viability, morphology, total or grade A motility, or sperm DNA fragmentation. A short (24-hour) abstinence period negatively influenced chromatin quality[107]. It seems that looking for the optimal time of abstinence is not very important in IUI programs, and is probably valuable only in selected male subfertility cases.

Immunological male subfertility   The clinical significance of antisperm antibodies in male subfertility remains unclear[108,109], and the importance of circulating antisperm antibodies is probably low[110,111]. However, most studies demonstrate a clear association between sperm surface antibodies and the fertility potential of the male[112–114].

In 1997 we published a prospective study comparing the effectiveness of the first-line IUI approach versus IVF for male immunological subfertility[16]. The objective of this prospective study was to compare success rates after two different treatment protocols, COH–IUI versus IVF. Both IUI and IVF yielded unexpectedly high pregnancy rates in this selected group of patients with long-standing subfertility due to sperm surface antibodies. Since cost–benefit analysis comparing COH–IUI with IVF may favor a course of four IUI cycles, we concluded that IUI could be used as first-line therapy in male immunological subfertility. Although most fertility centers use

IVF/ICSI in cases of immunological male subfertility[115,116], a well-organized prospective study is mandatory to examine the real value of IUI for this specific indication.

Other factors: number of inseminations   Theoretically, improved chances for conception may be expected when two consecutive inseminations are performed, since ovulation does not occur in a synchronized pattern but rather in waves of release after hCG administration[117]. Another appeal of double IUI (DIUI) is the attrition phenomenon, by which IUI bypasses the cervical mucus. In the natural cycle the cervical mucus acts as a reservoir for sperm at mid-cycle, and a single IUI (SIUI) might miss later-released cohorts of oocytes. Ransom *et al.*[118] could not demonstrate an increase in pregnancy rates after DIUI in a prospective randomized trial using hMG stimulation for ovarian hyperstimulation. This study was contradictory to results previously reported[119]. These authors described a major increase in cycle fecundity when a DIUI (18 and 42 hours after hCG) was performed. Ng *et al.*[120], however, found no difference in pregnancy outcome between SIUI and DIUI.

The GIFT center organized a randomized prospective cross-over study to compare the pregnancy rates between single versus double IUI cycles using two different regimens of ovarian stimulation. In this study, 113 subfertile couples were followed during 203 IUI cycles. In 156 cycles (76.5%), a male factor was involved. Increasing the frequency of insemination provided significantly better cycle fecundity after superovulation with clomiphene citrate–hMG–hCG (0.30 vs. 0.13, $p < 0.05$), but not after ovarian stimulation with clomiphene citrate–hCG (0.13 vs. 0.12)[63]. In a Cochrane review based on the results of two trials, double intrauterine insemination showed no significant benefit[63] over SIUI in the treatment of subfertile couples with partner's semen[121]. The authors admitted that there are no meaningful data to offer advice on the basis of this review. According to this report, a large randomized controlled trial of SIUI versus DIUI is mandatory.

Other factors: number of IUI treatment cycles   A significant decline in cycle fecundity after the third or fourth IUI cycle was reported in several studies[122–128]. The remaining couples do not seem to benefit from this method of treatment when compared with other methods of assisted reproduction.

CONCLUSIONS

IUI should be promoted as the best first-line treatment in most cases of subfertility, provided that at least one tube is patent and an inseminating motile count after sperm preparation of more than 1 million can be obtained. In this selected group of patients, it is unwise to start with assisted reproductive techniques such as IVF and ICSI, since these techniques are more invasive, more expensive and more associated with risk for genetic disorders. Promoting IVF and ICSI to result in pregnancy 'as quickly as possible' ignores the advantages of IUI completely.

ACKNOWLEDGMENTS

We gratefully acknowledge Ingrid Jossa for her technical support in preparing this manuscript.

REFERENCES

1. Allen NC, et al. Intrauterine insemination: a critical review. Fertil Steril 1985; 44: 568
2. Aitken RJ, Clarkson JS. Cellular basis of defective sperm function and its association with the genesis of reactive oxygen species by human spermatozoa. J Reprod Fertil 1987; 81: 459
3. Goverde AJ, et al. Intrauterine insemination or in-vitro-fertilisation in idiopathic subfertility and male subfertility: a randomised trial and cost-effectiveness analysis. Lancet 2000; 355: 13

4. Philips Z, Barraza-Llorens M, Posnett J. Evaluation of the relative cost-effectiveness of treatments for infertility in the UK. Hum Reprod 2000; 15: 95

5. Garceau L, et al. Economic implications of assisted reproductive techniques: a systematic review. Hum Reprod 2002; 17: 3090

6. Stone BA, et al. Determinants of the outcome of intrauterine insemination: analysis of outcomes of 9963 consecutive cycles. Am J Obstet Gynecol 1999; 180: 1522

7. Palermo G, et al. Pregnancies after intracytoplasmic injection of single spermatozoon into an oocyte. Lancet 1992; 340: 17

8. Vernaeve V, et al. Reproductive decisions by couples undergoing artificial insemination with donor sperm for severe male infertility: implications for medical counselling. Int J Androl 2005; 28: 22

9. Barratt C, et al. Gamete donation guidelines. The Corsendonk consensus document for the European Union. Hum Reprod 1998; 13: 500

10. Nijs M, Ombelet W. Cryopreservation of human sperm. Hum Fertil 2001; 4: 158

11. Cohlen BJ. Should we continue performing intrauterine inseminations in the year 2004? Gynecol Obstet Invest 2005; 59: 3

12. Peterson CM, et al. Ovulation induction with gonadotropins and intrauterine insemination compared with in vitro fertilization and no therapy: a prospective, nonrandomized, cohort study and meta-analysis. Fertil Steril 1994; 62: 535

13. Collins JA, Burrows EA, Wilan AR. The prognosis for live birth among untreated infertile couples. Fertil Steril 1995; 64: 22

14. Ombelet W, et al. Artificial Insemination (AIH). Artificial insemination 2: using the husband's sperm. In Acosta AA, Kruger TF, eds. Diagnosis and Therapy of Male Factor in Assisted Reproduction. Carnforth: Parthenon Publishing, 1996: 397

15. Cohlen BJ, et al. Timed intercourse versus intrauterine insemination with or without ovarian hyperstimulation for subfertility in men. Cochrane Database Syst Rev 2000; (2): CD000360

16. Ombelet W, et al. Intrauterine insemination after ovarian stimulation with clomiphene citrate: predictive potential of inseminating motile count and sperm morphology. Hum Reprod 1997; 12: 1458

17. Ombelet W, et al. Semen quality and intrauterine insemination. Reprod Biomed Online 2003; 7: 485

18. Duran EH, et al. Intrauterine insemination: a systematic review on determinants of success. Hum Reprod Update 2002; 8: 373

19. Brasch JG, et al. The relationship between total motile sperm count and the success of intrauterine insemination. Fertil Steril 1994; 62: 150

20. van der Westerlaken LA, Naaktgeboren N, Helmerhorst FM. Evaluation of pregnancy rates after intrauterine insemination according to indication, age, and sperm parameters. J Assist Reprod Genet 1998; 15: 359

21. Branigan EF, Estes MA, Muller CH. Advanced semen analysis: a simple screening test to predict intrauterine insemination success. Fertil Steril 1999; 71: 547

22. Miller DC, et al. Processed total motile count correlates with pregnancy outcome after intrauterine insemination. Urology 2002; 60: 497

23. Van Waart J, et al. Predictive value of normal sperm morphology in intrauterine insemination (IUI): a structured literature review. Hum Reprod 2001; 7: 495

24. Horvath PM, et al. The relationship of sperm parameters to cycle fecundity in superovulated women undergoing intrauterine insemination. Fertil Steril 1989; 52: 288

25. Toner JP, et al. Value of sperm morphology assessed by strict criteria for prediction of the outcome of artificial (intrauterine) insemination. Andrologia 1994; 27: 143

26. Campana A, et al. Intrauterine insemination: evaluation of the results according to the woman's age, sperm quality, total sperm count per insemination and life table analysis. Hum Reprod 1996; 11: 732

27. Lindheim SR, et al. Abnormal sperm morphology is highly predictive of pregnancy outcome during controlled ovarian hyperstimulation and intrauterine insemination. J Assist Reprod Genet 1996; 13: 569

28. Hauser R, et al. Intrauterine insemination in male factor subfertility: significance of sperm motility and morphology assessed by strict criteria. Andrologia 2001; 33: 13

29. Montanaro GM, et al. Stepwise regression analysis to study male and female factors impacting on pregnancy rate in an intrauterine insemination programme. Andrologia 2001; 33: 135

30. Lee RK, et al. Sperm morphology analysis using strict criteria as a prognostic factor in intrauterine insemination. Int J Androl 2002; 25: 277

31. Lee VMS, et al. Sperm motility in the semen analysis affects the outcome of superovulation intrauterine insemination in the treatment of infertile Asian couples with male factor infertility. Br J Obstet Gynaecol 2002; 109: 115

32. Dickey RP, et al. Comparison of the sperm quality necessary for successful intrauterine insemination with World Health Organization threshold values for normal sperm. Fertil Steril 1999; 71: 684

33. Tartagni M, et al. Usefulness of the hypo-osmotic swelling test in predicting pregnancy rate and outcome in couples undergoing intrauterine insemination. J Androl 2002; 23: 498

34. Duran EH, et al. Sperm DNA quality predicts intrauterine insemination outcome: a prospective cohort study. Hum Reprod 2002; 17: 3122

35. Zayed F, Lenton EA, Cooke ID. Comparison between stimulated in-vitro fertilization and stimulated intrauterine insemination for the treatment of unexplained and mild male factor infertility. Hum Reprod 1997; 12: 2408

36. Van Voorhis BJ, et al. Effect of the total motile sperm count on the efficacy and cost-effectiveness of intrauterine insemination and in vitro fertilization. Fertil Steril 2001; 75: 661

37. Comhaire F. Economic strategies in modern male subfertility treatment. Hum Reprod 1995; 10 (Suppl 1): 103

38. Dodson WC. Is superovulation and intrauterine insemination really an alternative to assisted reproductive technology? Semin Reprod Endocrinol 1995; 13: 85

39. Robinson D, Syrop CH, Hammitt DG. After superovulation–intrauterine insemination fails: the prognosis for treatment by gamete intrafallopian transfer/pronuclear stage transfer. Fertil Steril 1992; 57: 606

40. Dodson WC, Haney AF. Controlled ovarian hyperstimulation and intrauterine insemination for treatment of infertility. Fertil Steril 1991; 55: 457

41. Bergh T, Lundkvist O. Clinical complications during in-vitro fertilization treatment. Hum Reprod 1992; 7: 625

42. Rizk B, Smitz J. Ovarian hyperstimulation syndrome after superovulation using GnRH agonists for IVF and related procedures. Hum Reprod 1992; 7: 320

43. Ombelet W, Puttemans P, Brosens I. Intrauterine insemination: a first-step procedure in the algorithm of male subfertility treatment. Hum Reprod 1995; 10: 90

44. Ombelet W, et al. Multiple gestation and infertility treatment: registration, reflection and reaction: the Belgian project. Hum Reprod Update 2005; 11: 3

45. De Geyter C, De Geyter M, Nieschlag E. Low multiple pregnancy rates and reduced frequency of cancellation after ovulation induction with gonadotropins, if eventual supernumerary follicles are aspirated to prevent polyovulation. J Assist Reprod Genet 1998; 15: 111

46. Albano C, et al. Avoidance of multiple pregnancies after ovulation induction by supernumerary preovulatory follicular reduction. Fertil Steril 2001; 76: 820

47. Nuojua-Huttunen S, et al. Obstetric and perinatal outcome of pregnancies after intrauterine insemination. Hum Reprod 1999; 14: 2110

48. Wang JX, Norman RJ, Kristiansson P. The effect of various infertility treatments on the risk of preterm birth. Hum Reprod 2002; 17: 945

49. Gaudoin M, et al. Ovulation induction/intrauterine insemination in infertile couples is associated with low-birth-weight infants. Am J Obstet Gynecol 2003; 188: 611

50. Ombelet W, et al. Perinatal outcome of 12 021 singleton and 3,108 twin births after non-IVF assisted reproduction: a cohort study. Hum Reprod 2006; 21: 1025

51. Ombelet W, et al. Pros and cons of IUI in male subfertility treatment. Reprod Biomed Online 2003; 7 (Compendium 1): 66

52. Ombelet W, et al. Semen quality and intrauterine insemination. Reprod Biomed Online 2003; 7: 485

53. Crosignani PG, Walters DE. Clinical pregnancy and male subfertility; the ESHRE multicentre trial on the treatment of male subfertility. European Society of Human Reproduction and Embryology. Hum Reprod 1994; 9: 1112

54. Steures P, et al. Prediction of an ongoing pregnancy after intrauterine insemination. Fertil Steril 2004; 82: 45

55. Iberico G, et al. Analysis of factors influencing pregnancy rates in homologous intrauterine insemination. Fertil Steril 2004; 8: 1308

56. Hurd WW, et al. Comparison of intracervical, intrauterine, and intratubal techniques for donor insemination. Fertil Steril 1993; 59: 339

57. Ripps BA, et al. Intrauterine insemination in fertile women delivers larger numbers of sperm to the peritoneal fluid than intracervical insemination. Fertil Steril 1994; 61: 398

58. Williams DB, et al. Does intrauterine insemination offer an advantage to cervical cap insemination in a donor insemination program? Fertil Steril 1995; 63: 295

59. Oei ML, et al. A prospective, randomized study of pregnancy rates after transuterotubal and intrauterine insemination. Fertil Steril 1992; 58: 167

60. Guzick DS, et al. Efficacy of superovulation and intrauterine insemination in the treatment of infertility. National Cooperative Reproductive Medicine Network. N Engl J Med 1999; 340: 177

61. Arici A, et al. Evaluation of clomiphene citrate and human chorionic gonadotropin treatment: a prospective, randomized, crossover study during intrauterine insemination cycles. Fertil Steril 1999; 61: 314

62. Cohlen BJ, et al. Controlled ovarian hyperstimulation and intrauterine insemination for treating male subfertility: a controlled study. Hum Reprod 1998; 13: 1553

63. Ombelet W, et al. Intrauterine insemination (IUI) following superovulation: pregnancy rates after single versus repeated inseminations. A prospective randomized study in Proceedings of the 11th meeting of ESHRE. Hum Reprod (Abstract book 2) 1995; 10: 134

64. Cohlen BJ, et al. The pattern of the luteinizing hormone surge in spontaneous cycles is related to the probability of conception. Fertil Steril 1993; 60: 413

65. Zreik TG, et al. Prospective, randomized, cross-over study to evaluate the benefit of human chorionic gonadotrophin-timed versus urinary luteinizing hormone-timed intrauterine inseminations in clomiphene citrate-stimulated treatment cycles. Fertil Steril 1999; 71: 1070

66. Awonuga A, Govindbhai J. Is waiting for an endogenous luteinizing hormone surge and/or administration of human chorionic gonadotrophin of benefit in intrauterine insemination? Hum Reprod 1999; 14: 1765

67. Chiu D, et al. Follicular vascularity – the predictive value of transvaginal power doppler ultrasonography in an in vitro fertilization program. A preliminary study. Hum Reprod 1997; 12: 191

68. Bhal P, et al. Perifollicular vascularity as a potential variable affecting outcome in stimulated intrauterine insemination treatment cycles, a study using transvaginal power Doppler. Hum Reprod 1999; 16: 1682

69. Bhal PS, et al. Perifollicular vascularity as a potential variable affecting outcome in stimulated intrauterine insemination treatment cycles: a study using transvaginal power Doppler. Hum Reprod 2001; 16: 1682

70. Gregory L. Peri-follicular vascularity: a marker of follicular heterogeneity and oocyte competence and a predictor of implantation in assisted conception cycles. In Van Blerkom J, Gregory L, eds. Essential IVF. Boston: Kluwer Academic Publishers, 2004: Ch 3

71. Tarin J, et al. Effects of maternal ageing and dietary antioxidant supplementation on ovulation, fertilisation and embryo development in vitro in the mouse. Reprod Nutr Dev 1998; 38: 499

72. Aitken J, Fisher H. Reactive oxygen species generation and human spermatozoa: the balance of benefit and risk. Bioessays 1994; 16: 259

73. Tsai HD, et al. Artificial insemination; role of endometrial thickness and pattern, of vascular impedance of the spiral and uterine arteries, and of the dominant follicle. J Reprod Med 2000; 45: 195

74. Hock DL, et al. Sonographic assessment of endometrial pattern and thickness in patients treated with clomiphene citrate, human menopausal gonadotropins and intrauterine insemination. Fertil Steril 1997; 68: 242

75. De Geyter C, et al. Prospective evaluation of the ultrasound appearance of the endometrium in a cohort of 1,186 infertile women. Fertil Steril 2000; 73: 106

76. Gerli S, et al. Use of ethinyl estradiol to reverse the antiestrogenic effects of clomiphene citrate in patients undergoing intrauterine insemination: a comparative, randomized study. Fertil Steril 2000; 73: 85

77. Perez-Medina T, et al. Endometrial polyps and their implication in the pregnancy rates of patients undergoing intrauterine insemination: a prospective, randomized study. Hum Reprod 2005; 20: 1632

78. Wood EG, et al. Ultrasound-guided soft catheter embryo transfers will improve pregnancy rates in in-vitro fertilization. Hum Reprod 2000; 15: 107

79. Lindheim SR, Cohen MA, Sauer MV. Ultrasound guided embryo transfer significantly improves pregnancy rates in women undergoing oocyte donation. Int J Gynaecol Obstet 2000; 66: 281

80. Burke LM, et al. Predictors of success after embryo-transfer: experience from a single provider. Am J Obstet Gynecol 2000; 182: 1001

81. Ghazzawi IM, et al. Transfer technique and catheter choice influence the incidence of transcervical embryo expulsion and the outcome of IVF. Hum Reprod 1999; 14: 677

82. Smith KL, et al. Does catheter type affect pregnancy rate in intrauterine insemination cycles? J Assist Reprod Genet 2002; 19: 49

83. Lavie O, et al. Ultrasonographic endometrial changes after intrauterine insemination: a comparison of two catheters. Fertil Steril 1997; 68: 731

84. Fancsovits P, et al. Catheter type does not affect the outcome of intrauterine insemination treatment: a prospective randomized study. Fertil Steril 2005; 83: 699

85. Sanmay S, Atasu T, Karacan I. The effect of intrauterine insemination on uterine activity. Int J Fertil 1990; 35: 310

86. Sakkas D, et al. The use of two density gradient centrifugation techniques and the swim-up method to separate spermatozoa with chromatin and nuclear DNA anomalies. Hum Reprod 2000; 15: 1112

87. Hammadeh M, et al. Comparison of sperm preparation methods; effect on chromatin and morphology recovery rates and their consequences on the clinical outcome after in vitro fertilization embryo transfer. Int J Androl 2001; 24: 36

88. Nijs M, Ombelet W. Sperm analysis and preparation update. In Van Blerkom J, Gregory L, eds. Essential IVF. Boston: Kluwer Academic Publishers, 2004: Ch 6

89. Ren SS, et al. Comparison of four methods for sperm preparation for IUI. Arch Androl 2004; 50: 139

90. Dodson WC, et al. A randomized comparison of the methods of sperm preparation for intrauterine insemination. Fertil Steril 1998; 70: 574

91. Boomsma CM, et al. Semen preparation techniques for intrauterine insemination. Cochrane Database Syst Rev 2004; (3): CD004507

92. McKinney KA, Lewis SE, Thompson W. The effects of pentoxifylline on the generation of reactive oxygen species and lipid peroxidation in human spermatozoa. Andrologia 1996; 28: 15

93. Grigoriou O, et al. Effect of sperm treatment with exogenous platelet-activating factor on the outcome of intrauterine insemination. Fertil Steril 2005; 83: 618

94. Rondebush WE, et al. Platelet-activating factor significantly enhances intrauterine insemination pregnancy rates in non-male factor infertility. Fertil Steril 2004; 82: 52

95. Brown SE, Toner JP, Schnorr JA. Vaginal misoprostol enhances intrauterine insemination. Hum Reprod 2001; 16: 96

96. Barroso G, et al. A prospective randomized trial of the impact of misoprostol (PgE1) on pregnancy rate after intrauterine insemination (IUI) therapy: a preliminary report. Ginecol Obstet Mex 2001; 69: 346

97. Goldenberg M, et al. Intra-uterine insemination with prepared sperm vs. unprepared split ejaculates. Andrologia 1992; 24: 135

98. Kahn JA, et al. Fallopian tube perfusion: first clinical experience. Hum Reprod 1992; 7: 19

99. Kahn JA, et al. Fallopian tube sperm perfusion (FSP) versus intra-uterine insemination (IUI) in the treatment of unexplained infertility: a prospective randomized study. Hum Reprod 1993; 8: 890

100. Kahn JA, et al. Fallopian tube sperm perfusion used in a donor insemination programme. Hum Reprod 1992; 7: 806

101. Trout SW, Kemmann E. Fallopian sperm perfusion versus intrauterine insemination: a randomized controlled trial and metaanalysis of the literature. Fertil Steril 1999; 71: 881

102. Cantineau AE, et al. Intrauterine insemination versus Fallopian tube sperm perfusion in non-tubal subfertility: a systematic review based on a Cochrane review. Hum Reprod 2004; 19: 2721

103. Biacchiardi CP, et al. Fallopian tube sperm perfusion versus intrauterine insemination in unexplained infertility: a randomized, prospective, crossover trial. Fertil Steril 2004; 81: 448

104. Matilsky M, et al. The effect of ejaculatory frequency on semen characteristics of normozoospermic and oligozoospermic men from an infertile population. Hum Reprod 1993; 8: 71

105. Pellestor F, Girardet A, Andreo B. Effect of long abstinence periods on human sperm quality. Int J Fertil Menopausal Stud 1994; 39: 278

106. Baker HW, et al. Factors affecting the variability of semen analysis results in infertile men. Int J Androl 1981; 4: 609

107. De Jonge C, et al. Influence of the abstinence period on human sperm quality. Fertil Steril 2004; 82: 57

108. Barratt CLR, et al. The poor prognostic value of low to moderate levels of sperm surface-bound antibodies. Hum Reprod 1992; 7: 95

109. Jarow JP, Sanzone JJ. Risk factors for male partner antisperm antibodies. J Urology 1992; 148: 1805

110. Eggert-Kruse W, et al. Circulating antisperm antibodies and fertility prognosis: a prospective study. Hum Reprod 1989; 4: 513

111. Marshburn PB, Kutteh WH. The role of antisperm antibodies in infertility. Fertil Steril 1994; 61: 799

112. Adeghe J-HA. Male subfertility due to sperm antibodies: a clinical overview. Obstet Gynecol Surv 1992; 48: 1

113. Matson PL, et al. Effects of antisperm antibodies in seminal plasma upon sperm function. Int J Androl 1988; 11: 101

114. Acosta AA, et al. Fertilization efficiency of morphologically abnormal spermatozoa in assisted reproduction is further impaired by antisperm antibodies on the male partner's sperm. Fertil Steril 1994; 62: 826

115. Lombardo F, et al. Antisperm immunity in natural and assisted reproduction. Hum Reprod Update 2001; 7: 450

116. Lombardo F, et al. Antisperm immunity in assisted reproduction. J Reprod Immunol 2004; 62: 101

117. Abbasi R, et al. Cumulative ovulation rate in human menopausal/human chorionic gonadotropin-treated monkeys: 'step-up' versus 'step-down' dose regimens. Fertil Steril 1987; 47: 1019

118. Ransom MX, et al. Does increasing frequency of intrauterine insemination improve pregnancy rates significantly during superovulation cycles? Fertil Steril 1994; 61: 303

119. Silverberg KM, et al. A prospective, randomized trial comparing two different intrauterine insemination regimens in controlled ovarian hyperstimulation cycles. Fertil Steril 1992; 57: 357

120. Ng EH, et al. A randomized comparison of three insemination methods in an artificial insemination program using husbands' semen. J Reprod Med 2003; 48: 542

121. Cantineau AE, Heineman MJ, Cohlen BJ. Single versus double intrauterine insemination in stimulated cycles for subfertile couples: a systematic review based on a Cochrane review. Hum Reprod 2003; 18: 941

122. Comhaire F, et al. The effective cumulative pregnancy rate of different modes of treatment of male infertility. Andrologia 1994; 27: 217

123. Dodson WC, Haney AF. Controlled ovarian hyperstimulation and intrauterine insemination for treatment of infertility. Fertil Steril 1991; 55: 457

124. Friedman AJ, et al. Life table analysis of intrauterine insemination pregancy rates for couples with cervical factor, male factor, and idiopathic infertility. Fertil Steril 1992; 55: 1005

125. Kirby CA, et al. A prospective trial of intrauterine insemination of motile spermatozoa versus timed intercourse. Fertil Steril 1991; 56: 102

126. Nan PM, et al. Intra-uterine insemination or timed intercourse after ovarian stimulation for male subfertility. A controlled study. Hum Reprod 1994; 9: 2022

127. Plosker SM, Jacobson W, Amato P. Prediction and optimizing success in an intra-uterine insemination programme. Hum Reprod 1994; 9: 2014

128. Yang JH, et al. Two-day IUI treatment cycles are more successful than one-day IUI cycles when using frozen–thawed donor sperm. J Androl 1998; 19: 603

28

Intracytoplasmic sperm injection: current status of the technique and outcome

André Van Steirteghem

INTRODUCTION

Since the birth of Louise Brown in 1978[1], *in vitro* fertilization (IVF) has proved to be an efficient treatment to alleviate female factor infertility (tubal infertility and endometriosis) and unexplained infertility. When IVF was applied in couples with male infertility, it became apparent for all groups that the results were much less efficient. The normal fertilization rate of inseminated oocytes was significantly lower, resulting in the formation of many fewer embryos, which meant that embryos were not available for transfer in a substantial number of cycles[2].

Therefore, at the end of the 1980s, several procedures of assisted fertilization were developed and applied in couples where conventional IVF could not be used. The initial assisted fertilization procedures, partial zona dissection (PZD) and subzonal insemination (SUZI), gave some positive results, but overall experience with PZD and SUZI was that the percentage of normal fertilization was low and inconsistent, and the percentages of pregnancies and deliveries were too low to consider PZD and SUZI for routine clinical application. In July 1992, our group reported the first pregnancies and deliveries following the replacement of embryos generated after intracytoplasmic sperm injection (ICSI), an assisted fertilization procedure whereby a single spermatozoon is microinjected into the oocyte[3]. The initial observations with ICSI demonstrated that fertilization was significantly better after ICSI than after SUZI, and more embryos for transfer were obtained[4]. As a consequence of these findings, since July 1992, only ICSI has been applied in our center when assisted fertilization has been indicated[5]. Subsequently, the number of centers worldwide offering ICSI has increased tremendously, as has the number of treatment cycles per year[6]. ICSI has been used successfully worldwide to treat infertility due to severe oligoasthenoteratozoospermia, or azoospermia caused by impaired testicular function or obstructed excretory ducts[7,8].

The first part of this chapter reviews the current practice of ICSI, emphasizing indications, the ICSI procedure and the outcome parameters (fertilization and embryo cleavage as well as pregnancy and delivery). The second part reviews the pregnancy outcome and children's health after ICSI in relation to other forms of assisted reproductive technology.

393

CURRENT PRACTICE OF INTRACYTOPLASMIC SPERM INJECTION

Indications for ICSI

ICSI has clearly overshadowed the use of modified IVF procedures (including high insemination concentration) for the treatment of severe male factor infertility. ICSI requires only one spermatozoon with a functional genome and centrosome for the fertilization of each oocyte. Indications for ICSI are not restricted to impaired morphology of the spermatozoa, but also include low sperm counts and impaired kinetic quality of the sperm cells. ICSI can also be used with spermatozoa from the epididymis or testis when there is an obstruction in the excretory ducts. Azoospermia caused by testicular failure can be treated by ICSI if enough spermatozoa can be retrieved in testicular tissue samples. Table 28.1 gives an overview of the indications for ICSI[9,10]. To avoid contamination with extraneous DNA such as sperm DNA, ICSI is used as the insemination procedure in preimplantation genetic diagnosis, especially when polymerase chain reaction is the diagnostic procedure. Before its first clinical application, the ICSI procedure was evaluated and approved by the Ethics Committee of the Medical Campus of the Vrije Universiteit Brussel. Before starting treatment, couples were informed about the novel aspects of the treatment, the available data on ICSI treatment and the so far unknown possible later risks. Patients were asked to have prenatal diagnosis, and to participate in a prospective follow-up study of the children born[11].

ICSI procedure and results

Ovarian stimulation and oocyte retrieval for ICSI is similar to that for conventional IVF. In the majority of cases, the combination of a gonadotropin-releasing hormone (GnRH) agonist/antagonist and urinary or recombinant gonadotropins is used. Ovulation induction is usually done using urinary human chorionic

Table 28.1   Indications for intracytoplasmic sperm injection (ICSI)

Ejaculated spermatozoa

Oligozoospermia
Asthenozoospermia (caveat for 100% immotile spermatozoa)
Teratozoospermia ($\leq$ 4% normal morphology using strict criteria – caveat for globozoospermia)
High titers of antisperm antibodies
Repeated fertilization failure after conventional *in vitro* fertilization
Autoconserved frozen sperm from cancer patients in remission
Ejaculatory disorders (e.g. electroejaculation, retrograde ejaculation)

Epididymal spermatozoa

Congenital bilateral absence of the vas deferens (CBAVD)
Young's syndrome
Failed vasoepididymostomy
Failed vasovasostomy
Obstruction of both ejaculatory ducts

Testicular spermatozoa

All indications for epididymal sperm
Failure of epididymal sperm recovery because of fibrosis
Azoospermia caused by testicular failure (maturation arrest, germ-cell aplasia)
Necrozoospermia

gonadotropin (hCG). Reviewing a large number of cycles, the following outcome can be expected. Approximately 12 cumulus–oocyte complexes (COCs) are retrieved. Cumulus oophorus and corona radiata cells are removed by mechanical and enzymatic procedures. Microscopic evaluation reveals, on average, that 95% of COCs contain oocytes with an intact zona pellucida; 82% of COCs have metaphase II oocytes with one polar body, 10% of COCs contain germinal vesicle-stage oocytes and 3% metaphase I oocytes. ICSI is carried out only on metaphase II oocytes[12].

For the ICSI procedure, the oocyte is immobilized using a holding pipette; an injection pipette with an internal diameter of 6 μm is used to aspirate a single spermatozoon. These micropipettes are commercially available and can also be made in the laboratory. Before aspiration, the sperm is immobilized in polyvinylpyrrolidone. A morphologically normal sperm is aspirated into the injection needle, tail first. Immobilization of the sperm can also be achieved by crushing the tail with the injection pipette. The injection pipette is passed through the zona pellucida and the membrane of the oocyte into the cytoplasm in a position sufficiently distant from the first polar body.

After ICSI with ejaculated sperm, more than two-thirds of injected oocytes become normally fertilized. The fertilization rate with surgically retrieved sperm in non-obstructive azoospermia is less than with ejaculated sperm but still > 50%[13–14]. Further development of the normally fertilized oocytes after ICSI has been evaluated in a similar fashion to that for IVF. More than 80% of normally fertilized oocytes develop further to embryos of sufficient morphological quality to be replaced. For all types of sperm, the percentage of embryos replaced or frozen is between 60 and 65% of the normally fertilized oocytes. In the case of non-obstructive azoospermia, normal fertilization is compromised[15]. Also in non-obstructive azoospermia, testicular tissue can be damaged after repeated surgery[16].

Absence of fertilization occurs after ICSI when only a few oocytes are available, only totally immotile sperm are present, all sperm have no acrosome and/or all oocytes have abnormal morphology and are damaged by the injection itself. Fertilization occurs mostly in a subsequent cycle[17–19]. According to the published reports from IVF/ICSI registries, in a substantial proportion of assisted reproductive technology cycles, ICSI is applied as the procedure of fertilization. It has become apparent that, worldwide, a number of groups have abandoned conventional IVF, and use ICSI as a standard procedure even when sperm parameters are normal[7,20]. As indicated in Table 28.2, extracted from the European registry on IVF and ICSI[7], there are about the same number of oocyte retrievals per started cycle in the ICSI group, more embryo transfers per oocyte retrieval

Table 28.2 *In vitro* fertilization (IVF) and intracytoplasmic sperm injection (ICSI) results in Europe in 2001[7]

	IVF	ICSI
Treatment cycles (n)	120 946	114 378
Aspirations (n)	107 823	103 538
Aspirations/cycle started (%)	89.1	90.5
Embryo transfers (n)	93 482	95 919
Embryo transfers/aspirations (%)	86.7	92.6
Pregnancies/embryo transfers (%)	29.0	28.3

and a similar number of pregnancies per embryo transfer. The fact that most patients reach oocyte retrieval in the ICSI group may reflect the unimpaired fertility of the female partner. There are fewer unexpected fertilization failures in the ICSI group, but if embryos are obtained, ICSI embryos generate a similar percentage of pregnancies to that with IVF embryos[21].

A meta-analysis of sibling oocytes studied in patients with moderate oligoasthenoteratozoospermia (OAT) revealed that the odds of fertilization after ICSI are 3.9-fold greater than after IVF. The number needed to treat (NNT) in order to prevent one complete fertilization failure after IVF could be three, indicating that three ICSI procedures would have to be performed instead of conventional IVF in couples with moderate OAT, to prevent one complete fertilization failure[22]. A large randomized controlled trial (RCT) from the UK of 435 treatment cycles in 415 couples with non-male factor subfertility (IVF, $n = 224$; ICSI, $n = 211$) showed that the implantation rate was higher in the IVF group than in the ICSI group (95/318 (30%) vs. 72/325 (22%); relative risk (RR) 1.35 (95% confidence interval (CI) 1.04–7.6)). The pregnancy rate per cycle started was also higher after IVF (72 (33%) versus 53 (26%); RR 1.17 (0.97–1.35)). The authors concluded that ICSI offers no advantage over IVF in terms of clinical outcome in cases of non-male factor subfertility. They support the current practice that ICSI should be reserved only for severe male factor problems[20,23]. It has been suggested that ICSI should be the treatment of choice in all assisted reproduction cycles. If this were to be introduced without further studies, such a policy could have a serious impact on laboratory time, on medical resources and, above all perhaps, on overall safety because of bypassing the natural selection mechanisms of the gametes and because of the invasiveness of the technique itself[24].

OUTCOME AND CHILDREN'S HEALTH

For all forms of assisted reproductive technologies (ART), the most important outcome parameter is the health of the children born after ART, and especially the birth of a healthy singleton[25]. Even after several decades of ART practice, one has to realize that it is impossible to give an answer with regard to risks for pregnancy and birth complications for ovarian stimulation in view of timed intercourse and intrauterine insemination. Only in IVF and ICSI have enough data been collected to provide a valid estimation of the risks. Even then, there are limitations in the design of IVF and ICSI follow-up studies which make it impossible to estimate whether it is the ART procedure or the underlying infertility of the treated couples that influences the oucome[26]. Several aspects of ART outcome are reviewed here: pregnancy complications, major malformations and possible reasons for an adverse outcome as well as the increase of multiple ART pregnancies.

Pregnancy complications

The perinatal outcomes of singletons born after IVF have recently been assessed in a meta-analysis[27]. For the period 1978–2002, the study compared a cohort of 12 283 IVF and ICSI singletons with a control cohort of 1.9 million spontaneously conceived singletons, matched for maternal age and parity. In comparison with spontaneous

conceptions, IVF and ICSI pregnancies were associated with significantly higher odds of each of the perinatal outcome parameters studied: perinatal mortality, preterm delivery, low birth weight, very low birth weight and small for gestational age. In the ART singletons, the prevalence was higher for early preterm delivery, spontaneous preterm delivery, placenta previa, gestational diabetes, preeclampsia and neonatal intensive care admission. IVF patients must be counseled about these adverse perinatal outcomes, and obstetricians should manage these pregnancies as high-risk.

A systematic review by Helmerhorst et al. of the perinatal outcomes of singletons and twins after ART confirmed the data for singletons of the above meta-analysis[28]. The systematic review comprised 25 studies (17 with matched and eight with non-matched controls) published between 1985 and 2002. For singletons, the review indicated a significant increased relative risk for very preterm (< 32 weeks) and preterm (< 37 weeks) deliveries. The relative risks were also increased for very low birth weight (< 1500 g), low birth weight (< 2500 g), small for gestational age, Cesarean section, admission to the neonatal intensive care unit and perinatal mortality. Matched and non-matched studies gave similar results. For matched and non-matched studies of twin gestations, the above-mentioned outcome parameters were similar between ART and control pregnancies. Perinatal mortality was lower in assisted-conception twins compared with natural conception twins.

Major malformations

The question whether there is an increased risk for major congenital malformations after IVF or ICSI was recently reviewed in two meta-analyses[29,30]. The meta-analysis by Hansen et al.[29] indicated an overall increase after IVF and ICSI. This was also the case when only singletons, IVF children or ICSI children were analyzed separately. The pooled odds ratio risk for major birth defects was 1.32 (95% CI 1.20–1.45). A meta-analysis by Lie et al.[31] compared major malformations in 5935

ICSI children with those in 13 086 conventional IVF children. The relative risk for a major malformation after ICSI was 1.2 (95% CI 0.97–1.28). The meta-analysis by Rimm *et al.*[30] confirmed the higher risk of major malformations in IVF and ICSI children in comparison with spontaneously conceived children. There was no significant difference in the risk when IVF and ICSI were compared.

A multicentric cohort study[32] of the physical health of 5-year-old children conceived after ICSI ($n = 540$), IVF ($n = 538$) or natural conception ($n = 437$) indicated that in comparison with natural conception, the odds ratio for major malformations was 2.77 (95% CI 1.41–5.46) for ICSI and 1.80 (95% CI 0.85–3.81) for IVF children. Sociodemographic factors did not affect these results. The higher rate observed in the ICSI group was partially due to an excess in the (boys') urogenital system. In addition, IVF and ICSI children were more likely than naturally conceived children to have had a significant childhood illness, to have had a surgical operation, to require medical therapy and to be admitted to hospital. It will be important to continue monitoring these children. As reported by Ludwig[33], there are major gaps in valid data to assess major malformations after the different ART procedures as compared with spontaneously conceived children from fertile couples. This is the case for ovarian stimulation and intrauterine insemination. The major limitations of studies of major malformation rates include the absence of a control cohort, the use of historical controls with unclear definitions and the data collection in the control and study groups, as well as in the definitions of the term 'major malformation'[34].

Possible causes of adverse outcome

As indicated by Ludwig[35], factors involved at different steps of the ART treatment may lead to an increased risk of adverse outcome (Figure 28.1).

The genetics of the male and female partner may influence the outcome. It has been well established that there are more constitutional abnormal karyotypes in infertile males and females. Several studies have also indicated that abnormal sperm have more chromosomal abnormalities. In a cohort of 1298 ICSI parents seen for genetic counseling, it was concluded that there was an increased genetic risk for 557 of these children[12]. This increased risk was due to maternal or paternal age, chromosomal aberrations, monogenic or multifactorial disease and consanguinity. Slightly fewer than 5% of infertile males and 1.5% of tested females had an abnormal karyotype.

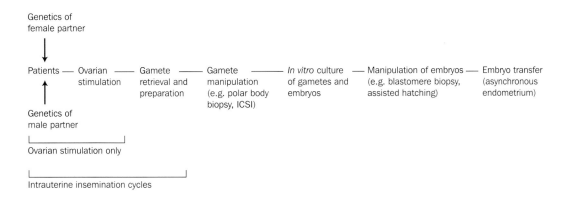

Figure 28.1 Possible influences during different steps of the treatment course in ovarian stimulation and assisted reproduction treatments. ICSI, intracytoplasmic sperm injection. From reference 35, with permission

With regard to fetal karyotypes after ART, there are only systematic data available for ICSI[36]. Results for 1586 fetal karyotypes indicated an increased risk related to chromosomal anomalies in the parents. The majority of cases (17/22) were paternally inherited. There were significantly more *de novo* anomalies (1.6%), but the absolute risk was low. More anomalies were observed when the sperm concentration was $< 20 \times 10^6$ sperm/ml and when sperm motility was impaired.

Although the ICSI procedure is much more invasive than conventional IVF, there is no difference in outcome between ICSI and IVF[29–31,37]. This contrasts with observations of abnormalities in the fertilization process after ICSI as compared with IVF in rhesus monkeys[38].

In theory, all manipulations of gametes and embryos such as gamete preparation and manipulation, *in vitro* culture, blastomere biopsy and assisted hatching could influence the constitution of embryos and ultimately the health of fetuses and children. Efforts should be pursued to establish multinational registries to collect data on the offspring, as has been done by the European Society for Human Reproduction and Embryology (ESHRE) Consortium on Preimplantation Genetic Diagnosis[39]. Strict quality management in the IVF laboratory (such as strict temperature control) is indicated because of its influence on outcome.

In the recent literature, case reports and case–control studies have been published on the occurrence of imprinting disorders in ART children. There are cases of Angelman's syndrome[40] and Beckwith–Wiedeman syndrome[41,42]. The absolute risk for these imprinting disorders in ART remains low, and so far the reason for an increased risk of imprinting errors remains unknown.

As outlined by Buck Louis *et al.*[26], a major drawback of all outcome studies is that the control group is fertile and the study group is infertile. It is therefore indicated that a comparison should be made between ART conceptions and spontaneous conceptions in a subfertile population. With regard to pregnancy complications, a study from the UK[43] indicated that there is an increased incidence of abruptio placentae, pre-eclampsia and Cesarean section in couples with idiopathic infertility, compared with fertile couples, whether conception is spontaneous or after infertility treatment. Similar observations were made in the USA, Denmark and Sweden[44–47]. The question remains unanswered why the risks are increased: is it due to *in vitro* culture conditions or to infertility status *per se*? To assess the contribution of *in vitro* handling, risk assessment for malformations could be done comparing ovarian stimulation alone or in combination with intrauterine insemination.

Multiple pregnancies after ART

There is increasing evidence that the major outcome risk after all forms of ART is the occurrence of multiple pregnancies and births. This is the case for ovulation induction, ovarian hyperstimulation with or without intrauterine insemination and IVF or ICSI[48]. For IVF–ICSI, the number of children born has been estimated to be about two million. This positive observation is overshadowed by the fact that at least half of these children are not from singleton pregnancies. The occurrence of multiple IVF–ICSI pregnancies and births is of course due to the replacement of more than one embryo. There is extensive evidence that multiple pregnancies and births generate more problems not only during pregnancy and delivery but also later in life (see literature in reference 48). Therefore, the prevention of multiple ART gestations should be considered a top priority for all infertility treatments. It is obvious that the practice of single embryo transfer may be the answer to this epidemic of multiple births.

REFERENCES

1. Steptoe PC, Edwards RG. Birth after the re-implantation of a human embryo. Lancet 1978; 2: 366

2. Tournaye H, et al. Comparison of in-vitro fertilization in male and tubal infertility: a 3 year survey. Hum Reprod 1992; 7: 218

3. Palermo GP, et al. Pregnancies after intracytoplasmic sperm injection of single spermatozoon into an oocyte. Lancet 1992; 340: 17

4. Van Steirteghem AC, et al. Higher success rate by intracytoplasmic sperm injection than by subzonal insemination. Report of a second series of 300 consecutive treatment cycles. Hum Reprod 1993; 8: 1055

5. Van Steirteghem AC, et al. High fertilization and implantation rates after intracytoplasmic sperm injection. Hum Reprod 1993; 8: 1061

6. Tarlatzis BC, Bili H. Intracytoplasmic sperm injection: survey of world results. Ann NY Acad Sci 2000; 900: 336

7. Nybo Andersen A, et al. Assisted reproductive technology in Europe, 2001. Results generated from European registers by ESHRE. Hum Reprod 2005; 20: 1158

8. Wright VC, et al. Division of Reproductive Health, National Center for Chronic Disease Prevention and Health Promotion, Centers for Disease Control and Prevention (CDC). Assisted reproductive technology surveillance – United States, 2002. MMWR Surveill Summ 2005; 54: 1

9. De Vos A, Van Steirteghem A. Gamete and embryo manipulation. In Strauss JF, Barbieri R, eds. Yen and Jaffe's Reproductive Endocrinology; Physiology, Pathophysiology, and Clinical Management. Philadelphia: Elsevier Saunders, 2004: 875

10. Devroey P, Van Steirteghem A. A review of ten years experience of ICSI. Hum Reprod Update 2004; 10: 19

11. Bonduelle M, et al. Pregnancy: prospective follow-up study of 55 children born after subzonal insemination and intracytoplasmic sperm injection. Hum Reprod 1994; 9: 1765

12. Bonduelle M, et al. Seven years of intracytoplasmic sperm injection and follow-up of 1987 subsequent children. Hum Reprod 1999; 14 (Suppl 1): 243

13. Joris H, et al. Intracytoplasmic sperm injection: laboratory set-up and injection procedure. Hum Reprod 1998; 13 (Suppl 1): 76

14. Van Steirteghem AC, et al. Results of intracytoplasmic sperm injection with ejaculated, fresh and frozen–thawed epididymal and testicular spermatozoa. Hum Reprod 1998; 13 (Suppl 1): 134

15. Vernaeve V, et al. Intracytoplasmic sperm injection with testicular spermatozoa is less successful in men with non-obstructive azoospermia than in men with obstructive azoospermia. Fertil Steril 2003; 79: 429

16. Schlegel PN, Su LM. Physiological consequences of testicular sperm extraction. Hum Reprod 1997; 13: 1688

17. Liu J, et al. Analysis of 76 total fertilization failure cycles out of 2732 intracytoplasmic sperm injection cycles. Hum Reprod 1995; 10: 2630

18. Staessen C, et al. One year's experience with elective transfer of two good quality embryos in the human in-vitro fertilization and intracytoplasmic sperm injection programmes. Hum Reprod 1995; 10: 3305

19. Vandervorst M, et al. Patients with absolutely immotile spermatozoa and intracytoplasmic sperm injection. Hum Reprod 1997; 12: 2429

20. Bhattacharya S, et al. Conventional in-vitro fertilisation versus intracytoplasmic sperm injection for the treatment of non-male-factor infertility: a randomised controlled trial. Lancet 2001; 357: 2075

21. Staessen C, et al. Conventional in-vitro fertilization versus intracytoplasmic sperm injection in sibling oocytes from couples with tubal infertility and normozoospermic semen. Hum Reprod 1999; 14: 2474

22. Tournaye H. Management of male infertility by assisted reproductive technologies. Bailliéres Best Pract Res Clin Endocrinol Metab 2000; 14: 423

23. Van Steirteghem A, Collins J. Evidence-based medicine for treatment: an in vitro fertilization trial. Semin Reprod Med 2003; 21: 49

24. Oehninger S. Place of intracytoplasmic sperm injection in management of male infertility. Lancet 2001; 357: 2068

25. Wennerholm UB, Bergh C. What is the most relevant standard of success in assisted reproduction? Singleton live births should also include preterm births. Hum Reprod 2004; 19: 1943

26. Buck Louis GM, et al. Research hurdles complicating the analysis of infertility treatment and child health. Hum Reprod 2005; 20: 12

27. Jackson RA, et al. Perinatal outcomes in singletons following in vitro fertilization: a metaanalysis. Obstet Gynecol 2004; 103: 551

28. Helmerhorst FM, et al. Perinatal outcome of singletons and twins after assisted conception: a systematic review of controlled studies. Br Med J 2004; 328: 261

29. Hansen M, et al. Assisted reproductive technologies and the risk of birth defects – a systematic review. Hum Reprod 2005; 20: 328

30. Rimm AA, et al. A metaanalysis of controlled studies comparing major malformation rates in IVF and

ICSI infants with naturally conceived children. J Assist Reprod Genet 2004; 21: 437

31. Lie RT, et al. Birth defects in children conceived by ICSI compared with children conceived by other IVF-methods; a meta-analysis. Int J Epidemiol 2005; 34: 696

32. Bonduelle M, et al. A multi-centre cohort study of the physical health of 5-year-old children conceived after intracytoplasmic sperm injection, in vitro fertilization and natural conception. Hum Reprod 2005; 20: 413

33. Ludwig M. Development of children born after IVF and ICSI. Reprod Biomed Online 2004; 9: 10

34. Kurinczuk JJ, Bower C. Birth defects in infants conceived by intracytoplasmic sperm injection: an alternative interpretation. Br Med J 1997; 315: 1260

35. Ludwig M. Is there an increased risk of malformations afer assisted reproductive technologies? Reprod Biomed Online 2005; 10 (Suppl 3): 83

36. Bonduelle M, et al. Prenatal testing in ICSI pregnancies: incidence of chromosomal anomalies in 1586 karyotypes and relation to sperm parameters. Hum Reprod 2002; 17: 2600

37. Bonduelle M, et al. Neonatal data on a cohort of 2889 infants born after ICSI (1991–1999) and of 2995 infants born after IVF (1983–1999). Hum Reprod 2002; 17: 671

38. Hewitson L, et al. Unique checkpoints during the first cell cycle of fertilization after intracytoplasmic sperm injection in rhesus monkeys. Nat Med 1999; 5: 431

39. Sermon K, et al. ESHRE PGD Consortium data collection IV: May–December 2001. Hum Reprod 2005; 20: 19

40. Ludwig M, et al. Increased prevalence of imprinting defects in patients with Angelman syndrome born to subfertile couples. J Med Genet 2005; 42: 289

41. Chang AS, et al. Association between Beckwith–Wiedemann syndrome and assisted reproductive technology: a case series of 19 patients. Fertil Steril 2005; 83: 349

42. Halliday J, et al. Beckwith–Wiedemann syndrome and IVF: a case–control study. Am J Hum Genet 2004; 75: 526

43. Pandian Z, Bhattacharya S, Templeton A. Review of unexplained infertility and obstetric outcome: a 10 year review. Hum Reprod 2001; 16: 2593

44. Williams MA, et al. Subfertility and the risk of low birth weight. Fertil Steril 1991; 56: 668

45. Henriksen TB, et al. Time to pregnancy and preterm delivery. Obstet Gynecol 1997; 89: 594

46. Basso O, et al. Subfecundity as a correlate of preeclampsia: a study within the Danish National Birth Cohort. Am J Epidemiol 2003; 157: 195

47. Ghazi HA, Spielberger C, Kallen B. Delivery outcome after infertility – a registry study. Fertil Steril 1991; 55: 726

48. Fauser CJM, Devroey P, Macklon NS. Multiple birth resulting from ovarian stimulation for subfertility treatment. Lancet 2005; 365: 1807

29

Sperm retrieval techniques for intracytoplasmic sperm injection

Valérie Vernaeve, Herman Tournaye

INTRODUCTION

Since its introduction in 1992, intracytoplasmic sperm injection (ICSI) has dramatically changed the treatment of severe male infertility[1]. This technique was initially introduced as a treatment for severe oligoasthenoteratozoospermia (OAT). Later, it also became a treatment option for those patients with azoospermia due to an obstruction of the vas deferens where surgery had failed or was not indicated. Both epididymal and testicular sperm were used with success[2–4]. Thereafter, testicular sperm from patients with severe testicular failure was also used with success[5–8].

According to the World Health Organization (WHO) manual, the diagnosis of azoospermia is made after standard evaluation of at least two semen samples[9]. In 454 men with azoospermia on their first semen analysis, 23 were found to be oligozoospermic in their second semen analysis[10]. Even men with repeated absence of spermatozoa in their semen analysis performed according to these standard guidelines may still have some spermatozoa in their ejaculates, which can only be observed after extended preparation, including centrifugation of the semen at $1000g$ for at least 15 min. Ron-El et al.[11] reported that in 49 patients with azoospermia, 17 patients (35%) had spermatozoa in their ejaculates that could be used for ICSI. It is therefore important to perform an extended semen preparation before embarking on testicular recovery techniques, especially in patients with non-obstructive azoospermia (NOA).

Azoospermia is present in about 8% of males with a fertility problem[10]. It is caused by genital tract obstruction, deficient spermatogenesis or hypogonadotropic hypogonadism. The last category is extremely rare: in a study comprising 3555 men with a male factor causing subfertility or infertility, only two cases were observed[10]. Although not completely correct, the terms obstructive azoospermia (OA) and NOA are frequently used, because azoospermia secondary to hypogonadotropic hypogonadism is so rare. A study carried out in 102 men with azoospermia showed that 46% had primary testicular failure with no evidence of obstruction at clinical work-up, 13% had primary testicular failure because of 47,XXY Klinefelter's syndrome and 14% had OA with evidence of obstruction and normal spermatogenesis at testicular biopsy, while 27% had no clinical signs of obstruction according to the classical work-up, including vasography; however, these men showed normal spermatogenesis[12]. These results show that combining clinical findings with histopathology of the testes is the only way of making a proper diagnosis.

In OA, complete spermatogenesis, i.e. normal spermatogenesis or hypospermatogenesis, is found at histology[13]. In NOA, testicular histology may show maturation arrest with or without focal spermatogenesis, germ-cell aplasia (Sertoli cell-only syndrome) with or without focal spermatogenesis, or tubular sclerosis and atrophy.

The therapeutic approach to infertility because of azoospermia is shown in Figure 29.1.

SURGICAL SPERM RETRIEVAL IN PATIENTS WITH OBSTRUCTIVE AZOOSPERMIA

In obstructive azoospermia, the epididymis is the preferred site for sperm retrieval. Motile epididymal sperm show very low levels of DNA damage, and can be retrieved in sufficient numbers to ensure cryopreservation[14]. There are no differences in outcome after ICSI using either fresh or frozen–thawed epididymal spermatozoa[15]. Different techniques are available to retrieve epididymal sperm. The main techniques are microsurgical epididymal sperm aspiration (MESA) and percutaneous epididymal sperm aspiration (PESA), of which the latter has to be preferred. However, when the cause or the site of suspected obstruction is unknown, a scrotal exploration is recommended. This procedure is of diagnostic value and offers an opportunity to perform reconstructive surgery such as vasovasostomy or epididymovasostomy[16]. If reconstruction is not feasible, MESA can still be performed during the exploration, and high numbers of retrieved epididymal spermatozoa can be frozen for later use. PESA has to be performed when microsurgical reconstruction is not possible or not indicated. This procedure is less invasive than MESA and can be performed repeatedly under local anesthesia[17–19]. Theoretically, PESA may cause more epididymal damage and fibrosis than MESA, but this issue is not relevant where reconstruction is not possible. The quantity of spermatozoa recovered may be lower than with MESA, and at least 20% of attempts are unsuccessful and may require MESA or testicular sperm retrieval[20,21]. In cases with obstructive azoospermia, testicular sperm can easily be obtained with testicular fine-needle aspiration (FNA), which has a high success rate of sperm retrieval in men with normal spermatogenesis[22]. Nevertheless, even in cases of obstructive azoospermia, testicular sperm extraction (TESE) may be preferred over FNA whenever cryopreservation is an option and epididymal sperm has not been obtained. If testicular aspiration is performed

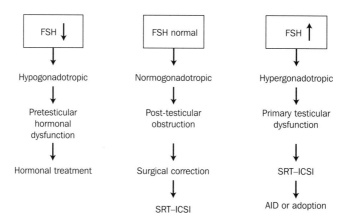

Figure 29.1 Management of azoospermia. FSH, follicle stimulating hormone; SRT, sperm recovery technique; ICSI, intracytoplasmic sperm injection; AID, artificial insemination with donor sperm

with a needle with a larger diameter, tissue cylinders may be obtained, which facilitate cryopreservation[23,24]. Unfortunately, these alternative methods are less patient-friendly than fine-needle aspiration and require loco-regional anesthesia.

SURGICAL SPERM RETRIEVAL IN PATIENTS WITH NON-OBSTRUCTIVE AZOOSPERMIA

Can we predict successful sperm retrieval?

As TESE is successful only in about 50% of patients with NOA, it is very important to determine those factors that may predict a successful recovery procedure[25]. ICSI using testicular spermatozoa from azoospermic patients involves treatment for both partners, i.e. the husband undergoes surgery for testicular sperm recovery and his wife undergoes ovarian stimulation and possibly oocyte retrieval. An unsuccessful sperm recovery procedure therefore has important emotional and financial implications. Objective counseling based on predictive factors may offer realistic expectations for both the couple and the physician.

Tournaye et al.[25] investigated different potential predictive parameters, i.e. the presence of at least one single spermatozoon in at least one preliminary semen analysis, maximum testicular volume, serum follicle stimulating hormone (FSH) and the presence of spermatozoa on histology of a randomly taken testicular biopsy. They found that none of these examined parameters could be used to predict the outcome of a TESE procedure. The findings from semen analysis turned out to be the weakest predictor, and the presence of spermatozoa on histology to be the only parameter that had a limited clinical value in predicting sperm recovery during TESE. A study performed by Ezeh et al.[26] corroborated these findings by establishing that the age of the men, body mass index, luteinizing hormone (LH), FSH or testicular volume could not be used to predict successful TESE.

They also found that the presence of spermatids at testicular histopathology was the best predictor. Other studies, too, corroborate these findings[27–30]. The predictive value of serum inhibin B, a direct product of the Sertoli cells, has been investigated[31]. This hormone also failed, alone or in combination with serum FSH, to predict the presence of sperm in men with NOA.

Brandell et al.[32] investigated the predictive power of genetic markers. They reported a limited series of patients in whom the presence of azoospermia factor b (AZFb) microdeletions of the Y chromosome indicated unsuccessful TESE. Unfortunately, only about 5% of NOA patients show Yq microdeletions, and mostly in the AZFc region. Amer et al.[33] reported that the detection of round spermatids in semen by May–Grünwald–Giemsa stain had a predictive power for successful testicular sperm retrieval. Other authors have also suggested that seminal plasma levels of antimullerian hormone, as well as telomerase assays of testicular tissue, may predict the presence of spermatids in cases of Sertoli cell-only syndrome[34–36]. Even the ratio of second (2D) to fourth digit (4D) length as a predictor for successful sperm retrieval has been reported[37]. The conclusion of this study was that in NOA there was a significantly lower 2D/4D ratio on the left side in men who had had successful retrieval than in those in whom retrieval had been unsuccessful. Thus, with some of the currently available parameters, the probability or rate of successful sperm retrieval may be predicted to some extent, but not accurately enough for an individual patient.

Testicular sperm extraction by open biopsy or percutaneous fine-needle aspiration?

In the case of NOA (included in frequently encountered subpopulations such as non-mosaic Klinefelter's patients and patients with a history of cryptorchidism), sperm will be recovered in about half of the patients by open TESE[25,38,39]. Taking open biopsies, however, may have severe adverse effects, including hematoma, inflammation and devascularization[40–42]. Consequently, less invasive recovery techniques such as FNA have also been carried out in patients with defective spermatogenesis. In 1996, Lewin et al.[43] reported a delivery following ICSI with spermatozoa recovered by FNA in a man with hypergonadotropic azoospermia that showed maturation arrest. A prospective open study in 85 couples further confirmed the feasibility of this technique, with a sperm recovery rate in 58.5% of attempts[44]. A high predictive value of the first FNA for sperm recovery at the subsequent attempt was reported by the same group[45]. Two other groups also showed the reliability of this technique in patients with NOA[18,46]. However, other groups have failed to corroborate these results. A controlled study by Friedler et al.[47] demonstrated that sperm retrieval by FNA is a less efficient method than TESE in NOA, with a sperm retrieval rate of 11% achieved by FNA vs. 43% by TESE. Two other controlled studies also reported a significantly lower recovery rate by retrieval with multiple needle biopsies compared with open biopsies[48,49]. Differences in the definition of NOA, i.e. defined on a clinical basis only, without histopathology, the subselection of patients or the inclusion of patients with hypospermatogenesis may account for these contradictory findings.

Multiple testicular biopsies or a single testicular biopsy?

Based on the assumption that a multifocal distribution of spermatogenesis throughout the entire testis is present in patients with NOA, some authors advocate taking only a single biopsy to control the adverse effects on testicular function[50,51]. The absence of spermatozoa in one single testicular biopsy, however, does not preclude the presence of some spermatozoa in the rest of the testes[52]. Therefore, multiple biopsies may be recommended for achieving high recovery rates[6,53]. Hauser et al.[54] showed that in about 46% of NOA patients, spermatozoa could only be recovered by multiple biopsies.

Microsurgical or conventional testicular sperm extraction?

In order to minimize testicular damage, enhance the sperm recovery rate and diminish the need for an extensive search for spermatozoa in the laboratory, the use of an operating microscope or optical loupe magnification has been proposed[55–57]. The results of these techniques, in terms of recovery and complication rate, are encouraging in cases where enlarged spermatozoa-containing tubules can be identified, i.e. when a Sertoli cell-only pattern predominates throughout the testis[55,57,58]. However, it is not evident whether these techniques will improve recovery rates when enlarged tubules are not present, such as in cases with maturation arrest. More prospective randomized studies, in well-defined populations of NOA patients, should be recommended before proposing this strategy as a gold standard.

How many TESE procedures?

In the literature, information regarding the outcome of repetitive TESE procedures is scarce. Schlegel and Su[40] recommended that TESE should be repeated at an interval of ≥6 months, because the chances of retrieving sperm went up to 80% compared with 25% when TESE was repeated after a shorter interval. Amer et al.[53] also found a higher sperm recovery rate (94.7%) if the sperm recovery procedure was performed at ≥3 months, compared with 75% if performed at <3 months. Another publication evaluated the outcome of 2–5 repetitive TESE procedures. They concluded that the outcome of repeated TESE cycles, up to the fourth trial, justifies the procedure, as pregnancies occurred in each trial up to the fourth but no pregnancies occurred in the fifth trial[59].

ICSI OUTCOME AFTER THE USE OF TESTICULAR SPERM

In patients with obstructive azoospermia, fertilization rate and pregnancy outcome after the use of epididymal sperm compare favorably with those of ICSI using ejaculated sperm[60]. Furthermore, pregnancy rates after ICSI using testicular spermatozoa from patients with normal spermatogenesis have been shown to be comparable to those obtained after ICSI using epididymal spermatozoa[61,62]. ICSI outcome after using frozen–thawed epididymal spermatozoa is comparable in many reports to that after using freshly retrieved spermatozoa[15,62–66].

As for epididymal spermatozoa, the outcome after ICSI with either fresh or frozen–thawed testicular spermatozoa is comparable as well[67,68]. In one small study, however, the outcome after using frozen–thawed testicular sperm was significantly lower[69]. We may therefore conclude that in men with OA, the choice between fresh or frozen epididymal or testicular sperm will be based on convenience rather than on conclusive medical grounds.

Several publications about the outcome of ICSI using testicular sperm in men with NOA have been published. Many studies, mostly dealing with small series, have reported acceptable fertilization and pregnancy rates in patients in whom azoospermia results from primary testicular failure[8,44,51,70–77]. Other studies have found acceptable pregnancy rates, but lower fertilization rates compared with OA[78–81]. Ubaldi et al.[83] found acceptable fertilization and pregnancy rates in NOA compared with OA or ejaculated sperm, but found a significant decrease in implantation rate in NOA patients. Ghazzawi et al.[84] found both high fertilization and pregnancy rates, but a high abortion rate, resulting in a low live-birth rate among NOA couples.

Other authors too have reported lower fertilization and/or pregnancy rates in this patient population[85–92]. A recent meta-analysis showed a significantly improved fertilization rate (relative risk (RR) 1.18, 95% confidence interval (CI) 1.13–1.23) and clinical pregnancy rate (RR 1.36, 95% CI 1.10–1.69) in men with OA as compared with NOA, with a non-significant increase in ongoing pregnancy rate[62]. This meta-analysis did not find any difference in either implantation rate or miscarriage rate between the two groups. These differences among the published reports can easily be explained given the heterogeneity of the patient population examined. In many of these reports, patient selection was performed after a preliminary biopsy[44,73–75,77,79,84,85,89]. In some series, a large group of patients with NOA showed hypospermatogenesis at testicular histology[44,72–75,83], and some of these publications dealt with small case-series[7,8,70,85,86,88,89]. The definition of NOA is often unclear and based only on clinical parameters, while no proper histological diagnosis is present[78,81,87,90].

A large study, not included in the meta-analysis of Nicopoullos et al.[62], analyzed the outcome of a consecutive series of 306 cycles in 235 patients with a well-defined (clinically and histologically) NOA[93]. The control group comprised 605 cycles performed in 360 azoospermic men with normal spermatogenesis. In this larger series, a significantly lower fertilization rate was observed, 48.5% vs. 59.7%, in men with NOA compared with men with OA. Both the clinical implantation rate and the clinical pregnancy rate per cycle were significantly lower in the NOA group compared with the OA group: 8.6% vs. 12.5% and 15.4% vs. 24%, respectively. If this series had been included in the meta-analysis, the conclusion would probably have been different, given that this study outnumbers the other series included. Furthermore, the meta-analysis considers different papers relating to the same patient series (repeated publications from the same group on extended patient series).

In order to counsel patients more adequately, Osmanagaoglu et al.[94] calculated life-table statistics in couples undergoing ICSI with testicular sperm from azoospermic men with NOA. It was observed that after three cycles, the expected chance of fathering a child was 31% in the NOA group compared with 48% in the OA group. Again, these data corroborate the finding that NOA patients perform less well than OA patients after ICSI.

Initially, mainly fresh testicular sperm was used in patients with NOA undergoing ICSI. Freezing testicular sperm may theoretically render multiple biopsies unnecessary. As TESE will not be successful in all NOA patients, a preliminary testicular biopsy with freezing of the tissue for later use may avoid pointless ovarian stimulation of the female partner in many NOA couples. However, insufficient data are available in the literature that focuses on this particular subgroup of azoospermic patients[95–99]. A recent study evaluated the outcome of 97 ICSI cycles scheduled with frozen–thawed testicular sperm in 69 histologically defined NOA patients[100]. Results were comparable to those of ICSI with fresh testicular sperm: clinical pregnancy rates per embryo transfer of 25% and 17.9%, respectively, in cycles using frozen–thawed and fresh testicular sperm. The implantation rate per replaced embryo was 11.3%, compared with 8.6% using fresh testicular sperm. The observed tendency towards better results with frozen–thawed spermatozoa may be explained by patient selection: the frozen–thawed group represents a subgroup of patients for whom the quality of testicular biopsies was sufficient to allow cryopreservation.

However, this approach involving preliminary freezing of testicular samples has an important disadvantage when all tissue samples with at least one spermatozoon observed are frozen. In approximately 20% of such patients, no spermatozoa can be recovered for ICSI. Yet, a successful back-up fresh retrieval can be performed in most of these couples. Patients should be informed about the advantages and disadvantages of performing a preliminary biopsy followed by cryopreservation whenever spermatozoa are successfully recovered, especially when the numbers of spermatozoa are limited.

PREGNANCIES AND CHILDREN OBTAINED AFTER TESE–ICSI

A possible explanation for the observed lower fertilization and pregnancy rates in patients with severe testicular failure may be the use of immature gametes. As a result, there have been concerns regarding possible adverse effects on children born after TESE–ICSI, especially in NOA. The spermatozoa from NOA men are known to show higher chromosomal aneuploidy rates[101–104]. Furthermore, the aneuploidy frequency in embryos obtained from NOA as well as OA is very high, 53% vs. 60%, respectively[105]. It is also assumed that genomic imprinting may be incomplete or deficient[106]. As a result, the use of testicular spermatozoa from men with NOA has been banned in The Netherlands.

So far, few publications have focused on the obstetric and neonatal outcome of children born after ICSI using testicular sperm, and registries on the outcome of ICSI pregnancies obtained with testicular sperm do not differentiate between OA and NOA. We therefore examined the outcome of 70 pregnancies and neonatal data concerning 61 children born after ICSI using testicular sperm from men with clinically and histologically defined NOA[107]. The results were compared with those of 204 pregnancies and 196 children born after TESE–ICSI in OA men. There were no statistically significant differences with respect to the outcome of pregnancy between the two groups studied. No differences were observed between the two groups regarding the birth weight of the children or the early perinatal mortality rate. Major malformations were present in 4% of the live-born children obtained with testicular sperm of NOA men, compared with 3% in the children of OA men.

These rates are comparable to the rates observed in ICSI children after the use of ejaculated sperm, using the same methodology and definitions as in a further study, where a 3.4% major malformation rate was found[108]. Other groups did not report an increased malformation rate after the use of testicular sperm, either[79,109,110]. In these studies, however, the subgroups of testicular sperm were small, and unfortunately, no distinction was made between obstructive and non-obstructive azoospermia. Only the report by Palermo et al.[79] also made this distinction, although it is not clear whether this was based on histopathology, which is an important prerequisite for categorizing the type of azoospermia[111]. So far, from these limited data, we may conclude that the results in terms of pregnancy and child outcome are rather reassuring. However, since the published studies include only a small number of patients, further study is certainly recommended.

ADVERSE EFFECTS OF TESTICULAR SPERM EXTRACTIONS

Spermatogenesis is a process that takes about 74 days, and it is highly sensitive to toxic effects and minor changes in temperature. Inflammatory changes in the testis following testicular surgery may thus have an adverse effect. According to Schlegel and Su[40], 82% of patients who have had testicular biopsy show intratesticular abnormalities on scrotal ultrasound, suggesting persistent hematoma and/or inflammation even as long as 3 months after TESE. The majority of these ultrasound abnormalities are resolved within 6 months after TESE, leaving linear scars or calcifications[40–42]. There is little evidence that multiple, blind testicular needle aspirations carry any less risk of testicular injury than an open biopsy with identification of testicular vessels. The use of microsurgical sperm retrieval procedures may further minimize the risk of inadvertent vascular injury to the testis[57,112]. This, however, needs to be examined.

Another concern is the occurrence of antigenic stimulation after testis biopsy. Hjort et al.[113] found the presence of antisperm antibodies in 31% of patients who had undergone a previous testicular biopsy 10 days to 5 weeks before analysis of their sera. However, Komori et al.[114] evaluated the presence of antisperm antibodies before and 1 year after TESE in patients with non-obstructive azoospermia and found no incidence of new antisperm antibody formation.

One investigation assessed serum concentrations of testosterone after multiple testicular biopsies in 15 patients. A significant decrease in the testosterone value was observed up until 6 months after surgery. The decline in testosterone was, to a certain extent, found to be reversible within the first year of follow-up, but not entirely[115]. However, two other studies did not reveal this decline in testosterone level. Komori et al.[114] assayed the serum testosterone concentrations before operation and at 1, 6 and 12 months after conventional multiple TESE or microdissection TESE in NOA patients. They found no significant postoperative decrease in serum total and free testosterone concentrations in all patients in both groups. A study by Schill et al.[42] evaluated the pre- and postoperative values of basal testosterone, up until 18 months after surgery. Their study found no statistically significant difference between testosterone values before and after testicular biopsies. These data suggest that it is unlikely that testicular biopsy has any longer-term negative effect on blood testosterone levels.

REFERENCES

1. Palermo G, et al. Pregnancies after intracytoplasmic sperm injection of single spermatozoon into an oocyte. Lancet 1992; 340: 17

2. Tournaye H, et al. Microsurgical epididymal sperm aspiration and intracytoplasmic sperm injection: a new effective approach to infertility as a result of congenital bilateral absence of the vas deferens. Fertil Steril 1994; 61: 1445

3. Craft I, Bennett V, Nicholson N. Fertilizing ability of testicular spermatozoa [Letter]. Lancet 1993; 342: 864

4. Schoysman R, et al. Pregnancy after fertilization with human testicular spermatozoa. Lancet 1993; 342: 1237

5. Devroey P, et al. Pregnancies after testicular sperm extraction and intracytoplasmic sperm injection in non-obstructive azoospermia. Hum Reprod 1995; 10: 1457

6. Tournaye H, et al. Recent concepts in the management of infertility because of non-obstructive azoospermia. Hum Reprod 1995; 10 (Suppl 1): 115

7. Silber S, et al. Normal pregnancies resulting from testicular sperm extraction and intracytoplasmic sperm injection for azoospermia due to maturation arrest. Fertil Steril 1996; 55: 110

8. Schlegel PN, et al. Testicular sperm extraction with intracytoplasmic sperm injection for non-obstructive azoospermia. Urology 1997; 49: 435

9. World Health Organization. WHO Laboratory Manual for the Examination of Human Semen and Sperm–Cervical Mucus Interaction, 4th edn. Cambridge: Cambridge University Press, 1999

10. World Health Organization. Towards more objectivity in diagnosis and management of male infertility. Results of a World Health Organization Multicentre Study. Int J Androl 1987; 7 (Suppl): 1

11. Ron-El R, et al. Extended sperm preparation: an alternative to testicular sperm extraction in non-obstructive azoospermia. Hum Reprod 1997; 12: 1222

12. Matsumiya K, et al. Clinical study of azoospermia. Int J Androl 1994; 17: 140

13. Jow WW, et al. Motile sperm in human testis biopsy specimens. J Androl 1993; 14: 194

14. Ramos L, et al. Assessment of DNA fragmentation of spermatozoa that were surgically retrieved from men with obstructive azoospermia. Fertil Steril 2002; 77: 233

15. Tournaye H, et al. No differences in outcome after intracytoplasmic sperm injection with fresh or with frozen–thawed epididymal spermatozoa. Hum Reprod 1999; 14: 90

16. Heidenreich A, Altmann P, Engelmann UH. Micorsurgical vasovasostomy versus microsurgical epididymal sperm aspiration/testicular extraction of sperm combined with intracytoplasmic sperm injection. A cost–benefit analysis. Eur Urol 2000; 37: 609

17. Tsirigotis M, et al. Cumulative experience of percutaneous epididymal sperm aspiration (PESA) with intracytoplasmic sperm injection. J Assist Reprod Genet 1996; 13: 315

18. Rosenlund B, et al. A comparison between open and percutaneous needle biopsies in men with azoospermia. Hum Reprod 1998; 13: 1266

19. Gorgy A. The efficacy of local anesthesia for percutaneous epididymal sperm aspiration and testicular sperm aspiration. Hum Reprod 1998; 13: 646

20. Girardi SK, Schlegel PN. Techniques for sperm recovery in assisted reproduction. Reprod Med Rev 1999; 7: 131

21. Lin YM, et al. Percutaneous epididymal sperm aspiration versus microsurgical epididymal sperm aspiration for irreparable obstructive azoospermia – experience with 100 cases. J Formos Med Assoc 2000; 99: 459

22. Tournaye H, et al. Fine needle aspiration versus open biopsy for testicular sperm recovery: a controlled study in azoospermic patients with normal spermatogenesis. Hum Reprod 1998; 13: 901

23. Sheynkin YR, et al. Controlled comparison of percutaneous and microsurgical sperm retrieval in men with obstructive azoospermia. Hum Reprod 1998; 13: 3086

24. Tuuri T, et al. Testicular biopsy gun needle biopsy in collecting spermatozoa for intracytoplasmic injection, cryopreservation and histology. Hum Reprod 1998; 14: 1274

25. Tournaye H, et al. Are there any predictive factors for successful testicular sperm recovery in azoospermic patients? Hum Reprod 1997; 12: 80

26. Ezeh UIO, et al. Establishment of predictive variables associated with testicular sperm retrieval in men with non-obstructive azoospermia. Hum Reprod 1999; 14: 1005

27. Chen CS, et al. Reconsideration of testicular biopsy and follicle-stimulating hormone measurement in the era of intracytoplasmic sperm injection for non-obstructive azoospermia? Hum Reprod 1996; 11: 2176

28. Mulhall JP, et al. Presence of mature sperm in testicular parenchyma of men with non-obstructive azoospermia: prevalence and predictive factors. Urol 1997; 49: 91

29. Seo JT, Ko WJ. Predictive factors of successful testicular sperm recovery in non-obstructive azoospermia patients. Int J Androl 2001; 24: 306

30. Schulze W, Thoms F, Knuth UA. Testicular sperm extraction: comprehensive analysis with simultaneously performed histology in 1418 biopsies from 766 subfertile men. Hum Reprod 1999; 14 (Suppl 1): 82

31. Vernaeve V, et al. Serum inhibin B cannot predict testicular sperm retrieval in patients with non-obstructive azoospermia. Hum Reprod 2002; 17: 971

32. Brandell RA, et al. AZFb deletions predict the absence of spermatozoa with testicular sperm extraction: preliminary report of a prognostic genetic test. Hum Reprod 1998; 13: 2812

33. Amer M, et al. May–Grunwald–Giemsa stain for detection of spermatogenic cells in the ejaculate: a simple predictive parameter for successful testicular sperm retrieval. Hum Reprod 2001; 16: 1427

34. Fénichel P, et al. Anti-Mullerian hormone as a seminal marker for spermatogenesis in non-obstructive azoospermia. Hum Reprod 1999; 14: 2020

35. Yamamoto Y, et al. Morphometric and cytogenetic characteristics of testicular germ cells and Sertoli cell secretory function in men with non-mosaic Klinefelter's syndrome. Hum Reprod 2002; 17: 886

36. Schrader M, et al. Telomerase activity and expression of telomerase subunits in the testicular tissue of infertile patients. Fertil Steril 2000; 73: 706

37. Wood S, et al. The ratio of second to fourth digit length in azoospermic males undergoing surgical sperm retrieval: predictive value for sperm retrieval and on subsequent fertilization and pregnancy rates in IVF/ICSI cycles. J Androl 2003; 24: 871

38. Vernaeve V, et al. Can biological or clinical parameters predict testicular sperm recovery in 47,XXY Klinefelter's patients? Hum Reprod 2004; 19: 1135

39. Vernaeve V, et al. Testicular sperm recovery and ICSI in patients with non-obstructive azoospermia with a history of orchidopexia. Hum Reprod 2004; 19: 2307

40. Schlegel P, Su L. Physiological consequences of testicular sperm extraction. Hum Reprod 1997; 12: 1688

41. Ron-El R, et al. Serial sonography and colour flow doppler imaging following testicular and epididymal sperm extraction. Hum Reprod 1998; 13: 3390

42. Schill T, et al. Clinical and endocrine follow-up of patients after testicular sperm extraction. Fertil Steril 2003; 79: 281

43. Lewin A, et al. Delivery following intracytoplasmic injection of mature sperm cells recovered by testicular fine needle aspiration in a case of hypergonadotropic azoospermia due to maturation arrest. Hum Reprod 1996; 11: 769

44. Lewin A, et al. Testicular fine needle aspiration: the alternative method for sperm retrieval in non-obstructive azoospermia. Hum Reprod 1999; 14: 1785

45. Fasouliotis SJ, et al. A high predictive value of the first testicular fine needle aspiration in patients with non-obstructive azoospermia for sperm recovery at the subsequent attempt. Hum Reprod 2002; 17: 139

46. Westlander G, et al. Sperm retrieval, fertilization, and pregnancy outcome in repeated testicular sperm aspiration. J Assist Reprod Genet 2001; 18: 171

47. Friedler S, et al. Testicular sperm retrieval by percutaneous fine needle sperm aspiration compared with testicular sperm extraction by open biopsy in men with non-obstructive azoospermia. Hum Reprod 1997; 12: 1488

48. Ezeh UI, Moore HD, Cooke ID. A prospective study of multiple needle biopsies versus a single open biopsy for testicular sperm extraction in men with non-obstructive azoospermia. Hum Reprod 1998; 13: 3075

49. Tournaye H. Surgical sperm recovery for intracytoplasmic sperm injection: which method is to be preferred? Hum Reprod 1999; 14: 71

50. Silber SJ, et al. High fertilization and pregnancy rate after intracytoplasmic sperm injection with spermatozoa obtained from testicle biopsy. Hum Reprod 1995; 10: 148

51. Silber SJ, et al. Distribution of spermatogenesis in the testicles of azoospermic men: the presence or absence of spermatids in the testes of men with germinal failure. Hum Reprod 1997; 12: 2422

52. Gottschalk-Sabag S, et al. Is one testicular specimen sufficient for quantitative evaluation of spermatogenesis? Fertil Steril 1995; 64: 399

53. Amer M, et al. Testicular sperm extraction: impact of testicular histology on outcome, number of biopsies to be performed and optimal time for repetition. Hum Reprod 1999; 14: 3030

54. Hauser R, et al. Multiple testicular sampling in non-obstructive azoospermia: is it necessary? Hum Reprod 1998; 13: 3081

55. Schlegel P. Testicular sperm extraction: microdissection improves sperm yield with minimal tissue excision. Hum Reprod 1999; 14: 131

56. Mulhall JP. The utility of optical loupe magnification for testis sperm extraction in men with nonobstructive azoospermia. J Androl 2005; 26: 178

57. Amer M, et al. Prospective comparative study between microsurgical and conventional testicular sperm extraction in non-obstructive azoospermia:

follow-up by serial ultrasound examinations. Hum Reprod 2000; 15: 653

58. Tsujimura A, et al. Conventional multiple or microdissection testicular sperm extraction: a comparative study. Hum Reprod 2002; 17: 2924

59. Friedler S, et al. Outcome of first and repeated testicular sperm extraction and ICSI in patients with non-obstructive azoospermia. Hum Reprod 2002; 17: 2356

60. Meniru GI, et al. Studies of percutaneous epididymal sperm aspiration (PESA) and intracytoplasmic sperm injection. Hum Reprod Update 1998; 4: 57

61. Nagy Z, et al. Comparison of fertilization, embryo development and pregnancy rates after intracytoplasmic sperm injection using ejaculated, fresh and frozen–thawed epididymal and testicular spermatozoa. Fertil Steril 1995; 63: 808

62. Nicopoullos JD, et al. Use of surgical sperm retrieval in azoospermic men: a meta-analysis. Fertil Steril 2004; 82: 691

63. Janzen N, et al. Use of electively cryopreserved microsurgically aspirated epididymal sperm with IVF and intracytoplasmic sperm injection. Fertil Steril 2000; 74: 696

64. Cayan S, et al. A comparison of ICSI outcomes with fresh and cryopreserved epididymal spermatozoa from the same couples. Hum Reprod 2001; 16: 495

65. Griffiths M, et al. Should cryopreserved epididymal or testicular sperm be recovered from obstructive azoospermic men for ICSI? Br J Obstet Gynaecol 2004; 111: 1289

66. Lin YH, et al. Intentional cryopreservation of epididymal spermatozoa from percutaneous aspiration for dissociated intracytoplasmic sperm injection cycles. Acta Obstet Gynecol Scand 2004; 83: 745

67. Habermann H, et al. In vitro fertilization outcomes after intracytoplasmic sperm injection with fresh or frozen–thawed testicular spermatozoa. Fertil Steril 2000; 5: 955

68. Gil-Salom M, et al. Intracytoplasmic sperm injection with cryopreserved testicular spermatozoa. Mol Cell Endocrinol 2000; 27: 15

69. De Croo I, et al. Fertilization, pregnancy and embryo implantation rates after ICSI with fresh or frozen–thawed testicular spermatozoa. Hum Reprod 1998; 13: 1893

70. Devroey P, et al. Outcome of intracytoplasmic sperm injection with testicular spermatozoa in obstructive and non-obstructive azoospermia. Hum Reprod 1996; 11: 1015

71. Madgar I, et al. Outcome of in vitro fertilization and intracytoplasmic injection of epididymal and testicular sperm extracted from patients with obstructive and nonobstructive azoospermia. Fertil Steril 1998; 69: 1080

72. Su LM, et al. Testicular sperm extraction with intracytoplasmic sperm injection for nonobstructive azoospermia: testicular histology can predict success of sperm retrieval. J Urol 1999; 161: 112

73. Mercan R, Urman B, Alatas C. Outcome of testicular sperm retrieval procedures in non-obstructive azoospermia: percutaneous aspiration versus open biopsy. Hum Reprod 2000; 15: 1548

74. Bukulmez O, et al. The origin of spermatozoa does not affect intracytoplasmic sperm injection outcome. Eur J Obstet Gynecol Reprod Biol 2001; 94: 250

75. Sousa M, et al. Predictive value of testicular histology in secretory azoospermic subgroups and clinical outcome after microinjection of fresh and frozen–thawed sperm and spermatids. Hum Reprod 2002; 17: 1800

76. Windt ML, et al. Intracytoplasmic sperm injection with testicular spermatozoa in men with azoospermia. J Assist Reprod Genet 2002; 19: 53

77. Levine LA, Dimitriou RJ, Fakouri B. Testicular and epididymal percutaneous sperm aspiration in men with either obstructive or nonobstructive azoospermia. Urology 2003; 62: 328

78. Aboulghar MA, et al. Fertilization and pregnancy rates after intracytoplasmic sperm injection using ejaculate semen and surgically retrieved sperm. Fertil Steril 1997; 68: 108

79. Palermo GD, et al. Fertilization and pregnancy outcome with intracytoplasmic sperm injection for azoospermic men. Hum Reprod 1999; 14: 741

80. De Croo I, et al. Fertilization, pregnancy and embryo implantation rates after ICSI in cases of obstructive and non-obstructive azoospermia. Hum Reprod 2000; 15: 1383

81. Balaban B, et al. Blastocyst transfer following intracytoplasmic injection of ejaculated, epididymal or testicular spermatozoa. Hum Reprod 2001; 16: 125

82. Ghanem M, et al. Comparison of the outcome of intracytoplasmic sperm injection in obstructive and non-obstructive azoospermia in the first cycle: a report of case series and meta-analysis. Int J Androl 2005; 28: 16

83. Ubaldi F, et al. Reproductive capacity of spermatozoa from men with testicular failure. Hum Reprod 1999; 14: 2796

84. Ghazzawi IM, et al. Comparison of the fertilizing capability of spermatozoa from ejaculates, epididymal aspirates and testicular biopsies using intracytoplasmic sperm injection. Hum Reprod 1998; 13: 348

85. Kahraman S, et al. High implantation and pregnancy rates with testicular sperm extraction and intracytoplasmic sperm injection in obstructive and non-obstructive azoospermia. Hum Reprod 1996; 11: 673

86. Fahmy I, et al. Intracytoplasmic sperm injection using surgically retrieved epididymal and testicular spermatozoa in cases of obstructive and non-obstructive azoospermia. Int J Androl 1997; 20: 37

87. Mansour RT, et al. Intracytoplasmic sperm injection in obstructive and non-obstructive azoospermia. Hum Reprod 1997; 12: 1974

88. Monzo A, et al. Outcome of intracytoplasmic sperm injection in azoospermic patients: stressing the liaison between the urologist and reproductive medicine specialist. Urology 2001; 58: 69

89. Goker EN, et al. Comparison of the ICSI outcome of ejaculated sperm with normal, abnormal parameters and testicular sperm. Eur J Obstet Gynecol Reprod Biol 2002; 104: 129

90. Pasqualotto FF, et al. Outcome of in vitro fertilization and intracytoplasmic injection of epididymal and testicular sperm obtained from patients with obstructive and nonobstructive azoospermia. J Urol 2002; 167: 1753

91. Schwarzer JU, et al. Male factors determining the outcome of intracytoplasmic sperm injection with epididymal and testicular spermatozoa. Andrologia 2003; 35: 220

92. Schwarzer JU, et al. Sperm retrieval procedures and intracytoplasmatic spermatozoa injection with epididymal and testicular sperms. Urol Int 2003; 70: 119

93. Vernaeve V, et al. Intracytoplasmic sperm injection with testicular spermatozoa is less successful in men with nonobstructive azoospermia than in men with obstructive azoospermia. Fertil Steril 2003; 79: 529

94. Osmanagaoglu K, et al. Cumulative delivery rates after intracytoplasmic sperm injection in women older than 37 years. Hum Reprod 2003; 17: 940

95. Friedler S, et al. Intracytoplasmic injection of fresh and cryopreserved testicular spermatozoa in patients with nonobstructive azoospermia: a comparative study. Fertil Steril 1997; 68: 892

96. Oates RD, et al. Fertilization and pregnancy using intentionally cryopreserved testicular tissue as the sperm source for intracytoplasmic sperm injection in 10 men with non-obstructive azoospermia. Hum Reprod 1997; 12: 734

97. Ben-Yosef D, et al. Testicular sperm retrieval and cryopreservation prior to initiating ovarian stimulation as the first line approach in patients with non-obstructive azoospermia. Hum Reprod 1999; 14: 1794

98. Gianaroli L, et al. Diagnostic testicular biopsy and cryopreservation of testicular tissue as an alternative to repeated surgical openings in the treatment of azoospermic men. Hum Reprod 1999; 14: 1034

99. Kupker W, et al. Use of frozen–thawed testicular sperm for intracytoplasmic sperm injection. Fertil Steril 2000; 73: 453

100. Verheyen G, et al. Should diagnostic testicular sperm retrieval followed by cryopreservation for later ICSI be the procedure of choice for all patients with non-obstructive azoospermia? Hum Reprod 2004; 19: 2822

101. Bernardini L, et al. Frequency of hyper-, hypohaploidy and diploidy in ejaculated, epididymal and testicular germ cells of infertile patients. Hum Reprod 2000; 15: 2165

102. Martin RH, et al. Chromosome analysis of spermatozoa extracted from testes of men with non-obstructive azoospermia. Hum Reprod 2000; 15: 1121

103. Levron J, et al. Sperm chromosome abnormalities in men with severe male factor infertility who are undergoing in-vitro fertilization with intracytoplasmic sperm injection. Fertil Steril 2001; 76: 479

104. Mateizel I, et al. Fish analysis of chromosome X, Y and 18 abnormalities in testicular sperm from azoospermic patients. Hum Reprod 2002; 17: 2249

105. Platteau P, et al. Comparison of the aneuploidy frequency in embryos derived from testicular sperm extraction in obstructive and non-obstructive azoospermia. Hum Reprod 2004; 19: 1570

106. Tesarik J, Mendoza C. Genomic imprinting abnormalities: a new potential risk of assisted reproduction. Mol Hum Reprod 1996; 2: 295

107. Vernaeve V, et al. Pregnancy outcome and neonatal data of children born after ICSI using testicular sperm in obstructive and non-obstructive azoospermia. Hum Reprod 2003; 18: 2093

108. Bonduelle M, et al. Neonatal data on a cohort of 2889 infants born after ICSI (1991–1999) and of 2995 infants born after IVF (1983–1999). Hum Reprod 2002; 17: 671

109. Wennerholm U-B, et al. Obstetric outcome of pregnancies following ICSI, classified according to sperm origin and quality. Hum Reprod 2000; 15: 1189

110. Ludwig M, Katalinic A. Malformation rate in fetuses and children conceived after ICSI: results of a prospective cohort study. Reprod Biomed Online 2002; 5: 171

111. Tournaye H. Gamete source and manipulation. In Vayena E, Rowe P, Griffin D, eds. Current Practices and Controversies in Assisted Reproduction: a WHO Report. Geneva: World Health Organization, 2002: 83

112. Okada, et al. Conventional versus microdissection testicular sperm extraction for nonobstructive azoospermia. J Urol 2002; 168: 1063

113. Hjort T, Husted S, Linnet-Jepsen P. The effect of testis biopsy on autosensitization against spermatozoal antigens. Clin Exp Immunol 1974; 18: 201

114. Komori K, et al. Serial follow-up study of serum testosterone and antisperm antibodies in patients with non-obstructive azoospermia after conventional or microdissection testicular sperm extraction. Int J Androl 2004; 27: 32

115. Manning M, Jünemann KP, Alken P. Decrease in testosterone blood concentrations after testicular sperm extraction for intracytoplasmic sperm injection in azoospermic men. Lancet 1998; 352: 37

30

Hyaluronic acid binding by sperm: andrology evaluation of male fertility and sperm selection for intracytoplasmic sperm injection

Gabor Huszar, Attila Jakab, Ciler Celik-Ozenci, G Leyla Sati

CYTOPLASMIC RETENTION AND OTHER BIOCHEMICAL MARKERS OF SPERM CELLULAR MATURITY

The primary interest of our laboratory has been the development of objective biochemical markers of human sperm maturity and function, which would predict male fertility independently from the traditional semen criteria of sperm concentration and motility. In measurements of sperm creatine-N-phosphotransferase or creatine kinase (CK), we found significantly higher sperm CK contents in men with diminished fertility[1,2]. The sperm CK immunostaining patterns indicated (Figure 30.1a) that the high sperm CK activity was a direct consequence of increased cytoplasmic protein and CK concentrations in the spermatozoon[3]. This suggested that we had identified a sperm developmental defect in the last phase of spermiogenesis when the surplus cytoplasm (unnecessary for mature sperm) is normally extruded and left in the adluminal area as 'residual bodies'[4].

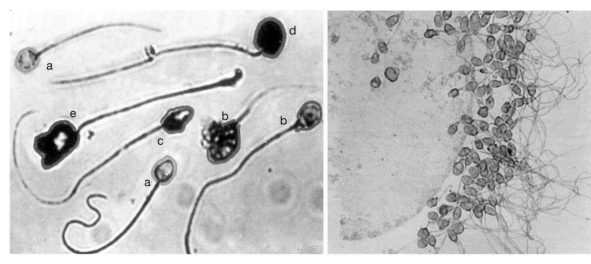

Figure 30.1   Left panel: Mature (a) and diminished-maturity sperm with cytoplasmic retention (b–e) after creatine kinase (CK) immunostaining. Right panel: CK-immunostained sperm–hemizona complex. Observe that only the clear-headed mature spermatozoa without cytoplasmic retention are able to bind. See also Color plate 4 on page xxvi

In addition to the CK-B isoform, we found another adenosine triphosphate (ATP)-containing protein, which was proportional to the incidence of mature sperm, characterized by lack of cytoplasmic retention[5]. We have identified this developmentally regulated protein as the 70-kDa testis-expressed chaperone protein, which in man is called HspA2[6].

We have further shown that mature and diminished-maturity sperm are different with respect to HspA2 levels, as expressed by concentrations of sperm CK and HspA2 (% HspA2/(HspA2 + CK-B)), morphological and morphometric attributes, zona pellucida-binding properties and fertility[7,8]. Furthermore, we have established that in spermiogenesis, simultaneously with cytoplasmic extrusion and the commencement of HspA2 synthesis, the sperm plasma membrane also undergoes maturation-related remodeling. This remodeling step facilitates formation of the sites for zona pellucida binding and, very important from the point of view of andrology testing and selection of sperm for intracytoplasmic sperm injection (ICSI), for hyaluronic acid binding in mature sperm[9]. Finally, we demonstrated that all sperm maturational events related to the decline of CK activity and increase in HspA2 expression are completed by the time that the sperm enter the caput epididymis[10].

SPERM MATURITY AND FERTILITY

The predictive value of sperm HspA2 levels in the assessment of male fertility was tested in two blinded studies of couples undergoing *in vitro* fertilization (IVF). In the first, we classified 84 husbands from two different IVF centers (with no information on their semen parameters or reproductive histories) based only on their sperm HspA2 ratios into 'high likelihood' (> 10% HspA2 ratio) and 'low likelihood' (< 10% HspA2 ratio) for fertility groups[8]. All pregnancies occurred in the 'high likelihood' group. No

pregnancy occurred in the 'low likelihood' group. In the 'high likelihood' group, if at least one oocyte was fertilized, the predictive rate of the HspA2 ratio for pregnancy was very high at 30.4% per cycle. An additional important utility of the HspA2 ratio became apparent: nine of the 22 'low likelihood' men were normospermic but had diminished fertility. Thus, the HspA2 ratio provided, for the first time, a diagnostic tool for unexplained male infertility (infertile men with normal semen)[7]. In a recent second study, we re-examined the utility of HspA2 ratios in 194 couples treated at Yale. The receiver operating characteristic (ROC) curve analysis indicated a 100% predictive value for failure to achieve pregnancy below the 10.4% HspA2 threshold. Similar to the 1992 study, nine of the 15 men with < 10% HspA2 ratio and pregnancy failure were normospermic[11].

To identify the steps of the fertilization process at which the low-HspA2 immature sperm are deficient, we explored human sperm–oocyte binding. With the study of sperm–hemizona complexes, we established that only the clear-headed (low CK) mature sperm were able to bind to the zona (Figure 30.1b)[7]. Sperm with retained cytoplasm were deficient in the oocyte-binding site, the formation of which may occur with plasma membrane remodeling simultaneously with cytoplasmic extrusion[9].

From the perspective of male infertility, it is important that synthesis of the HSP70 family of proteins is developmentally regulated and that they appear during meiotic prophase as a component of the synaptonemal complexes[12]. An apparent function of HSP70-2 in mice is maintaining the synaptonemal complex and assisting chromosome crossing-over during meiosis and spermatocyte development. Accordingly, the targeted disruption of the *hsp70-2* gene causes arrested sperm maturation and azoospermia[13]. These events could be related to faulty meiotic recombination in spermatocytes, to disruption of the meiotic cell-cycle regulatory machinery or perhaps to triggering of the apoptotic machinery in spermatocytes, or even

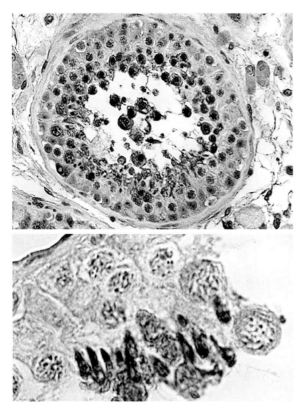

Figure 30.2 Human testicular biopsy tissues immunostained with HspA2 antiserum. Sections represent lower (upper panel) and high (lower panel) magnifications to illustrate the tubular structure, and staining pattern of the adluminal area. HspA2 expression begins in meiotic spermatocytes, but is predominant during terminal spermiogenesis in elongated spermatids and spermatozoa. See also Color plate 5 on page xxvii

in spermatids or ejaculated immature sperm. Regarding human sperm, our laboratory was the first to demonstrate the expression pattern of the HspA2 protein in the human testis and sperm, and to correlate the expression level of HspA2 to sperm function[6]. Figure 30.2 clearly demonstrates the two-wave expression of HspA2, first in spermatocytes related to meiosis, and then at the time of terminal spermiogenesis in elongated spermatids.

In general, chaperone proteins facilitate the assembly and intracellular transport of proteins. Indeed, the second wave of HspA2 expression is simultaneous with major sperm protein movements underlying cytoplasmic extrusion and

remodeling of the human sperm plasma membrane. We believe that retention of the cytoplasm, and the lack of zona-binding sites in immature sperm, are likely related to the diminished expression of HspA2, and also to diminished DNA integrity as a consequence of the impaired delivery of DNA-repair enzymes during and following meiosis[2-6].

GENETIC ASPECTS OF DIMINISHED SPERM MATURITY

Assuming that HspA2 is a component of the synaptonemal complex in man as well as in rodents, we hypothesized that the frequency of chromosomal aneuploidies will be higher in immature versus mature sperm[14]. We have examined this question in sperm arising from semen and from 80% Percoll pellets (enhanced in mature sperm) of the same ejaculate in ten oligozoospermic men. Immature sperm with retained cytoplasm, which signifies spermiogenetic arrest, were identified by immunocytochemistry. We have evaluated with fluorescence *in situ* hybridization (FISH) approximately 7000 sperm nuclei in each of the 20 fractions (142 086 sperm in all) using centromeric probes for the X, Y and 17 chromosomes. The proportions of immature sperm (as detected by cytoplasmic retention) were $45.4 \pm 3.4\%$ vs. $26.6 \pm 2.2\%$ in the two groups (median 48.2% vs. 25%, $p < 0.001$; $n = 300$ sperm evaluated per fraction, 6000 sperm in all). There was also a concomitant decline in total disomy, total diploidy and total aneuploidy frequencies with respect to the tested chromosomes in the 80% Percoll versus semen sperm fractions (0.17 vs. 0.54%, 0.14 vs. 0.26% and 0.31 vs. 0.81%, respectively; $p < 0.001$ in all comparisons). The mean decline in aneuploidies was 2.7-fold. Regarding our hypothesis that aneuploidies are related to sperm immaturity, there was a close correlation between the incidence of immature sperm with cytoplasmic retention and disomies ($r = 0.7$ with all chromosomes, and $r = 0.76$ in case of the

Y disomy; $p < 0.001$ in both), indicating that disomies originate primarily in immature sperm. Thus, the idea that the common factor underlying sperm immaturity and aneuploidies is the diminished expression of HspA2 appears to be valid[14]. However, there was no relationship with diploidies ($r < 0.1$). Thus, in agreement with the ideas presented by Egozcue *et al.*, chromosomal diploidy is likely to arise by diverse cellular mechanisms[15].

SPERM HEAD SHAPE AND SPERM MATURITY

The relationship between abnormal sperm morphology and chromosomal aberrations has been of long-term interest[16,17]. Although there are data supporting this association, studies prior to our recent work regarding this relationship were based on the frequency of abnormal or aneuploid sperm in semen samples, but not on the examination of the same individual sperm for both attributes. The study of the direct relationship between sperm shape and numerical chromosomal aneuploidies was made possible because we determined that sperm preserve their shape after undergoing the decondensation and denaturation steps that are a prerequisite for performing FISH[18].

In a subsequent project, we examined the potential relationship between numerical chromosomal aberrations and sperm shape, as well as the applicability of such data to sperm selection for ICSI[19]. In order to accomplish this goal, we studied the post-FISH status of sperm whether haploid, disomic or diploid, and also evaluated the shape and dimensions of the same spermatozoa by their corresponding phase-contrast microscopy images in a selected sperm population. (The selected sperm population had much higher proportions of disomic and diploid spermatozoa than occur physiologically.)

First, using objective shape measurements, we evaluated 1286 individual sperm from 15 men: 900 haploid, 256 disomic and 130 diploid sperm,

using centromeric FISH probes for the X, Y, 10, 11 and 17 chromosomes. We studied normal, disomic and diploid genotypes in sperm images utilizing three-color FISH (17, X and Y) and two-color FISH for the 10 and 11 chromosomes (60 sperm from each man; 30 sperm with X, Y, 17 chromosomes, and 30 sperm with 10, 11 chromosomes).

In another approach, we sorted the 900 non-aneuploid sperm and classified them into 'small head', 'intermediate head' and 'large head' groups. Further, we sorted the 256 aneuploid and 130 diploid sperm according to the head size parameter ranges established in the non-aneuploid sperm, and determined the frequencies of disomies and diploidies within the three head-size groups.

Aneuploidies and diploidies were present within all three groups. The frequency of chromosomal aberrations correlated positively with sperm head size, as size reflects cytoplasmic retention and immaturity. The frequency of chromosomal aneuploidies was also related to the other sperm head parameters, including head area, perimeter and long and short axes, indicating that the study of any of the four sperm head parameters is relevant to the relationship between sperm shape and disomies or diploidies. The mean percentages of disomies in small, intermediate and large sperm head categories were $27 \pm 2\%$, $23 \pm 1\%$ and $50 \pm 2\%$, respectively. Moreover, the mean percentages of diploidies in the three sperm head categories were $3 \pm 1\%$, $8 \pm 1\%$ and $89 \pm 2\%$, respectively.

When we asked the question, 'How many of the disomic or diploid sperm will fall within the lowest third of the 900 non-aneuploid sperm, the 'most normal' sperm category?', we found that sperm of any head size or shape may have chromosomal aberrations. Furthermore, about 27% of sperm with disomy and 3% with diploidy of the 386 sperm selected for this analysis were among the 300 sperm within the most normal third of the study population, whether we considered one or any of the four basic morphometric parameters.

In another analysis, we classified the same 1286 sperm according to their shape characteristics as normal ($n = 367$), intermediate ($n = 368$), abnormal ($n = 504$) and amorphous ($n = 47$). Disomic and diploid sperm were present in all four groups with an increasing frequency of 18%, 18%, 41% and 98%, respectively, in line with the severity of the sperm shape abnormality, which was most apparent in the abnormal and amorphous sperm shape categories[19].

Finally, we classified the 1286 spermatozoa according to the Kruger strict morphology method as normal and abnormal. The normal strict morphology scores of the haploid ($n = 900$), disomic ($n = 256$) and diploid ($n = 130$) sperm were 24%, 10% and 1%, respectively. These values are also in accordance with the morphometric results, which indicate that the haploid, disomic and diploid sperm are different from each other, not only in genetic or morphometric aspects but also in morphology. We have also evaluated our sperm shape classification with the Kruger method, in order to compare objective morphometry based on the biochemical marker approach with strict morphology. We found good agreement: the Kruger normal scores in the symmetrical, asymmetrical, irregular and amorphous groups were 26%, 3%, 1% and 0%, respectively. However, it was also clear that there were aneuploid sperm in the normal group, demonstrating that the strict morphology evaluation is not discriminatory with respect to the identification of haploid spermatozoa.

Using all three shape-directed approaches, our results support a relationship between abnormal sperm shape and disomies/diploidies, as the combined rates of disomy and diploidy increased within each morphological category from small head size to large head size, from normal to amorphous and from Kruger normal to abnormal, reflecting the direction of declining sperm maturity. Moreover, with the exception of the amorphous class, all classes (normal, intermediate and even abnormal) showed similar disomy frequencies. Thus, these data further confirmed that shape assessment is an unreliable method for the selection of non-aneuploid sperm.

We can conclude that: (1) there is an overall relationship between sperm shape abnormalities and frequencies of chromosomal aneuploidies in spermatozoa; this relationship is likely based on the common upstream events of diminished maturation that affect both meiotic events and cytoplasmic extrusion during late spermiogenesis; (2) shape characteristics are not predictive for ploidy in individual spermatozoa; and (3) thus, visual shape assessment, i.e. choosing the 'best-looking' sperm, is an unreliable method for ICSI selection of normal spermatozoa.

SPERM MATURITY TESTING BY HYALURONIC ACID BINDING

Concurrently with the sperm maturation studies, we investigated the effects of hyaluronic acid (HA) or hyaluronan, which is a linear repeating polymer of disaccharides, on human sperm function. HA in the medium increased the velocity, retention of motility and viability of freshly ejaculated, as well as cryopreserved–thawed, human spermatozoa[20,21]. The enhancement of sperm motility and velocity occurred as a direct response to HA, as indicated by two observations: (1) there was an instantaneous increase in sperm tail cross-beat frequency and sperm velocity upon HA exposure; (2) when we transferred the HA-exposed sperm after density gradient centrifugation to a regular medium, the motility and velocity properties returned to those of the control sperm. We concluded that HA effects on sperm are receptor-mediated. Indeed, the presence of the HA receptor in human sperm has been established by three laboratories[22–24].

Recognizing the association between the presence of plasma-membrane HA receptors and the various upstream features of sperm maturity, we were interested to develop the sperm HA-binding assay to a clinical andrology test, as well as a device for the selection of mature sperm for ICSI[25]. We hypothesized that (1) mature sperm would selectively bind to solid-state HA; this assumption has recently been proved by studies using the various cytoplasmic and nuclear biochemical markers: HA-bound sperm are devoid of cytoplasmic retention and caspase-3, which signifies an ongoing apoptotic process[26]; (2) diminished-maturity spermatozoa, having low HspA2 ratios, chromosomal aberrations and lack of spermatogenetic membrane remodeling, will not bind to solid-state HA, and thus HA binding would facilitate the selection of individual mature sperm with low levels of chromosomal aneuploidies.

Our current ideas on sperm maturation in men are summarized in Figure 30.3. In seeking the underlying mechanism for diminished zona binding by immature sperm, we have established that in spermiogenesis, simultaneously with cytoplasmic extrusion and the commencement of HspA2 synthesis, the sperm plasma membrane also undergoes a maturation-related remodeling that promotes formation of the zona-binding and HA-binding sites. Thus, in immature sperm with cytoplasmic retention, there are low densities of zona-binding sites and also of HA receptors[6,7,20,25].

Based on the concepts of Figure 30.3, we have examined three issues:

- *Whether, via the HA receptors, sperm would permanently bind to solid-state hyaluronic acid.* Indeed, sperm bind to HA. There are three sperm populations: (1) sperm that bind permanently to HA; (2) sperm that exhibit no binding; (3) a small proportion of sperm (< 5%) that initially bind to HA but are soon released, and then rebind. We interpreted these three patterns as mature sperm with a high density of HA receptors, immature sperm with deficient maturity and plasma membrane remodeling, and sperm of intermediate maturity with a low density of HA receptors.

- *The diagnostic utility of sperm binding to HA was tested in a chamber device that is coated with HA in order to examine what proportion of mature sperm exhibit HA binding (Figure 30.4).* It is of note that the HA-binding assay has been approved by the Food and Drug Administration (FDA) for andrology testing.

We found that sperm HA-binding has diagnostic utility. We evaluated the percentage binding of sperm to HA-coated slides in 56 men. With respect to binding, we classified the sperm populations as follows: > 85% ($n = 32$), excellent binding: these men do not require intervention; binding between 65 and 85% ($n = 14$), intermediate: these couples may benefit from intrauterine insemination (IUI); diminished sperm-binding properties, < 60–65% ($n = 10$): these men should be retested, and if the low binding score is confirmed, they should be treated with IVF or ICSI. In line with our previous findings, binding scores were largely independent of sperm concentrations. Among men within the < 20 million sperm/ml concentration range ($n = 18$ of 56 men), we identified three excellent, seven moderate and eight diminished HA-binders.

SELECTION OF SPERM WITH LOW ANEUPLOIDY FREQUENCIES FOR ICSI

The third issue:

- *Whether, due to the relationship between sperm maturity and the meiotic process, sperm with low levels of chromosomal aberrations would preferentially bind to HA*

is addressed in the experiments described below.

The development of this novel sperm selection method using HA binding, in line with concepts presented in Figure 30.3, is based on the recognition that, during spermatogenesis, formation of the zona pellucida-binding and HA-binding sites is commonly regulated. Indeed, we have found a close correlation ($r = 0.73$, $p < 0.001$; $n = 54$) between sperm-binding scores either to HA or to the zona of bisected human oocytes[27]. Thus, HA-selected mature sperm have frequencies of chromosomal aberrations comparable with those of sperm selected by the zona pellucida in conventional fertilization. This relationship is based on the dual role of the HspA2 chaperone, which

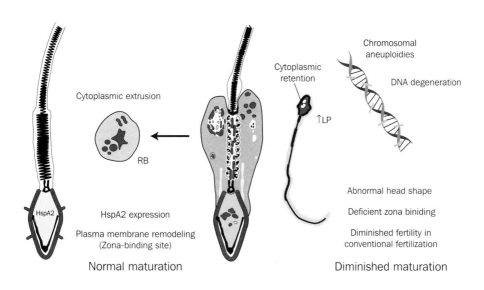

Figure 30.3 A model of normal and diminished maturation of human sperm. In *normal* sperm, maturation HspA2 is expressed in the synaptonemal complex of spermatocytes, supporting meiosis. HspA2 is likely also involved in the processes of late spermiogenesis, such as cytoplasmic extrusion (represented by loss of the residual body, RB), plasma membrane remodeling and formation of the zona pellucida- and hyaluronic acid-binding sites (change from blue to red membrane and stubs). *Diminished-maturity* sperm lack HspA2 expression, which causes meiotic defects and a higher rate of retention of creatine kinase (CK) and other cytoplasmic enzymes, increased levels of lipid peroxidation (LP) and consequent DNA fragmentation, abnormal sperm morphology and deficiency in zona and hyaluronic acid binding. See also Color plate 6 on page xxvii

supports meiosis as a component of the synaptonemal complex, and facilitates plasma membrane remodeling as well as the formation of the zona pellucida- and hyaluronic acid (HA)-binding sites during spermiogenesis[6].

The increased rate of chromosomal aberrations and other potential consequences of using immature sperm for ICSI are of major concern. Based on the association between sperm maturation and plasma membrane remodeling, we formulated the hypothesis that the presence of the HA receptor in mature but not in immature sperm, and a respective device with an HA-coated surface, will facilitate the selection of single, mature sperm with high DNA integrity and a low frequency of chromosomal aneuploidies for ICSI. The HA-selected mature sperm, in addition to having low levels of meiotic errors, are also devoid of cytoplasmic retention, persistent histones, the apoptotic process and DNA fragmentation, factors that would adversely affect the paternal contribution of sperm to the zygote[9,14,25,28–30]. The five-fold decline of sex-chromosome disomies is consistent with the increase of chromosomal aberrations in ICSI children conceived with visually selected sperm. Since HA is a normally occurring component of the female reproductive tract, there should be no ethical concerns[31–34].

In these experiments, we used sperm-selection platforms, Falcon Petri dishes that have spots of immobilized bacterial hyaluronic acid that were prepared using proprietary coating technology (Biocoat Inc., Fort Washington, PA). The sperm–hyaluronic acid binding-assay slides are based on Cell-VU® disposable glass sperm-counting chambers that are treated with a bilaminar hyaluronan coating. The coating consists of hyaluronan grafted to a base-coat, cross-linked with a polyfunctional isocyanate. Total coating depth is less than a micrometer.

We have tested the efficiency of sperm selection with respect to elimination of sperm with chromosomal aneuploidies and diploidies[35]. Washed sperm of 34 moderately oligospermic men were studied. After incubation for 15 min, the HA-attached sperm were collected using an ICSI micropipette. Both HA-selected and unselected sperm were subjected to FISH, using centromeric probes for the X, Y and 17 chromosomes. The control sperm population comprised the unselected sperm. Aliquots of the initial unselected sperm suspension and HA-bound sperm were examined after FISH. Data were analyzed by χ^2 analysis.

In experiments 1 and 2, washed sperm were prepared by dilution of semen with 3–5 volumes of human tubal fluid 0.5% BSA (HTF; Irvine Scientific Co., Irvine, CA). The diluted semen was centrifuged at 1200 g for 15 min, at room temperature. The sperm pellet was resuspended in 0.5 ml HTF to approximately 30 million sperm/ml. In the second experiment, the sperm suspension was also subjected to centrifugation on a discontinuous 45%/90% ISolate® gradient.

With the use of the Falcon Petri dishes with an immobilized HA spot, a drop of sperm suspension was placed close to the edge of the HA spot, and the sperm were allowed to migrate spontaneously. The mature sperm that had completed plasma membrane remodeling bound to the HA, while immature sperm with diminished HA receptor concentrations moved freely over the HA (Figure 30.4). The HA-bound sperm also exhibited vigorous beating with increased tail cross-beat frequency[20,21]. After 15 min (twice the maximum binding period)[25], the bound sperm were collected with the ICSI micropipette, fixed with methanol–acetic acid and subjected to FISH. The control for the selection experiments was always the respective unselected sperm suspension, also treated with FISH (Figure 30.5).

In experiment 3, 5–10-μl drops of sperm suspension were placed on HA-coated glass slides. After a 5-min HA-binding period, the slide was placed at a slight angle and the unbound sperm were eliminated by slowly applying and removing drops of HTF until no free sperm were visible. The HA-bound sperm were removed one-by-one by micropipette and placed in a hydrophobic pen-circled area wetted with HTF, fixed and subjected to FISH.

From the semen fraction of each man we analyzed a mean of 4770 sperm, or 162 210 sperm in the 34 men. In the HA-bound and micropipette-collected sperm fractions, due to the burdens of the task, we studied fewer sperm. In the first experiment, we evaluated 7530 sperm (range 224–1142 per man) and in the second experiment, 9720 sperm (range 373–1955 sperm per man). In the third experiment of individually selected sperm, we evaluated 24 420 sperm (range 1086–3973 per man).

For the HA-bound sperm (495–2079 per man, 41 670 in all) versus unselected sperm (4770 sperm per man, or 162 210 in all), the chromosomal disomy frequencies, with the three probes studied, were reduced to 0.16 from 0.52%, diploidy to 0.09 from 0.51% and sex-chromosome disomy to 0.05 from 0.27% (a 5.4-fold reduction, vs. four-fold respective increase in ICSI offspring).

Our HA–sperm selection method provides a technique for reducing the genetic impact of ICSI fertilization at the traditional evolutionary level by introducing only mature spermatozoa that would have been part of the physiological fertilization pool. In light of our data and of the adverse ICSI consequences reviewed, it is of interest to define the expected advantages of HA-mediated sperm selection in improving ICSI outcome:

• In sperm selected by HA binding, the frequencies of chromosomal disomies and diploidies are in the normal range, independent of the aneuploidy frequencies of the initial semen. In this respect, the sperm selection properties of HA are similar to those of the zona pellucida.

• Mature sperm selected by virtue of HA binding are also viable, and devoid of persistent histones and apoptosis, as evidenced by aniline

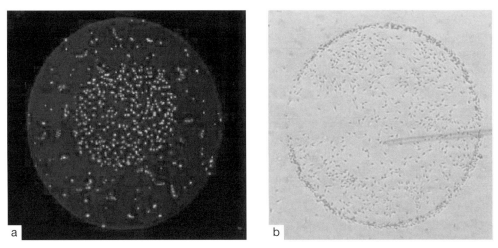

Figure 30.4   Sperm movement patterns on the hyaluronic acid-coated spots used for sperm selection. Mature sperm are bound, and diminished-maturity sperm remain motile. Sperm are stained with cyber green DNA stain (Molecular Probes, Eugene, OR) that permeates viable sperm. See Color plate 7 on page xxviii

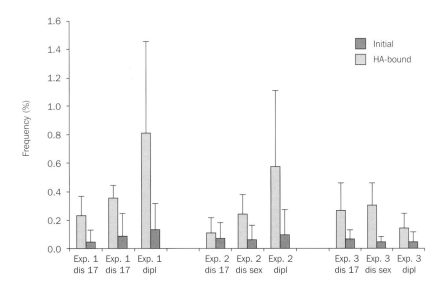

Figure 30.5   Disomy (dis) and diploidy (dipl) frequencies in semen and hyaluronic acid (HA)-selected sperm fractions in the three experiments

blue staining and the absence of active caspase-3, respectively[25,26]. Thus, the paternal contribution of HA-selected sperm will be improved, and we would expect a lower rate of miscarriages following ICSI with HA-selected sperm.

• HA-selected mature sperm do not exhibit DNA fragmentation, as tested by the comet assay and DNA-nick translation[30,36]. This should alleviate concerns related to the potential deterioration of individual development and the increase in cancer rates following ICSI fertilization.

- HA-selection of sperm will allow lesser exposure to toxic polyvinylpyrrolidone.

ACKNOWLEDGMENT

This research was supported by the National Institutes of Health (NIH) (HD-19505, HD-32902, OH-04061).

REFERENCES

1. Huszar G, Corrales M, Vigue L. Correlation between sperm creatine phosphokinase activity and sperm concentrations in normospermic and oligospermic men. Gamete Res 1988; 19: 67
2. Cayli S, et al. Biochemical markers of sperm function: male fertility and sperm selection for ICSI. Reprod Biomed Online 2003; 7: 462
3. Huszar G, Vigue L. Incomplete development of human spermatozoa is associated with increased creatine phosphokinase concentration and abnormal head morphology. Mol Reprod Dev 1993; 34: 292
4. Clermont Y. The cycle of the seminiferous epithelium in man. Am J Anat 1963; 112: 35
5. Huszar G, Vigue L. Spermatogenesis-related change in the synthesis of the creatine kinase B-type and M-type isoforms in human spermatozoa. Mol Reprod Dev 1990; 25: 258
6. Huszar G, et al. Putative creatine kinase M-isoform in human sperm is identified as the 70-kilodalton heat shock protein HspA2. Biol Reprod 2000; 63: 925
7. Huszar G, Vigue L, Oehninger S. Creatine kinase immunocytochemistry of human sperm–hemizona complexes: selective binding of sperm with mature creatine kinase-staining pattern. Fertil Steril 1994; 61: 136
8. Huszar G, Vigue L, Morshedi M. Sperm creatine phosphokinase M-isoform ratios and fertilizing potential of men: a blinded study of 84 couples treated with in vitro fertilization. Fertil Steril 1992; 57: 882
9. Huszar G, et al. Sperm plasma membrane remodeling during spermiogenetic maturation in men: relationship among plasma membrane beta 1,4-galactosyl-transferase, cytoplasmic creatine phosphokinase, and

creatine phosphokinase isoform ratios. Biol Reprod 1997; 56: 1020
10. Huszar G, et al. Cytoplasmic extrusion and the switch from creatine kinase B to M isoform are completed by the commencement of epididymal transport in human and stallion spermatozoa. J Androl 1998; 19: 11
11. Ergur AR, et al. Sperm maturity and treatment choice of IVF or ICSI: diminished sperm HspA2 chaperone levels predict IVF failure. Fertil Steril 2002; 77: 910
12. Allen JW, et al. HSP70-2 is part of the synaptonemal complex in mouse and hamster spermatocytes. Chromosoma 1996; 104: 414
13. Dix DJ, et al. Targeted gene disruption of Hsp70-2 results in failed meiosis, germ cell apoptosis, and male infertility. Proc Natl Acad Sci USA 1996; 93: 3264
14. Kovanci E, et al. FISH assessment of aneuploidy frequencies in mature and immature human spermatozoa classified by the absence or presence of cytoplasmic retention. Hum Reprod 2001; 16: 1209
15. Egozcue S, et al. Diploid sperm and the origin of triploidy. Hum Reprod 2002; 17: 5
16. Bernardini L, et al. Study of aneuploidy in normal and abnormal germ cells from semen of fertile and infertile men. Hum Reprod 1998; 13: 3406
17. Templado C, et al. Aneuploid spermatozoa in infertile men: teratozoospermia. Mol Reprod Dev 2002; 61: 200
18. Celik-Ozenci C, et al. Human sperm maintain their shape following decondensation and denaturation for fluorescent in situ hybridization: shape analysis and objective morphometry. Biol Reprod 2003; 69: 1347
19. Celik-Ozenci C, et al. Sperm selection for ICSI: shape properties do not predict the absence or presence of numerical chromosomal aberrations. Hum Reprod 2004; 19: 2052
20. Huszar G, Willetts M, Corrales M. Hyaluronic acid (Sperm Select) improves retention of sperm motility and velocity in normospermic and oligospermic specimens. Fertil Steril 1990; 54: 1127
21. Sbracia M, et al. Hyaluronic acid substantially increases the retention of motility in cryopreserved/thawed human spermatozoa. Hum Reprod 1997; 12: 1949
22. Kornovski BS, et al. The regulation of sperm motility by a novel hyaluronan receptor. Fertil Steril 1994; 61: 935
23. Ranganathan S, Ganguly AK, Datta K. Evidence for presence of hyaluronan binding protein on spermatozoa and its possible involvement in sperm function. Mol Reprod Dev 1994; 38: 69

24. Cherr GN, et al. Hyaluronic acid and the cumulus extracellular matrix induce increases in intracellular calcium in macaque sperm via the plasma membrane protein PH-20. Zygote 1999; 7: 211

25. Huszar G, et al. Hyaluronic acid binding by human sperm indicates cellular maturity, viability, and unreacted acrosomal status. Fertil Steril 2003; 79 (Suppl 3): 1616

26. Cayli S, et al. Cellular maturity and apoptosis in human sperm: creatine kinase, caspase-3 and Bclx expression in mature and diminished maturity spermatozoa. Mol Human Reprod 2004; 10: 365

27. Cayli S, et al. Hyaluronic acid binding is a test of human sperm maturity and function: correlation between the hyaluronic acid binding and hemizona binding tests. Presented at the 19th Annual Meeting of the European Society for Human Reproduction and Embryology, Madrid, Spain, 2003

28. Seli E, Sakkas D. Spermatozoal nuclear determinants of reproductive outcome: implications for ART. Hum Reprod Update 2005; 11: 337

31. Simpson JL, Lamb DJ. Genetic effects of intracytoplasmic sperm injection. Semin Reprod Med 2001; 19: 239

32. Bonduelle M, et al. Prenatal testing in ICSI pregnancies: incidence of chromosomal anomalies in 1586 karyotypes and relation to sperm parameters. Hum Reprod 2002; 17: 2600

33. Van Steirteghem A, et al. Follow-up of children born after ICSI. Hum Reprod Update 2002; 8: 111

34. Bonduelle M, et al. A multi-centre cohort study of the physical health of 5-year-old children conceived after intracytoplasmic sperm injection, in vitro fertilization and natural conception. Hum Reprod 2005; 20: 413

29. Sakkas D, Mariethoz E, St John JC. Abnormal sperm parameters in humans are indicative of an abortive apoptotic mechanism linked to the Fas-mediated pathway. Exp Cell Res 1999; 251: 350

35. Jakab A, et al. Intracytoplasmic sperm injection: a novel selection method for sperm with normal frequency of chromosomal aneuploidies. Fertil Steril 2005; 84: 1665

36. Huszar GB, et al. Absence of DNA cleavage in mature human sperm selected by their surface membrane receptors. Presented at the 54th Annual Meeting of the American Society for Reproductive Medicine, San Francisco, CA, 1998

30. Sati L, et al. Persistent histones in immature sperm are associated with DNA fragmentation and affect paternal contribution of sperm: a study of aniline blue staining, fluorescence in situ hybridization and DNA nick translation. Presented at the 60th Annual Meeting of the American Society for Reproductive Medicine, Philadelphia, PA, 2004

31

In vitro maturation of spermatozoa

Rosália Sá, Mário Sousa, Nieves Cremades, Cláudia Alves, Joaquina Silva, Alberto Barros

SPERMIOGENESIS *IN VITRO*: ANIMAL STUDIES

The development of methods for the *in vitro* study of mammalian spermatogenesis faces problems due to tissue specificities that are difficult to attain under culture conditions. These problems arise because spermatogenesis depends strongly on the compartmentalization of cellular associations, for example topographic arrangements that determine spatial and temporal relationships between gene expression and specific signal molecules. Even if stable somatic cell populations such as peritubular cells, Leydig cells and Sertoli cells, and stem/progenitor germ cells such as mitotic dividing spermatogonia, can be maintained, this is very difficult to achieve with differentiated germ cells such as meiosis-driven spermatocytes and spermatids. Hence, at present, the major goal of somatic cell–germ cell coculture systems is to establish a minimum of conditions that can artificially keep alive a more or less functional epithelium for a reasonable period of time (2–3 weeks).

These objectives are directed not only towards producing gametes *in vitro* for those cases where no spermatids are found, but also towards enabling a more controlled study of the mechanism of action of toxins, hormones and signal molecules on the seminiferous epithelium. These *in vitro* systems may allow the development of more efficient culture media, and may serve as a unique model to facilitate the isolation of highly purified cell populations in order to study gene expression and signal pathways of stage-specific germ cells. Finally, these systems may also provide an alternative tool for developing gene therapy strategies that could bypass the need for animal experimentation or preliminary *in vivo* clinical trials. This is especially important for those patients showing maturation arrest due to a genetic cause, in whom gene transfer *in vitro* could be used to overcome the defect and thus to produce *in vitro* gametes for treatment.

Amphibians, insects and fishes

Amphibians and insects show a single spermatogenic cell lineage of interconnected cells confined to a germ-line cyst. Although they contain Sertoli-like nurse cells, the development of germ cells is not dependent on contact with Sertoli cells. These specificities enable cysts to evolve individually, which explains why they can be maintained in culture so efficiently. In fact, culture of cell suspensions in media supplemented with follicle stimulating hormone (FSH) has shown that, in *Xenopus*, the newt and *Drosophila*, spermatogonia and primary spermatocytes can divide, complete meiosis and then evolve into elongated spermatids, although not into spermatozoa. In the animal kingdom, the complete *in vitro* differentiation from spermatogonia to spermatozoa has only been achieved in the eel, after 21 days of culture in the presence of testosterone[1].

Rodents

In contrast, restoration of the spermatogenic cycle *in vitro* remains to be successfully achieved in mammals. This can be explained by the existence of very complex mixtures of germ cells at different stages, and of complex intercellular relationships between Sertoli cells, basement lamina and germ cells, with germ cell development appearing also to be dependent on numerous hormones, growth factors and interleukins secreted by intraepithelial cells, and by cells located in the surrounding connective tissue[2–21].

In rodents, seminiferous tubule fragments, which preserve Sertoli cell and germ cell contacts, can be maintained viable for several months if cultured under conditions of 32°C, 5% CO_2 in air, pH 7.2, in the presence of vitamins, amino acids, sodium pyruvate and 10% fetal calf serum. However, after 3 weeks, only Sertoli cells remained alive, spermatogonia and spermatocytes degenerated and no round spermatids were ever formed *in vitro*[22]. Later experiments, using *in vitro* culture of rat seminiferous tubule segments, then showed that late-pachytene spermatocytes could end meiosis I in 2–4 days and form secondary spermatocytes. Secondary spermatocytes then ended meiosis II in 2–3 further days, giving origin to round spermatids. As these experiments were conducted in the absence of hormones, it was suggested that late-pachytene spermatocytes have all the information required for both meiotic divisions and early spermiogenesis[23]. These experiments were further expanded to show that preleptotene spermatocytes could evolve after 3 days into zygotene spermatocytes, and these into late-pachytene spermatocytes after 7 more days in organ culture. They also confirmed the need for about 7 days to develop from the late-pachytene stage to the round spermatid stage. Curiously, it

was shown that meiosis I and meiosis II could be spontaneously accelerated, thus originating round spermatids in only 2 days of culture. Unfortunately, the process of round spermatid maturation into elongating spermatids, which took 4 days, ended in the production of highly abnormal cells[24].

By using mouse premeiotic germ cells cocultured on Sertoli cell-like feeder layers, it was shown that it was even possible to obtain round spermatids from spermatogonia in about 10–12 days, although this pace of spermatogenesis was very accelerated. However, these haploid germ cells then became arrested[25]. Also, using rodent germ cell suspensions, preleptotene spermatocytes were shown to evolve to the zygotene stage in about 3 days, the latter into late-pachytene spermatocytes in 7 days and these into round spermatids in 2–7 days, thus completing the two meiotic divisions *in vitro* in about 12–17 days. However, round spermatids were also unable to differentiate into normal elongating spermatids. The ability of spermatocytes to differentiate into round spermatids *in vitro* was suggested to be due to primary spermatocytes receiving the information needed for completion of the meiotic divisions at the mid- and late-pachytene stages, at which time RNA transcription is activated and formation of the chromatoid body is begun. Further studies then showed, using organ culture without hormonal supplementation and with only 0.2% fetal calf serum, an accelerated process (21 days) of proliferation and differentiation from the spermatogonia up to the round spermatid stage. Unfortunately, these round spermatids also remained arrested[26]. The *in vitro* culture of mouse premeiotic germ cells using cell suspensions and a complex medium containing growth factors, FSH and testosterone was also shown to enable the production of round spermatids after 7–10 days. These were microinjected into oocytes, and fertile normal offspring were obtained, thus suggesting that round spermatids produced *in vitro* from normal seminiferous tubules keep all their normal developmental potential[27].

Overall, experiments with rodent spermatogenesis *in vitro* revealed that most of the cells degenerate rapidly in the first 2 days, especially if contacts with Sertoli cells are lost, with successful preparation of Sertoli–spermatogenic cell cocultures depending on minimal cell-junction disruption during enzymatic dissociation, cell-plating at maximum density, supplementation with hormones (FSH and testosterone), growth factors and vitamins, frequent replenishment of the culture medium and simultaneous removal of metabolic waste products.

The action of hormones

Spermatogenesis is a hormone-sensitive process, with FSH being especially critical for the initiation of spermatogenesis and both FSH and testosterone being needed to support germ cell differentiation. FSH and testosterone exert direct and indirect actions on Sertoli cells. Acting on Sertoli cells, FSH causes cyclic adenosine monophosphate (cAMP) accumulation (cAMP crosses gap junctions and activates germ-cell gene transcription), protein kinase activation, production of lactate (essential for spermatocyte RNA synthesis), synthesis of transferrin and androgen-binding protein (essential to mediate testosterone action on germ cells) and RNA and protein synthesis, including the expression of stem cell factor (SCF). On spermatocytogenesis, FSH was suggested to play a determinant role in preventing cell degeneration, to stimulate spermatogonia proliferation (through binding of SCF to c-Kit receptor in A spermatogonia) and spermatogonia conversion to preleptotene spermatocytes and to modulate meiotic divisions. Regarding its actions on spermiogenesis, contradictory roles have been ascribed to FSH, with some authors observing a stimulatory action on round spermatid differentiation[28,29], and others demonstrating that it inhibits the spermiogenic process[30].

Under luteinizing hormone (LH) influence, testosterone is secreted by Leydig cells and binds to intracellular cytoplasmic androgen receptors of Sertoli cells. These then translocate to the nucleus and stimulate transcription. Testosterone is 50–100 times more concentrated in the testis than in serum, with lower or intermittent levels inhibiting spermatogenesis. The effectiveness of testosterone also declines with time, which explains the need for supraphysiological levels to maintain spermatogenesis. However, there is no absolute need for the presence of high levels of testosterone to stimulate spermiogenesis. This was demonstrated by using knock-out mice with absent LH receptors. In this situation, LH is unable to stimulate Leydig cells, causing a very low level of intratesticular testosterone. These animals showed the presence of conserved spermatogenesis, but quantitative analysis demonstrated that if spermiogenesis proceeds qualitatively it is decreased quantitatively[31]. Thus, if spermatogenesis can be maintained in the presence of low testosterone levels, higher concentrations of testosterone are needed to sustain quantitative spermatogenesis, possibly by the induction of high levels of androgen receptors or growth factors. These observations also explain how low levels of testosterone appear to be sufficient to stimulate the proliferation of spermatogonia and meiosis, although inducing round spermatid apoptosis and spermiogenesis decline[32]. However, the addition of normal testosterone concentrations failed to restore a normal germ cell number in those cases where spermiogenesis was inhibited due to absent or low testosterone levels, which suggests a need for other factors in stimulating quantitative spermatogenesis[33]. Like FSH, testosterone has been implicated in germ cell survival, the induction of spermatogonia proliferation, spermatocyte differentiation and meiosis. The main action of testosterone is, however, to induce and control round spermatid maturation and conversion to elongated spermatids[34–38].

Both FSH and testosterone thus act synergistically, and most of their actions also appear to be mediated by intermediates secreted by androgen-sensitive extratesticular tissues, local steroids or other paracrine factors produced in response to pituitary hormones. Paracrine effects have been described for diverse growth factors, cytokines, vasoactive peptides, hormones, endogenous opioid peptides and neuropeptides[5,7,8,11,18].

SPERMIOGENESIS *IN VITRO*: EXPERIMENTAL STUDIES IN THE HUMAN

Initial trials

The use of human adult whole testicular tissue or whole testicular tissue cell suspensions for the study of spermatogenesis *in vitro* raises the problem that it is impossible to assure a complete absence of spermatids in such samples. To study whether the human spermatogenic cycle can be restored *in vitro*, it is thus necessary to avoid any possible contamination by a hidden focus of elongating or elongated spermatids. For this, experiments must be carried out with round spermatids or mixtures of round spermatids, diploid germ cells and Sertoli cells, after careful isolation of each cell type[39–41].

In some patients with spermacytogenesis and absent spermiogenesis, a few round spermatids might escape meiotic arrest and be isolated. Because of the rather disappointing results with round spermatid injection, in vitro culture of round spermatids was initiated in an effort to try to overcome the poor clinical outcomes obtained with the use of such immature haploid germ cells. The correct identification of round spermatids is technically difficult, and an inappropriate option could have a detrimental effect on the outcome of round spermatid injection. Although guidelines have emerged on how to recognize correctly and test these cells, flagellar growth by in vitro culture of round spermatids could help further in the correct identification of live and viable round spermatids[41–48].

In cocultures of Sertoli cells with primary spermatocytes, round spermatids and elongating spermatids, at 32°C in media supplemented with serum, no meiosis resumption or elongating spermatid maturation was observed at up to 4 days. This temperature was chosen based on mouse experiments that had demonstrated an inhibition of protein synthesis when male germ cells were submitted to temperatures higher than 32–34°C[49]. In contrast, about 22% of cultured isolated round spermatids grew flagella in 1–2 days. However, these late round spermatids became arrested, and were incapable of inducing normal embryo development[50–52]. This type of experiment was also clinically applied in the absence of serum supplementation and at 37°C, but no beneficial effects could be obtained; besides a small improvement noticed in the fertilization rate after round spermatid microinjection, none of the *in vitro* cultured round spermatids developed a flagellum after 3 days of culture[53].

Vero cell monolayers

In order to try to improve the above-reported results, it was hypothesized that round spermatids could be better matured using Vero cell cocultures, as these cells secrete interleukins, growth factors and detoxicating substances[54]. By using cocultures on Vero cell monolayers at 37°C, isolated human round spermatids were able to mature into late spermatids and spermatozoa in about 5 days[39], although this was far more rapid than the expected physiological pace of *in vivo* spermiogenesis that takes about 16–22 days[55,56]. Although most of the mature gametes displayed abnormal nuclei and were not used for clinical treatments, these were the very first experiments in mammals that demonstrated it might be possible to attain the complete spermatid differentiation process *in vitro*, from the round spermatid to the spermatozoon stage, using Vero cell cocultures in the absence of hormonal supplementation.

In these experiments, testicular samples from three patients with normal karyotypes and secretory azoospermia (SAZ) were used. The testicular diagnostic biopsy (TDB) showed two cases with complete maturation arrest at the primary spermatocyte stage (cMA) and one case with incomplete MA (iMA: presence of at least one seminiferous tubule section containing spermiogenesis up to the late spermatid or spermatozoa stage). At the open-treatment testicular biopsy (testicular sperm extraction, TESE), samples with cMA showed a few early round spermatids (Sa1: without flagellum, at the Golgi phase) escaping meiotic block (cases 1, 2), whereas the sample with iMA enabled the recovery of spermatozoa (case 3). Round spermatids were isolated from all these cases by micromanipulation and *in vitro* cultured on Vero cell monolayers. Spermiogenesis was achieved in 5 days only in case 1 (1/3, 33%), thus demonstrating that round spermatids escaping from meiotic block can contain normal spermiogenic potential. In contrast, the failure of round spermatid maturation in case 3 (with conserved spermiogenesis) suggests that the culture medium was not optimized for germ cell differentiation *in vitro*, or that SAZ samples show different genetic causes, with some cases of meiosis arrest eliciting normal spermatid development and some cases with decreased spermiogenesis not eliciting such a differentiation process.

Overall, only 18% of early round spermatids (Sa1) were capable of extruding a flagellum (Sa2), 11% attained the early elongating stage (Sb2) and the early elongated stage (Sd1), and 2% differentiated into late elongated spermatids (Sd2) or spermatozoa (Sz), although with morphological head defects. Analysis of spermatid differentiation and arrest rates in relation to the previous spermatid stage demonstrated that most Sa1 (82% aSa1) and Sd1 (86% aSd1) became arrested. On the other hand, maturation arrest was rather low at the other transition stages, with 36% of arrested Sa2 (aSa2) and 0% of arrested Sb2 (aSb2). Thus, most of the Sa2 evolved into Sb2 (64%) and all Sb2 differentiated into Sd1 (Table 31.1, Figure 31.1).

These results suggest that the most critical steps in spermiogenesis are extrusion of the flagellum, at the transition from Sa1 to Sa2, and the final maturation step of spermiogenesis where

Table 31.1   Spermatid maturation and arrest on Vero cell monolayers (*n*)

	Case 1	Case 2	Case 3	Total
Spermatid maturation				
Sa1	37	10	15	62
Sa2	11	0	0	11
Sb2	7	0	0	7
Sd1	7	0	0	7
Sd2/Sz	1	0	0	1
Spermatid arrest				
Total aSa1	26	10	15	51
aSa1	26	6	7	39
aSb1	0	4	8	12
aSa2	4			4
aSb2	0			0
aSd1	6			6

Sa1, early round spermatids; Sa2, late round spermatids (with flagellum); Sb2, early elongating spermatids; Sd1, early elongated spermatids; Sd2, late elongated spermatids; Sz, spermatozoa; a, arrested

nuclear elongation and condensation occur as Sd1 are transformed into Sd2/Sz. This was further proved by the observation that cytoplasm elongation, and nuclear elongation and condensation, occurred in the absence of flagellum extrusion (24% Sb1). The low rate of *in vitro* maturation of round spermatids into late elongated spermatids/spermatozoa (2%) might thus be attributed to failure of the culture medium in allowing efficient transition of Sa1 into Sa2 (82% aSa1) and of Sd1 into Sd2/Sz (86% aSd1), or to important genetic disturbances harbored by the majority of Sa1 from secretory azoospermia cases that hampered further development.

Vero cell-enriched conditioned medium

Although Vero cells were successfully employed in human embryo culture, with embryo transfer

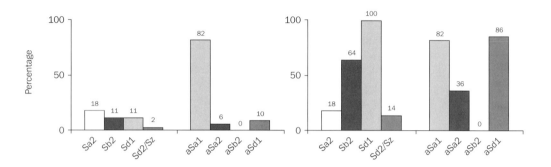

Figure 31.1   Vero cell monolayers. Percentage distribution of spermatid maturation and arrest relative to the initial number of early round spermatids (left) or number of spermatids present in the previous spermiogenic stage (right). See Table 31.1 for spermatid maturation stages

never causing transmission of any disease to the children born[57,58], cell monolayers should be avoided due to concerns about the exploitation of animal or human feeder layers with cells to be used in clinical treatments. Experiments were therein expanded using Vero cell-enriched conditioned medium (CM). This comprised the supernatant fluid covering Vero cell monolayers after 2 days of culture, thus containing all paracrine factors secreted by the cell monolayers. In these experiments, early round spermatids (Sa1: without flagellum) were isolated from cases with conserved and disrupted spermatogenesis and cultured, and spermatids matured *in vitro* were microinjected into donated oocytes, to study their developmental potential. Testicular samples from 12 patients with normal karyotypes were used, seven cases with secretory azoospermia (SAZ) and five cases with obstructive azoospermia (OAZ). The diagnostic histopathological testicular biopsy (TDB) showed two cases of incomplete Sertoli cell-only syndrome (iSO: at least one seminiferous tubule section showing round spermatids), one case of complete maturation arrest (cMA: arrest at meiosis I) and four cases with hypospermatogenesis (HP) in SAZ, whereas all OAZ cases had conserved spermiogenesis. At the treatment testicular biopsy (testicular sperm extraction, TESE), all samples enabled the recovery of spermatozoa, with the exception of one iSO case that showed a focus

of spermacytogenesis with a few Sa1 escaping meiotic arrest[40].

All patient samples showed the maturation of Sa1 into Sa2 (late round spermatids: with flagellum) and Sb2 (early elongating spermatids), but the number of cases with successful differentiation into early elongated spermatids (67% Sd1) and late elongated spermatids/spermatozoa (58% Sd2/Sz) progressively decreased (Table 31.2). In comparison with Vero cell monolayers[39], the relatively better results obtained with CM (33% vs. 58%; $p > 0.05$) may be related to the lower number of cases studied on feeder layers and to the predominance of complete spermiogenesis in CM cases, which gives a better genetic background to round spermatids. As complete spermiogenesis *in vitro* was achieved in 7/12 (58%) of the samples, it might be concluded that round spermatids isolated from cases with complete spermiogenesis and from one case with absent spermiogenesis (differentiation of Sd2 after 9 days of culture) had a similar spermiogenic potential. This suggests that although not all round spermatids will be able to differentiate *in vitro* and not all patient samples will present round spermatids with differentiation potential, it is worthwhile culturing immature haploid germ cells to study whether they can differentiate *in vitro* in patients with spermiogenesis failure. Because most SAZ (11/12, 92%) and all OAZ (5/11, 45%) cases presented complete

Table 31.2 Patients with successful spermatid maturation in Vero cell-enriched conditioned medium (*n* (%)). See Table 31.1 for spermatid maturation stages

	Sa1	*Sb2*	*Sd1*	*Sd2*	*Failures*
OAZ	5	5	3 (60)	3 (60)	2 (40)
HP	4	4	3 (75)	2 (50)	2 (50)
MA	1	1	1 (100)	1 (100)	0
SO	2	2	1 (50)	1 (50)	1 (50)
MA + SO	3	3	2 (67)	2 (67)	1 (33)
SAZ	7	7	5 (71)	4 (57)	3 (43)
Total	12	12	8 (67)	7 (58)	5 (42)

OAZ, obstructive azoospermia; HP, hypospermatogenesis; MA, maturation arrest; SO, Sertoli cell-only syndrome; SAZ, secretory azoospermia

spermiogenesis, the high rate of early round spermatid differentiation arrest, especially in cases with obstructive azoospermia (40%) and hypospermatogenesis (50%), seems not to be related to the presence of important background genetic disturbances of Sa1 but rather is dependent on limitations of the culture system and culture medium.

Under culture, Sa1 extruded a flagellum and transformed into Sb2 after 2–3 days, Sb2 matured into Sd1 in 3–4 further days and Sd1 differentiated into Sd2 in 2 more days. This gave a total duration of *in vitro* spermiogenesis of 7–9 days, which is an improvement regarding the more accelerated *in vitro* maturation process (5 days) observed with Vero cell monolayers[39], as it approaches the physiological *in vivo* process of human spermiogenesis that lasts for about 16–22 days[55,56].

Overall, 25% of Sa1 were capable of extruding a flagellum and attaining the Sb2 stage, 11% differentiated into Sd1 and 5% matured into Sd2 (Table 31.3, Figure 31.2). Although OAZ cases showed a much better *in vitro* differentiation efficiency, differences were not significant (9% in OAZ vs. 4% in SAZ; $p > 0.05$). These results confirm those obtained with Vero cell monolayers (11% Sb2, 11% Sd1, 2% Sd2)[39], although CM

seems to allow better early and late spermiogenesis maturation rates. Analysis of spermatid arrest rates in relation to the previous cell stage gave a similar picture. Transition from Sa1 into Sb2 was the main step of differentiation arrest (75% of arrest at the Sa1 stage, aSa1), with transition from Sb2 to Sd1 (58% of arrest at the Sb2 stage, aSb2) and from Sd1 to Sd2 (48% of arrest at the Sd1 stage, aSd1) being less affected. Although no significant differences were found between obstructive and non-obstructive azoospermia, OAZ cases showed a lower rate of Sd1 arrest (29% in OAZ vs. 56% in SAZ; $p > 0.05$). In comparison, Vero cell monolayers showed a similar rate of Sa1 arrest (82% vs. 75% aSa1), better progression from Sa2 into Sb2 (36% vs. 0% aSa2), a worse maturation rate of Sb2 into Sd1 (0% vs. 58% aSb2) and better differentiation from Sd1 into Sd2 (86% vs. 48% aSd1)[39]. Results in CM thus confirm that the most critical stages in spermiogenesis are extrusion of the flagellum, at the transition from Sa1 to Sa2, and the final nuclear elongation and condensation maturation step during Sd1 and Sd2 formation. This was further proved by the observation that cytoplasm elongation and nuclear elongation and condensation were able to occur in the absence of flagellum extrusion (Sb1). In fact, of the 178/238

Table 31.3 Spermatid maturation and arrest in Vero cell-enriched conditioned medium (*n*). See Table 31.1 for spermatid maturation stages

	OAZ	HP	MA + SO	SAZ	Total
Cases	5	4	3	7	12
Spermatid maturation					
Sa1	54	94	90	184	238
Sb2	17	25	18	43	60
Sd1	7	9	9	18	25
Sd2/Sz	5	4	4	8	13
Spermatid arrest					
aSa1	37	69	72	141	178
aSb2	10	16	9	25	35
aSd1	2	5	5	10	12

OAZ, obstructive azoospermia; HP, hypospermatogenesis; MA, maturation arrest; SO, Sertoli cell-only syndrome; SAZ, secretory azoospermia

aSa1, 83 (35%) remained as aSa1, whereas 95 (40%) evolved into Sb1.

All *in vitro* differentiated late spermatids (Sd2) and arrested early-elongating spermatids (aSb2) were used in experimental oocyte microinjections in order to evaluate their developmental potential (Table 31.4). For this, 24 donated excess oocytes were used, 12 mature meiosis II (MII) oocytes, and 12 immature meiosis I (MI) oocytes that spontaneously matured to the MII stage in less than 6 h[40]. No significant differences were found between microinjection cycles using Sd2 or aSb2. Despite the lower fertilization rate (41%), the embryo cleavage (78%), high-quality embryo morphology (71%) and blastocyst formation (60%) rates appeared normal, thus suggesting that *in vitro*-matured spermatids are capable of sustaining normal embryo development, at least when using round spermatids retrieved from testicular samples with conserved spermatogenesis[40]. Data on embryo development did not include the developmental potential of unipronuclear zygotes (one pronucleus and two polar bodies). If these had been used, the fertilization rate would be near

normal (64%). Although unipronuclear zygotes may be euploid (due to karyosyngamy) or haploid (due to oocyte activation with failure of male pronucleus formation), clinical microinjection cycles using round spermatids from patients with conserved spermiogenesis have suggested that unipronuclear zygotes might result from karyosyngamy, as they have enabled term pregnancies and the birth of normal children[48].

Hormonal supplementation

To analyze further the spermiogenic potential of round spermatids, studies based on Vero cell monolayers and Vero cell-enriched conditioned medium were expanded to 61 patients with secretory azoospermia. In these experiments, the effect of coculturing round spermatids with diploid germ cells and Sertoli cells (autologous coculture system) was studied. For this, cells were isolated by micromanipulation and then mixed in culture microdrops (Figure 31.3): 10–30 spermatogonia A (SGA: fusiform shape), 200 primary spermato-

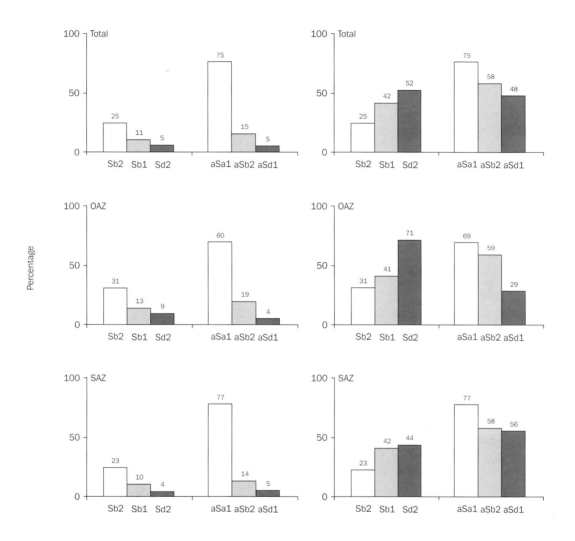

Figure 31.2   Vero cell-enriched conditioned medium. Percentage distribution of spermatid maturation and arrest relative to the initial number of early round spermatids (left) or number of spermatids present in the previous spermiogenic stage (right). See Table 31.1 for spermatid maturation stages. OAZ, obstructive azoospermia; SAZ, secretory azoospermia

cytes (ST1: 19–24 μm in diameter), 10–20 secondary spermatocytes, when available (ST2: polarized cytoplasm and nucleus, 14 μm in diameter), variable amounts of early round spermatids, when available (Sa1: 8–10 μm in diameter), and 30–80 Sertoli cells (SC: cytoplasm filled with dense lipid droplets and lysosomes, nucleus with a raised border and a large nucleolus). To confirm the purity of the cell populations, isolated germ cells were analyzed by fluorescence *in situ* hybridization (FISH) using DNA fluorescent probes to the centromeric regions of chromosomes X, Y and 18 (Figure 31.4). The potential beneficial effect of supplementing the culture medium with hormones was also assessed, using 25 U/l recombinant follicle stimulating hormone (rFSH) or rFSH and 1 μmol/l testosterone (T). The developmental potential of sper-

Table 31.4 Spermatid microinjection outcome after maturation in Vero cell-enriched conditioned medium (*n* (%))

	IVMO			MII			All oocytes		
	Sd2	aSb2	Total	Sd2	aSb2	Total	Sd2	aSb2	Total
MII injected	10	2	12	2	10	12	12	12	24
Degenerated	0	1 (50)	1 (8)	0	1 (10)	1 (8)	0	2 (17)	2 (8)
Intact	10 (100)	1 (50)	11 (92)	2 (100)	9 (90)	11 (92)	12 (100)	10 (83)	22 (92)
non-fertilized (0PN1PB)	3 (30)	1 (100)	4 (36)	0	1 (11)	1 (9)	3 (25)	2 (20)	5 (23)
activated (0PN2PB)	1 (10)	0	1 (9)	0	2 (22)	2 (18)	1 (8)	2 (20)	3 (14)
abnormal fertilization (1PN2PB)	2 (20)	0	2 (18)	1 (50)	2 (22)	3 (27)	3 (25)	2 (20)	5 (23)
normal fertilization (2PN2PB)	4 (40)	0	4 (36)	1 (50)	4 (44)	5 (45)	5 (42)	4 (40)	9 (41)
Embryo cleavage	2 (50)		2 (50)	1 (100)	4 (100)	5 (100)	3 (60)	4 (100)	7 (78)
Grade A/B embryos	0		0	1 (100)	4 (100)	5 (100)	1 (33)	4 (100)	5 (71)
Blastocysts	0		0	1 (100)	2 (50)	3 (60)	1 (100)	2 (50)	3 (60)
High-grade blastocysts				1 (100)	2 (100)	3 (100)	1 (100)	2 (100)	3 (100)

aSb2, arrested early elongating spermatids; Sd2, late elongated spermatids; IVMO, *in vitro*-matured (MI) oocytes; MII, mature meiosis II oocytes; PN, pronuclei; PB, polar bodies

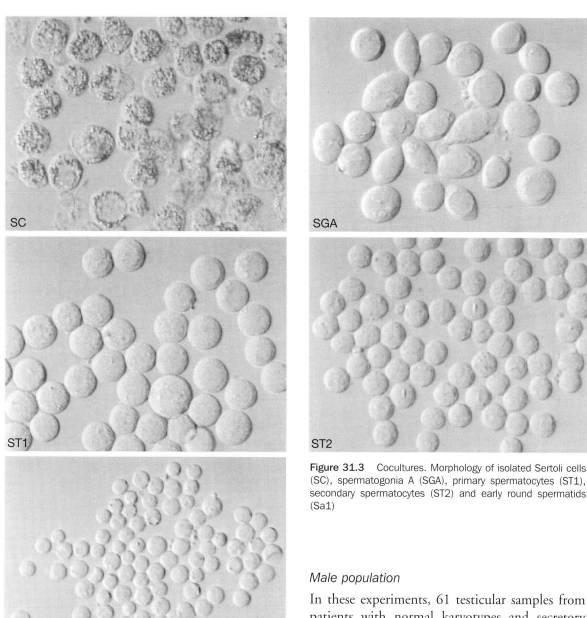

Figure 31.3 Cocultures. Morphology of isolated Sertoli cells (SC), spermatogonia A (SGA), primary spermatocytes (ST1), secondary spermatocytes (ST2) and early round spermatids (Sa1)

Male population

In these experiments, 61 testicular samples from patients with normal karyotypes and secretory azoospermia were used (Figure 31.5)[41]. The testicular diagnostic biopsy (TDB) showed nine cases with Sertoli cell-only syndrome (15% SO), 23 cases with maturation arrest (38% MA) and 29 cases with hypospermatogenesis (48% HP). At TESE, all HP samples enabled the recovery of late elongated spermatids (Sd2) and spermatozoa (Sz); three SO cases had conserved spermiogenesis (Sd2/Sz), two SO samples enabled the recovery of early round spermatids (Sa1) and four SO cases

matids obtained after maturation *in vitro* was studied by microinjection into donated surplus MII oocytes, with the chromosome constitution of the embryos being thereafter analyzed by FISH[41].

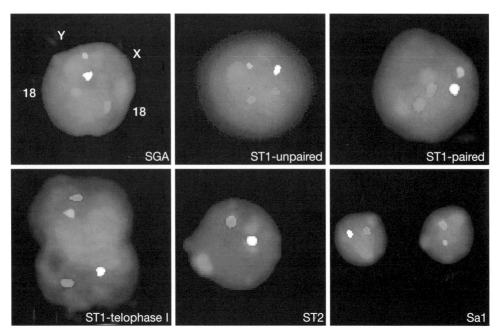

Figure 31.4   Cocultures. Fluorescence *in situ* hybridization (FISH) analysis of spermatogonia A (SGA), primary spermatocytes (ST1), secondary spermatocytes (ST2) and early round spermatids (Sa1). 18 = violet, X = yellow, Y = red. See also Color plate 8 on page xxviii

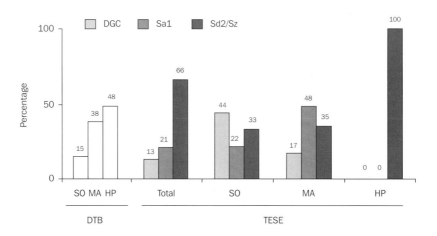

Figure 31.5   Cocultures. Percentage distribution of patients in terms of histopathology at testicular diagnostic biopsy (TDB) and type of cells found at treatment biopsy (testicular sperm extraction, TESE). SO, Sertoli cell-only syndrome; MA, maturation arrest; HP, hypospermatogenesis; DGC, diploid germ cells; Sa1, early round spermatids; Sd2/Sz, late elongated spermatids/spermatazoa

had only diploid germ cells (DGCs); eight MA cases had Sd2/Sz, 11 MA samples had Sa1 and four MA cases had DGCs. Sertoli cells, DGCs and Sa1 retrieved from cases showing Sd2/Sz at TESE were used as controls (29 HP, eight MA and three SO cases). DGCs and Sa1 retrieved from

Table 31.5   Spermatid maturation and arrest in cocultures (*n*). See Table 31.1 for spermatid maturation stages

	Controls			Cases		
	CM	FSH	FSH + T	CM	FSH	FSH + T
Cases	11	13	16	8	4	9
Mean culture days	12	6	7	10	11	8
range	5–20	3–9	4–11	8–12		6–12
Spermatid maturation						
Sa1	203	273	286	201	59	194
Sa2	32	71	110	15	9	62
Sb2	19	54	91	11	6	44
Sd1	11	6	35	3	1	25
Sd2	2	0	22	0	0	16
Spermatid arrest						
Total aSa1	171	202	176	186	50	132
aSa1	126	126	65	156	39	57
aSb1	45	76	111	30	11	75
aSa2	13	17	19	4	3	18
aSb2	8	48	56	8	5	19
aSd1	9	6	13	3	1	9

CM, conditioned medium; FSH, follicle stimulating hormone; T, testosterone

cases with absent spermiogenesis at TESE were used as case studies (six SO and 15 MA cases).

Pace of spermiogenesis

Under *in vitro* culture, early round spermatids (Sa1) extruded a flagellum (Sa2) after 1–2 days, Sa2 transformed into early elongating spermatids (Sb2) in 2–3 days, Sb2 matured into early elongated spermatids (Sd1) in 3–4 further days and Sd1 differentiated into late elongated spermatids (Sd2) in 2–3 more days. The total duration of *in vitro* spermiogenesis was thus about 8–12 days[41], which is an improvement regarding the more accelerated *in vitro* maturation process observed with Vero cell monolayers (5 days)[39] or with Vero cell-enriched conditioned medium (7–9 days)[40], approaching the physiological *in vivo* process of human spermiogenesis that lasts for about 16–22 days[55,56].

Regarding the mean culture days needed to reach the early spermatid elongated stage (Table 31.5), no significant differences were observed between control and case groups within each culture medium (non-supplemented medium, CM: $p = 0.554$; FSH: $p = 0.512$; FSH + T: $p = 0.635$). In contrast, comparisons between different culture media within the control and case groups revealed significant differences. In controls, no significant differences were found for CM/FSH ($p = 0.153$) and FSH/FSH + T ($p = 0.545$), but significant differences were found for CM/FSH + T ($p = 0.019$). In cases, no significant differences were found for CM/FSH ($p = 0.821$), FSH/FSH + T ($p = 0.395$) and CM/FSH + T ($p = 0.447$).

Rates of spermatid maturation and arrest by testicular phenotype

In controls (conserved spermiogenesis, with Sd2/Sz at TESE), the rates of patients whose testicular samples enabled successful *in vitro* maturation of spermatids showed that the spermiogenic potential of early round spermatids appeared to be higher in HP than in SO/MA, that the best maturation results were obtained with CM + FSH + T and that FSH inhibited late spermatid differentiation (Table 31.6, Figure 31.6). However, even in CM + FSH + T, only 25% of SO/MA patients and 38% of HP patients reached the Sd2 stage. In comparison, Vero cell-enriched conditioned medium allowed better results, as 60% of OAZ ($n = 5$), 50% of HP ($n = 4$), 67% of SO/MA ($n = 3$) and 57% of SAZ ($n = 7$) cases elicited the *in vitro* differentiation of Sa1 into Sd2[40]. Although no significant differences were found related to the present rates[41], the above tendencies need some specific comments: (1) better rates of spermatid differentiation are obtained with essential paracrine factors secreted by Vero cells than with hormone supplementation; (2) the present series is much larger (61 vs. 12 cases) and thus more consistent with reality; (3) round spermatids from different azoospermic patients do not exhibit similar spermiogenic differentiation potential, even when retrieved from patients with the same testicular phenotype. For this reason, the rates of maturation appear to be quite variable due to the individual nature of the process, and thus are not consistent and reprodutible.

In cases (absent spermiogenesis, with DGCs or Sa1 at TESE), the rates of patients whose testicular samples enabled successful *in vitro* maturation of spermatids (Table 31.6, Figure 31.6) suggest that early round spermatids exhibit a lower differentiation potential in non-supplemented media regarding controls, that early round spermatids appear to be more resistant to FSH actions regarding controls in relation to early (Sa1 into Sa2) and mid- (Sa2 into Sb2) spermiogenesis and that testosterone is especially capable of stimulating term spermiogenesis (Sd1 into Sd2) in comparison with controls. Although no significant differences were found with regard to control cases, results indicate that early round spermatids retrieved from cases with absent spermiogenesis are inhibited by FSH or need higher, pharmacological FSH concentrations.

Comparisons between controls and cases within the same culture medium

Comparisons between controls (Sd2/Sz at TESE) and cases (DGCs/Sa1 at TESE) within the same culture medium regarding rates of spermatid maturation and arrest in relation to the number of early round spermatids (Table 31.5, Figure 31.7) revealed that in CM, controls achieved significantly higher maturation rates of Sa2 ($p = 0.009$) and Sd1 ($p = 0.031$), with no significant differences for Sb2 ($p = 0.136$) and Sd2 ($p = 0.158$). On the other hand, no significant differences were found in medium supplemented with FSH, for the transition from Sa1 to Sa2 (early spermiogenesis; $p = 0.080$), Sa2 to Sb2 (mid-spermiogenesis; $p = 0.082$), Sb2 to Sd1 (late spermiogenesis; $p = 0.0807$) or Sd1 to Sd2 (term spermiogenesis; $p > 1$). In medium supplemented with FSH + T, controls presented significantly higher maturation rates of Sb2 ($p = 0.029$), with no differences found for Sa2 ($p = 0.145$), Sd1 ($p = 0.833$) and Sd2 ($p = 0.825$). In contrast, comparisons with cells present in the previous spermiogenic stage (Table 31.5, Figure 31.8) showed that the rates of Sd1 in CM and of Sb2 in FSH + T were in fact not decreased in cases, and that the rates of Sd1 were increased in FSH + T. In comparison with previous studies using Vero cell-enriched conditioned medium (HP: 27% Sb2, 10% Sd1, 4% Sd2; OAZ: 31% Sb2, 13% Sd1, 9% Sd2)[40], the present *in vitro* maturation rates were lower, being rescued only to similar or higher levels when the medium was supplemented with FSH + T[41].

Comparisons between different media within the same patient group

Comparisons between the different culture media (CM, FSH, FSH + T) in relation to the number of Sa1 present at the beginning of the cultures (Table 31.5, Figure 31.7), showed, in controls, significantly ($p < 0.000$) higher maturation rates of Sa2 and Sb2 with FSH and especially with FSH + T, and of Sd1 and Sd2 with FSH + T. These results indicate that in samples with conserved spermiogenesis (control group), early spermiogen-

Table 31.6 Patients with successful spermatid maturation in cocultures (n). See Table 31.1 for spermatid maturation stages

| | Controls | | | | | | | | | Cases | | |
| | SO/MA | | | HP | | | Total | | | SO/MA | | |
	CM	FSH	FSH + T	CM	FSH	FSH + T	CM	FSH	FSH + T	CM	FSH	FSH + T
Cases	1	2	8	10	11	8	11	13	16	8	4	9
Sa2	1	2	4	9	11	8	10	13	12	7	2	6
Sb2	1	2	4	9	9	7	10	11	11	6	2	6
Sd1	1	0	3	7	2	6	8	2	9	2	1	4
Sd2	0	0	2	2	0	3	2	0	5	0	0	4

SO, Sertoli cell-only syndrome; MA, maturation arrest; HP, hypospermatogenesis; CM, conditioned medium; FSH, follicle stimulating hormone; T, testosterone

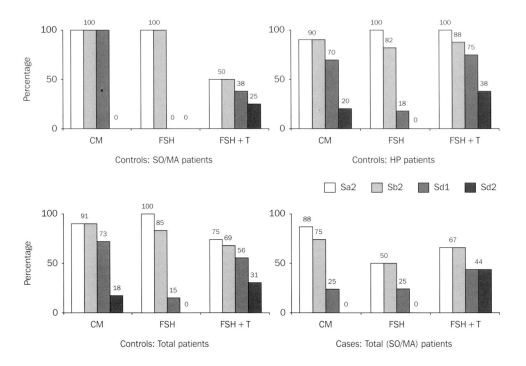

Figure 31.6 Cocultures. Percentage distribution of patients whose testicular tissue samples enabled successful *in vitro* maturation of early round spermatids. SO, Sertoli cell-only syndrome; MA, maturation arrest; HP, hypospermatogenesis; CM, conditioned medium; FSH, follicle stimulating hormone; T, testosterone. See Table 31.1 for spermatid maturation stages

esis (Sa1–Sa2: flagellum extrusion) and midspermiogenesis (Sa2–Sb2) are stimulated by FSH and potentiated by testosterone, whereas late spermiogenesis (Sb2–Sd1) and term spermiogenesis (Sd1–Sd2) tend to be inhibited by FSH and highly stimulated by testosterone, thus suggesting that FSH and testosterone show a synergic action in the early steps and an antagonistic action at the late stages of spermiogenesis. In relation to the *in vitro* maturation potential of early round spermatids in cases, no significant differences were found for the transition Sa1–Sa2 ($p = 0.069$), Sa2–Sb2 ($p = 0.199$), Sb2–Sd1 ($p = 0.912$) or Sd1–Sd2/Sz ($p > 1$) in the presence of FSH. On the other hand, all spermatid maturation steps were significantly stimulated ($p < 0.000$) by FSH + T. These results show that in testicular samples with absent spermiogenesis, early

spermiogenesis (Sa1–Sa2: flagellum extrusion) and midspermiogenesis (Sa2–Sb2) tend to be stimulated by FSH and highly potentiated by testosterone, whereas late spermiogenesis (Sb2–Sd1) and term spermiogenesis (Sd1–Sd2) are highly stimulated by testosterone. This testosterone effect was so strong that the yield of spermiogenesis in FSH + T attained the same level for all spermiogenic stages as that observed in controls[41], as well as in cases with OAZ[40]. If results demonstrate that FSH and testosterone show a synergic action in the early steps of spermiogenesis and an antagonistic action at the late stages of spermiogenesis, in either controls or cases, they also suggest that Sa1 from cases appear to be more resistant to FSH and that *in vitro* spermiogenesis might benefit from higher, pharmacological FSH concentrations.

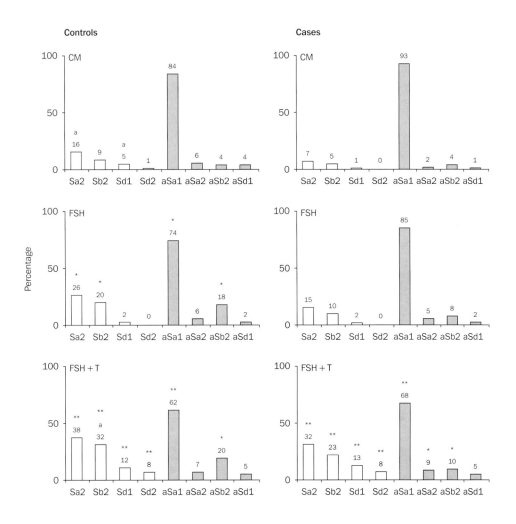

Figure 31.7   Cocultures. Percentage distribution of spermatid maturation and arrest relative to the initial number of early round spermatids. Significant differences between controls/cases (a) within the same culture medium. Significant differences versus CM or CM/FSH within the same patient group. CM, conditioned medium; FSH, follicle stimulating hormone; T, testosterone. See Table 31.1 for spermatid maturation stages

A different picture was found when data were analyzed regarding rates of spermatid *in vitro* maturation in relation to the number of cells present in the previous stage (Table 31.5, Figure 31.8). In controls, Sa2 were stimulated by FSH and potentiated by testosterone, Sb2 only tended to be stimulated by FSH and were highly stimulated by testosterone, Sd1 were inhibited by FSH and partially rescued by testosterone, and differentiation of Sd2 tended to be inhibited by FSH but was highly stimulated by testosterone. In contrast, in cases, the transition from Sa1 to Sa2 tended to be stimulated by FSH but was potentiated by testosterone, conversion from Sa2 to Sb2 was not affected by hormones, maturation from Sb2 to Sd1 tended to be inhibited by FSH and was stimulated by testosterone, and differentiation of Sd1 into Sd2 tended to be inhibited by FSH and was

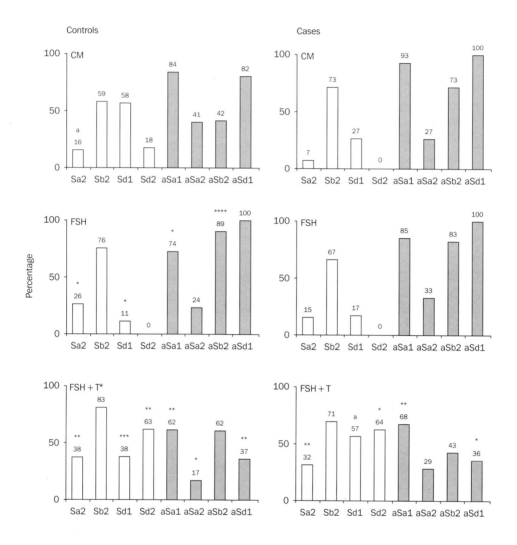

Figure 31.8 Cocultures. Percentage distribution of spermatid maturation and arrest relative to the number of spermatids present in the previous spermiogenic stage. Significant differences between controls/cases (a) within the same culture medium. Significant differences versus CM (*), CM/FSH (**), FSH (***) or CM/FSH + T (****) within the same patient group. CM, conditioned medium; FSH, follicle stimulating hormone; T, testosterone. See Table 31.1 for spermatid maturation stages

highly stimulated by testosterone. Data thus suggest that FSH stimulates early spermiogenesis in controls and cases (with Sa1 from cases being more resistant to FSH action), stimulates midspermiogenesis in controls but not in cases, and inhibits late and term spermiogenesis in both controls and cases. Correspondingly, testosterone potentiates FSH action on early spermiogenesis in controls and cases, potentiates FSH in midspermiogenesis only in controls, and stimulates late and especially term spermiogenesis in controls and cases[41].

Analysis of spermatid arrest rates confirmed the previous observations (Table 31.5, Figure 31.7)[41]. In controls, the large majority of Sa1 became arrested (aSa1), with aSa1 rates being significantly decreased with FSH ($p = 0.007$ compared with CM) and FSH + T ($p = 0.000$ compared with CM; $p = 0.002$ compared with FSH). Maturation arrest at Sa2 (aSa2) was not affected by hormones ($p = 0.937$, FSH/CM; $p = 0.916$, FSH + T/CM; $p = 0.841$, FSH + T/FSH). However, comparisons with the number of cells present in the previous spermiogenic stage demonstrated that in fact aSa2 rates tended to be decreased by FSH and were significantly decreased by testosterone (Figure 31.8). Arrest at Sb2 (aSb2) was significantly increased under both hormone supplementations ($p = 0.000$, FSH/CM and FSH + T/CM; $p = 0.544$, FSH + T/FSH), but this effect was caused by FSH, as shown by comparisons with the number of cells present in the previous spermiogenic stage (Figure 31.8). Finally, although no significant differences were found between media in relation to the rates of arrest at Sd1 (aSd1: $p = 0.167$, FSH/CM; $p = 0.953$, FSH + T/CM; $p = 0.126$, FSH + T/FSH), comparisons with the number of cells present in the previous spermatid stage demonstrated that aSd1 rates were significantly decreased by testosterone (Figure 31.8). In cases, the large majority of the Sa1 also became arrested, with rates of aSa1 tending to be decreased by FSH and being significantly decreased by testosterone ($p = 0.069$, FSH/CM; $p = 0.000$, FSH + T/CM; $p = 0.012$, FSH + T/FSH). Although maturation arrest at Sa2 showed a tendency to be increased by FSH and appeared to be significantly increased by testosterone ($p = 0.197$, FSH/CM; $p = 0.002$, FSH + T/CM; $p = 0.307$, FSH + T/FSH), this was only due to the presence of a higher number of cells in the previous spermatid stage (Figure 31.8). The same was observed regarding arrest at Sb2 ($p = 0.164$, FSH/CM; $p = 0.022$, FSH + T/CM; $p = 0.762$, FSH + T/FSH), although in reality testosterone decreased the rates of aSb2 (Figure 31.8). Finally, although FSH and testosterone tended to increase the rates of Sd1 arrest (aSd1: $p = 0.912$, FSH/CM; $p = 0.069$, FSH + T/CM; $p = 0.309$, FSH + T/FSH), aSd1 rates were significantly decreased by testosterone (Figure 31.8).

In conclusion, experimental data on spermiogenesis *in vitro* using isolated early round spermatids showed that: (1) early spermiogenesis, characterized by the maturation of early round spermatids to late round spermatids (Sa1 to Sa2, flagellum extrusion), and midspermiogenesis, characterized by the maturation of late round spermatids to early elongating spermatids (Sa2 to Sb2), are stimulated by FSH and potentiated by testosterone, in controls (conserved spermiogenesis) and cases (absent spermiogenesis), although Sa1 and Sa2 from cases exhibit FSH resistance; (2) late spermiogenesis, characterized by the transition of elongating spermatids to early elongated spermatids (Sb2 to Sd1), and especially term spermiogenesis, characterized by the maturation of early elongated spermatids to late elongated spermatids and spermatozoa (Sd1 to Sd2/Sz), are highly stimulated by testosterone and inhibited by FSH.

In comparison with results obtained with Vero cell-enriched conditioned medium[40], spermatid arrest at all stages was decreased with FSH + T, eliciting figures similar to OAZ cases. These results thus suggest that the most critical steps in spermiogenesis are extrusion of the flagellum, at the transition from Sa1 to Sa2, and the final maturation step of spermiogenesis, where nuclear elongation and condensation are observed during Sd1 and Sd2/Sz formation. This was further confirmed (Table 31.5) by the fact that in controls, of all aSa1, 62% in CM, 46% in FSH and 23% in FSH + T remained as aSa1 (cases: 78% in CM, 66% in FSH and 29% in FSH + T), whereas 22% in CM, 28% in FSH and 39% in FSH + T (cases: 15% in CM, 19% in FSH and 39% in FSH + T) developed cytoplasm elongation and nuclear condensation and elongation (Sb1). This suggests that both hormones act to promote cytoplasm elongation and nuclear elongation and condensation even in the absence of flagellum extrusion. Notwithstanding, even in the presence of FSH + T, the rate of *in vitro* maturation from early round spermatids to late elongated spermatids/spermatozoa remained low (8%). This can probably be

Table 31.7   Spermatid microinjection outcome after maturation in cocultures (n (%))

	Sa1	Sa2	Sa1 + Sa2	Sb2 + Sd1	Sb1	abnSd2
Cases	6	2	8	8	9	5
MII injected	23	3	26	50	27	14
Degenerated	2 (9)	0	2 (8)	2 (4)	3 (11)	3 (31)
Intact	21	3	24	48	24	11
non-fertilized (0PN1PB)	15 (71)	0	15 (63)	32 (67)	22 (92)	8 (73)
activated (0PN2PB)	0	0	0	1 (2)	0	0
abnormal fertilization (1PN2PB)	6 (29)	3 (100)	9 (38)	12 (25)	0	2 (18)
normal fertilization (2PN2PB)	0	0	0	3 (6)	2 (8)	1 (9)
Embryo cleavage	6 (100)	3 (100)	9 (100)	14 (93)	2 (100)	3 (100)
Grade A/B embryos	4 (67)	3 (100)	7 (78)	13 (93)	2 (100)	1 (33)
Morulae	1 (17)	1 (33)	2 (22)	6 (46)	0	0

Sa1, early round spermatids; Sa2, late round spermatids (with flagellum); Sb2, early elongating spermatids; Sd1, early elongated spermatids; Sb1, abnormally matured early elongating spermatids (without flagellum); abnSd2, late elongated spermatids with abnormal head morphology; MII, meiosis II (mature) oocytes; PN, pronuclei; PB, polar bodies

attributed to insufficiencies of the culture medium that did not allow efficient early spermiogenesis (Sa1–Sa2: 62–68% aSa1), although late spermiogenesis (Sb2–Sd1: 43–62% aSb2) and term spermiogenesis (Sd1–Sd2/Sz: 36–37% aSd1) were also affected.

Microinjection outcome

Whenever excess donated oocytes were available, *in vitro* differentiated spermatids were used for experimental microinjections to evaluate their developmental potential (Table 31.7)[41]. After microinjection of morphologically normal spermatids, most of the oocytes did not fertilize (63% Sa1/Sa2; 67% Sb2/Sd1) or formed unipronuclear zygotes (38% Sa1/Sa2; 25% Sb2/Sd1), whereas the rates of normal fertilization (2PN2PB: two pronuclei and two polar bodies) were very low (0% Sa1/Sa2; 6% Sb2/Sd1). On the other hand, the rates of embryo cleavage (93–100%), high-quality embryos (78–93%) and morula formation (22–46%) were quite regular. FISH analysis was performed in 12/23 (52%) of the embryos, 7/9 (78%) from Sa1/Sa2 and 5/14 (36%) from

Sb2/Sd1 microinjection. In the case of Sa1/Sa2, all seven embryos were from 1PN2PB zygotes. The cytogenetic data showed that 6/7 (86%) of the embryos were mosaic aneuploid (most of the blastomeres were aneuploid), whereas 1/7 (14%) were mosaic euploid (64% of the blastomeres euploid and 36% of the blastomeres aneuploid). Of the two morulae analyzed, 1/2 (50%) was the mosaic euploid case. In the case of Sb2/Sd1, five embryos were analyzed. One embryo was derived from a 2PN2PB zygote, but it was haploid at FISH. Four embryos were derived from 1PN2PB zygotes, of which two were mosaic aneuploid or chaotic, whereas the other two were morulae with euploid mosaicism (79% euploid and 21% aneuploid; 69% euploid and 31% aneuploid). Thus, with Sb2/Sd1, 2/5 (40%) of the embryos were euploid (morulae). These results thus suggest that: (1) unipronuclear zygotes derived from *in vitro*-matured spermatids are almost always diploid, (2) *in vitro*-matured round spermatids give a low fertilization and embryo developmental potential, with only 14% of embryos being euploid, and (3) *in vitro* matured elongating and elongated spermatids elicit low fertilization rates but show normal rates (40%) of euploid embryo development.

Abnormally matured spermatids were also microinjected to study their developmental potential (Table 31.7)[41]. Elongating spermatids without a flagellum (Sb1) gave high rates of non-fertilization (92%), but could induce 8% of 2PN2PB zygotes. These cleaved normally, although they did not reach the morula stage, and FISH analysis revealed that one was haploid and the other mosaic aneuploid. Although we cannot be sure about the normality of the nucleus, it is tentative to speculate that the absence of a normal flagellum somehow hampers normal fertilization and embryo development due to the presence of a disrupted male centrosome. The developmental potential of spermatids that had reached the late elongated stage but displayed abnormal head morphology was also studied. These experiments were very important, because the last step of spermiogenesis *in vitro* was the one with the worst results and in which most of the cells developed structural defects. The rate of non-fertilization (73%) was very high, with corresponding low rates of 1PN2PB zygotes (18%) and 2PN2PB zygotes (9%), although similar to those obtained with morphologically normal Sb2/Sd1. In comparison with normal elongating/elongated spermatids, the rate of embryo cleavage was also similar (100%), the rate of high-quality grade embryos was lower (33%) and no morulae were obtained. FISH analysis of the single embryo obtained from a 2PN2PB zygote revealed a chaotic chromosome constitution. These results are quite disappointing, and clearly demonstrate that the *in vitro* culture medium still does not offer the best conditions to allow proper early round spermatid maturation up to the terminal stage of spermiogenesis.

Methodological problems

Experiments with isolated round spermatids revealed that the optimized culture conditions have not yet been met[39–41]. In fact, most cases were unable to progress through complete spermiogenesis *in vitro*, which suggests that the process is still not entirely reproducible and seems to vary individually from patient to patient. The absence of late elongated spermatid differentiation from early round spermatids isolated from cases with conserved spermatogenesis also points to important deficiencies of the *in vitro* culture medium, whose consequences still remain to be ascertained. Possible causes could be the need for specific factors secreted by connective-tissue cells that surround the seminiferous epithelium, loss of the basal lamina, the rupture of cell connections during cell dissociation, loss of compartmentalization into apical and basal systems as determined by Sertoli cells *in vivo* and absence of renewal of the culture medium.

Growth factors and hormones

The antiapoptotic action of FSH and the FSH-inhibiting action on spermiogenesis, as well as the antiapoptotic action of testosterone and the testosterone-stimulating action on spermiogenesis, were already known from animal studies[28,32,33,38,59,60]. Under organ culture and in the absence of serum and testosterone, the rates of apoptosis in human seminiferous tubules also appeared to be increased[61,62], with the addition of FSH being able to stimulate spermatogonia proliferation and increase the number of spermatocytes, the rate of meiosis and the number of round spermatids[59]. Similarly, in experiments conducted with testicular tissue cell suspensions, which included Sertoli cells and all types of germ cells, testosterone was shown to inhibit Sertoli cell apoptosis, potentiate the stimulatory action of FSH on premeiotic germ cells and stimulate spermiogenesis, whereas FSH inhibited spermatid differentiation[63–70]. These antagonistic actions of FSH and testosterone in spermiogenesis were further studied in later experiments. FSH was shown to stimulate early (early round spermatids into late round spermatids) and mid- (late round spermatids into early elongating spermatids) spermiogenesis, and inhibit late (elongating spermatids into early elongated spermatids) and especially term (early elongated spermatids into late elongated spermatids/spermatozoa) spermiogenesis. On the other hand, testosterone was demonstrated to potentiate the effects of FSH in early and midspermiogenesis, and stimulate the final spermiogenic maturation steps[41].

Regarding future improvement of the *in vitro* maturation medium, experiments have demonstrated that several human-specific growth factors might be added to cultures to decrease the rate of apoptosis and increase the genetic potential of *in vitro* matured spermatids. The experimental results have also suggested that the culture medium might be improved by using sequential media. Thus, high pharmacological FSH (500 U/l) and low testosterone (1 µmol/l) concentrations should be used in the first 2–4 days of culture to favor early round spermatid maturation into late round spermatids, and then replaced by low/absent FSH and high testosterone (10 µmol/l) concentrations to elicit *in vitro* maturation to elongating and elongated spermatids. This is especially true for clinical cases with absent spermiogenesis in the original testicular biopsy, whose early round spermatids appear to be highly insensitive to FSH. In this sense, it would also be worthwhile studying FSH receptor gene mutations, mRNA transcription and protein translation in these testicular samples, including isolated Sertoli cells and early germ cells, as cell insensitivity might also be due to absent or abnormal FSH receptors[41,71].

Sertoli cell–germ cell contacts

Cell contacts are essential for inhibiting apoptosis, inducing proliferation of spermatogonia, germ-cell gene expression and the sharing of gene products such as mRNAs encoded by the sex chromosomes[5,7,8,11,72]. Cell junctions and intercellular bridges depend on the presence of FSH and testosterone, on several growth factors and on high densities of cells. Furthermore, FSH, as potentiated by testosterone, renders Sertoli cells competent to bind round spermatids[11,38].

Although Sertoli cell and diploid germ cell connections are partially reacquired during *in vitro* cocultures, these appear to be absent between Sertoli cells and round spermatids despite the presence of FSH and testosterone[71]. This might explain why, in the above experiments, most round spermatids and differentiated elongating and elongated spermatids remained arrested or showed an absence of tails, short tails or abnormal head configurations[39–41].

Paracrine factors, cell densities and medium renewal

Although investigations conducted with dissociated and isolated cells assure that no elongating or elongated spermatids are hidden in the testicular tissue samples[39–41], this type of culture system has an absence of critical limiting factors, such as specific paracrine factors (minimized by the presence of Sertoli cells in cocultures, which under FSH and testosterone stimulation secrete growth factors critical for germ cell survival and differentiation), renewal of the culture medium (the study of individual cell fates needs microdrops) and high cell densities (due to inherent difficulties in the long-duration micromanipulation method used for cell isolation). To overcome this problem, new methods should first be developed to purify Sertoli cells, diploid germ cells and early round spermatids to give high purity and concentration[71].

Chromosome aberrations

In patients with obstructive azoospermia, conserved spermatogenesis and normal karyotypes, the rates of late spermatid/spermatozoa aneuploidy were found to be normal, whereas in cases with disrupted spermiogenesis these rates appeared to be increased[73–76]. Cases with abnormal karyotypes frequently show meiotic arrest due to errors of homolog pairing and segregation, although spermatids escaping from meiotic block might display a normal chromosomal constitution through a positive mechanism of selection[77,78]. Abnormal synapsis and chromosomal segregation could also be key determinants of impaired spermiogenesis *in vitro*[5,11,62]. However, experimental data have suggested that early round spermatids from patients with secretory azoospermia do not harbor an increased rate of chromosome aberrations[41] and that spermatid development *in vitro* seems not to be related to aneuploidy[71], which was confirmed by microinjection experiments with *in vitro* differentiated spermatids showing that about 40% of morulae were euploid[41].

Apoptosis and methylation errors

Apoptosis has been implicated as a key regulator of normal spermatogenesis, adapting the number of germ cells to the number of Sertoli cells available[79]. In this mechanism, Sertoli cells secrete Fas ligand (FasL) that binds to the Fas receptor (FasR) on germ cells, triggering the activation of initiator procaspase-2, -8 and -10[80,81]. Germ cells may also enter apoptosis via endogenous stimuli that act through mitochondria injury and activation of initiator procaspase-9. Both extrinsic and intrinsic apoptotic pathways then end on a common activation of effector procaspase-3, -6 and -7, which trigger DNA fragmentation and cell death[82,83]. The action of caspases appears to be modulated by several Bcl-2 gene products, both proapoptotic (Bax) and antiapoptotic (Bcl-2), which display preferential germ cell-stage targets. Bax seems to be restricted to spermatogonia and preleptotene spermatocytes, and is responsible for the normal degeneration of premeiotic germ cells associated with adult ages. In contrast, Bcl-2 and Bcl-xL antagonize the action of Bax. The same occurs with Bcl-w, which predominates in spermatogonia[11,62].

In animals, *in vivo*, classical signs of apoptosis were described in premeiotic germ cells but not in Sertoli cells, whereas both cell types exhibited evident degeneration during *in vitro* cultures[6,84]. In humans, in cases of pathology or during *in vitro* cultures, the absence of specific growth factors, hormones and nutrients also activates the FasL–FasR system, up-regulates Bax and decreases Bcl-2 levels, thus triggering the apoptosis of germ cells[78,85–87]. Sertoli cell phagocytosis is then responsible for the clearance of apoptotic germ cells, as shown *in vivo* after the injection of apoptotic cells into the seminiferous tubules of rodents[88] and *in vitro* during cocultures[71,78].

In azoospermic patients showing increased levels of apoptosis, DNA fragmentation was found in the nuclei of spermatids and sperm, whereas annexin-V labeling was negative in round spermatids but positive in sperm[65,67,70,87]. Although caspases were indicated as inoperant in elongated spermatids and sperm[11,62], other results demonstrated that caspase-3 activity is present in the sperm midpiece of ejaculated sperm, being quantitatively correlated with decreased sperm motility and teratozoospermia[89]. Experimental studies using isolated germ cells also suggested that cocultures *in vitro* appear to be mainly limited by germ cell apoptosis[39–41,71]. In fact, premeiotic germ cells not only exhibited the classical morphological signs of apoptosis but also showed caspase-3 activation in nuclei. Similarly, *in vitro*-formed spermatids arrested in development, or abnormally matured, displayed caspase-3-like activity in the cytoplasm, nucleus, acrosome and/or midpiece. In these studies, FasR, caspase-8, -9 and -3, Bcl-2 and Bax were shown to be expressed in all germ-cell stages[71].

Studies have also demonstrated that *in vitro*-cultured mouse testicular spermatids show abnormal DNA methylation and abnormal chromatin remodeling[11,62]. Because genomic imprinting errors in the male germ line of patients with severe oligozoospermia were described, spermatids from azoospermic patients might also carry a substantial risk for transmitting severe methylation defects[90]. Spermatids from testicular samples showing Y chromosome deletions[91–93], CFTR (cystic fibrosis transmembrane conductance regulator gene) mutations[94,95] and chromosomal aberrations[77,78] have also been observed to display low *in vitro* spermiogenic potential[40,78].

However, because developmentally arrested cells are unable to mature normally and abnormal spermatid maturation can be easily diagnosed, it is possible that *in vitro*-differentiated spermatids with normal morphology are viable and show a normal genetic constitution[39–41]. This also applies to genomic imprinting, which has been shown to be fully established by the time mouse round spermatids are formed[96]. That the maturation of germ cells into late elongated spermatids and sperm with normal morphology may reflect a correct genetic constitution of the gametes is also supported by clinical studies in which normal viable pregnancies, without fetal abnormalities, were obtained after selection of male haploid gametes with strict normal morphology from testicular biopsies[44,47,48,97,98].

CLINICAL TRIALS

Experimental efforts to develop adequate *in vitro* culture systems capable of sustaining *in vitro* spermiogenesis culminated on 21 May 2000, with the first term delivery of two normal healthy male twins (2.8 kg, 3 kg), after Cesarean section at 37 weeks of gestation. In this particular case, the male patient had secretory azoospermia, a normal karyotype and a diagnostic testicular biopsy showing maturation arrest. At TESE, a focus of conserved spermiogenesis was retrieved, but only morphologically abnormal late elongated spermatids could be found after extensive search. Microinjection was performed using these gametes, but of the five MII oocytes available, only one grade-B embryo was obtained and transferred, without an ensuing pregnancy. A second attempt at TESE was then scheduled 6 months later, 5 days before oocyte pick-up. Early elongating spermatids, with normal morphology, were isolated and transferred to microdrops of Vero cell-enriched conditioned medium. After 4–5 days of culture, three had differentiated into late elongated spermatids with normal morphology. Of the nine MII oocytes available, three were microinjected with *in vitro*-matured gametes, and six were microinjected with abnormal elongated spermatids retrieved from the original testicular sample. Only the first three

oocytes fertilized and cleaved normally, having been transferred (4B, 6B, 4C). The following pregnancy was normal, without complications, and at the present age of 5 years old, both children are healthy, without physical or psychological constraints (personal communication).

A similar case was published in November 2000, in which only abnormal late elongated spermatids were found at TESE, and whose microinjection elicited poor fertilization and embryo development rates, and no pregnancy. In a second TESE attempt, the authors cultured whole testicular cell suspensions for 1–2 days and then injected late elongated spermatids with normal morphology. A pregnancy ensued that gave rise to the birth of healthy twins[66]. Similar attempts were performed by the same authors, with seven more children having been born[68,99], from cases with either only diploid germ cells or the presence of complete spermiogenesis and abnormal elongated spermatids. In these cases, no conclusive individual cell fate can be defined, as normal spermatids could be hidden in the tissue. In addition, the very short culture period (1–2 days) contrasts highly with the normal testicular cycle that needs more than 1 month to proceed through meiosis and spermiogenesis, and 16 days to evolve from the late-pachytene or secondary spermatocyte stage to elongated spermatids[55,56,100]. Finally, early elongated spermatids might be safely used for clinical treatments without *in vitro* culture, as the fertilization, embryo cleavage and pregnancy rates using these haploid germ cells are normal[44,47,53].

In conclusion, if patients have no spermatozoa/elongated spermatids in the treatment testicular biopsy, most probably there will also be no elongating spermatids. One should then carefully search for round spermatids. If these are found, most probably there will be no severe meiotic arrest and thus round haploid germ cells might be safely used for treatments, either without or with concomitant artificial oocyte activation[48]. However, preimplantation genetic diagnosis, prenatal diagnosis and children follow-up should be strictly applied to all still experimental treatment cycles[101–103]. Alternatively, and due to the very high rate of fertilization and embryo development failures, round spermatids might be cultured in medium supplemented with synthetic serum substitute, hormones and growth factors, and if evolved into mature spermatids with normal morphology then they might be used for clinical treatment[48,71].

ACKNOWLEDGMENTS

We would like to acknowledge the following members of the Center for Reproductive Genetics A Barros, Porto: C Oliveira, J Teixeira da Silva, J Beires (Gynecology), L Ferrás (Urology), P Viana, S Sousa and A Gonçalves (Embryology), and members of the Department of Genetics, Faculty of Medicine, University of Porto: R Neves (apoptosis gene expression), C Ferrás, J Marques, S Fernandes (Y chromosome), A. Grangeia, F Carvalho (CFTR), S Dória, MJ Pinho, C Almeida and MS Fernandes (karyotypes and FISH). This research was partially financially supported by Governmental and European funds through FCT (POCTI/SAU-MMO/60709/04, 60555/04, 59997/04, UMIB).

REFERENCES

1. Miura T, et al. Spermatogenesis-preventing substance in Japanese eel. Development 2002; 129: 2689
2. Russell LD, Alger LE, Nequin LG. Hormonal control of pubertal spermatogenesis. Endocrinology 1987; 120: 1615
3. Hilscher W. Review. The genetic control and germ cell kinetics of the female and male germ line in mammals including man. Hum Reprod 1991; 6: 1416
4. Spiteri-Grech J, Nieschlag E. Paracrine factors relevant to the regulation of spermatogenesis – a review. J Reprod Fertil 1993; 98: 1
5. Kierszenbaum AL. Mammalian spermatogenesis in vivo and in vitro: a partnership of spermatogenic and somatic cell lineages. Endocr Rev 1994; 15: 116
6. Dirami G, et al. Evidence that basement membrane prevents apoptosis of Sertoli cells in vitro in the absence of known regulators of Sertoli cell function. Endocrinology 1995; 136: 4439
7. Gnessi L, Fabbri A, Spera G. Gonadal peptides as mediators of development and functional control of the testis: an integrated system with hormones and local environment. Endocr Rev 1997; 18: 541
8. Schlatt S, Meinhardt A, Nieschlag E. Paracrine regulation of cellular interactions in the testis: factors in search of a function. Eur J Endocrinol 1997; 137: 107
9. Bellvé AR. The male germ cell; origin, migration, proliferation and differentiation. Cell Dev Biol 1999; 9: 379
10. De Rooij DG. Stem cell review. Stem cells in the testis. Int J Exp Pathol 1998; 79: 67
11. De Rooij DG. Proliferation and differentiation of spermatogonial stem cells. Reproduction 2001; 121: 247
12. Setchell BP. The Parkes Lecture. Heat and the testis. J Reprod Fertil 1998; 114: 179
13. Zirkin BR. Spermatogenesis: its regulation by testosterone and FSH. Cell Dev Biol 1998; 9: 417
14. Lunenfeld E, Zeyse D, Huleihel M. Cytokines in the testis, human sperm cells, and semen. Assist Reprod 1999; 9: 157
15. Weinbauer GF, Wessels J. Review. Paracrine control of spermatogenesis. Andrologia 1999; 31: 249
16. Gazvani MR, et al. Role of mitotic control in spermatogenesis. Fertil Steril 2000; 74: 251
17. Sutton KA. Molecular mechanims involved in the differentiation of spermatogenic stem cells. Rev Reprod 2000; 5: 93
18. O'Donnell L, et al. Estrogen and spermatogenesis. Endocr Rev 2001; 22: 289
19. Kleene KC. Review. A possible meiotic function of the peculiar patterns of gene expression in mammalian spermatogenic cells. Mech Dev 2001; 106: 3
20. Kleene KC. Review. Sexual selection, genetic conflict, selfish genes, and the atypical patterns of gene expression in spermatogenic cells. Dev Biol 2005; 277: 16
21. Sofikitis N, et al. Efforts to create an artificial testis: culture systems of male germ cells under biochemical conditions resembling the seminiferous tubular biochemical environment. Hum Reprod Update 2005; 11: 229
22. Steinberger A, Steinberger E, Perloff W. Mammalian testes in organ culture. Exp Cell Res 1964; 36: 19

23. Parvinen M, et al. Spermatogenesis in vitro: completion of meiosis and early spermiogenesis. Endocrinology 1983; 112: 1150

24. Toppari J, Parvinen M. In vitro differentiation of rat seminiferous tubular segments from defined stages of the epithelial cycle morphologic and immunolocalization analysis. J Androl 1985; 6: 334

25. Rassoulzadegan M, et al. Transmeiotic differentiation of male germ cells in culture. Cell 1993; 75: 997

26. Staub C, et al. The whole meiotic process can occur in vitro in untransformed rat spermatogenic cells. Exp Cell Res 2000; 260: 85

27. Marh J, et al. Mouse round spermatids developed in vitro from preexisting spermatocytes can produce normal offspring by nuclear injection into in vivo developed mature oocytes. Biol Reprod 2003; 69: 169

28. Hikim APS, Swerdloff RS. Temporal and stage-specific effects of recombinant human follicle-stimulating hormone on the maintenance of spermatogenesis in gonadotropin-releasing hormone antagonist-treated rat. Endocrinology 1995; 136: 253

29. Sairam MR, Krishnamurthy H. The role of follicle-stimulating hormone in spermatogenesis: lessons from knockout animal models. Arch Med Res 2001; 32: 601

30. McLachlan RI, et al. The effects of recombinant follicle-stimulating hormone on the restoration of spermatogenesis in the gonadotropin-releasing hormone-immunized adult rat. Endrocrinology 1995; 136: 4035

31. Zhang F-P, et al. The low gonadotropin-independent constitutive production of testicular testosterone is sufficient to maintain spermatogenesis. Proc Natl Acad Sci USA 2003; 100: 13692

32. Mclachlan RI, et al. Effects of testosterone on spermatogenic cell populations in the adult rat. Biol Reprod 1994; 51: 945

33. Huang HFS, et al. Restoration of spermatogenesis by high levels of testosterone in hypophysectomized rats after long-term regression. Acta Endocrinol 1987; 116: 433

34. Sun Y-T, et al. The effects of exogenously administered testosterone on spermatogenesis in intact and hypophysectomized rats. Endocrinology 1989; 125: 1000

35. Sun Y-T, et al. Quantitative cytological studies of spermatogenesis in intact and hypophysectomized rats: identification of androgen-dependent stages. Endocrinology 1990; 127: 1215

36. Awoniyi CA, et al. Exogenously administered testosterone maintains spermatogenesis quantitatively in adult rats actively immunized against gonadotropin-releasing hormone. Endocrinology 1992; 130: 3283

37. O'Donnell L, et al. Testosterone promotes the conversion of round spermatids between stages VII and VIII of the rat spermatogenic cycle. Endocrinology 1994; 135: 2608

38. O'Donnell L, et al. Testosterone withdrawal promotes stage specific detachment of round spermatids from the rat seminiferous epithelium. Biol Reprod 1996; 55: 895

39. Cremades N, et al. In-vitro maturation of round spermatids using coculture on Vero cells. Hum Reprod 1999; 14: 1287

40. Cremades N, et al. Developmental potential of elongating and elongated spermatids obtained after in-vitro maturation of isolated round spermatids. Hum Reprod 2001; 16: 1938

41. Sousa M, et al. Developmental potential of human spermatogenic cells cocultured with Sertoli cells. Hum Reprod 2002; 17: 161

42. Sousa M, Barros A, Tesarik K. Human oocyte activation after intracytoplasmic injection of leucocytes, spermatocytes and round spermatids: comparison of calcium responses. Mol Hum Reprod 1996; 2: 853

43. Sousa M, Barros A, Tesarik J. Current problems with spermatid conception. Hum Reprod 1998; 13: 255

44. Sousa M, et al. Clinical efficacy of spermatid conception. Analysis using a new spermatid classification scheme. Hum Reprod 1999; 14: 1279

45. Sousa M, Barros A, El Shafie M. Failed fertilization in vitro: principles and evaluation of transmission electron microscopic images. In El Shafie M, et al., eds. Ultrastructure of Human Oocytes. New York: Parthenon Publishing, 2000: 65

46. Sousa M, Fernandes S, Barros A. Prognostic factors for successful testicle spermatid retrieval. Mol Cell Endocrinol 2000; 166: 37

47. Sousa M, et al. Predictive value of testicular histology in secretory azoospermic subgroups and clinical outcome after microinjection of fresh and frozen–thawed sperm and spermatids. Hum Reprod 2002; 17: 1800

48. Sousa M, et al. Spermatid injection and beyond. In Gurgan T, Demirol A, eds. 13th World Congress on In Vitro Fertilization: Assisted Reproduction & Genetics. Bologna: Medimond, 2005: 83

49. Nakamura M, Romrell LJ, Hall PF. The effects of temperature and glucose on protein biosynthesis by immature (round) spermatids from rat testes. J Cell Biol 1978; 79: 1

50. Aslam I, Fishel S. Short-term in-vitro culture and cryopreservation of spermatogenetic cells used for human in-vitro conception. Hum Reprod 1998; 13: 634

51. Aslam I, Fishel S. Evaluation of the fertilization potential of freshly isolated, in vitro cultured and cryopreserved human spermatids by injection into hamster oocytes. Hum Reprod 1999; 14: 1528

52. Balaban B, et al. Progression to the blastocyst stage of embryos derived from testicular round spermatids. Hum Reprod 2000; 15: 1377

53. Bernabeu R, et al. Successful pregnancy after spermatid injection. Hum Reprod 1998; 13: 1898

54. Desai N, Goldfarb J. Cocultured human embryos may be subjected to widely different microenvironments: pattern of growth factor/cytokine release by Vero cells during the coculture interval. Hum Reprod 1998; 13: 1600

55. Heller CG, Clermont Y. Spermatogenesis in man: an estimate of its duration. Science 1963; 140: 184

56. Heller CG, Clermont Y. Kinetics of the germinal epithelium in man. Recent Prog Horm Res 1964; 20: 545

57. Ménézo YJR, Guerin J-F, Czyba J-C. Improvement of human early embryo development in vitro by coculture on monolayers of Vero cells. Biol Reprod 1990; 42: 301

58. Ménézo YJR, et al. Coculture of embryos on Vero cells and transfer of blastocysts in humans. Hum Reprod 1992; 7 (Suppl): 101

59. Foresta C, et al. Evidence for a stimulatory role of follicle-stimulating hormone on the spermatogonial population in adult males. Fertil Steril 1998; 69: 636

60. Baarends WM, Grootegoed JA. Male gametogenesis. In Fauser BCJM, ed. Reproductive Medicine. Molecular, Cellular and Genetic Fundamentals. New York: Parthenon Publishing, 2003: 381

61. Erkkila K, et al. Testosterone regulates apoptosis in adult human seminiferous tubules in vitro. J Clin Endocrinol Metabol 1997; 82: 2314

62. Print CG, Loveland KL. Germ cell suicide: new insights into apoptosis during spermatogenesis. BioEssays 2000; 22: 423

63. Tesarik J, et al. Human spermatogenesis in vitro: respective effects of follicle stimulating hormone and testosterone on meiosis, spermiogenesis, and Sertoli cell apoptosis. J Clin Endocrinol Metab 1998; 83: 4467

64. Tesarik J, et al. Differentiation of spermatogenic cells during in vitro culture of testicular biopsy samples from patients with obstructive azoospermia: effect of recombinant follicle stimulating hormone. Hum Reprod 1998; 13: 2772

65. Tesarik J, et al. Germ cell apoptosis in men with complete and incomplete spermiogenesis failure. Mol Hum Reprod 1998; 4: 757

66. Tesarik J, et al. Birth of healthy twins after fertilization with in vitro cultured spermatids from a patient with massive in vivo apoptosis of postmeiotic germ cells. Fertil Steril 2000; 74: 1044

67. Tesarik J, et al. In-vitro spermatogenesis resumption in men with maturation arrest: relationship with in-vivo blocking stage and serum FSH. Hum Reprod 2000; 15: 1350

68. Tesarik J, et al. Pharmacological concentrations of follicle-stimulating hormone and testosterone improve the efficacy of in vitro germ cell differentiation in men with maturation arrest. Fertil Steril 2002; 77: 245

69. Tesarik J, et al. In-vitro effects of FSH and testosterone withdrawal on caspase activation and DNA fragmentation in different cell types of human seminiferous epithelium. Hum Reprod 2002; 17: 1811

70. Tesarik J, et al. Caspase-dependent and -independent DNA fragmentation in Sertoli and germ cells from men with primary testicular failure: relationship with histological diagnosis. Hum Reprod 2004; 19: 254

71. Sá R, et al. In vitro maturation of sperm. In Gurgan T, Demirol A, eds. 13th World Congress on In Vitro Fertilization: Assisted Reproduction & Genetics. Bologna: Medimond, 2005: 79

72. Morales CR, Wu XQ, Hecht NB. The DNA/RNA-binding protein, TB-RBP, moves from the nucleus to the cytoplasm and through intercellular bridges in male germ cells. Dev Biol 1998; 201: 113

73. Egozcue S, et al. Human male infertility: chromosome anomalies, meiotic disorders, abnormal spermatozoa and recurrent abortion. Hum Reprod Update 2000; 6: 93

74. Sun F, et al. Meiotic defects in a man with non-obstructive azoospermia: case report. Hum Reprod 2004; 19: 1770

75. Guichaoua MR, et al. Meiotic anomalies in infertile men with severe spermatogenic defects. Hum Reprod 2005; 20: 1897

76. Pang M-G, et al. The high incidence of meiotic errors increases with decreased sperm count in severe male factor infertilities. Hum Reprod 2005; 20: 1688

77. Alves C, et al. Unique (Y;13) translocation in a male with oligozoospermia. Cytogenetic and molecular studies. Eur J Hum Genet 2002; 10: 467

78. Pinho MJ, et al. Unique (Yq12;1q12) translocation with loss of the heterochromatic region of chromosome 1 in a male with azoospermia due to meiotic arrest. Hum Reprod 2005; 20: 689

79. Rodriguez I, et al. An early and massive wave of germinal cell apoptosis is required for the development of functional spermatogenesis. EMBO J 1997; 16: 2262

80. Lee J, et al. The Fas system, a regulator of testicular germ cell apoptosis, is differentially up-regulated in Sertoli cell versus germ cell injury of the testis. Endocrinology 1999; 140: 852

81. Pentikainen V, Erkkila K, Dunkel L. Fas regulates germ cell apoptosis in the human testis in vitro. Am J Physiol 1999; 276: E310

82. Nicholson DW. Caspase structure, proteolytic substrates, and function during apoptotic cell death. Cell Death Differ 1999; 6: 1028

83. Kroemer G, Martin SJ. Review. Caspase-independent cell death. Nat Med 2005; 11: 725

84. Woolveridge I, et al. Apoptosis in the rat spermatogenic epithelium following androgen withdrawal: changes in apoptosis related genes. Biol Reprod 1999; 60: 461

85. Lin WW, et al. In situ end-labeling of human testicular tissue demonstrates increased apoptosis in conditions of abnormal spermatogenesis. Fertil Steril 1997; 68: 1065

86. Hikim AP, et al. Spontaneous germ cell apoptosis in humans: evidence for ethnic differences in the susceptibility of germ cells to programmed cell death. J Clin Endocrinol Metabol 1998; 83: 152

87. Steele EK, et al. A comparison of DNA damage in testicular and proximal epididymal spermatozoa in obstructive azoospermia. Mol Hum Reprod 1999; 5: 831

88. Nakagawa A, et al. In vivo analysis of phagocytosis of apoptotic cells by testicular sertoli cells. Mol Reprod Dev 2005; 71: 166

89. Almeida C, et al. Quantitative study of caspase-3 activity in the ejaculate and swim-up regarding semen quality. Hum Reprod 2005; 20: 1307

90. Marques CJ, et al. Altered genomic imprinting in disruptive spermatogenesis. Lancet 2004; 363: 1700

91. Kamp C, et al. High deletion frequency of the complete AZFa sequence occurs only in men with Sertoli-cell-only-syndrome. Mol Hum Reprod 2001; 7: 987

92. Fernandes S, et al. High frequency of DAZ1/DAZ2 gene deletions in patients with severe oligozoospermia. Mol Hum Reprod 2002; 8: 286

93. Ferrás C, et al. AZF and DAZ gene copy specific deletion analysis in maturation arrest and Sertoli cell only syndrome. Mol Hum Reprod 2004; 10: 755

94. Grangeia A, et al. Characterization of CFTR mutations and IVS8-T variants in Portuguese patients with CAVD. Hum Reprod 2004; 19: 2502

95. Grangeia A, et al. A novel missense mutation P1290S at exon 20 of the CFTR gene in a Portuguese patient with congenital bilateral absence of the vas deferens. Fertil Steril 2005; 83: 448

96. Shamanski FL, et al. Status of genomic imprinting in mouse spermatids. Hum Reprod 1999; 14: 1050

97. Van Steirteghem AC, et al. Follow-up of children born after ICSI. Hum Reprod Update 2002; 8: 111

98. Lidegaard O, Pinborg A, Andersen AN. Imprinting diseases and IVF: Danish National IVF cohort study. Hum Reprod 2005; 20: 950

99. Tesarik J, et al. Restoration of fertility by in vitro spermatogenesis. Lancet 1999; 353: 555

100. Steele EK, Lewis SEM, McClure N. Science versus clinical adventurism in treatment of azoospermia. Lancet 1999; 353: 516

101. Carvalho F, et al. Preimplantation genetic diagnosis for familial amyloidotic polyneuropathy (FAP). Prenat Diagn 2001; 21: 1093

102. Alves C, et al. Preimplantation genetic diagnosis using FISH for carriers of Robertsonian translocations: the Portuguese experience. Prenat Diagn 2002; 22: 1153

103. Sousa M, Barros A. Ethics, social, legal, counselling. A moral case study for discussion: designer babies and tissue typing. Reprod Biomed Online 2004; 9: 596

32

New developments in the evaluation and management of the infertile male

Darius A Paduch, Marc Goldstein, Zev Rosenwaks

INTRODUCTION

The development of intracytoplasmic sperm injection (ICSI) has been the major breakthrough in male infertility treatment since the introduction of *in vitro* fertilization (IVF) itself. This novel technique has made it possible successfully to treat men with severe oligospermia or azoospermia who were otherwise doomed to permanent sterility. Perhaps the greatest measure of the success of this procedure has been its application – in combination with microsurgical testicular sperm extraction (TESE) – in men with non-obstructive azoospermia and in men with Klinefelter's syndrome[1,2].

GENETICS AND MALE INFERTILITY

While it is tempting to regard the male simply as a provider of enough haploid germ cells to be used for ICSI, we must not give up the pursuit of understanding the underpinnings of male reproductive physiology and evaluation of the underlying pathophysiology. Only by unraveling the basic science and genetic basis of male infertility can we ensure future innovations in this important area.

This chapter illustrates how a better understanding of the physiological and genetic basis of male infertility has helped in providing not only

innovative therapy but also optimal counseling for our patients.

An example of the critical importance of a thorough work-up of the male is seen in the area of Y microdeletions. Hopps *et al.*[3], among others, showed that Y-microdeletions screening has significant prognostic value, since no spermatozoa are ever recovered during TESE in men with AZFa or AZFb (azoospermia factors) deletions. Recently, two groups independently showed that mutations in ubiquitin-specific protease-26, which results in spermatogenic arrest and Sertoli cell-only syndrome, occurs in over 10% of men with non-obstructive azoospermia (NOA)[4,5].

Similarly, new discoveries in the genetics of hypogonadotropic hypogonadism have expanded our understanding of the hypothalamus–pituitary–testis axis. Kallmann's syndrome is a common form of hypogonadotropic hypogonadism. Typically, patients with Kallmann's syndrome present with delayed puberty, short stature, anosmia and, later in life, infertility[6]. Genetic studies have revealed that mutations in two genes are responsible for the spontaneous and hereditary forms of Kallmann's syndrome: KAL-1 and FGFR-1[7]. KAL-1 is located on the X chromosome (Xp22.3), and mutations or deletions in this gene result in the X-linked form of the disease. Mutations in fibroblast growth factor receptor 1 (FGFR-1), also known as KAL-2, on 8p11.2–12 occur in the autosomal dominant form of the disease. KAL-1 encodes a protein that is necessary for normal migration of gonadotropin releasing hormone (GnRH) primitive cells from the olfactory placode to the hypothalamus, while FGFR-1 is necessary for initial evagination of the olfactory bulbs.

Identification of these mutations has clinical value, since the presence of each mutation is associated with different associated syndromes. The KAL-1 mutation is associated with renal defects, whereas FGFR-1 heterozygous loss of function mutation is associated with hearing problems and cleft palate. The FGFR-1 mutation has also been identified in patients with spontaneous resolution of idiopathic hypogonadotropic hypogonadism (IHH)[8]. Treatment with human chorionic gonadotropin (hCG) and follicle stimulating hormone (FSH) in men with Kallmann's syndrome results in the initiation of sperm production, allowing men with Kallmann's syndrome to father children[9]. Since the KAL-1 gene is located on the X chromosome, the KAL-1 mutation will be transferred to daughters of men with the mutation and will be phenotypically present in the next generation. Thus, knowing that the mutation is present may affect the decision about reproductive choices and may dictate the length of hCG and FSH replacement[10].

Men with Kallmann's syndrome should be evaluated by a urologist. Measurement of testicular volume has significant prognostic value. Men with a testicular volume of less than 4 ml responded poorly to hCG and FSH treatment (sperm appeared in the ejaculate in 36% of such men), whereas 71% of men with testicular volumes above 4 ml presented with sperm in the ejaculate after hormonal therapy[11]. There were no significant differences in hormone levels before and after treatment in men with small versus larger testes. Recently, there has been renewed interest in idiopathic hypogonadotropic hypogonadism as it was shown that mutations in the GPR54 receptor, a player in the KiSS-1 pathway of GnRH regulation, could cause non-anosmic hypogonadotropic hypogonadism[12]. Since intraventricular infusion

of KiSS-1 stimulates the release of gonadotropins, one can easily envision the use of KiSS homologs in the future pharmacotherapy of hypogonadism.

ONCOLOGY AND MALE INFERTILITY

Basic science and clinical advances in oncology have significantly improved the overall survival of patients with childhood and adult malignancies. These advances in survival most often require the use of aggressive chemotherapeutic agents, bone marrow transplants and total body irradiation. It has long been established that chemotherapy, especially the use of alkylating agents in high doses, or irradiation results in permanent azoospermia in 20–50% of patients[13]. In many others, treatment results in oligospermia[14]. Although Leydig cells are quite resistant to radio/chemotherapy, children and adults undergoing such treatments[15] can suffer from delayed puberty and can exhibit low testosterone production. Pharmacological prevention of germinal cell damage during chemotherapy or radiation treatment has been extensively evaluated in animals. The intuitive choice would be to arrest germinal proliferation for the duration of chemotherapy with GnRH agonists. A beneficial effect of GnRH agonist suppression on the post-treatment recovery of spermatogenesis after radiotherapy and chemotherapy has been shown in rodents but not in non-human primates[16]. Although several centers are currently investigating this in humans, thus far there are no human data to support concomitant use of GnRH agonists to prevent testicular damage during radio/chemotherapy. With a better understanding of spermatogenesis, we may be able to offer chemoprevention in the future[17].

Every attempt should be made at sperm cryopreservation prior to chemo- or radiotherapy. Many men, especially those with testicular tumors, will have poor sperm quality for cryopreservation. Children and early adolescents are usually azoospermic[18,19]. The poor sperm quality prior to cancer treatment may be caused by paraneoplastic syndromes and mediated by cytokines, tumor necrosis factor (TNF) and other molecules affecting sperm production[20]. In selected cases with severe oligospermia, testicular sperm procurement should be considered prior to chemotherapy[18]. Similarly, if an adolescent male is not able to deliver a semen sample, vibratory stimulation or electroejaculation can be used[21]. In prepubertal adolescents, immature testicular tissue can be cryopreserved, but this approach should be considered experimental since, at present, there are no techniques available to induce the maturation of immature human germ cells *in vitro*, for subsequent use for IVF/ICSI[22,23]. It is important to consider that a 12–14-year-old boy who is to undergo total body irradiation will likely have no chance of spermatogenesis in the future and will not enter the reproductive age for another decade. Current developments in sperm maturation *in vitro* promise at least some hope for these boys[19]. Three approaches have been successful in animals: (1) transplantation of germ stem cells in rodents with successful restoration of qualitative spermatogenesis, (2) maturation of germ stem cells *in vitro* and (3) transplantation of mature germ cell tissue back into the germ cell-depleted testis[22–25]. The success of these experiments in rodents and primates probably justifies the cryopreservation of testicular tissue in children and adolescents who will undergo cancer treatments which have a high likelihood of resulting in azoospermia. This is an exciting area of research, and since this approach requires surgical retrieval of testicular tissue, together with extensive knowledge of the biology of male reproduction, it underscores the importance of the participation of male infertility specialists in the care of cancer patients.

One of the more interesting questions pertinent to oncology and male fertility is the safety of using sperm from men who have undergone chemotherapy or radiation treatment. Can the use of such sperm increase the risk of genetic abnormalities in the offspring? Is the risk indefinite, or is there a wash-out period after which the use of sperm from cancer survivors is acceptable? Is

preimplantation genetic diagnosis (PGD) required for embryos created using sperm from fathers who are cancer survivors? There is an increased risk of sperm aneuploidy immediately after chemotherapy, but this risk decreases with time[26,27]. Currently, most authorities agree that couples should use birth control for 18–24 months after the last cycle of therapy. This area, however, requires further study. Follow-up of offspring conceived by men post-chemo/radiotherapy has failed to detect an increased risk of gross chromosomal aberrations in the offspring[28].

MEDICAL TREATMENT IN MALE INFERTILITY

Advances in the medical treatment of men with idiopathic oligoasthenoteratospermia have been limited. The use of clomiphene citrate, tamoxifen and aromatase inhibitors may be helpful in carefully selected cases. Aromatase inhibitors have a role in men with hyperestrogenemia. Patients with Klinefelter's syndrome may benefit from treatment with aromatase inhibitors[29–31]. Tamoxifen (20 mg taken orally twice daily) can increase sperm density and motility in oligospermic patients with normal gonadotropins, but seems to have no effect in patients with high FSH and luteinizing hormone (LH)[32]. The addition of testosterone to tamoxifen may have beneficial effects[33,34]. Testosterone alone suppresses spermatogenesis and should never be given to infertile men. Clomiphene citrate may be helpful in selected men with oligospermia. It results in increased testosterone levels and sperm density, but, thus far, there is no evidence that treatment with clomiphene citrate results in improved pregnancy rates[35,36]. The potential long-term effect of estrogen feedback and estrogen production in men is unknown.

There is no evidence that treatment with hCG and/or FSH in men with idiopathic normo-gonadotropic oligospermia is effective. However, recently it has been shown that some men with idiopathic oligospermia have an abnormal pulsatile release of LH[37]. Foresta *et al.* showed that the suppression of high circulating FSH levels improves Sertoli cell function[38]. Further advances in our understanding of the hypothalamus–pituitary–testis axis may allow the optimization of protocols for hormonal manipulation in infertile men.

In at least 30% of infertile men, no etiology is found after thorough evaluation. Considering the limited success of the available pharmacological treatment of idiopathic male infertility, it is no surprise that many infertile men seek alternative remedies[39].

Vitamins and minerals play an important regulatory function in multiple biochemical pathways in cells, and as cofactors they are believed to have an impact on the quality of sperm and sperm DNA integrity. Multiple studies have shown that an increase in oxidative stress in semen contributes to defects in sperm chromatin[40–42]. This provides a rationale for treating infertile men with antioxidants and supplements such as vitamins and minerals in the hope of improving sperm quality, and increasing fertilization rates. L-carnitine supplementation has resulted in improved sperm density and motility using 2 g a day for 3–6 months in small randomized studies. Other studies have shown no benefit[43]. Vitamin E, A and C supplementation in men with infertility may improve semen parameters, but there are no studies documenting on improvement in fertility[44]. Supplementation with vitamins E, A and C does not improve the sperm chromatin structure as evaluated by the sperm chromatin structure assay (SCSA)[45]. Thus, vitamin and mineral supplementation should be considered as non-specific or empirical therapies, which may be helpful in some patients.

SURGICAL EXTRACTION OF SPERM

Because no successful therapy exists for men with idiopathic non-obstructive azoospermia, the surgical extraction of sperm for use with ICSI is the mainstay of therapy for these men. In experienced hands, sperm can be extracted from more than 50% of men with NOA using microsurgical techniques (Table 32.1)[1,2,46]. Thus far there are no reliable tests to predict which patients will have sperm present in the testes. Turek *et al.* proposed fine-needle mapping as an adjunct method to verify the presence of sperm in men with NOA; however, this method is operator-dependent[47,48]. Magnetic resonance spectroscopy using new algorithms and 3T MRI (three-tesla magnetic resonance imaging) is being evaluated in our and other centers, and hopefully will allow us to identify patients who will benefit from testicular sperm extraction (TESE). It remains to be seen whether hormonal manipulation prior to TESE will improve recovery rates and fertilization rates.

In our hands, the use of fresh testicular sperm yields better pregnancy and fertilization rates when compared with frozen testicular sperm. Other centers claim that using frozen testicular tissue yields equally good results. For unreconstructable obstructive azoospermia, such as in men with congenital absence of the vas deferens, the use of cryopreserved epididymal sperm yields results equal to those with fresh spermatozoa (Table 32.2). For reconstructable obstructive azoospermia, such as vasectomy reversal, technical advances have yielded success rates which make microsurgical repair the most cost-effective option for initial treatment[48–55].

The development of artery- and lymphatic-sparing microsurgical techniques of varicocele repair has resulted in improved outcomes and minimal morbidity in men with varicocele-associated infertility and adolescents with varicocele[56–59]. Although controversy exists regarding the benefits of varicocelectomy, several studies have shown that varicocele repair in men with non-obstructive azoospermia or severe oligoasthenospermia may improve spermatogenesis sufficiently to allow IVF/ICSI with ejaculated instead of testicular sperm[60–64]. Recent data suggest that varicocele repair may improve the sperm

Table 32.1 Sperm parameters and intracytoplasmic sperm injection (ICSI) outcome with testicular spermatozoa. Extended from reference 46

	Azoospermia	
	Obstructive	Non-obstructive
Cycles (n)	156	457
Mean concentration $\pm$ SD ($\times 10^6$/ml)	0.4 ± 1	0.3 ± 2
Mean motility $\pm$ SD (%)	4.3 ± 8	2.5 ± 7
Fertilization (n (%))	918/1318 (69.6)*	2395/4380 (54.7)*
Clinical pregnancies (n (%))	70 (44.9)	181 (39.6)

*χ^2 test, 2×2, 1 df; effect of etiology of azoospermia on fertilization rate, $p = 0.0001$

Table 32.2 First-attempt *in vitro* fertilization/intracytoplasmic sperm injection (IVF/ICSI): fresh vs. cryopreserved epididymal sperm. Results are given as mean $\pm$ SD unless otherwise indicated. Adapted from reference 49

	Fresh (n = 108)	Cryopreserved (n = 33)
Male age (years)	38.3 ± 8.8	38.2 ± 11.1
Female age (years)	33.2 ± 5.1	33.1 ± 5.5
Total number of sperm aspirated (n)	99×10^6	$82 \times 10^6 \pm 110$
Number of vials stored (n)	5.5	4.7 ± 2.5
Number of oocytes injected (n)	10.8 ± 5.5	10.1 ± 5.3
Number of oocytes fertilized (n)	8.2 ± 5.1	7.9 ± 4.6
Number of embryos per transfer (n)	3.3 ± 1.0	3.2 ± 0.8
Number of pregnant couples per total number of couples (n (%))	72/108 (66.7)	20/33 (60.6)

chromatin structure[65]. Varicocele repair in adolescents may also prevent both future infertility and androgen deficiency in aging men. If this hypothesis is confirmed, varicocele repair will be employed not only to improve sperm production but also to prevent or even treat hypogonadism[59,66,67].

Evaluating and instituting specific treatments in the infertile male are critical for optimizing the medical care of the infertile couple. Furthermore, recent data showing a 20-fold increase in the incidence of testicular cancer in infertile men mandates male partner evaluation[68]. Over the next decade, further developments in our understanding of the genetics and physiology of male reproduction, advances in stem cell research and better ways of measuring outcomes of surgical techniques[69,70], as well as other novel therapeutic options, will allow us to offer treatment to patients who are considered sterile by today's standards.

REFERENCES

1. Schlegel PTN, et al. Fresh testicular sperm from men with nonobstructive azoospermia works best for ICSI. Urology 2004; 64: 1069

2. Schiff JD, et al. Success of testicular sperm injection and intracytoplasmic sperm injection in men with Klinefelter syndrome. J Clin Endocrinol Metab 2005; 90: 6263

3. Hopps CV, et al. Detection of sperm in men with Y chromosome microdeletions of the AZFa, AZFb and AZFc regions. Hum Reprod 2003; 18: 1660

4. Stouffs K, et al. Possible role of USP26 in patients with severely impaired spermatogenesis. Eur J Hum Genet 2005; 13: 336

5. Paduch DA, Mielnik A, Schlegel PN. Novel mutations in testis-specific ubiquitin protease 26 gene may cause male infertility and hypogonadism. Reprod Biomed Online 2005; 10: 747

6. Karges B, de Roux N. Molecular genetics of isolated hypogonadotropic hypogonadism and Kallmann syndrome. Endocr Dev 2005; 8: 67

7. Gonzalez-Martinez D, Hu Y, Bouloux PM. Ontogeny of GnRH and olfactory neuronal systems in man: novel insights from the investigation of inherited forms of Kallmann's syndrome. Front Neuroendocrinol 2004; 25: 108

8. Pitteloud N, et al. Reversible Kallmann syndrome, delayed puberty, and isolated anosmia occurring in a single family with a mutation in the fibroblast growth factor receptor 1 gene. J Clin Endocrinol Metab 2005; 90: 1317

9. Szilagyi A, et al. Kallmann's syndrome: pregnancy through intracytoplasmic sperm injection and complicated by gestational diabetes. Gynecol Endocrinol 2001; 15: 325

10. Abujbara MA, et al. Clinical and inheritance profiles of Kallmann syndrome in Jordan. Reprod Health 2004; 1: 5

11. Miyagawa Y, et al. Outcome of gonadotropin therapy for male hypogonadotropic hypogonadism at university affiliated male infertility centers: a 30-year retrospective study. J Urol 2005; 173: 2072

12. Kaiser UB, Kuohung W. KiSS-1 and GPR54 as new players in gonadotropin regulation and puberty. Endocrine 2005; 26: 277

13. Agarwal A, Allamaneni SS. Disruption of spermatogenesis by the cancer disease process. J Natl Cancer Inst Monogr 2005; (34): 9

14. Humpl T, Schramm P, Gutjahr P. Male fertility in long-term survivors of childhood ALL. Arch Androl 1999; 43: 123

15. Alves CH, et al. Growth and puberty after treatment for acute lymphoblastic leukemia. Rev Hosp Clin Fac Med Sao Paulo 2004; 59: 67

16. Shetty G, Meistrich ML. Hormonal approaches to preservation and restoration of male fertility after cancer treatment. J Natl Cancer Inst Monogr 2005; (34): 36

17. Meistrich ML, Shetty G. Suppression of testosterone stimulates recovery of spermatogenesis after cancer treatment. Int J Androl 2003; 26: 141

18. Shin D, Lo KC, Lipshultz LI. Treatment options for the infertile male with cancer. J Natl Cancer Inst Monogr 2005; (34): 48

19. Tournaye H, Goossens E, Verheyen G, et al. Preserving the reproductive potential of men and boys with cancer: current concepts and future prospects. Hum Reprod Update 2004; 10: 525

20. Bussen S, et al. Semen parameters in patients with unilateral testicular cancer compared to patients with other malignancies. Arch Gynecol Obstet 2004; 269: 196

21. Muller J, et al. Cryopreservation of semen from pubertal boys with cancer. Med Pediatr Oncol 2000; 34: 191

22. Schlatt S, et al. Progeny from sperm obtained after ectopic grafting of neonatal mouse testes. Biol Reprod 2003; 68: 2331

23. Schlatt S, von Schonfeldt V, Schepers AG. Male germ cell transplantation: an experimental approach with a clinical perspective. Br Med Bull 2000; 56: 824

24. Zhang X, Ebata KT, Nagano MC. Genetic analysis of the clonal origin of regenerating mouse spermatogenesis following transplantation. Biol Reprod 2003; 69: 1872

25. Feng LX, et al. Generation and in vitro differentiation of a spermatogonial cell line. Science 2002; 297: 392

26. Martin RH, et al. Analysis of sperm chromosome complements before, during, and after chemotherapy. Cancer Genet Cytogenet 1999; 108: 133

27. De Mas P, et al. Increased aneuploidy in spermatozoa from testicular tumour patients after chemotherapy with cisplatin, etoposide and bleomycin. Hum Reprod 2001; 16: 1204

28. Meistrich ML, Byrne J. Genetic disease in offspring of long-term survivors of childhood and adolescent cancer treated with potentially mutagenic therapies. Am J Hum Genet 2002; 70: 1069

29. Raman JD, Schlegel PN. Aromatase inhibitors for male infertility. J Urol 2002; 167: 624

30. Karaer O, Oruc S, Koyuncu FM. Aromatase inhibitors: possible future applications. Acta Obstet Gynecol Scand 2004; 83: 699

31. Kawakami E, et al. Improvement in spermatogenic function after subcutaneous implantation of a capsule containing an aromatase inhibitor in four oligozoospermic dogs and one azoospermic dog with high plasma estradiol-17beta concentrations. Theriogenology 2004; 62: 165

32. Kadioglu TC, et al. Treatment of idiopathic and postvaricocelectomy oligozoospermia with oral tamoxifen citrate. BJU Int 1999; 83: 646

33. Adamopoulos DA, et al. Effectiveness of combined tamoxifen citrate and testosterone undecanoate treatment in men with idiopathic oligozoospermia. Fertil Steril 2003; 80: 914

34. Adamopoulos DA. Present and future therapeutic strategies for idiopathic oligozoospermia. Int J Androl 2000; 23: 320

35. Siddiq FM, Sigman M. A new look at the medical management of infertility. Urol Clin North Am 2002; 29: 949

36. Vandekerckhove P, et al. Clomiphene or tamoxifen for idiopathic oligo/asthenospermia. Cochrane Database Syst Rev 2000; (2): CD000151

37. Scaglia HE, et al. Altered testicular hormone production in infertile patients with idiopathic oligoasthenospermia. J Androl 1991; 12: 273

38. Foresta C, et al. Suppression of the high endogenous levels of plasma FSH in infertile men are associated with improved Sertoli cell function as reflected by elevated levels of plasma inhibin B. Hum Reprod 2004; 19: 1431

39. Zini A, et al. Use of alternative and hormonal therapies in male infertility. Urology 2004; 63: 141

40. Sharma RK, Said T, Agarwal A. Sperm DNA damage and its clinical relevance in assessing reproductive outcome. Asian J Androl 2004; 6: 139

41. Saleh RA, et al. Effect of cigarette smoking on levels of seminal oxidative stress in infertile men: a prospective study. Fertil Steril 2002; 78: 491

42. Saleh RA, et al. Leukocytospermia is associated with increased reactive oxygen species production by human spermatozoa. Fertil Steril 2002; 78: 1215

43. Agarwal A, Said TM. Carnitines and male infertility. Reprod Biomed Online 2004; 8: 376

44. Eskenazi B, et al. Antioxidant intake is associated with semen quality in healthy men. Hum Reprod 2005; 20: 1006

45. Silver EW, et al. Effect of antioxidant intake on sperm chromatin stability in healthy nonsmoking men. J Androl 2005; 26: 550

46. Palermo GD, et al. Fertilization and pregnancy outcome with intracytoplasmic sperm injection for azoospermic men. Hum Reprod 1999; 14: 741

47. Turek PJ, et al. Diagnostic findings from testis fine needle aspiration mapping in obstructed and nonobstructed azoospermic men. J Urol 2000; 163: 1709

48. Turek PJ, et al. Testis sperm extraction and intracytoplasmic sperm injection guided by prior fine-needle aspiration mapping in patients with nonobstructive azoospermia. Fertil Steril 1999; 71: 552

49. Janzen N, et al. Use of electively cryopreserved microsurgically aspirated epididymal sperm with IVF and ICSI for unreconstructable azoospermia. Fertil Steril 2000; 74: 696

50. Tournaye H, et al. No differences in outcome after intracytoplasmic sperm injection with fresh or with frozen–thawed epididymal spermatozoa. Hum Reprod 1999; 14: 90

51. Anger JT, et al. Sperm cryopreservation and in vitro fertilization/intracytoplasmic sperm injection in men with congenital bilateral absence of the vas deferens: a success story. Fertil Steril 2004; 82: 1452

52. Fukunaga N, et al. Efficiency of using frozen–thawed testicular sperm for multiple intracytoplasmic sperm injections. J Assist Reprod Genet 2001; 18: 634

53. Nikolettos N, et al. Outcome of anticipated ICSI cycles using intentionally frozen–thawed testicular spermatozoa according to the spouse's response to ovarian stimulation. Clin Exp Obstet Gynecol 2002; 29: 126

54. Nikolettos N, et al. Outcome of ICSI cycles using frozen–thawed surgically obtained spermatozoa in poor responders to ovarian stimulation: cancellation or proceeding to ICSI? Eur J Obstet Gynecol Reprod Biol 2000; 92: 259

55. Oates RD, et al. Fertilization and pregnancy using intentionally cryopreserved testicular tissue as the sperm source for intracytoplasmic sperm injection in 10 men with non-obstructive azoospermia. Hum Reprod 1997; 12: 734

56. Matthews GJ, Matthews ED, Goldstein M. Induction of spermatogenesis and achievement of pregnancy after microsurgical varicocelectomy in men with azoospermia and severe oligoasthenospermia. Fertil Steril 1998; 70: 71

57. Goldstein M, et al. Microsurgical inguinal varicocelectomy with delivery of the testis: an artery and lymphatic sparing technique. J Urol 1992; 148: 1808

58. Marmar JL, Kim Y. Subinguinal microsurgical varicocelectomy: a technical critique and statistical analysis of semen and pregnancy data. J Urol 1994; 152: 1127

59. Schiff J, et al. Managing varicoceles in children: results with microsurgical varicocelectomy. BJU Int 2005; 95: 399

60. Raman JD, Walmsley K, Goldstein M. Inheritance of varicoceles. Urology 2005; 65: 1186

61. Gat Y, et al. Induction of spermatogenesis in azoospermic men after internal spermatic vein embolization for the treatment of varicocele. Hum Reprod 2005; 20: 1013

62. Schlegel PN, Kaufmann J. Role of varicocelectomy in men with nonobstructive azoospermia. Fertil Steril 2004; 81: 1585

63. Cakan M, Altug U. Induction of spermatogenesis by inguinal varicocele repair in azoospermic men. Arch Androl 2004; 50: 145

64. Pasqualotto FF, et al. Induction of spermatogenesis in azoospermic men after varicocele repair. Hum Reprod 2003; 18: 108

65. Zini A, et al. Beneficial effect of microsurgical varicocelectomy on human sperm DNA integrity. Hum Reprod 2005; 20: 1018

66. Su LM, Goldstein M, Schlegel PN. The effect of varicocelectomy on serum testosterone levels in infertile men with varicoceles. J Urol 1995; 154: 1752

67. Cayan S, et al. The effect of microsurgical varicocelectomy on serum follicle stimulating hormone, testosterone and free testosterone levels in infertile men with varicocele. BJU Int 1999; 84: 1046

68. Raman J, Norbert C, Goldstein M. Increased incidence of testicular cancer in men presenting with infertility and an abnormal semen analysis. J Urol 2005; 174: 1819

69. Goldstein M, Li PS, Matthews GJ. Microsurgical vasovasostomy: The microdot technique of precision suture placement. J Urol 1998; 159: 188

70. Chan PTK, Brandell RA, Goldstein M. Prospective analysis of outcomes after microsurgical intussusception vaso-epididymostomy. BJU Int 2005; 96: 598

Index

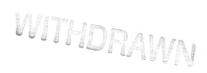